Infertility in Practice

Second Edition

Commissioning Editor: *Stephanie Donley*
Project Development Manager: *Louise Cook, Joanne Scott*
Project Manager: *Jess Thompson*
Illustration Manager: *Mick Ruddy*
Design: *Jayne Jones and Andy Chapman*
Illustrator: *Martin Woodward*

Infertility in Practice

Second Edition

Adam H Balen MD, FRCOG

Consultant Obstetrician and Gynecologist
Subspecialist in Reproductive Medicine and Surgery
Department of Obstetrics and Gynecology
Leeds General Infirmary
Leeds, UK

Honorary Senior Lecturer
Leeds Medical School
University of Leeds

And

Howard S Jacobs MD, FRCP FRCOG

Emeritus Professor of Reproductive Endocrinology
The Middlesex Hospitals
London, UK

Forewords by Ian D Cooke and Alan DeChorney

Churchill Livingstone

An imprint of Elsevier

Infertility in Practice, 2/e
Balen & Jacobs

Churchill Livingstone
An Imprint of Elsevier
Robert Stevenson House, 1-3 Baxter's Place
Leith Walk, Edinburgh EH1 3AF

Original ISBN : 0-4430-7165-9

First Printed in India 2004
Reprinted 2006

Indian Reprint ISBN-13 : 978-81-8147-250-2
Indian Reprint ISBN-10 : 81-8147-250-0

Published by Elsevier, a division of Reed Elsevier India Private Limited,
Shri Pratap Udyog, 274, Captain Gaur Marg, Sriniwaspuri, New Delhi-110065 (India).

Printed and bound at Saurabh Printers Pvt. Ltd.
A-16, Sector IV, NOIDA 201 301.

Contents

Foreword

to the first edition

Adam Balen and Howard Jacobs have written a significant and practical exposition on fertility. The key factor in any infertility dissertation is measuring results, not only in regards to pregnancy rates, but also to patient selection and precision of treatment. This is best illustrated in Chapter 2, "Prevention of Infertility", which evaluates aging related to fecundity. The graphic illustrations in this text are helpful, well constructed and emphatically make the point. Other information is supplemented, for example: male infertility and the debate concerning falling sperm count in developed countries.

Chapter 4, "Investigating Infertility", is a well-honed and quick approach that addresses economies of scale and includes a sensitive and compassionate discussion for counseling patients in regards to psychosexual issues, phobias, work issues and religious aspects. Many years ago, I wrote a paper discussing the stress on care providers of infertility and did this in the pique of group dynamics. Interestingly, Balen and Jacobs have picked up on this theme as well. Their book is the only other place I have seen this issue addressed.

Throughout the book are segments entitled "Advice" which respond to the many difficult questions infertility patients pose as well as adding a pragmatic facet unparalleled elsewhere. A unique contribution is "Planning a Pregnancy" (Ch. 3) which provides valuable preconception advice for patients. Clinicians who deal with patients with infertility problems are frequently asked questions about the effects of various drugs and environmental situations on the first trimester, including the pre-embryonic stage. The authors provide information on counseling these patients.

It is tempting for books to take an encyclopedic and focused approach to polycystic ovary disease when discussing fertility. This is an extremely strong part of this contribution as well, which is not surprising as it is an area of expertise of the authors. An endocrinologic approach is most apparent and to which an old quote of Sir William Oslers, "to know syphilis is to know medicine", can be applied – "to know polycysitc ovary is to know endocrinology". All aspects are evaluated in depth, with insights provided along the way, including servoregulatory mechanisms and ovulation induction protocols in the special group of patients. Long-standing effects on the patients' health are also addressed with wisdom.

The chapter on endometriosis (Ch. 9) presents a balanced view in regards to surgery versus medical therapy. If you were to choose an area of mystery, it would be the patient with unexplained fertility (Ch. 12). Although many etiologies have been proposed, nevertheless this is an area where many therapies seem to work with no satisfactory explanation. The discussion of super-ovulation and intrauterine insemination are handled fairly, as is the section on assisted reproductive technologies. In this area, the graphic information is especially helpful.

The book ends with a discussion of ethical issues touching on all of the different controversies in a provocative manner. Questions such as, does everyone have the right to treatment? Are experiments on pre-embryos appropriate? Is the role of sex selection unethical? Should older women (greater than 50) receive treatment via the new reproductive technologies?

This book is unique in that it contains a series of chapters on complications of therapy including hyperstimulation syndrome, ovarian carcinoma (Ch. 17) and ectopic pregnancy (Ch. 21). It is rare to find such a complete body of knowledge in regards to complications. There is no doubt that this adds to the practicality of this offering. The book ends with the "testy" question of when therapy should be stopped. This allows the authors to show their sensibility as well as their breadth of knowledge. This essay discusses the pros and cons of therapy as well as efficacy and risk; it includes the difficult realization that the couple may not have a child. Advice on adoption and foster homes is also presented.

This book is very much like being on a long trip with a well informed travelling companion who speaks so well on every topic that you query, that you wish that each fact could have been written down.

However, if you are concerned with the infertility workup, management, treatment, epidemiology, psychological complications or problems with early pregnancy, Balen and Jacobs have done the job for you.

I appreciated the integration of clinical medicine with basic science and clinical research. In this day of information overload, for bright people to take information and integrate it into a practice management plan that is both rational and logical is rewarding for the reader. Congratulations to Balen and Jacobs on a job well done.

Alan DeCherney
Department of Obstetrics and Gynecology
University College of Los Angeles School of Medicine
California and Past President of the American Society of Reproductive Medicine, 1997.

Foreword

to the second edition

Being asked to write the foreword has given me a chance to read this second edition carefully. I have appreciated its emphasis on the epidemiological, community and medical aspects as well as the pharmacology and therapeutics.

This volume is an important contribution to the literature on infertility. Reproductive medicine has emerged from gynaecological endocrinology, but has lost much of its familiarity with general endocrinology, which is done here so well. It has, however, also been broadened by a great explosion of reproductive biology, molecular biology and genetics, not least in andrology. These are directions in which the field will develop still further, making it the most exciting and intellectually demanding area of obstetrics and gynaecology. This book is directed at subspecialty trainees, but also to those gynaecologists with a special interest in the field. It is a compendium of information enabling the generalist to keep up with the field, to be excited by it and enthused by its broad expanse.

The new chapters in this edition have paid even more attention to the authors' interests and expertise in PCO, POF and egg donation, which are important and welcome; the practitioner also needs to have his/her horizons extended in these areas. Of particular relevance are the chapters on the HFEA and on Ethics. The concluding words in the last chapter which encourage the reader to "consider the ethical implications before such problems feature in the next consultation" sound a timely warning. As there is now a greater awareness of patient autonomy the practitioner needs to understand the ethical principles which apply to each clinical scenario and a rehearsal of the relevant issues is a helpful exercise. Clinical practice is also tightly controlled within a legal framework and the practising specialist must be familiar with that framework and its ethical basis.

Throughout the book there is a humanity that thinks of the patient, his/her response to infertility and to the effects of treatment. There is a concern about the future impact of current treatment, such as ovarian stimulation and its potential for malignancy, as well as genetic change, possibly influencing imprinting. The longer term consequences of decisions made now, the use of donor gametes or ICSI, are also highlighted, contributing to a thoughtful dissertation that extends the boundaries of the science yet avoids developing the technology for its own sake.

It has been a privilege to have the opportunity to write this foreword and I hope that the reader will enjoy the book as much as I have.

Ian D Cooke
Emeritus Professor of Obstetrics and Gynaecology, Sheffield University
President of the British Fertility Society, 2003.

Preface

to the second edition

In the five years since we first published *Infertility in Practice*, fertility therapy continues to expand most rapidly. A great deal of public attention has focused on the "high-tech" advances in assisted conception therapies. IVF itself has been available for a quarter of a century and in many European countries 1 – 2% of babies now born result from IVF therapy. Recent innovations, such as micromanipulation of gametes for therapy (e.g. intracytoplasmic sperm injection (ICSI)) and biopsy of embryos for pre-implantation genetic diagnosis (PGD) have broadened the applications for IVF technology. Some recent advances, for example cryopreservation of ovarian tissue, have generated great excitement, because of the prospect of preserving fertility prior to sterilising therapy for cancer. Other developments, such as cloning and stem cell research, have created concerns about the potential abuse of such technology. Whilst the scientists have been busy improving the prospects for women with ovarian failure and for men with very low sperm counts, the clinical approach to investigation and therapy has also made great strides to minimize the time taken to reach diagnosis and direct a couple to appropriate treatment.

Infertility in Practice has been written as a practical guide and is based on the authors' experience of daily clinical practice. The aim of the book is to place the modern approach to the management of infertility in the context of sound theory and evidence-based therapy. We have striven to provide the reader with a comprehensive classification of the causes of infertility, their investigation and management. In the second edition we have extended the chapter on ovulation induction and included a chapter on all aspects of polycystic ovary syndrome – subjects in which we have developed particular interest. We have also addressed the important issues of counseling, ethics and the regulation of fertility therapies. A glimpse into the future is provided in a new chapter on emerging technologies some of which are already being incorporated into daily practice.

The treatments for most causes of infertility provide very satisfactory cumulative chances of conception and of birth of a healthy child. However, the side effects must be borne in mind, whether this is the immediate risk of ovarian hyperstimulation syndrome and multiple pregnancy or the long term possibility of ovarian cancer. In this edition we discuss the outcome for the children born as a result of assisted reproduction technology. The cost of treatment must also be considered.

References for further reading are provided throughout the book. The list is, however, not exhaustive as the book is written as a practical guide rather than a highly academic work of reference. Many of the references are of contemporary reviews which will enable the interested reader to explore the literature further.

We hope that, whatever your expertise, *Infertility in Practice*, will help with the management of couples attending your clinic.

Adam H Balen
Howard S Jacobs
Leeds and London, 2003.

Dedicated to Frances, Sandra
and our children.

SECTION 1

Infertility – background, diagnosis, and counseling

Chapter 1

Introduction

Infertility is common. Approximately one sixth of marriages are involuntarily childless although the exact number inevitably depends on how the complaint is defined. Medical definitions of infertility tend to emphasize the immediate problem brought to the consultation, reflecting the typically short-term interaction of many doctors, particularly specialists, with their patients. Most accepted definitions therefore involve the number of months prior to the consultation during which the couple has been exposed to the chance of a pregnancy. When the lifetime experience of a couple's attempt to raise a family is considered, a quite different picture emerges: thus studies from Oxford and Copenhagen revealed that at least a quarter of all couples experience unexpected delays in achieving their desired family size,[1,2] although only half may seek treatment.[2] In recent years there has been an increase in publicity about infertility and reproductive medicine technologies which has gone some way to reduce both the stigma of infertility and the reluctance of couples to seek advice.

For the purposes of this book we will be using definitions of infertility that are measured in terms of the duration of exposure to the chance of conceiving. It is important at the outset to acknowledge that the single most important determinant of a couple's fertility is the age of the female partner. Figure 1.1 shows that for women up to and including the age of 25 the cumulative conception rate (CCR – see below) is 60% at 6 months and 85% at a year – that is to say, of 100 couples trying to conceive, 40 will not be pregnant after 6 months and 15 will still not have conceived after a year of trying. For couples where the female partner is 35 years of age or older, the conception rates are 60% at a year and 85% at 2 years – i.e. their fertility has halved because of age alone.

The data shown in Figure 1.1 were taken from a study of the French national experience of donor insemination. The advantage of this study, which was undertaken before the AIDS epidemic prevented the use of fresh samples for insemination, is that the age of the donors is more or less fixed and therefore the age-related variation is essentially attributable to the women. It is worth reflecting on the reason for the strikingly different effects the passage of years has on fertility of the two sexes. In men the supply of sperm is continuous, the germ cells of the testis dividing all the time, so the average age of sperm in an ejaculate is measured in months. Women, however, are born with a

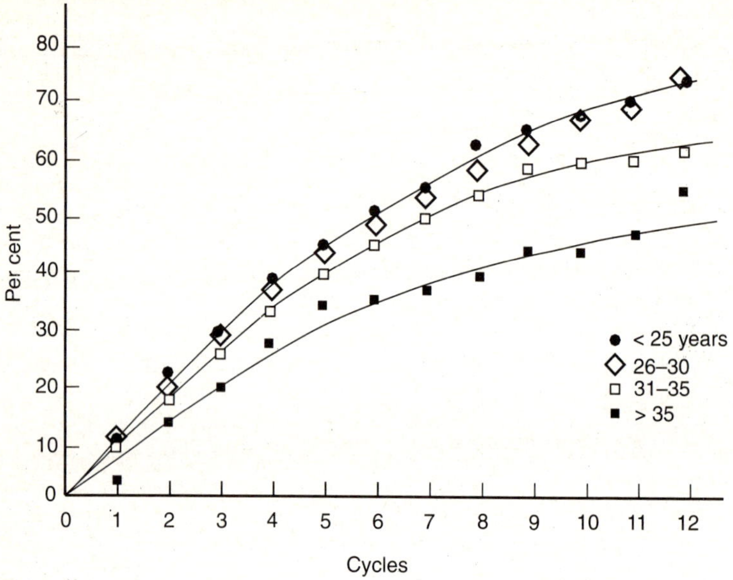

Figure 1.1 Female fecundity as a function of age. Results of donor insemination in 2193 nulliparous women with azoospermic husbands (Schwartz & Mayaux/ Fédération CECOS (1982) *N Engl J Med* **306**: 404, with permission).[5]

finite complement of eggs, which do not undergo further cell division until just after fertilization. Thus an oocyte ovulated today is pretty well the same age as the woman from whose ovary it came. Even DNA, the most stable molecule in biology, is not completely invulnerable to the passage of years; this impact of age on oocytes is consistent with its effect on the risk of congenital abnormalities, well known in many cases to increase with maternal age.

Measuring Infertility and the Reponse to Treatment

In trying to decide whether a couple should be investigated, and indeed in trying to formulate a prognosis for the success of treatment, the clinician needs a definition of normal fertility that is sensitive to the fact that in nature the highest rates of fertility do not exceed 30% conceptions per cycle. Using that figure, one can see that if 100 couples discontinue contraception, at the end of 1 month 30 can expect to be pregnant and 70 will need to try again next month. At the end of the second month, 70 ÷ 3 = 23 more will have conceived, giving a cumulative conception rate (CCR) of 30 + 23 = 53% at 2 months.

If we assume that the monthly rate of conception remains constant, it is easy to see how theoretical CCRs can be calculated for any infertility diagnosis and for any duration of treatment. In practice, monthly rates of conception do not remain constant because the more fertile couples conceive in the earlier months and, when we turn from theoretical examples to real clinical situations, follow-up is usually incomplete. The question then arises as to how to deal with the results of couples who leave a study before they have conceived or before their program of treatment has been completed. Moreover, couples leave treatment after different periods of time according to their own needs and circumstances, for example because of emotional stress or financial constraints.

By convention, in the calculation of CCR, the outcome for those leaving a program for reasons other than pregnancy is assumed to be the same as for those who remain in treatment. This assumption is the basis for the construction of CCR based on life table analysis, a method that was originally devised to describe survival from malignant disease. Figure 1.2 shows an example of a life table analysis of the fertility of a group of women treated by ovarian diathermy. This method of analysis can be easily adapted for use in a computer spreadsheet.

CCRs calculated from life tables have been used extensively to express fertility rates in relation to age and disease and to compare the results of treatment in different centers. An important extension of the CCR is the cumulative live birth rate (CLBR). Because the rates of miscarriage and several obstetric complications are closely influenced by maternal age, the fall-off with age of the CLBR is even more severe than that of the CCR. It is, however, the CLBR that our patients want to hear in answer to the question "What are our chances?" and so it behoves us to acknowledge certain limitations in its interpretation. The first is that it has been shown that as the number of drop-outs increases, the *calculated* conception or birth rate increases. This means that the more careless clinics are in obtaining follow-up information, the more this method of describing results exaggerates their success. The second important point to note is that drop-outs from treatment are not random: people leave a program largely because of their experience of it. One may safely assume the outcome of the whole group would have been worse if those who had dropped out because of their own, or the staff's, lack of confidence had stayed in and their results contributed directly to the determination of the group's response to treatment. Because of the free-market approach to infertility treatment patients may enter a given clinic's statistical record after already having had treatment elsewhere. Thus what may be recorded as a first cycle may actually only be the first in that clinic for the couple concerned. This is the case particularly in countries such as England, where the majority of

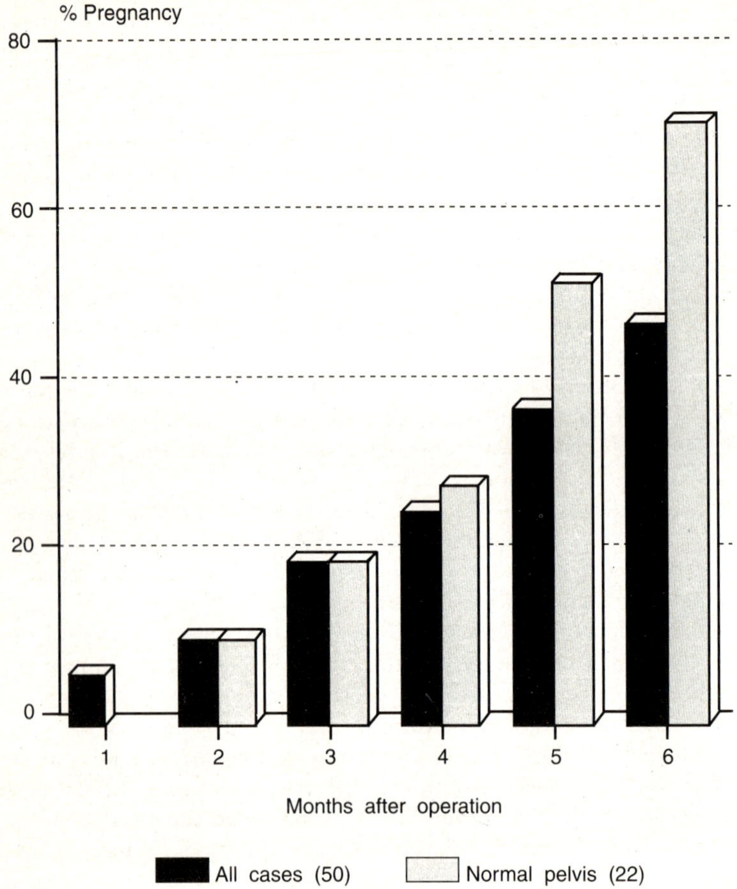

Figure 1.2 Cumulative conception rate – laparoscopic ovarian diathermy. (From Armar & Lachelin (1993) *Br J Obstet Gynaecol* **100**: 161)[6]. The filled bars refer to all cases treated by ovarian diathermy, the tinted bars to those who had a normal pelvis at laparoscopy.

patients have been forced to fund their own treatment and many travel between clinics.

Definition of Infertilty

The live birth rate (or "take-home baby rate") clearly depends on both the rate of conception and the survival of the pregnancy, which in infertility practice is largely determined by the miscarriage rate. By convention, when one refers to a patient as being infertile one is referring to a slow rate of conception – infertility is rarely absolute. As mentioned above, in normal people age is the most important determinant of the conception rate. All other things being equal, a couple in which the female partner is aged 25 or below stands a 5 out of 6 chance of conceiving in the year after discontinuing contraception. If, despite a regular menstrual cycle and a normal sex life, pregnancy has not occurred by then, most authorities would accept that that couple has a fertility problem and would offer investigation and treatment. If there is a history of a menstrual disturbance, assessment of the woman's fertility should take into account how long it will take her to accumulate the 12 or 13 ovulations that women with normal cycles have in one year. Clearly if a woman ovulates only four times a year, it will take her three times as long as a woman with a regular cycle to accumulate the same chance of getting pregnant. In that situation it makes no sense to defer investigation for a year. Similarly if there is a history of pelvic inflammatory disease, of a severe attack of appendicitis (particularly if there has been peritonitis), or in the male partner an attack of orchitis or a history of cryptorchidism, investigation should begin sooner rather than later.

A more difficult problem is defining infertility in the couple with an older female partner. In one way one might consider delaying investigation because it takes longer for a woman of 35 years and older to achieve a particular conception rate. On the other hand, the slope of the line relating the risk of childlessness to age gets much steeper as one approaches the age of 40. Furthermore, the prospects of achieving a pregnancy with treatment is parallel to this curve. There is therefore little time to lose in such couples and in our practice we are more active in advising investigation and treatment as the female partner passes her 35th birthday. There seems little point in waiting beyond a year and in many women (particularly those with some diagnostic clue in their history) we recommend initiating investigation after 6 months of unprotected intercourse.

Is Infertility Becoming More Common?

According to the UK Government Statistical Services there is a steadily rising proportion of women in the UK who have never had a child.[3] Among women who were born in 1948, 13% were childless at the age of 35; this proportion had almost doubled for women born 10 years later. Figure 1.3, taken from the OPCS publication on birth statistics, shows that this trend is likely to continue.[4]

Infertility as a complaint brought to medical attention is also on the increase. There are several reasons. The first is a secular change in family planning. Among married women, the mean age of mothers at

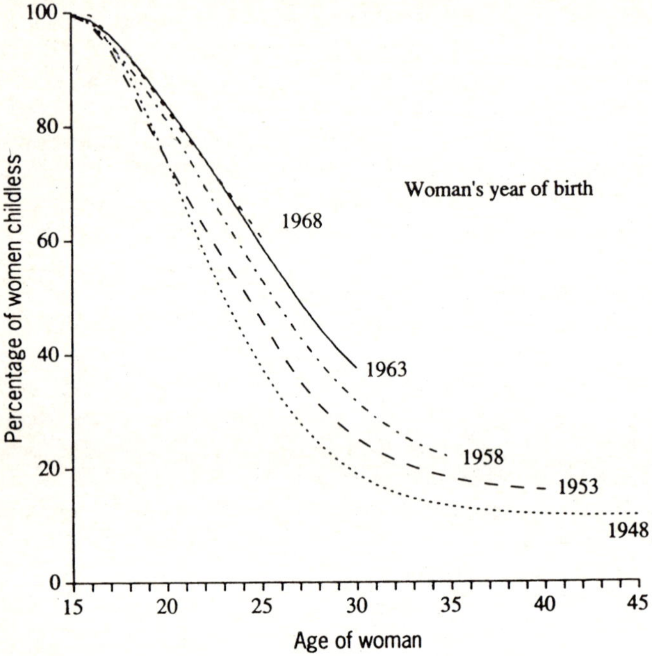

Figure 1.3 Percentage of women childless at successive ages in England and Wales.

first birth in the UK was 28 years in 1993, as opposed to 25 years in 1983 (Fig. 1.4). This change seems to be a feature of the demography of many first-world countries. In France, for example, the proportion of women giving birth after the age of 30 has doubled since 1972; in the USA between 1980 and 1986 the rate of primigravidae between 35 and 39 years of age increased by 81% and it doubled for women over the age of 39. As emphasized earlier, age is so crucial a determinant of fertility that the increasing age at which many women now choose to start their family means that fertility problems feature more in their lives than ever before. In the USA women over the age of 35 now account for more than 50% of all presentations for infertility. It is naturally particularly galling for a woman to have conscientiously pursued safe contraception for many years only to find that when she does plan to start a family, fertility eludes her.

Another important change that seems to be occurring in several European countries and in the USA is a decline in male fertility. Several studies have described a fall in the average sperm density of both patients and donors in donor insemination programs (see Ch. 2). Environmental pollution arising from estrogenic industrial waste is thought the most likely cause. The decline in sperm density seems to

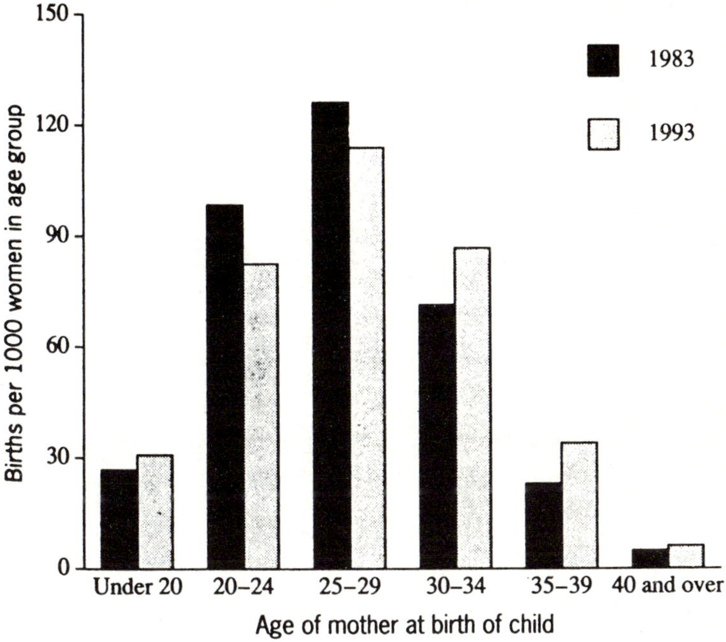

Figure 1.4 Age-specific fertility rates in England and Wales 1983 and 1993.

be occurring at a time when there is an increase in the incidence of testicular cancer and the frequency of hypospadias and cryptorchidism (p. 15). Clinically, the changes are very noticeable. In our own ovulation induction program increasing numbers of couples are now also requiring treatment for the male partner. Ten years ago the need appeared to be low – now almost 40% of the couples we treat need assistance on the male side.

Finally, people's expectations of fertility treatment are steadily rising, fed no doubt by charismatic doctors, exciting technology, and a culture in which everyone is clear about "rights," even if a little vague about responsibilities and obligations. Moreover, people from all walks of life now bring their infertility problems to medical clinics; for example, lesbian couples, hitherto regarded as having chosen an inevitably childless partnership, not infrequently now seek treatment for infertility. Quite apart from any value judgments one might make, such requests illustrate the gray zone between the use of biological technology for medical and for social reasons. But whatever one's attitude – and we return to this area in Chapter 15 – the high expectations most people now have mean that, for some couples, facing the possibility of not succeeding, and of not having children, is close to impossible. In these cost-containing days of efficiency-based medicine it is important to remember that for many people experience is the only tutor they believe. In the management of infertility, some treatment for the couple with a dismal prognosis may not be out of place.

Principles of Infertility Treatment

In an ideal world, the objective of treatment would be the reversal of the specific lesion causing childlessness, so permitting the couple to achieve the family size they would have chosen had they not suffered from infertility. The reality is that a single reversible cause is not all that common, and there are biological, social, and financial constraints to be considered. One can none the less formulate certain principles. The first principle, and probably one that commands the widest agreement, is that the interests of the unborn child must be foremost. Accepting this means that at the infertility consultation one will also need to consider preparation for pregnancy, both physical (diet, smoking, etc., see Ch. 3) and mental (the need for counseling, see Ch. 5). Since multiple pregnancy can have such devastating effects, in terms of both the obstetric outcome and the life of the family, we consider that as much effort should be invested in the safety of treatment as in its efficacy. For the correction of anovulatory infertility, a single dominant follicle producing a single fetus and a singleton full-term normal delivery must be the target to aim for. We therefore do not consider that ovulation induction should be undertaken in units where the ultrasound facilities are inadequate to diagnose polycystic ovaries or to track follicle and endometrial growth accurately. Despite the disappointment of having to discontinue treatment when the ovaries over respond (Ch. 6), one should never be tempted to administer human chorionic gonadotropin (hCG) because of pressure from the patient. It is to everyone's advantage to have the criteria for administering hCG clearly understood when treatment is first discussed so if treatment does have to be discontinued, disappointment is not compounded by misunderstanding.

In couples in whom assisted fertility therapy is required, it goes without saying that the financial implications need to be clearly stated at the outset, that the cost and availability of drugs need to be explored, and that the stressful nature of the procedure should be openly acknowledged. The impact of age and the duration of infertility must be explained very fully. The role of counselors and the availability of quick and efficient communication are very important.

Finally, some thoughts about the safety of infertility treatment. The risks of treatment can be thought of as immediate, for example technical problems caused by procedures (e.g. trauma and penetration of pelvic structures, anesthetic hazards, etc.), ovarian hyperstimulation

(Ch. 17), and multiple pregnancy (Ch. 17). Concern has also been expressed over long-term hazards, for example the development of ovarian cancer, in relation to infertility treatment (Ch. 17). We cannot know at present how real these risks will prove to be but we need to inform our patients about them and not to allow treatment with such apparently innocuous drugs as clomiphene to go unsupervised month after month.

Since the first edition of *Infertility in Practice* was published 5 years ago there have been many advances in the understanding and management of infertility and these will be discussed in this second edition. They include, for example: greater understanding of the pathophysiology of the polycystic ovary syndrome combined with the use of insulin sensitizing agents in its management; further refinement of regimens for superovulation including the use of gonadotropin releasing hormone antagonists; pre-implantation genetic diagnosis (PGD) as a therapeutic tool, opening up the possibility for aneuploidy screening and many other updates to practice that will run through this edition. We have also seen evidence-based guidelines for investigation and management published variously by the Royal College of Obstetricians and Gynaecologists (RCOG), the European Society of Human Reproduction and Embryology (ESHRE) and the American Society of Reproductive Medicine (ASRM). It is reassuring to see a consolidation of knowledge in an attempt to ensure evidence-based practice, which, certainly in the UK, is being used to state the case for adequate funding of fertility care.

References

1. Green E & Vessey M (1990) The prevalence of subfertility: a review of the current confusion and a report of two new studies. *Fertil Steril* **54**: 978–983.
2. Schmidt L, Munster K & Helm P (1995) Infertility and the seeking of infertility treatment in a representative population. *Br J Obstet Gynaeçol* **102**: 978–984.
3. OPCS (1994) *Fertility trends in England and Wales: 1984–94*. Birth statistics. OPCS, HMSO, London.
4. UK Government Statistics (1990–2000) *Mean age of mothers at livebirth, 1990–2000*. www.statistics.gov.uk/downloads/theme_population/Fm1_29/Fm1_29_v3.pdf (Table 1.6).
5. Schwartz D & Mayaux MJ (1982) Female fecundity as a function of age: results of artificial insemination in 2193 nulliparous women with azoospermic husbands. Fédération CECOS. *N Engl J Med* **306**: 404.
6. Armar NA & Lachelin GCL (1993) Laparoscopic ovarian diathermy: an effective treatment for anti-oestrogen resistant anovulatory infertility in women with the polycystic ovary syndrome. *Br J Obstet Gynaecol* **100**: 161–164.

Chapter 2

Prevention of infertility

If the numbers of couples seeking investigation and treatment of subfertility is on the increase, is fertility declining? If so, is this a global problem or unique to developing countries – and then, is it secondary to the older age at which women, in particular, are choosing to start a family or is it caused by environmental problems? Globally there is undoubtedly a problem with overpopulation and there are those who raise this as an issue when considering funding infertility therapy. In global terms, however, the number of children conceived as a result of infertility therapy is tiny, as is the final family size of couples who undergo treatment. In this chapter we do not deal with the broader ethical debate but outline some of the preventable causes of infertility.

Male Infertility

Falling Sperm Counts

There has been a growing literature in recent years concerning the possible effects of environmental pollutants (possibly estrogens) on the increasing rates of cryptorchidism and germ cell tumors and the decline in sperm concentrations over the last 20–50 years. However, few of the studies were performed prospectively and most observed either sperm donors or men undergoing vasectomy. In many of the studies important factors such as age, ejaculatory frequency, and period of abstinence were not controlled for. Single samples from men are also misleading as there can be huge variations in the same individual.

Carlsen *et al.*'s study,[1] which reviewed 61 papers from 1938 to 1990, provided semen analyses of nearly 1500 men and concluded that there was a 40% decline in sperm concentration over the period studied, from 113×10^6/ml to 66×10^6/ml (Fig. 2.1). Yet when Brake & Krause[2] reanalyzed the data from 48 of the papers that covered the last 20 years there was a significant increase in sperm concentration. Furthermore it has been suggested that the statistical analysis should take into consideration the fact that the distribution of sperm concentrations is heavily skewed towards lower values and that nearly all of the observed decline in mean sperm count might actually be a consequence of the reduction in the lower reference range of normal from 60×10^6/ml in the 1940s to the present value of 20×10^6/ml.[3] Despite criticisms of meta-analyses there is a body evidence that points to a real decline not only in sperm concentration but also in its

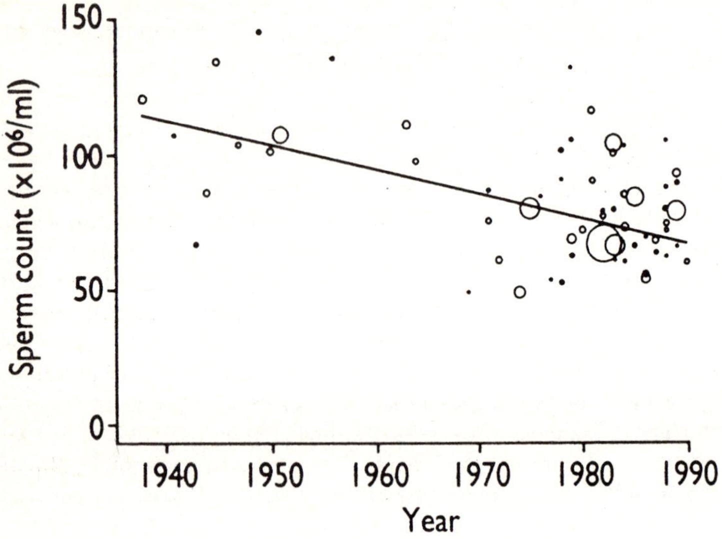

Figure 2.1 Linear regression of mean sperm density reported in 61 publications from 1938 to 1990 (represented by circles whose area is proportional to the number of subjects in study), each weighted according to the number of subjects. (From Keiding & Skakkebaek (1995) **311**: 570, with permission.)[38]

quality.[4,5,6,7] A more recent study by Irvine *et al.*[8] has provided stronger evidence of a decline in semen quality by examining the samples of 577 volunteer semen donors who donated samples for research to a single laboratory over an 11 year period. The donors were divided into four birth cohorts (born before 1959, 1960–64, 1965–69, and 1970–74) and it was found that the median sperm concentration fell from 98×10^6/ml in those born before 1959 to 78×10^6/ml in those born after 1970 ($p = 0.002$). Both the total number of sperm and motile sperm fell significantly, by 29% and 24%, respectively.

In contrast to these seemingly convincing data are those from the USA that have been published separately by Fisch[9,10] and Paulsen,[11] neither of whom were able to demonstrate a decline in sperm counts in North American populations. Furthermore, we failed to demonstrate a fall in sperm density in men donating sperm to a London sperm bank over the last 20 years. These conflicting data have led to the suggestion that there are significant geographical variations in sperm quality. The finding of higher sperm concentrations in North America (in particular New York) is not only difficult to explain but also impacts on the linear regression analyses that have been performed to describe temporal changes of semen quality, as the majority of the studies in the early part of the period studied were from New York, while later data were from Europe and developing countries.

A paper by Bahadur *et al.*[12] reanalyzed the data published in Carlsen's report and included three new European reports. Two models were used to calculate the trend in sperm counts: a linear regression and a quadratic model analysis. The quadratic model actually suggested an upward rise in sperm count since 1975. This paper suggests that the change in sperm counts in the USA over time is greater than in European, Asian, African, and South American communities and again that it is demography that accounts for the fluctuations in values with time. Further data have indicated significant regional differences between European cities and also seasonal variations, with higher counts in winter months.[13] Overall there remains controversy[14] and clearly longitudinal studies are required, particularly in those countries where concerns have been expressed.

In addition to the concerns about deteriorating semen quality the incidence of hypospadias, cryptorchidism and testicular cancer is rising.[15] It has been suggested that environmental estrogenic pollutants are to blame. There are a large number of estrogenic chemicals which might accumulate in our ecosystem (organochlorine pesticides (including DDT), polychlorinated biphenyls (PCBs), surfactants, products of combustion). The Western diet is high in animal fats, proteins and refined carbohydrates and leads to an increase in endogenous estrogen concentrations, which might affect the developing male fetus.[16] Cow's milk contains substantial amounts of estrogens, and indeed more than half of British cows that are farmed for their milk are pregnant. In addition, a number of plant foods (e.g., soya) contain weak estrogens (phytoestrogens). Synthetic estrogens such as diethylstilbestrol and ethinylestradiol have not only been ingested by mothers but may also find their way into drinking water. Estrogens in river water have been detected by the large increases in the yolk protein vitellogen whose secretion is normally only induced by estrogen. The finding of hermaphroditic fish in British rivers has been used to monitor estrogenic pollution. Organic farmers who were asked to provide semen samples when attending a conference were found to have significantly higher sperm concentrations than printers, electricians, or metal workers ,[17] which lends further credence to the possible effects of environmental toxins on spermatogenesis.

Undescended Testes (Cryptorchidism)

The gonad differentiates into the testis during week 8 of intrauterine life, at which time the gubernaculum has developed through a gap in the anterior abdominal wall to the genital swellings (the future scrotum). Between weeks 8 and 12 the cremasteric muscle develops and the processus vaginalis herniates from the peritoneum ventral to the gubernaculum. The testes continue to develop and at 28 weeks the processus vaginalis extends to the scrotum, the gubernaculum swells and the epididymis and testes descend rapidly, with the epididymis descending first. The gubernaculum atrophies and the upper part of the processus vaginalis should close but if it does not a hernia or hydrocele may result. Testicular descent is dependent on testosterone and its active metabolite dihydrotestosterone. Mullerian inhibitory factor (MIF) may also play a role.

Boys with undescended testes have a 40% rate of epididymal and vasal abnormalities, compared with 0.5–1% in the normal population. These abnormalities may have resulted from the failure of testicular descent, ductal immaturity, or an abnormal hormonal environment. Ipsilateral testicular testosterone is necessary for normal ductal development.

By the age of 6 months the gonadocytes have usually developed into adult spermatogonia, which in turn start to mature into primary spermatocytes by the age of 3 years. This process is delayed and arrested in boys with testes undescended after the age of 1 year.

Retractile testes occur four times as often as undescended testes and do not require surgery. The testis can be milked into the scrotum, where it remains for a few seconds, whereas if the cryptorchid testis can be brought down it quickly springs back. Intramuscular injections of human chorionic gonadotropin (hCG) invariably cause retractile testes to descend but not the cryptorchid testis.

Most men with unilateral undescended testes are fertile but with a reduced sperm count. The undescended testis produces few, if any sperm after orchidopexy as the shrunken testis is largely fibrotic. Bilateral undescended testes in adulthood carry a very poor prognosis for fertility. While it is thought that orchidopexy should be performed at a young age, there is actually no difference in subsequent fertility when the procedure is performed either early or late in the age range 4–14 years. Hormonal therapy, instituted at any age, does not appear to help.

Carcinoma in situ has been found in cryptorchid testes that have not been brought down before the age of 10 years and if left, this is likely to develop into testicular cancer. Men with undescended testes have a relative risk of developing a testicular germ cell cancer of 5.9 compared with controls; the relative risk on the ipsilateral side in unilateral cryptorchidism is 8.0 and 1.6 in the contralateral descended side. Early orchidopexy, before the age of 5 years, may decrease this risk.[18]

Orchidopexy

This is important in order to prevent recurrent testicular torsion. If surgery in the inguinal region is required it is vital to avoid accidental, or unwitting, injury to the vas deferens or testicular vessels, which can be a particular risk of inguinal herniorrhaphy.

Prophylactic MMR (Mumps, Measles, Rubella) Vaccination

This protects against the development of mumps orchitis, which after puberty may significantly affect spermatogenesis. Chickenpox can also cause a severe orchitis. Viral oophoritis is an uncommon cause of female sterility; it is usually secondary to mumps and so should also be prevented by the MMR vaccination in childhood.

Orchitis

If orchitis occurs it is essential to try to minimize testicular atrophy, which is secondary to raised intratesticular pressure. Steroids should be administered (prednisolone 40–60 mg per day). In those not responding, surgery can be performed to relieve pressure necrosis by placing incisions in the tunica albuginea.

Sexually Transmitted Diseases

Gonorrhea causes irreversible obstruction of the spermatic ducts but is much less prevalent in the West than 30–40 years ago. *Chlamydia trachomatis* is now the most common sexually transmitted pathogen in developed countries, causing urethritis and epididymitis. Young men and women should be advised about the use of barrier methods of contraception and men urged to use condoms until they are in a stable relationship in which they wish to start a family.

Injuries

Trauma to the testes can result in permanent damage and also increase the risk of the subsequent production of antisperm antibodies. Men should therefore be advised to wear appropriate protection when participating in contact sports.

Varicocele Ligation

In some countries varicocele ligation is performed in teenagers to prevent subsequent infertility. There is controversy surrounding the role of varicocele ligation in male infertility and therefore no justification for performing prophylactic ligation in childhood or adolescence at the present time (see also Ch. 11).

Occupational Factors

Men who have to work in the presence of environmental toxins should be made aware that these can affect fertility. Some metals are toxic to spermatogenesis, for example lead, cadmium, and mercury;[19] metal welders have been observed to have fertility problems as have workers with a number of chemicals (pesticides: dibromochloropropane, chlordecone, ethylene dibromide; glycol ethers – used in inks, paint and adhesives).

Drugs

While the effects of many drugs on spermatogenesis are reversible, some can have a permanent effect; for example, spermatogenesis does not always make a full recovery after therapy with sulfasalazine, which is used in the treatment of inflammatory bowel diseases. Olsalazine, which can be used instead of sulfasalazine, does not appear to have an adverse effect on fertility. Sometimes the side-effects of drug therapy have to be weighed against their therapeutic benefits but there are often alternative preparations – for example, many antihypertensives cause impotence (beta-blockers, methyldopa, captopril) while others do not (calcium channel blockers).

Chemotherapy/Radiotherapy

Men should be made aware of the possibility of freezing sperm before chemotherapy or radiotherapy. Alkylating agents (cyclophosphamide, procarbazine, cisplatin) are particularly damaging to gonadal function. Unfortunately we still see cases where this risk was not discussed before treatment. Men who are about to undergo chemo/radiotherapy are often severely debilitated and may have difficulty producing a sperm sample. Furthermore the quality of the sample may be very poor. Since the advent of IVF with micromanipulation of gametes (see Ch. 13) it is now possible to provide treatment for men for whom donor insemination was the only option in the past. Thus any sperm that can be produced before spermatotoxic therapy is initiated should be frozen for future use.

Advice About Age

Fecundity declines with age, primarily that of the woman. Men have fathered children into their nineties, although there is an increase in the rate of fresh mutations with increasing paternal age that can lead to dominantly inherited congenital defects such as Marfan's syndrome, Alpert's syndrome and achondroplasia. Sperm numbers and function do tend to decline with age although there is no predictable pattern.[20,21] A study from Bristol identified a correlation between increased time to conception and paternal age, after taking account of other variables such as female age and other factors that affect fertility.[22] The reasons for this are unclear and may be due to a combination of factors including declining testicular endocrine function, reduced coital frequency, and declining spermatozoal function.

Women are born with a fixed number of oocytes (about 1 million per ovary), although fewer than 500 ovulate and the remainder degenerate. In the Oxford Family Planning survey[23] it was found that parous women who stopped contraception experienced a significant decline in fertility after the age of 37, while in nulliparous women there was a significant decrease in fertility from the age of 28 onward. Smoking accelerates the age of the menopause by up to 2 years (see Ch. 8). Nulliparity also brings forward the age of the menopause. It is a decline in oocyte quality rather than uterine receptivity that accounts for the age-related decline in infertility, as evidenced by the high pregnancy rates that are achieved in older, sometimes postmenopausal women, who undergo oocyte donation receiving eggs donated by women who may be 10–30 years younger than themselves.[24] The decline in oocyte quality with age, which is accompanied by an increase in the rate of chromosomal abnormalities, accelerates when the critical mass of follicles has declined to about 10 000 per ovary – usually around the age of 37 years.[25] A woman's fertility is therefore thought to decline significantly after the age of 37. Recent data have suggested that the decline in fertility starts much earlier, with women aged between 19 and 26 years having twice the chance of a spontaneous pregnancy compared with women aged from 35 to 39 years.[26] In this study fertility also declined in men after the age of 35 years.

It has been suggested that the increase in chromosomal abnormalities is not directly due to the chronological age of the oocyte and its prolonged state of meiotic arrest, but that the normal oocytes are ovulated and selected first. This would explain why women who have premature ovarian failure have an increased risk of chromosomally abnormal fetuses as they near the end of their reproductive life.[27] The best known association between maternal age and aneuploidy is for trisomy 21, Down's syndrome, yet a full understanding of the mechanism(s) remains elusive and trisomic chromosomal imbalance continues as a major cause of human genetic disease. To facilitate wider understanding of aneuploidy, its incidence has been studied cytogenetically at different developmental time-points, most commonly either on mature gametes or on tissues from clinically recognized pregnancies.

With the widespread introduction of IVF programs, a number of human cytogenetic studies have been performed on metaphase II oocytes which have failed to fertilize following insemination. Age-related increases in the incidence of aneuploidy have been found by some but not all investigators (see review by Nugent & Balen).[28] It is thought that anomalies in chromosome segregation arise most commonly during a dysfunctional first meiotic division.[29] Insights into potential mechanisms have been provided by Angell and colleagues[30] using *in vitro* culture and donated oocytes from women of different ages to examine the segregation of chromosomes during first meiosis compared with observations on metaphase II oocytes. They found that 64 of 179 meiosis II oocytes examined had an abnormal haploid complement but none involved a whole extra chromosome as would be predicted by the classical model of non-disjunction. These results suggested that premature division of the centromere at meiosis I may be the most important source of human trisomy.

While observations on human oocytes from failed IVF are of interest, they may not be an accurate reflection of the *in vivo* situation for a variety of reasons. The oocytes have usually been collected following superovulation regimens and will thus include oocytes from follicles otherwise destined to undergo atresia. Furthermore, they have failed to fertilize following insemination, have undergone prolonged periods in culture, and have predominantly been donated by older women undergoing IVF for diverse indications. Another factor which may influence interpretation of these studies is a significant inter-individual variation in non-disjunction, suggested by aneuploidy in multiple oocytes from some patients. Embryonic chromosomal abnormalities are a major cause of implantation failure and early pregnancy loss, thereby accounting for the relatively low rates of human fertility in spontaneous and assisted conceptions.[31]

Chromosomal aberrations for X, Y, 18, and 21 have been found in 70% of abnormally developing monospermic donated embryos in IVF. Aneuploidy rates have been reported of 13.5% for embryos from women below the age of 30 years, 19.8% for those aged 30–34 years and 23.1% for those aged 35–39 years.[32] More recently, when fluorescent *in situ* hybridization (FISH) was used, 3 and 1 of 64 embryos were aneuploid for chromosomes 16 and 18, respectively, in patients over 35 years of age.[31] These results suggest a relationship between maternal age and malsegregation of certain chromosomes during female meiosis, although we should recognize that these 'spare' embryos may not be representative of the *in vivo* situation. With an increasing number of studies becoming available, together with more reliable laboratory facilities, further insight into aneuploidy should become available. Furthermore, some clinics are beginning to offer aneuploidy screening of preimplantation embryos for older couples who would not otherwise require IVF. This procedure is not yet licenced in the UK.

There is a higher rate of spontaneous abortion with increased maternal age. Cytogenetic studies of several thousand first trimester abortuses from clinically recognized pregnancies found a total aneuploidy frequency of 35–40%.[33] Of those analyzed, trisomy 16 was the commonest, representing 20–35% of those observed. Aneuploidy of chromosomes 2, 13, 15, 18, 21, and 22 accounted for the remainder. Effects of maternal age on aneuploidy vary, with chromosome 16 showing a linear increase with maternal age whereas chromosome 21 shows an exponential rise towards the end of the reproductive life span.

Young men and women should be made aware of these issues. Unfortunately our society encourages career development for men and women without providing suitable flexibility for women and appropriate crèche facilities. Figure 2.2 suggests some measures for preventing infertility in both men and women.

Female Infertility

Contraception

Probably the most important advice that can be given to a young woman concerns appropriate methods of contraception. Pelvic infection, most commonly caused by *Chlamydia trachomatis*, results in severe tubal damage in 10–30% of women after a first attack, 30–60% after a second and 50–90% after a third. Chlamydial pelvic inflammatory disease (PID) is often "silent," with the patient having no notion that there was an infection until severe adhesions and pelvic damage are noted at laparoscopy during infertility investigations.

The combined oral contraceptive (COC) pill is the most efficacious contraceptive and also provides some protection against PID, reducing the risk of hospitalization with PID by 50%. The mechanism is by the effect of progestogens on thickening cervical mucus, thereby inhibiting penetration by spermatozoa and the bacteria that ride with them. The COC does not, however, confer complete protection from sexually transmitted diseases (STDs) and barrier methods of contraception should be used in addition to the COC, especially by women who are not in a stable relationship.

Prevention of infertility

Male		**Female**
Environmental	– reduce estrogenic pollutants – protect workers in chemical industries	Avoid unwanted pregnancies and TOPs
Undescended testes	– orchidopexy	
Surgery to testis	– avoid injury to vas, testicular vessels	Care of pelvic organs with abdominal surgery
Orchitis	– MMR vaccination	
Varicocele	– ligation?	

Both

Avoid STDs – barrier methods of contraception
Don't delay childbearing
Storage of sperm/oocytes (ovarian tissue) before chemo-/radiotherapy

Figure 2.2 Suggested measures for the prevention of infertility. TOPs, terminations of pregnancy; STDs, sexually transmitted diseases.

The COC has been associated with up to double the risk of developing cervical cancer,[34] while any barrier method of contraception that prevents STDs should also reduce the incidence of cervical dysplasia and the consequent need for cone biopsy of the cervix or diathermy loop excision (DLE) of the abnormal area. Surgery to the cervix can lead to disturbances in the production of cervical mucus or cervical stenosis and hence infertility or otherwise can result in cervical incompetence and miscarriage.

The intrauterine contraceptive device (IUCD) is thought to increase the risk of developing a clinical PID by 50–100% compared with non-users and certainly PID associated with the presence of an IUCD is often severe. The risk of PID is mostly related to lifestyle, with a very low rate of PID in IUCD users who are in long-term, stable, monogamous relationships. Of all the different types of IUCD, the progestogen-releasing IUCD (Mirena intrauterine system (IUS)) appears to minimize the risk of infection by its effect on the cervical mucus. We do not generally recommend the use of IUCDs in nulliparous women unless the woman anticipates being in a long-term relationship; however, an IUS could be offered.

A woman's fertility is put at significant risk when she undergoes a termination of pregnancy. Suction termination of pregnancy risks damage to the cervix, although this is reduced by cervical preparation with intravaginal prostaglandins preoperatively. Damage to the uterus by perforation may occur and pelvic infection, caused by introduction of infection during the procedure or secondary to retained products of conception, occurs after 5% of surgical terminations. There is debate about the routine use of antibiotic prophylaxis before termination of pregnancy, with conflicting evidence about its benefit because of the possible risk of inducing antibiotic resistance. The results of preoperative endocervical swabs are rarely available by the time of the procedure. On balance we consider it prudent to offer prophylaxis (in the form of a tetracycline and metronidazole or Augmentin) to nulliparous women having a surgical termination of pregnancy. Medical termination of pregnancy with the anti-progesterone RU486 also carries a 5% risk of retained products of conception and hence pelvic infection, although overall may lead to slightly fewer cases of subsequent infertility than surgical termination of pregnancy.

General Health Screening

Issues relating to women's health and prepregnancy screening are covered in Chapter 3. Family planning clinics should also provide general health screening and discuss issues such as weight, smoking, and alcohol consumption.

Young women with erratic menstrual cycles who are likely to have polycystic ovary syndrome, or who might have stigmata of the syndrome such as acne, should be warned against excessive weight gain as obesity worsens the endocrine profile of these women and increases the risk of infertility (see Chs 6 and 7).

Chemotherapy/Radiotherapy

The oocyte is more vulnerable to freezing than spermatozoa[35] and current work on oocyte cryopreservation is still largely at the research stage, with only a few successful pregnancies having been reported so far. In addition to oocyte cryopreservation, work is under way to try to preserve ovarian tissue for later use, either for ovarian autografting or for the *in vitro* culture of follicles, from which oocytes can be obtained for *in vitro* fertilization. This is an extremely exciting area of research in which considerable advances have taken place in the last 5 years (see Ch. 18).

Abdominal Surgery

Surgery for appendicitis should be performed swiftly, and preferably before peritonitis evolves. Pelvic structures should be left alone and if peritonitis has occurred, peritoneal lavage should be performed and antibiotics administered for at least 2 weeks. General surgeons should be trained to respect pelvic structures. If there is doubt about the diagnosis before performing a laparotomy a gynecological opinion should be sought and a laparoscopy performed, as all too often salpingo-oophorectomies have been performed through extended grid-iron or midline incisions for benign ovarian cysts that should have been managed conservatively. Gynecologists should be all too well aware of the care that should be taken when operating on young women in order to preserve fertility and avoid disrupting ovarian or tubal anatomy.

Environmental Pollutants

Environmental pollutants have not been thought to have an equivalent effect on female fertility as they have on male fertility.[36,37] There is some evidence from non-human primate studies that dioxins might induce endometriosis, but this is unproven in humans. This is a highly topical subject and further research is required before firm conclusions are drawn about the effects of environmental pollutants (other than cigarette smoke) on female reproductive health.[37]

References

1. Carlsen E, Giwercman A, Keiding N & Skakkebaek NE (1992) Evidence for decreasing quality of semen during the past 50 years. *Br Med J* **305**: 609–613.
2. Brake A & Krause W (1992) Decreasing quality of semen. *Br Med J* **305**: 1498.
3. Bromwich P, Cohen J, Stewart I & Walker A (1994) Decline in sperm counts: an artefact of changed reference range of "normal"? *Br Med J* **309**: 19–22.
4. Auger J, Kunstmann JM, Czyglik F & Jouannet P (1995) Decline in semen

quality among fertile men in Paris during the past 20 years. *N Engl J Med* **332**: 281–285.
5. Forti G & Serio M (1993) Male infertility: is its rising incidence due to better methodology of detection or an increasing frequency? *Hum Reprod* **8**: 1153–1154.
6. Sherins RJ (1995) Are semen quality and male fertility changing? *N Engl J Med* **332**: 327–328.
7. Skakkebaek NE & Keiding N (1994) Changes in semen and the testis. *Br Med J* **309**: 1316–1317.
8. Irvine S, Cawood E, Richardson D, MacDonald E & Aitken J (1996) Evidence of deteriorating semen quality in the United Kingdom: a birth cohort study of 577 men in Scotland over 11 years. *Br Med J* **312**: 467–471.
9. Fisch H, Goluboff ET, Olsen JH, Feldshuh J, Broder SJ & Barad DH (1996) Semen analyses in 1283 men from the United States over a 25 year period: no decline in quality. *Fertil Steril* **65**: 1009–1014.
10. Fisch H & Goluboff ET (1996) Geographic variations in sperm counts: a potential cause of bias in studies of semen quality. *Fertil Steril* **65**: 1044–1047.
11. Paulsen CA, Berman NG & Wang C (1996) Data from men in greater Seattle area reveals no downward trend in semen quality: further evidence that deterioration of semen quality is not geographically uniform. *Fertil Steril* **65**: 1015–1021.
12. Bahadur G, Ling KLE & Katz M (1996) Statistical modelling reveals demography and time are the main contributing factors in global sperm count changes between 1938–1996. *Hum Reprod* **11**: 2635–2639.
13. Jorgensen N, Andersen A-G, Eustache F *et al.* (2001) Regional differences in semen quality in Europe. *Hum Reprod* **16**: 1012–1019.
14. Irvine DS (1997) Declining sperm quality: a review of facts and hypotheses. *Baillière's Clin Obstet Gynaecol* **11**: 655–671.
15. Sharp L, Black RJ, Muir CS, Warner J & Clarke JA (1993) Trends in cancer of the testis in Scotland, 1961–90. *Health Bull* **51**: 255–267.
16. Sharpe RM & Skakkebaek NE (1992) Are oestrogens involved in falling sperm counts and disorders of the male reproductive tract? *Lancet* **341**: 1392–1395.
17. Abell A, Ernst E, Bonde JP (1994) High sperm density among members of organic farmers' association. *Lancet* **343**: 1498.
18. Kiely EA (1994) Scientific basis of testicular descent and management implications for cryptorchidism. *Br J Clin Practice* **48**: 37–41.
19. Bonde JPE (1993) The risk of male subfecundity attributable to welding of metals: studies of semen quality, infertility, fertility, adverse pregnancy outcome and childhood malignancy. *Int J Androl* **16**: 1–29.
20. Speroff L (1994) The effect of aging on fertility. *Curr Opin Obstet Gynecol* **6**: 115–120.
21. Vermeulen A (1993) Environment, human reproduction, menopause and andropause. *Envir Health Perspect* **101** (Suppl. 2): 91–100.
22. Ford WCL, North K, Taylor H, Farrow A, Hull MGR & Golding J (2000). Increasing paternal age is associated with delayed conception in a large population of fertile couples: evidence for declining fecundity in older men. *Hum Reprod* **15**: 1703–1708.
23. Howe G, Westhoff C, Vessey M & Yeates D (1985) Effects of age, cigarette smoking and other factors on fertility: findings in a large prospective study. *Br Med J* **290**: 1697–1700.
24. Abdalla HI, Burton G, Kirkland A, Johnson MR *et al.* (1993) Age, pregnancy and miscarriage: uterine versus ovarian factors. *Hum Reprod* **8**: 1512–1517.
25. Faddy MJ, Gosden RG, Gougeon A, Richardson SJ & Nelson JF (1992) Accelerated disappearance of ovarian follicles in mid life: implications for forecasting menopause. *Hum Reprod* **7**: 1342–1346.
26. Dunson DB, Colombo B & Baird DD (2002) Changes with age in the level and duration of fertility in the menstrual cycle. *Hum Reprod* **17**: 1399–1403.

27. Zheng CJ & Byers B (1992) Oocyte selection: a new model for the maternal-age dependence of Down syndrome. *Hum Genet* **90**: 1–6.
28. Nugent D & Balen AH (1999) Pregnancy in the older woman. *J Brit Menop Soc* **5**: 132–135.
29. Moore DP & Orr-Weaver TL (1998) Chromosome segregation during meiosis: building an unambivalent univalent. *Curr Topic Dev Biol* **37**: 263–299.
30. Angell RR, Xian J, Keith J, Ledger W & Baird DT (1994) First meiotic division abnormalities in human oocytes: mechanism of trisomy formation. *Cytogene Cell Genet* **65**: 194–202.
31. Munne S, Alikani M, Tomkin G, Grifo J & Cohen J (1995) Embryo morphology, developmental rates and maternal age are correlated with chromosome abnormalities. *Fertil Steril* **64**: 382–391.
32. Jamieson ME, Coutts JRT & Connor JM (1994) The chromosome constitution of human preimplantation embryos fertilized *in vitro*. *Hum Reprod* **9**: 709–715.
33. Hassold T, Hunt P & Sherman S (1993) Trisomy in humans: incidence, origin, and etiology. *Curr Opin Genet Dev* **3**: 398–403.
34. Moreno V, Bosch FX, Munoz N *et al.* (2002) Effect of oral contraceptives on risk of cervical cancer in women with human papillomavirus infection: the IARC multicentric case-control study. *Lancet* **359**: 1085–1101.
35. Newton H, Aubard Y, Rutherford AJ, Sharma V & Gosden R (1996) Low temperature storage and grafting of human ovarian tissue. *Hum Reprod* **11**: 487–1491.
36. Review Symposium (2001) Environmental effects on reproductive health. *Hum Reprod Update* **7**: no. 3.
37. Sharara FI, Seifer DB & Flaws JA (1998) Environmental toxicants and female reproduction. *Fertil Steril* **70**: 613–622.
38. Keiding N, Skakkebaek NE (1995) **311**: 570

Chapter 3

Planning a pregnancy

Introduction

Denial of fertility treatment because of problems with a couple's health (usually the woman's) or because of unhealthy habits such as smoking is a contentious issue. The debate concerns the reduced success of fertility treatments in couples with health problems and the increased risks during pregnancy and to the subsequent health of the newborn child. While the welfare of the child is of paramount importance, it is often argued by those seeking fertility treatment that fertile women with health problems similar to their own are neither forbidden from conceiving nor advised to terminate their pregnancy when they do conceive. Why, then, should we be selective in our choice of whom we treat? The two main reasons given are:

1. the fact that there are limitations on resources that encourage selection of those who are likely to become pregnant quickly
2. the fact that we are not very effective at preconception health screening and counseling for couples who have health problems but who do not have subfertility.

In most cases we advise *deferring* treatment until the patient's health has improved, rather than *denying* treatment. There are occasions, however, where the risks to the unborn child are such that we do not advise treatment (for example, use of crack cocaine) or where careful counseling and management are required (e.g. HIV infection of the potential mother).

Other Issues

Patients who attend fertility clinics often have problems in addition to the main cause of their subfertility. Before treatment is started one should address these issues in order to optimize the chances of conception and increase the probability of producing a healthy child who is developmentally normal. Most women appreciate that changes in lifestyle and diet are worthwhile if they are for the benefit of their unborn child. One should, however, try to avoid being too dogmatic or discriminatory, not least because denial of treatment increases stress and is self-limiting in what it can hope to achieve.

Weight

Women

Women who have a normal body mass index (BMI) are more likely to conceive and to have a normal pregnancy than those who are not of the correct weight for their height. The BMI is calculated by dividing the weight (in kilograms) by the height (in meters) squared. The normal range is 20–25 kg/m^2 (Fig. 3.1).

Women who are underweight become anovulatory and amenorrheic (see Ch. 6). It is usually easy to induce ovulation in underweight women, who then conceive readily. However, these pregnancies are more likely to miscarry or result in the premature delivery of growth-retarded babies. These babies are then at increased risk of problems in later life, such as cardiovascular disease and diabetes, because of programming during fetal life.[1] Thus, for the prospective mother, weight gain rather than ovulation induction is the correct management.

Obesity is the more likely problem in Western society, and the UK has one of the highest rates of obesity in Europe. Not only does obesity reduce fertility, but also obese women who conceive are at greater risk of miscarriage,[2] gestational diabetes, hypertension, thromboembolism, and complicated operative delivery. The nutritional status of the new-born is also thought to have a major influence on disease in

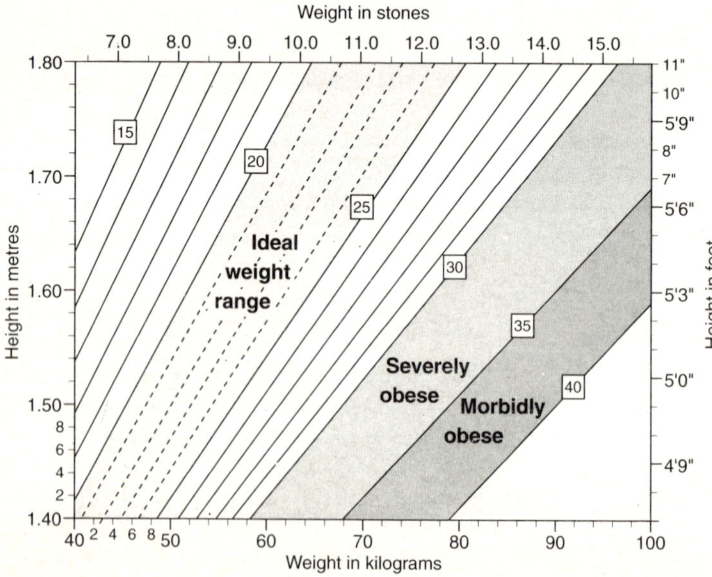

Figure 3.1 Body mass index (BMI) chart. Each diagonal line represents the BMI in kg/m^2 (chart devised by Dr G. Conway, Middlesex Hospital, London).

adulthood.[1] We are therefore reluctant to treat women who have a BMI greater than 30 kg/m^2 and would advise that the BMI should be less than 28 kg/m^2.[2] There is conclusive evidence that weight loss improves overall reproductive function, particularly in women with polycystic ovary syndrome (see Chs 6 and 7).[3,4] It can sometimes be difficult to explain this approach to overweight patients as many obese women ovulate and conceive, which makes it difficult to justify deferring treatment to their anovulatory peers until they have lost weight.

Men

Men who are significantly overweight might also be expected to have fertility problems since obesity in men is associated with reduced serum androgen concentrations and elevated serum estrogen concentrations. The hyperinsulinemia of obesity results in a fall in sex hormone binding globulin (SHBG) levels and so the free testosterone concentration stays in the normal male range.[5] Most obese men are therefore able to reproduce normally, provided there is no physical impediment to coitus. Extreme obesity in men, however, is sometimes associated with hypogonadotropic hypogonadism.[6]

Dietary Advice for Women Wishing to Conceive

Dietary advice for women wishing to conceive is shown in Tables 3.1 and 3.2. Women attending the fertility clinic should be given general advice about diet and exercise. A balanced diet should provide about 2000 kilocalories daily (a satisfactory range is 1500–2500 kilocalories), which increases by about 200 kilocalories during pregnancy. Some women like to have very specific advice about diet while others, if there are concerns, should be encouraged to keep a record of what they eat over 2 separate days and then discuss with a dietician how best to

Table 3.1 Recommended daily requirements

	Non-pregnant	Pregnant
Energy (kilocalories)	1940	2140
Protein (grams)	45	51
Folate (micrograms)	300	400
Iron (milligrams)	15	15
Calcium (milligrams)	1200	1700
Zinc (milligrams)	7	7
Iodine (micrograms)	140	140
Carbohydrate (grams)	250	275

Table 3.2 The energy values of the main energy-yielding compounds

	Kilojoules/gram	Kilocalories/gram
Fat	9	37
Alcohol	7	29
Protein	4	17
Carbohydrate	3.75	16

improve their diet. Specific diets have been recommended for women with polycystic ovary syndrome (PCOS)[7] and some women find them to be advantageous, although overall it is an achievable, sustainable diet that is important. In particular we do not favor low carbohydrate diets to the exclusion of all else, as recommended by some. A healthy diet requires the right amounts of the four main food groups (see Appendix 1). In general, it is unnecessary to take vitamin supplements, as long as the diet contains fresh fruit, vegetables (preferably lightly cooked), dairy products, and some fish and/or lean meat. The one exception is folic acid, which is now recommended for women who are trying to conceive.

Folic Acid (Folate)

Recent studies have shown that folic acid helps to reduce the risk of babies developing neural tube defects. Table 3.3 lists some useful sources of folate. Women who are planning a pregnancy are advised to consume additional folate prior to conception and to continue to do so during the first 12 weeks of pregnancy. The daily requirement is 400 micrograms. A higher dose (5 mg) is advised to prevent *recurrence* of a neural tube defect and for women on antiepileptic drugs. There are a number of tablets that contain both iron and folate and these are often recommended during pregnancy. Many multivitamin tablets also contain folic acid.

Special Diets for Sex Selection and Fertility

It has been suggested that changes in diet can both aid fertility and achieve sex selection, the latter by enhancing zona pellucida receptivity to either X- or Y-bearing spermatozoa.

Sex Selection

Advocates of sex selection have advised special diets, vaginal douches of differing pH, or intercourse at different times around the time of

Table 3.3 Useful sources of folate in a typical serving

Boiled broccoli	30 mg
Boiled sprouts	100 mg
Boiled cabbage	25 mg
Boiled carrots	10 mg
Boiled cauliflower	45 mg
Boiled green beans	50 mg
Peas	30 mg
Potatoes	45 mg
Spinach	80 mg
Folate is lost by overboiling vegetables	
Banana	15 mg
Grapefruit	20 mg
Orange	50 mg
Orange juice	40 mg
Bovril	95 mg per cup
Marmite	40 mg per serving
Milk	35 mg per pint
Boiled brown rice	15 mg
Boiled white rice	5 mg
2 slices white bread	25 mg
2 slices wholemeal bread	40 mg
Cornflakes (fortified)	100 mg

Liver is rich in folate but should be avoided by those trying to conceive because of the possible danger of consuming too much vitamin A

ovulation. Not only are there complete contrasts in opinion about these methods, there are no prospective randomized studies that support any of the practices. Similarly, while mechanical separation of spermatozoa is practiced by some clinics, the results have not stood up to scientific scrutiny. Sex selection to prevent the transmission of sex-linked congenital disease is possible after pre-embryo biopsy in the context of IVF treatment (or later in pregnancy by chorionic villus biopsy or amniocentesis).

Fertility

Some minerals and vitamins have been used in the treatment of male infertility. Zinc sulfate (120 mg twice daily) was found to increase sperm concentration and serum testosterone concentrations in a small study of men with oligospermia and low testosterone levels.[8] Vitamin

E, because of its antioxidant properties, has been advocated for use both orally (300–600 mg daily for at least 6 weeks)[9] and *in vitro*[10] in men with asthenozoospermia. Vitamin B_{12} has also been used for the treatment of oligozoospermia. There are, however, insufficient data from prospective studies of these therapies so, while not harmful, they are of uncertain benefit.

The "Foresight" program in Britain, in addition to giving sensible preconception advice about general health, advocates changes in diet to enhance fertility and reduce miscarriage. Patients are asked to send their hair for analysis of minerals, metals, and trace elements and advice is invariably given to take vitamin/mineral supplements. We are not aware of prospective randomized studies that have shown this approach to be of any clinical benefit and so do not recommend it.

Acquired Infections

Listeriosis can cause miscarriage and may be acquired from cooked–chilled foods that have not been adequately reheated. Cold meat pies, ready-to-eat poultry, unpasteurized milk, and soft ripened cheeses (Brie, Camembert, blue vein types) should be avoided by women who may be pregnant. When pregnant, women should also avoid contact with sheep at lambing time and handling silage because of the risk of contracting listeriosis, toxoplasmosis, or chlamydiosis. Toxoplasmosis can be caught from cats and dogs and so women should be advised to make sure that they wash their hands thoroughly after handling either pets or their food bowls.

Exercise

Regular physical exercise is an essential adjunct to a healthy diet and does not cause problems for women either trying to conceive or during pregnancy. Sudden changes in exercise patterns can be detrimental and should certainly be avoided during pregnancy. Excessive exercise can lead to hypothalamic dysfunction in women and men and weight loss can render women amenorrheic (see Ch. 6).

Alcohol

Alcohol has profound effects on Leydig cell function by reducing testosterone synthesis and its metabolite, acetaldehyde, causing membrane damage and the formation of Leydig cell autoantibodies, which persist long term. Excessive intake of alcohol also disturbs hypothalamic–pituitary function, further worsening testicular and sexual function. Impotence is a well-known effect of alcoholism, as are the signs of hyperestrogenism (gynecomastia, female escutcheon), which is probably secondary to disturbances of the metabolism of testosterone and estrogens in the cirrhotic liver.

Alcoholism can lead to amenorrhea and disorders of ovulation, probably by central effects rather than by acting on the ovary. Alcohol consumption during early pregnancy can lead to severe developmental abnormalities in the baby (growth retardation, mental retardation, physical malformations). A sensible limit while trying to conceive is less than 6 units of alcohol per week. There is some evidence that complete cessation of alcohol consumption is associated with improved fertility.[11] Alcohol should also be avoided during pregnancy, although small regular quantities are preferable to binge drinking, which some think is the main cause of the fetal alcohol syndrome.

Smoking

The metabolites of cigarette smoking are toxic to oocytes (causing oxidative damage to mitochondria), sperm (causing a higher percentage of morphological abnormalities), and embryos (causing miscarriage). Smoking reduces both the chance of getting pregnant and also the success of fertility treatments.

Lower Fertility

The Oxford Family Planning Association database permitted observation of over 17 000 women in the UK, of whom over 4000 stopped contraception to become pregnant.[12] There was a highly significant trend of decreasing fertility with increasing numbers of cigarettes smoked per day. It was estimated that 5 years after stopping contraception, approximately 11% of women who smoked more than 20 cigarettes a day, but only 5% of non-smokers, remained undelivered. A systematic review of published studies reported that the overall odds ratio for the risk of infertility was 1.60 (95% CI 1.34–1.91) for smokers compared with non-smokers.[13] The chance of conception in smokers undergoing IVF was 0.66 (95% CI 0.49–0.88).[13] There is some evidence that ex-smokers can expect a return to normal fecundity[14] although smoking brings forward the age of the menopause and so appears to have a direct effect on ovarian function. Even passive smoking may have an adverse effect on female fertility[15] and furthermore, while it was thought that smoking had no effect on male fertility, a recent study has suggested otherwise.[15]

Higher Risk of Miscarriage

Smoking during pregnancy doubles the risk of miscarriage, increases the risk of premature labor by 50%, doubles the rate of having a low

Table 3.4 Planning a pregnancy

Optimize health: normal BMI, exercise
Diet: folate, appropriately prepared food
Restrict alcohol < 6 units/week
Stop smoking
Optimize pre-existing medical conditions
Avoid teratogenic drugs

birthweight baby, and leads to intrauterine growth retardation and thus an increased perinatal mortality. There have been reports of an increased rate of congenital limb abnormalities, with terminal transverse defects, thought to be a result of vascular insufficiency. The restriction of the normal growth of the baby may in turn cause the child both physical and mental developmental problems in later life. Smoking is also associated with an increased risk of sudden infant death syndrome.

Table 3.4 shows what steps should be taken when planning a pregnancy.

Medical Conditions and Drugs

It is beyond the scope of this book to give an exhaustive account of the medical conditions that can occur in women of reproductive years. Any debilitating condition can lead to anovulatory infertility secondary to loss of hypothalamic pulsatility of gonadotropin releasing hormone (GnRH) or weight loss. Some conditions may be inherited and so prenatal genetic counseling would be appropriate. We describe some of the disorders that can affect fertility and the drugs that should be avoided because of teratogenicity. The period of greatest risk is from week 3 to week 11 of pregnancy, at a time when many women are initially unaware that they have conceived (although most women who are having fertility treatment perform a pregnancy test the day that their expected period is late). In general, it is advisable to avoid taking any drugs unless their need is proven. Many drugs have warnings against use in pregnancy because of the difficulties in testing new drugs during pregnancy. Thus cautions about the avoidance of drugs during pregnancy may be due to lack of data rather than proven teratogenicity.

> Prostaglandin synthetase inhibitors (indomethacin, mefenamic acid, naproxen, diclofenac, etc.) may inhibit ovulation and result in an increased chance of the formation of a "luteinized unruptured follicle" (LUF). Beware!

Psychiatric Disorders

Infertility can cause psychological distress, sexual dysfunction, and impotence but is not thought to cause psychiatric disease itself. Psychiatric illness, on the other hand, can result in infertility. Women with schizophrenia may have menstrual disturbances (often secondary to hypothalamic dysfunction or drug-induced hyperprolactinemia) and anorexia nervosa leads to weight-related amenorrhea. Bulimia nervosa often goes undetected and is usually denied by the patient, but can be a significant contributor to infertility because of its association with PCOS. Any psychiatric illness can cause hypothalamic dysfunction and anovulatory infertility. Major tranquilizers cause hyperprolactinemia and may result in amenorrhea.

Anxiety and depression

Infertility causes profound anxiety and may lead to clinical depression. Management should be in the form of supportive care with the aid of the clinic counselor and drug therapy should be avoided. If a patient is on sedatives or antidepressants she is probably better deferring pregnancy until her psychological state is stable and she is no longer taking drugs. It should be remembered that these women are prone to postnatal depression and, when they conceive, their obstetrician should be informed. Hypnotic drugs (benzodiazepines) should be avoided in women trying to conceive, although if absolutely necessary the shorter acting preparations (loprazolam, lormetazepam, and temazepam) can be used in a single dose. Barbiturates should also be avoided. Antidepressants are probably safe in pregnancy but, again, should be avoided unless absolutely necessary. Some antidepressants can interfere with sexual function (e.g. amitriptyline, clomipramine, dosulepin (dothiepin), imipramine, mianserin) or cause menstrual irregularities (e.g. amoxapine). Monoamine-oxidase inhibitors should be avoided in women wishing to conceive. Serotonin reuptake inhibitors (e.g. fluoxetine) have become very popular recently and are used in the treatment of depression, as appetite suppressants (although a combination of diet and exercise is a better approach in the management of obesity) and in the treatment of premenstrual syndrome. These drugs should also be avoided if there is a chance of a pregnancy.

Psychosis

Antipsychotic drugs can cause anovulatory infertility by effects on the hypothalamus and by causing hyperprolactinemia. They should also be used with caution in pregnancy as they can cause extrapyramidal signs in the neonate. Lithium, used in the treatment of mania and in the prophylaxis of manic depression, can lead to hypothyroidism; it is also teratogenic and should be avoided.

Clinicians working in fertility clinics have an overriding responsibility to the health of the unborn child. It is appropriate to hold a case conference with all the members of the team who care for a patient with psychiatric disease before embarking upon fertility treatment. It is therefore essential to liaise with the psychiatrist to help with the psychodynamics of impending pregnancy and parenthood as well as to advise on the use of specific medication (such as alternatives to lithium).

Neurological Disorders

Epilepsy

There is an increased risk of anomalies in the fetuses of epileptic women who are not taking antiepileptic drugs, possibly because of a genetic linkage between epilepsy and some fetal anomalies, for example facial clefts. Anticonvulsant drugs are teratogenic and so it is important to try to achieve adequate control of epilepsy in women who are trying to conceive with the lowest dose of a single drug. There is an increased risk of neural tube defects associated with the use of carbamazepine and sodium valproate and patients should be counseled and advised to have antenatal screening. Phenytoin increases the risk of facial clefts and can cause the fetal hydantoin syndrome (small digits, congenital heart defects, facial clefts, abnormalities of head and mental development). It is mandatory to seek the advice of a neurologist before a patient with epilepsy commences fertility therapy.

Myotonic dystrophy

This autosomal dominantly inherited condition often presents with infertility, due to either anovulation or testicular atrophy. The obstetric and genetic sequelae of this condition are so severe as to indicate caution before offering treatment to these patients.

Endocrine Disorders

All of the endocrinopathies can affect gonadal function either directly or by effects on the hypothalamic–pituitary axis. The common causes of anovulatory infertility and their treatments are discussed in detail in Chapter 6. Women with prolactinomas might not wish to conceive but if they do fall pregnant it is important to know the size and position of the tumor: lactotroph hyperplasia leads to a 10–20% increase in pituitary mass during pregnancy, although symptomatic expansion of treated macroprolactinomas occurs in only 7% of cases and the risk with microprolactinomas (< 1 cm diameter) is very small. Dopamine agonist therapy (e.g. bromocriptine, cabergoline) is usually discontinued during pregnancy unless the patient has a macroprolactinoma with suprasellar extension (in which case pregnancy should ideally be avoided) (see Ch. 6). Cabergoline is the drug of first choice for hyperprolactinemia but is not licenced for use in pregnancy and so patients wishing to conceive are usually switched to bromocriptine therapy.

Polycystic ovary syndrome (see also Chs 6 and 7)

Women with polycystic ovary syndrome who do not wish to conceive are often prescribed antiandrogen therapy to suppress unwanted acne and hirsutism. Antiandrogens such as cyproterone acetate are usually taken in combination with ethinylestradiol (e.g. as the preparation Dianette), which is contraceptive. If an accidental pregnancy should occur antiandrogens could theoretically affect development of the genitalia, although there have been over 16 million women-years of use of Dianette and approximately 40 pregnancies in which the preparation has been taken beyond the critical period of organogenesis but no adverse consequences have been reported. Strict contraceptive advice should be given to women using other non-contraceptive antiandrogen preparations, such as spironolactone, finasteride, or flutamide.

Congenital adrenal hyperplasia

Congenital adrenal hyperplasia (CAH) encompasses a number of disorders of steroidogenesis of differing degrees of severity. Patients with salt-losing 21 hydroxylase deficiency commonly require replacement therapy with glucocorticoids and fludrocortisone, which should be continued during pregnancy, although in our experience pregnancy is very uncommon in women with CAH.[16] Furthermore, there is a subgroup of women with CAH who have non-suppressible hypersecretion of progesterone which causes infertility due to failure of endometrial thickening. The control of progesterone secretion can be independent of the control of androgen levels, regardless of the type of steroid therapy used, and adrenalectomy is sometimes indicated if standard suppressive therapies do not restore a regular ovulatory cycle.

Cushing's syndrome

Cushing's syndrome causes menstrual irregularities and subfertility. Pregnancy should be avoided until treatment of Cushing's syndrome is complete although if a pregnancy should occur it has been suggested that termination is advisable because of the potential risks of the disease to the mother. Fetal virilization does not occur, little adrenocorticotropic hormone (ACTH) crosses the placenta, and the fetus is protected from cortisol as it is converted to cortisone by the placenta.

Acromegaly

Women with active acromegaly rarely conceive because of coexistent abnormalities in prolactin and gonadotropin secretion and most have

PCOS. Bromocriptine sometimes aids conception and, if pregnancy does occur, the fetus is not affected by acromegaly.

Thyroid disease

Thyroid disease is common in young women and affects fertility by both hyper- and hypothyroidism causing anovulatory cycles. The latter may be associated with hyperprolactinemia. Women with hyperthyroidism and amenorrhea have usually lost weight. Fertility is usually restored once the patient is rendered euthyroid. The fetus cannot synthesize thyroxine until 12 weeks' gestation and is dependent on placental transfer. Hypothyroidism in the first trimester can have a profound effect on fetal neurological development and so thyroid replacement therapy should be vigorously adhered to, with close monitoring of maternal thyroid stimulating hormone (TSH) and free thyroid hormone concentrations. Hyperthyroidism has the potential to affect the fetus by transplacental passage of thyroid-stimulating autoantibodies or TSH receptor binding antibodies (rendering the fetus thyrotoxic or hypothyroid, respectively), rather than as a result of high circulating concentrations of maternal thyroid hormones. Antithyroid drugs should be reduced to the lowest necessary dose and maternal thyroid function monitored regularly.

Pregnancy ameliorates autoimmune thyroid disease and drug therapy can sometimes be discontinued. Thyroid function should also be monitored closely postpartum because rebound thyroid disease can have a profound effect on maternal health. Hyperthyroidism should be managed with antithyroid drugs, and not radio-iodine, if there is any risk of pregnancy. Propylthiouracil is preferred to carbimazole as it inhibits peripheral conversion of thyroxine (T_4) to triiodothyronine (T_3) and causes a smaller risk of blood dyscrasia, although both drugs have been used safely during pregnancy. Carbimazole may rarely cause aplasia cutis in the neonate. Surgery should be considered if thyrotoxicosis is not controlled with 20 mg of carbimazole or 300 mg of propylthiouracil.

Diabetes

Both type 1 and type 2 diabetes are associated with disturbed ovarian function. If the diabetes is poorly controlled anovulatory infertility may occur. Type 1 diabetes can affect hypothalamic–pituitary function and may be associated with premature menopause due to ovarian autoimmunity. Women with type 2 diabetes are hyperinsulinemic and insulin increases ovarian steroidogenesis leading to hyperandrogenism and PCOS. Thus there is a close association between diabetes and PCOS. Women with PCOS are prone to develop gestational diabetes, especially if they are overweight. Women who are diabetic should be encouraged to have tight control over their blood sugar concentrations in order to enhance their fertility and to minimize the risks of congenital anomalies and pregnancy complications.

There have been conflicting reports about sexual dysfunction in women with diabetes and a suggestion of impaired sexual response, particularly in those with type 2 diabetes. Up to 25% of young men with long-standing (> 10 years) diabetes experience erectile dysfunction, due to both vascular and neurological sequelae of the disease, and the rate increases to 75% by the age of 60. Retrograde ejaculation has also been reported as a consequence of diabetic neuropathy. Diabetes is not thought to have a significant effect on the hypothalamic–pituitary–testicular axis or on spermatogenesis.

Gastrointestinal Disease

Celiac disease

Men and women with celiac disease (gluten-sensitive enteropathy) appear to have an increased rate of infertility due both to abnormalities of the hypothalamic–pituitary axis and, in men, impotence and disordered spermatogenesis. Gluten withdrawal should correct most abnormalities but does not always improve sperm function.

Inflammatory bowel disease

Inflammatory bowel disease can impair fertility but this depends largely on nutritional status, activity of the disease, and drug therapy. Surgery can cause pelvic damage and care should be taken when performing laparoscopic evaluation of the pelvis because of the risk of adhesions and damage to the bowel. Pyschosexual difficulties also occur due to altered perceptions of body image, particularly after resective surgery. Sulfasalazine causes reversible oligospermia but the newer preparation olsalazine is thought not to affect spermatogenesis. These drugs are probably safe in pregnancy, although folate supplementation is recommended in the third trimester.

Irritable bowel syndrome

Irritable bowel syndrome (IBS) is increasingly recognized in young women as a cause of pelvic and generalized abdominal pain. Women with IBS are often of an anxious disposition and their symptoms might be exacerbated by concerns about subfertility. Management is with a combination of high fiber diets, stool bulking agents and antispasmodics (anticholinergic drugs), although the latter should be avoided in pregnancy.

Peptic ulcers

Peptic ulceration can be treated successfully with H_2 receptor antagonists (ranitidine, cimetidine) which, however, can cause gynecomastia and impotence in men (less so with ranitidine than cimetidine). Omeprazole, a proton pump inhibitor, can, rarely, have similar effects and so should also be avoided in pregnancy.

Renal Disease

Adults with severe renal disease are unlikely to conceive.

In men

Men may have erectile dysfunction, primary hypogonadism and irreversible histological changes in the testes, with hyalinization of the tubular basement membranes and reduced numbers of Leydig cells. Uremia also leads to hypothalamic failure and hyperprolactinemia – the latter caused by both pituitary overproduction and reduced renal excretion of prolactin. Hypothalamic anovulatory infertility seems to respond better to hemodialysis than male infertility but both recover to a greater degree following successful renal transplantation.

In women

Pregnancy should only be contemplated in a woman with renal disease if her plasma creatinine concentration is less than 250 mmol/L and urea less than 10 mmol/L. Pregnancy can significantly worsen renal function and this, combined with the reduced life expectancy of these patients, must be discussed in depth in the pre-pregnancy clinic. Optimally, women who have had a renal transplant should have been in good health for 2 years with no evidence of graft rejection, proteinuria, or hypertension. Immunosuppressive drugs should be continued and teratogenesis is unlikely at the doses usually required by women who have stable renal function.

Cardiovascular Disease

Women with congenital or acquired heart disease should be evaluated by a cardiologist prior to conception and the risks of pregnancy discussed. Antiarrhythmic drugs are generally safe in women planning a pregnancy and their benefits outweigh the risks. Amiodarone can affect thyroid function and cause either hypo- or hyperthyroidism and secondary subfertility; serum total T_4 concentrations can be elevated in the absence of hyperthyroidism and it is necessary to measure T_3 and TSH. Disopyramide, flecainide, and procainamide should be used with caution in pregnancy and it is sometimes appropriate to change the antiarrhythmic preparation before trying to conceive.

Hypertension can be managed safely with a number of drugs in early and late pregnancy. Diuretics should be avoided not only because they affect electrolyte homeostasis and can cause hypovolemia and renal failure but also because they might reduce placental blood flow, particularly if the patient has pre-eclampsia. Beta-blockers appear to be safe, although they have been associated with intrauterine growth retardation. Adrenergic neurone blocking drugs, such as guanethidine, and alpha-blockers, such as phenoxybenzamine, should be avoided in women trying to conceive; they can also cause ejaculatory failure in men. Angiotensin-converting enzyme (ACE) inhibitors are effective and widely used; they may cause impotence in men and should not be given to women planning a pregnancy because of concerns about teratogenicity. Calcium channel blockers should also be avoided if there is a chance of pregnancy, as there are reports of teratogenicity in animals. Women who require antihypertensive therapy should therefore be stabilized on a preparation that is safe in pregnancy before trying to conceive (e.g. methyldopa, labetalol).

There are increasing numbers of women now reaching childbearing age who have severe cardiovascular disease and who in the past would have died at an early age. Many will have had extensive surgery and there are a few who have had heart transplants or, in the case of cystic fibrosis, heart–lung transplants. These individuals should be managed in conjunction with their cardiologists.

Respiratory Disease

Asthma

Asthma is the commonest respiratory disorder in women of reproductive years, affecting approximately 1%. Pregnancy itself places relatively little stress on the respiratory system and the effect of pregnancy on asthma is variable and unpredictable, with some women noticing an improvement and others a deterioration. As emotional stress affects asthma, infertility might cause a worsening of the condition, which is sometimes cyclical. Betasympathomimetic drugs, theophylline, steroids, and disodium cromoglicate are safe, whether taken by inhaler or orally.

Cystic fibrosis

The prognosis for patients with cystic fibrosis has improved tremendously over the last 20 years and many women with cystic fibrosis are now well enough to have a family. It is important that these women are as fit as possible before embarking on a pregnancy as they and their babies do better if they have good lung function and are free from chest infections. Pancreatin and mucolytics such as acetylcysteine are safe in pregnancy.

Women with cystic fibrosis who conceive have a similar rate of miscarriage but an increased risk of perinatal mortality and maternal mortality compared with normal women, although the latter is no greater than in women with cystic fibrosis of the same age who are not pregnant. Being underweight is probably the most significant problem for women with cystic fibrosis with respect to both fertility and risks during pregnancy. It has been reported that only 20% of women with cystic fibrosis are fertile as the remainder have abnormal cervical mucus with increased viscosity. This mechanical barrier to conception can in theory be overcome by intrauterine insemination (IUI).

Men with cystic fibrosis are usually, but not invariably, azoospermic due to abnormal development of the mesonephric ducts. Spermatogenesis is usually normal and sperm collected from the epididymis or testis can achieve IVF with the aid of intracytoplasmic injection of sperm (ICSI).

It is sensible to offer pre-conception genetic counseling to couples in which one or both partners have cystic fibrosis.

Tuberculosis

In recent years there has been an upswing in the incidence of tuberculosis, secondary to the immigration of non-immunized women of low socioeconomic status and to the immunosuppressive effects of HIV infection. Ethambutol and isoniazid appear not to cause terotogenicity and rifampicin appears to be safe but streptomycin should be avoided.

Antibiotics and Anti-infective Agents

We have listed the anti-infective agents in common use in the UK (see below). When caution is expressed it is sensible to advise the use of contraception until the infection has been treated. In any case, women with severe infections and debilitating illness are unlikely to conceive until they are better.

Antibiotics

Antibiotics thought to be safe in early pregnancy include:

- cephalosporins
- erythromycin
- fusidic acid
- nitrofurantoin
- penicillins.

Antibiotics that should be used with caution include:

- ciprofloxacin
- clindamycin
- gentamicin
- metronidazole

- nalidixic acid
- ofloxacin
- rifampicin
- spectinomycin
- vancomycin.

Antibiotics that should be avoided include:

- aminoglycosides (if absolutely necessary, gentamicin is probably the safest)
- chloramphenicol
- colistin
- co-trimoxazole
- dapsone
- fosfomycin
- sulfonamides
- tetracyclines.

Live vaccines

These include BCG, yellow fever, typhoid, cholera, measles, mumps, rubella, Sabin poliomyelitis; they should not be administered unless the risk of infection is so great as to outweigh any risk to the fetus.

Antifungals

Safe: nystatin.
Caution: amphotericin, fluconazole, flucytosine, griseofulvin, itraconazole, ketoconazole, terbinafine.

Antiviral agents

Aciclovir is probably safe, but only use if necessary.
Avoid: ganciclovir, ribavirin (tribavirin), podophyllin.

Human immunodeficiency virus

Women with HIV should be counseled carefully before trying to conceive (see below). Combination therapy for HIV is recommended during pregnancy and labor in order to reduce the risk of transmission of the virus to the baby. The various drugs used in combination include antiretroviral agents, such as zidovudine, together with two protease inhibitors (e.g., saquinavir, lopinavir, ritonavir, indinavir).[17]

Amebicides

Safe: diloxanide.
Caution: metronidazole.

Antimalarials

The benefits of prophylaxis and treatment outweigh the risk. Safe: chloroquine, proguanil, and pyrimethamine (with folate supplements). Avoid: Fansidar, halofantrine, Maloprim, mefloquine, primaquine, quinine.

Anthelmintics

Avoid: mebendazole, piperazine, pyrantel.

Human Immunodeficiency Virus

Men with acquired immunodeficiency syndrome (AIDS) have an increased rate of testicular atrophy, testosterone deficiency, and anti-sperm antibodies. It is debatable whether infected men should be encouraged to procreate because of sexual transmission of the virus and the high risk of infection of the partner.[18] There are reports of pregnancies which have not resulted in transmission of HIV to the mother after insemination with prepared samples of semen.[19]

HIV seroprevalence amongst pregnant women in Europe is between 1.5 and 5.5 per 1000 in urban areas. Women with AIDS who are fit enough to be ovulating are thought to have an approximately 15–20% chance of transmitting the virus to their child *in utero*. This risk does not appear to be increased if their partner is infected. The risk of materno–fetal transmission appears to be reduced by a combination of drug therapy (zidovudine (AZT) and/or didanosine or zalcitabine together with protease inhibitors such as saquinavir, lopinavir, ritonavir, and indinavir)[17] with elective cesarean section. While the immunosuppressive effects of pregnancy might precipitate deterioration of the disease, there are still insufficient data on the effects of pregnancy on maternal prognosis. Data from the European Collaborative Study[20] suggested that 5 years after delivery 14% of mothers will have died, 24% will have developed stage IV disease, and more than 60% will be without serious disease. In the past children born to infected parents were likely to become orphans in childhood or early adolescence but current combination therapy significantly reduces the likelihood of disease progression and the disease can be maintained in a quiescent state – perhaps indefinitely. Worldwide, of course, the situation varies greatly, with some developing countries experiencing an AIDS epidemic that is spiraling out of control.

Of great importance is the issue of handling blood, semen, and follicular fluid with possible infection of laboratory staff. Couples who seek advice about becoming pregnant where one or both partners have HIV should be counseled carefully. If they maintain their wish to conceive, they should be advised to have unprotected intercourse only around the time of ovulation. If the woman is HIV positive and the man negative, his sperm can be inseminated, thus avoiding the risk of his becoming infected. The converse situation requires IVF to minimize the risk to the woman, although, as already mentioned, there are reports of the use of prepared, washed sperm from HIV-positive men being used to inseminate their partners without transmission of the virus. The use of donated gametes by the non-infected partner can also be considered.

The extent to which couples with HIV should be investigated and treated by fertility clinics should be decided on an individual basis. The ethical issues raised are considerable.[18,19] There is a move in the UK to introduce blanket screening of all coupes undergoing IVF because of the putative risk of viral transmission (particularly hepatitis C) in liquid nitrogen during embryo cryopreservation.

Hematological Problems

Anemia

Anemia is common and worsens in pregnant women who have reduced stores of iron. The hemodilutional effect of pregnancy causes a "physiological anemia" but there is also evidence that the diet of most women contains insufficient iron to meet the demands of pregnancy and many women of reproductive age lack storage iron. Folic acid requirements also increase during pregnancy and there is evidence that folate supplementation reduces the risk of neural tube defects and other major developmental abnormalities in the developing fetus. In addition to the routine use of folic acid by all women wishing to conceive (see above), some women have an increased demand for folate, for example those requiring antiepileptic drugs. Vitamin B_{12} deficiency is rare in young women.

It is useful to perform a full blood count on women attending a fertility clinic as it is preferable not to become pregnant if anemic, although anemia itself does not cause infertility.

Sickle cell anemia

Women from high prevalence groups (Afro-Caribbean women and those from India and the Mediterranean countries) should be screened in the fertility clinic for hemoglobinopathies. They will already know if they have sickle cell anemia (HbSS). Sickling crises are more frequent during pregnancy and can be fatal; there is also an increased risk of miscarriage due to placental infarction. These patients should be counseled by their hematologist about the risks of becoming pregnant. Women with sickle cell trait (HbAS), on the other hand, are healthy and rarely have problems during pregnancy. Their partners should be screened for HbAS and the possibility of antenatal diagnosis discussed.

Thalassemia

Prospective parents with thalassemia should receive genetic counseling and be reviewed before they conceive by a hematologist with a special interest. Women with alpha thalassemia (α_1 or α_2, that is, with two or three alpha globin molecules) and beta thalassemia minor require close attention to iron and folate supplementation during pregnancy and should enter pregnancy in as healthy a condition as possible. Patients with beta thalassemia major often have severe problems and require regular blood transfusions throughout life. This can lead to iron overload and hemochromatosis, with endocrine dysfunction secondary to excess deposition of iron in the pituitary gland and gonads. Involvement of the liver and pancreas can contribute to the hormonal disturbances and these patients have delayed puberty and hypogonadal infertility. Testicular biopsy may demonstrate iron overload. Desferrioxamine can be used to chelate excess iron, although therapy has to be commenced prepubertally to prevent pituitary dysfunction.

Thrombophilic disorders

Women with thrombophilic disorders are at risk of thromboembolism during pregnancy and those with a history of thrombosis are often prescribed prophylactic anticoagulants for all or part of their pregnancy. The commonest practice is to commence heparin in labor and continue for 6 weeks postpartum. Women with prosthetic heart valves might be on long-term warfarin therapy and present particular dilemmas when trying to conceive. Warfarin should be avoided during the first trimester because of the risk of chondrodysplasia punctata, which results in abnormal bone and cartilage formation. Prolonged use of heparin can cause osteoporosis and this is of particular concern in women with infertility secondary to long-standing ovarian failure, who might already have compromised bone density caused by estrogen deficiency. The risk of osteoporosis appears to be reduced by the use of low molecular weight heparins, although these preparations have not yet been licenced for use in pregnancy. Careful consideration should be given to women at high risk of thromboembolism who are undergoing superovulation, as the resultant high serum concentrations of estradiol might put them at an increased risk of thrombosis and heparin prophylaxis is sometimes advisable. Therapy should therefore be coordinated with the advice of a thrombosis expert.

Antiphospholipid syndrome

The antiphospholipid syndrome is associated with recurrent miscarriage (see discussion in Ch. 20), although most women with the coagulation defects that constitute this disorder do not have overt signs or symptoms of connective tissue disease.

Connective Tissue Disorders

Systemic lupus erythematosus

Women with systemic lupus erythematosus (SLE) should be advised against conceiving during active phases of the disease as pregnancy can cause severe flare-ups. There is a high risk of miscarriage, which has been reported in up to 40% of pregnancies and can occur in the first or second trimesters. Strategies to prevent miscarriage include the use of aspirin, heparin, corticosteroids, and immunoglobulins.

Other connective tissue disorders, such as rheumatoid arthritis, do not appear to increase the risk of miscarriage. Prenatal counseling is important in order to rationalize drug therapy. Corticosteroids and chloroquine are safe in pregnancy, as is aspirin in low dose, but paracetamol is preferable as an analgesic. Indomethacin and other non-steroidal anti-inflammatory drugs should be avoided in pregnancy, as should gold and penicillamine.

Chemotherapy

Pregnancy should be avoided during chemotherapy.

Effect on Men

Regimens that contain alkylating agents (busulfan, carmustine, chlorambucil, cyclophosphamide, estramustine, ifosfamide, lomustine, melphalan, chlormethine (mustine), thiotepa, treosulfan) can severely affect gametogenesis and so men, if well enough, should be advised to produce sperm for cryopreservation. Since the advent of ICSI, this advice has assumed even greater importance than before (see Chs 11 and 13). Men can also be adversely affected by cytarabin, doxorubicin, procarbazine, and vinblastine. Chemotherapy predominantly affects seminiferous tubules but Leydig cell function may also be compromised.

Effect on Women

The effect of alkylating agents on women is variable. It is more dependent on age and dose, with women over the age of 30 being more likely to have premature ovarian failure. In the future it might be possible to freeze oocytes or ovarian biopsies containing primordial follicles, but in the meantime it is not usually feasible for women to undergo IVF before starting chemotherapy (see discussion in Ch. 18). Most other chemotherapeutic agents allow preservation of ovarian function once the patient has recovered from the underlying disease. Treatment with the oral contraceptive pill or GnRH analogs does not protect the oocytes. It is fortunate that methotrexate, which is used to treat choriocarcinoma and some women with ectopic pregnancy, does not affect fertility. If radiotherapy of the pelvic region is required oophoropexy will reduce the dose of radiation to the ovaries but cryopreservation of ovarian tissue should provide the solution for these patients in the future.

References

1. Barker DJP (1990) The fetal and infant origins of adult disease. *Br Med J* **301**: 111.
2. Hamilton-Fairley D, Kiddy D, Watson H, Paterson C & Franks S (1992) Association of moderate obesity with poor pregnancy outcome in women with polycystic ovary syndrome treated with low dose gonadotropins. *Br J Obstet Gynaecol* **99**: 128–131.
3. Clark AM, Thornley B, Tomlinson L, Galletley C & Norman RJ (1998) Weight loss in obese infertile women results in improvement in reproductive outcome for all forms of fertility treatment. *Hum Reprod* **13**: 1502–1505.
4. Wang JX, Davies M & Norman RJ (2000) Body mass and probability of pregnancy during assisted reproduction treatment: retrospective study. *Br Med J* **321**: 1320–1321.
5. Amatruda JM, Harman SM, Pourmotabbed G & Lockwood DH (1978) Depressed plasma testosterone and fractional binding of testosterone in obese males. *J Clin Endocrinol Metab* **47**: 268.
6. Glass AR, Burman KD, Dahms WT & Boehm TM (1981) Endocrine function in human obesity. *Metabolism* **30**: 89.
7. Harris C & Carey A (2000) *A Woman's Guide to Dealing with Polycystic Ovary Syndrome*. Thorsons, London.
8. Netter A, Hartoma R & Nahoul K (1981) Effect of zinc administration on plasma testosterone, dihydrotestosterone and sperm count. *Arch Androl* **7**: 69.
9. Engel S, Mockel C & Diezel W (1985) Der Einfluβ von α-Tokopherolazetat auf die Spermienmotilitat. *Dermatol Monatsschr* **171**: 800.
10. Aitken RH & Clarkson JS (1988) Significance of reactive oxygen species and antioxidants in defining the efficacy of sperm preparation techniques. *J Androl* **9**: 367.
11. Jensen TK, Hjollund NHI, Henriksen TB *et al.* (1988) Does moderate alcohol consumption affect fertility? Follow up study among couples planning first pregnancy. *Br Med J* **317**: 505–510.
12. Howe G, Westhoff C, Vessey M & Yeates D (1985) Effects of age cigarette smoking and other factors on fertility: findings in a large prospective study. *Br Med J* **290**: 1697–1700.
13. Augood C, Duckitt K & Templeton AA (1998) Smoking and female infertility: a systematic review and meta-analysis. *Hum Reprod* **13**: 1532–1539.
14. Hughes EG & Brennan BG (1996) Does cigarette smoking impair natural or assisted fecundity? *Fertil Steril* **66**: 679–689.
15. Hull MGR, North K, Taylor H, Farrow A & Ford WCL (2000) Delayed conception and active and passive smoking. *Fertil Steril* **74**: 725–733.
16. Holmes-Walker DJ, Conway GS, Honour JW, Rumsby G & Jacobs HS (1995) Menstrual disturbance and hypersecretion of progesterone in women with congenital adrenal hyperplasia due to 21- hydroxylase deficiency. *Clin Endocrinol* **43**: 291–296.
17. Jordan R, Gold L, Cummins C & Hyde C (2002) Systematic review and meta-analysis of evidence for increasing numbers of drugs in antiretroviral combination therapy. *Br Med J* **324**: 757–760.
18. Smith JR, Forster GE, Kitchen VS, Hooi YS, Munday PE & Paintin DB (1991) Infertility management in HIV positive couples: a dilemma. *Br Med J* **302**: 1447–1450.
19. Gilling-Smith C, Smith JR & Semprini AE (2001) HIV and infertility: time to treat. *Br Med J* **322**: 566–567.

20. Thorne C, Newell ML, Dunn D & Peckham C (1995) The European Collaborative Study: clinical and immunological characteristics of HIV-1 infected pregnant women. *Br J Obstet Gynaecol* **102**: 869–875.

Further Reading

De Swiet M (2002) *Medical disorders in obstetric practice*. Blackwell, Oxford.

Johnson MR & McGregor AM (1990) Endocrine disease and pregnancy. *Baillière's Clin Endocrinol and Metab* **4**: 313–322.

Liel Y, Harman-Boehm I, Arbelle JE & Glick SM (1993) Medical conditions leading to infertility. In: Insler V & Lunenfeld B (eds) *Infertility: male and female*. Churchill Livingstone, Edinburgh, pp 703–738.

Chapter 4

Investigating infertility

Introduction

Fertility investigations should normally be instigated as soon as the couple seeks help. Even if they have been trying for less than a year, it is worthwhile asking some general questions to ensure that major problems, such as irregularities of the menstrual cycle, a history of pelvic surgery, or orchidopexy have not been ignored. If the couple's medical history is normal the expected cumulative chance of conception over a period of time should be explained and investigations deferred until they have been trying for a year. When the female partner is aged 35 years or older, monthly fecundity is significantly reduced but we do not believe that investigations should be delayed proportionately because of the concomitant age-related decline in the success of treatment (see Ch. 1).

Once the decision has been taken to investigate, it should be possible to perform the basic screening tests within 3–4 months and provide the couple with a management plan, which may involve reassurance, more detailed investigations, or treatment. A pragmatic approach should be taken. Infertility is rarely absolute and treatment options may be discussed to enhance a couple's fertility even in the absence of a clear diagnosis. To quote from the European Society of Human Reproduction and Embryology (ESHRE) Capri Workshop Group: "Both old and new diagnostic tests must be considered, but to what degree is diagnostic certainty necessary? The science of infertility is uncertain and it is not a life-threatening condition. Testing until uncertainty vanishes may delay treatment (and if the delay is long enough, the female patient will become menopausal)."[1]

Couples usually attend the infertility clinic together but there are sometimes secrets between them that might yield clinically relevant information. We suggest that the physical examination of the individual is performed with the partner out of the room, as this is a good time to detect confidential information about previous pregnancies, illnesses, or sexually transmitted diseases. It is essential to remember that one is dealing both with the couple and with two individual patients, who often have separate general practitioners. It is of paramount importance not to convey confidential information to the wrong GP, as the issues that surround infertility are extremely sensitive. It is our practice to send patients copies of correspondence so that they have a written record of what has been discussed. Not only does this help to avoid confusion but it also increases confidence that everyone is included in the communication "loop."

General Investigations

The fertility clinic should be used for general health screening and preconception counseling. Particular attention should be paid to body weight, blood pressure, urinalysis, cervical cytology, and rubella immunity. Some clinics ascertain hepatitis B, C, and HIV status before offering assisted conception – this is becoming routine practice in the UK because of the putative risk of viral contamination of cryopreserved embros via liquid nitrogen.

Investigating the Female Partner

Examination

A calculation of the body mass index is made from the height and weight (kg/m^2) – the normal range is 20–25 kg/m^2 (see p. 28). The patient's general appearance may give clues about either systemic disease or endocrine problems. The presence of normal secondary sexual characteristics should be noted.

Signs of endocrine disorder

Signs of hyperandrogenism (acne, hirsutism, balding) are suggestive of the polycystic ovary syndrome (PCOS), although biochemical screening helps to differentiate other causes of androgen excess. Hirsutism can be graded and given a Ferriman Gallwey score (Fig. 4.1). It is useful to monitor the progress of hirsutism, or its response to treatment, by making serial records, either using a chart such as the one illustrated or by taking photographs of affected areas of the body. It is important to distinguish between hyperandrogenism and virilization (Table 4.1), which is associated with high circulating

Table 4.1 Hyperandrogenism versus virilization

Hyperandrogenism	Virilization
Acne	Acne
Hirsutism	Hirsutism
Male pattern balding	Male pattern balding
	Increased muscle mass
	Deep voice
	Clitoromegaly
	Breast atrophy

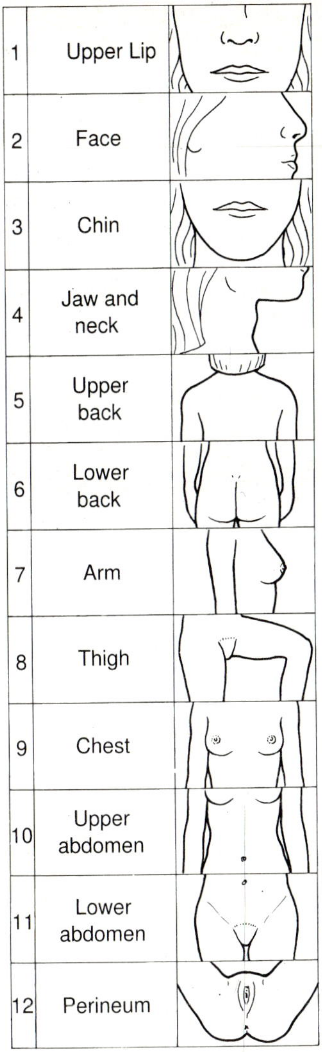

Figure 4.1 Ferriman Gallwey score. Each area is given a score from 1 to 4 (1 = mild, 2 = moderate, 3 = complete light coverage, 4 = heavy coverage).

androgen levels and causes deepening of the voice, increase in muscle bulk, and cliteromegaly. Virilization suggests a more profound disturbance of androgen secretion than usually seen with PCOS and indicates the need to exclude androgen secreting tumors, congenital adrenal hyperplasia (CAH), and Cushing's syndrome.

One should be aware of the possibility of Cushing's syndrome in women with stigmata of the PCOS and obesity as it is a disease of

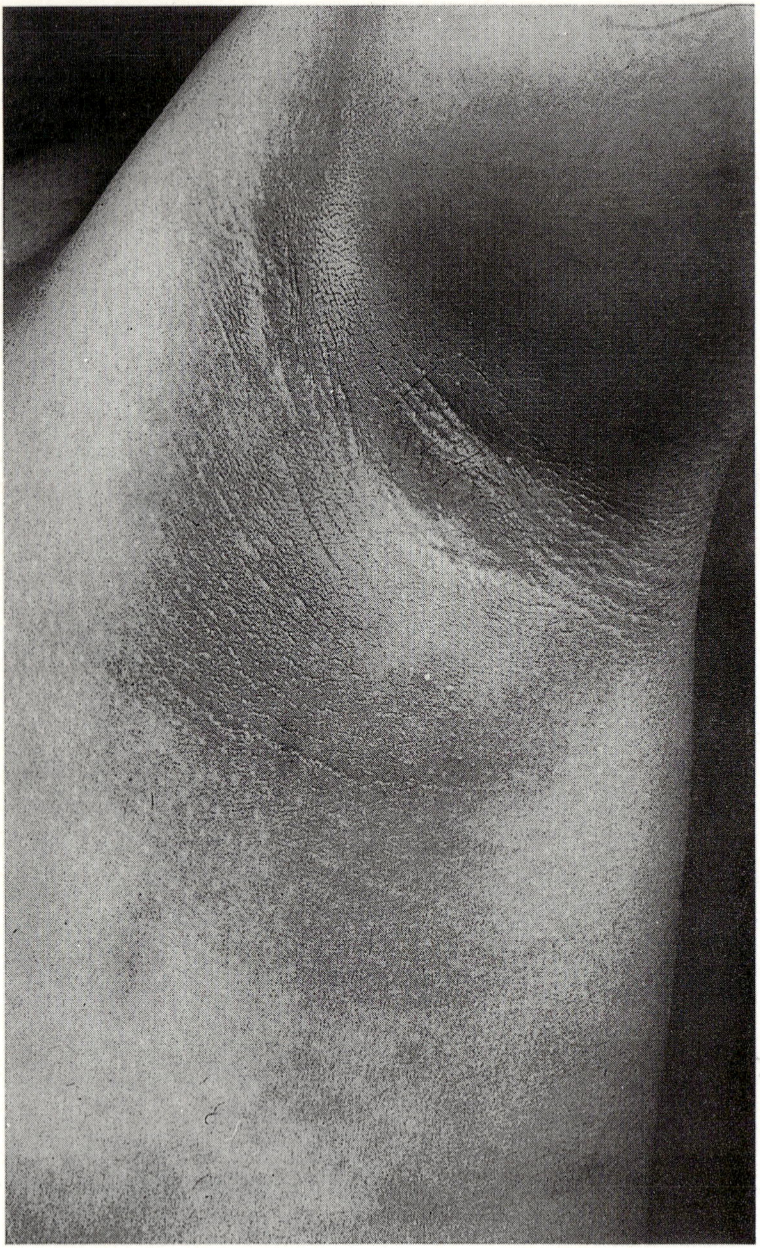

Figure 4.2a

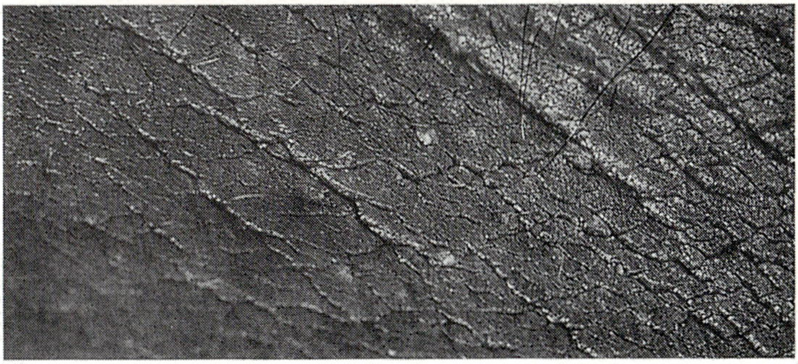

Figure 4.2b Acanthosis nigricans, as seen typically in the axilla or skin of the neck. (**a**) Axilla, (**b**) close-up, demonstrating hypertrophic and pigmented skin.

insidious onset and dire consequences; additional clues are the presence of central obesity, moon face, plethoric complexion, buffalo hump, proximal myopathy, thin skin, bruising, and abdominal striae (which alone are a common finding in obese individuals).

Acanthosis nigricans is a sign of profound insulin resistance and is usually visible as hyperpigmented thickening of the skin folds of the axilla and neck; it is associated with PCOS and obesity (Fig. 4.2a & b).

Amenorrheic women may have hyperprolactinemia and galactorrhea. It is important, however, not to examine the breasts before taking blood as the serum prolactin concentration may become falsely elevated. General, vaginal, and breast examinations and stress can all cause a temporary elevation in serum prolactin concentration. If there is suspicion of a pituitary tumor, the patient's visual fields should be checked, as bitemporal hemianopia secondary to pressure on the optic chiasm requires urgent attention.

Thyroid disease is common and the thyroid gland should be palpated and signs of hypothyroidism (dry thin hair, proximal myopathy, myotonia, slow-relaxing reflexes, mental slowness, bradycardia, etc.) or hyperthyroidism (goiter with bruit, tremor, weight loss, tachycardia, hyperreflexia, exophthalmos, conjunctival edema, ophthalmoplegia) elicited.

General examination

It is important to perform a general physical examination, including examination of the breasts. One should remember that the patient might require an anesthetic as part of investigations and so consideration of fitness for anesthesia is important (Table 4.2).

Table 4.2 General examination (female partner)	
Signs of endocrine disorders:	– acne, hirsutism, balding
	– acanthosis nigricans
	– virilization
	– visual field defects
	– goiter, signs of thyroid disease
BMI	
BP	
Fitness for possible anesthetic	
Urinalysis	
Breast examination: lumps, galactorrhea	
Cervical smear if required	
Abdominal examination: masses, scars, striae, hirsutism	
Pelvic examination:	– developmental anomalies
	– vaginal nodules of endometriosis
	– tenderness
	– mobility of uterus
	– masses
	– endocervical swab
	– rectal examination if indicated

Pelvic examination

A pelvic examination should be performed. Endometriosis is suggested by the presence of nodules in the vagina, thickening of the posterior fornix, tenderness, and fixity of the pelvic organs. If the examination is painful one should be alerted to the possibility of pelvic pathology and include a laparoscopy early in the course of investigations. Adnexal masses should be investigated by ultrasound in the first instance.

Endocervical swabs – *Chlamydia* detection

A controversial subject is the routine swabbing of the cervix for *Chlamydia trachomatis*. Chlamydial DNA has been recovered from 50% of women with tubal infertility compared with approximately 12% of pregnant women or women with non-tubal infertility. *Chlamydia* infection is the commonest cause of tubal infertility in developed countries and is the commonest sexually transmitted pathogen in the UK. It is thought that at least 1 in 20 women in the UK between the ages of 18 and 25 years may have undiagnosed infection. *Chlamydia trachomatis* causes urethritis and epididymitis in men and cervicitis, salpingitis, and endometritis in women, although symptoms can be mild and non-specific. It has both intracellular and extracellular forms and requires prompt transfer to the laboratory in a special transport medium for tissue culture. The antigen can be detected by enzyme linked immunosorbent assay (ELISA) of endocervical swabs. *Chlamydia* serology provides evidence of past infection and is a routine screening test in some clinics. The presence of chlamydial antibodies correctly predicts tubal damage in 90% of cases, of whom over half have no history of pelvic inflammatory disease. A sensitive urinary assay is now available for detection of previous *Chlamydia* infection. We advise the use of *Chlamydia* screening to help identify patients whose tubal status should be tested early in the investigative process. There is evidence, however, that screening tests may be negative in the presence of infection in the upper genital tract and so there is rationale for prophylactic antibiotics prior to any procedure that involves instrumentation of the cervix.

In recent years it has been suggested that pelvic infection with *Mycoplasma hominis* or *Ureaplasma urealyticum* accounts for some cases of tubal infertility. However, finding these organisms on routine swabs does not predict infertility because of their high prevalence in fertile women. Bacterial vaginosis causes up to 50% of vaginal infections, yet often goes unrecognized. The organisms responsible include *Gardnerella vaginalis*, *Mycoplasma hominis*, *Mobiluncus* spp., anaerobic gram-negative rods of the genera *Prevotella*, *Prophyromonas*, and *Bacteroides* and *Peptostreptococcus* spp. Coinfection with *Chlamydia*, gonorrhea, and *Trichomonas* is common. Bacterial vaginosis is associated with infective complications following gynecological surgery, second trimester miscarriage, and premature labor/delivery. Screening in the infertility clinic and treatment may be of benefit.[2]

Diagnosis of Anovulatory Infertility

Determining the cause of anovulatory infertility is the key to treatment as correction of the cause will result in cumulative conception rates that mimic those expected for normal women of the same age.

It is first necessary to ascertain whether ovulation is occurring (Table 4.3). Patients with anovulatory infertility will have oligomenorrhea or amenorrhea and a low luteal phase progesterone. A progesterone concentration of greater than 30 nmol/L suggests ovulation but it can be difficult to know when to take the blood if the patient has an erratic cycle – and impossible if she is amenorrheic. If the progesterone is 15–30 nmol/L the timing may have been incorrect. It is then necessary to check the timing of the blood test to subsequent menstruation and repeat the test in the following cycle (sometimes two progesterone measurements in the same cycle are helpful). The optimal way to assess ovulation in women with irregular cycles is by a combination of serial ultrasound scans and serum endocrine measurements (follicle stimulating hormone (FSH) and luteinizing hormone (LH) in the follicular phase and progesterone in the luteal phase).

Table 4.3 Assessment of ovulation

Ovulation can only be confirmed with certainty if a pregnancy occurs
Regular cycle with cycle variation no more than ± 2 days – 95% likely to be ovulatory
Mid-luteal serum progesterone > 30 nmol/L (see text)
(Day important – not necessarily day 21)
Ultrasound monitoring of folliculogenesis and ovulation
Detection of LH surge in urine (hard to use prospectively)
Basal body temperature (stressful)
Mittelschmerz
Thinning of cervical mucus
Mid-cycle bleed

Basal body temperature (BBT) charts (Fig. 4.3) provide an overview of the regularity of a woman's cycle and an assessment of coital frequency, as the couple are requested to encircle days when they have intercourse. Temperature charts are, however, a source of considerable stress and do not provide a prospective indication of the day of ovulation. The rationale behind the use of BBT measurements is that progesterone will raise the BBT by 0.2–0.5°C, although between 10% and 75% of ovulatory cycles fail to show an adequate rise in BBT. A "flat" chart therefore does not necessarily indicate anovulation.

Some women are aware of changes in the consistency of their cervical mucus and can assess for themselves when the mucus is receptive (the so-called Billing's method of family planning). Estrogenized cervical mucus will stretch either between the fingers of an individual who wishes to assess her own mucus or between two microscope slides at the time of a postcoital test (Spinnbarkeit). This can then be measured in centimeters (see postcoital test, p. 107) (Figs 4.4 and 4.5).

Commercially available kits that indicate the presence of LH in the urine are expensive and are also a cause of stress. Women with PCOS and a high serum concentration of LH can give false-positive results. The kits can also be affected by variations in ambient temperature. Women who are having regular menstrual cycles (frequency of 23–35 days, with no more than 2–3 days variation each month) have a greater than 95% chance that they are ovulating and up to 75% of women with an erratic cycle are also found to be ovulating. Women with regular cycles should be reassured and for them the value of BBT charts or urinary LH kits can be questioned. If they are aware of pelvic discomfort (*Mittelschmerz*) or cervical mucus changes around the time of ovulation then this can be used as a guide to when to have intercourse.

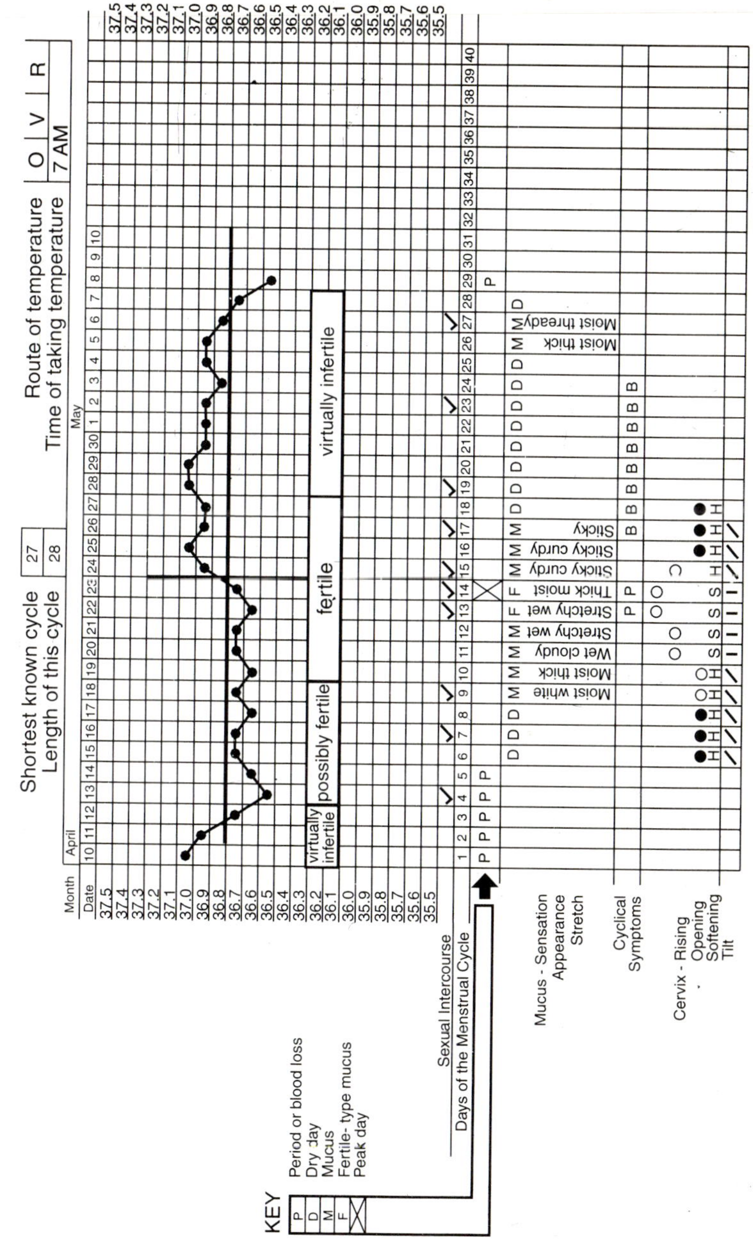

Figure 4.3 A rise of 0.2–0.5°C, secondary to progesterone secretion by the corpus luteum, suggests that ovulation has occurred.

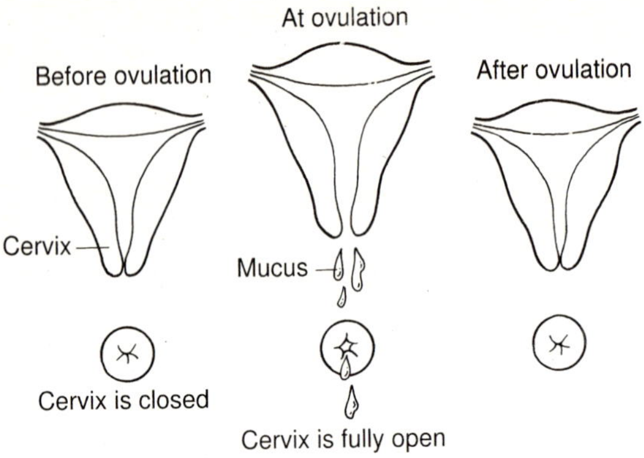

Figure 4.4 The production of cervical mucus at different times in the cycle.

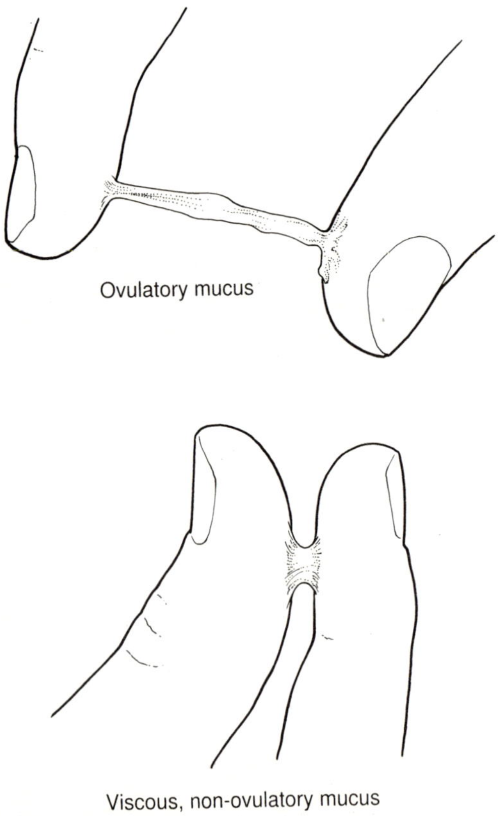

Figure 4.5 Self-assessment of Spinnbarkeit.

The optimal frequency of intercourse is every 2–3 days in the follicular phase of the cycle and, if possible, daily for 2–3 days at the predicted time of ovulation. Abstinence until the "day of ovulation" can be detrimental to sperm function (see also later Ch. 4 and 11). It is therefore important to advise couples about the frequency of intercourse and try to diffuse the tensions that often result from timed intercourse "to order."

The timing of sexual intercourse in relation to ovulation has a strong influence on the chance of conception (Fig. 4.6). The precise number of fertile days in a woman's menstrual cycle is uncertain and it has been estimated that conception only occurs when intercourse has taken place during a 6-day period that ends on the day of ovulation. A recent study demonstrated that the probability of conception was 10% when intercourse occurred 5 days before ovulation and 33% when it took place on the day of ovulation. The fertile period appears to last 6 days and ends on the day of ovulation. The rapid decline in the probability of conception after this time is due either to a short survival time of the oocyte or a swift change in the nature of the cervical mucus. This information has important implications for some fertility treatments which rely upon insemination after ovulation has been identified by using temperature charts. Furthermore, if commercially available kits for detecting the mid-cycle surge of LH in the urine are used to focus a couple to have intercourse on the day of the LH surge and the following day, they may be missing 3 or 4 fertile days prior to this and reducing their chance of conception.

With respect to the precise timing of the fertile "window" in the menstrual cycle, this occurs between days 10 and 17 in only about 30% of women.[3] Even in women with regular menstrual cycles, the timing of the fertile window can be highly variable. Wilcox *et al.*[3] estimated that 2% of women were in their fertile period by day 4 of their cycle, 17% by day 7 and 54% by day 12. Most women appear to reach their fertile window early in the cycle although a proportion do so much later, even past day 35.

In another study by Wilcox *et al.*[4] it was also found that 94% of pregnancies were attributed to sperm that were 1 or 2 days old, although sperm can retain their capacity to fertilize *in vitro* for 5 days and survive in estrogenized cervical mucus for 7 days. There is no evidence that closely spaced ejaculations are detrimental to fertility; in fact, the opposite applies in some cases (see Ch. 11). It is suggested that normal couples wishing to conceive should have intercourse frequently during the first part of the menstrual cycle up to the day of ovulation.

The luteal phase of the cycle normally lasts for between 10 and 17 days and the concept of "luteal phase deficiency" (LPD) is controversial. Probably the most convincing argument against the phenomenon of

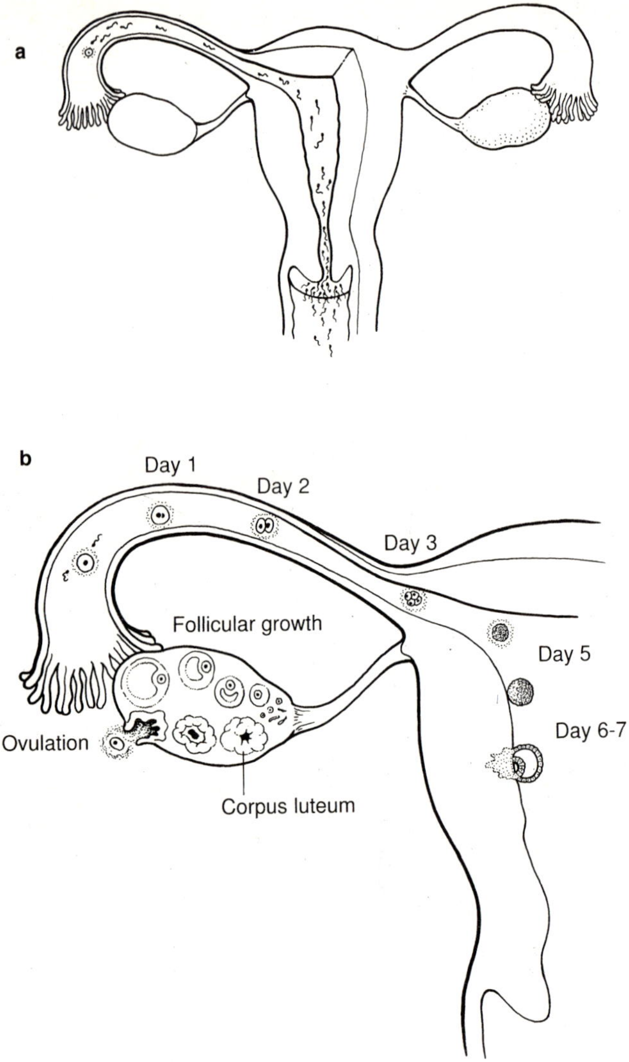

Figure 4.6 (**a**) The passage of sperm through the genital tract. (**b**) Ovulation, fertilization, and implantation.

LPD is the failure of luteal support – with either progesterone or human chorionic gonadotropin (hCG) – to improve pregnancy rates in spontaneous pregnancies. Endometrial biopsy has been used to assess the quality of ovulation further by equating histological changes with serum progesterone levels. Histological dating is, however, an unreliable indicator of the endometrial response to hormonal stimulation and is open to considerable biological variability and observer error. We do not recommend endometrial biopsy for determining whether the patient has ovulated.

Endocrine Profile

A baseline endocrine profile is optimally performed during the first 3 days of the cycle. It is essential to be aware of the normal reference range for the assay in the laboratory in which it is being performed. Reference ranges vary from laboratory to laboratory and can be quite different if different types of assay are used (e.g., radioimmunoassays and immunoradiometric assays give very different results for gonadotropin measurements).

It is essential that the date of the blood test is recorded carefully, as it is not uncommon for all hormones to be measured on the day of the luteal phase progesterone measurement – usually day 21 – which can be very misleading: for example, if the patient has a 35-day cycle, ovulation might be occurring on day 21 and the gonadotropin levels will be perceived to be in the menopausal range, because of the mid-cycle surge, while the progesterone will not yet have begun to rise (Fig. 4.7).

If the patient has amenorrhea or oligomenorrhea a random blood sample has to be taken and is best repeated a week later in order to get

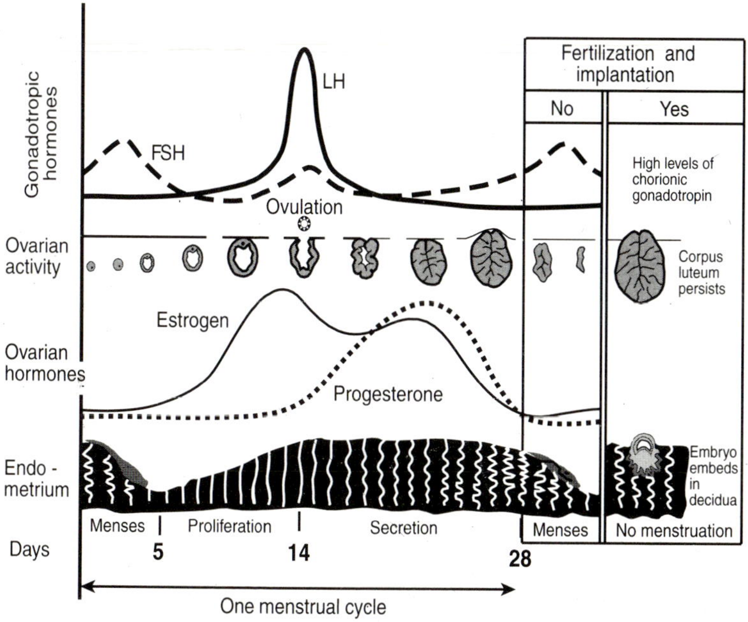

Figure 4.7 Schematic diagram of the menstrual cycle.

an impression of the underlying pathology. An assessment of endocrine status in these cases can usefully be performed in conjunction with a pelvic ultrasound scan to assess ovarian activity and endometrial thickness.

Progesterone

This should be measured in the mid-luteal phase, 7 days after ovulation and 7 days before the next expected period. An ovulatory concentration is one greater than 30 nmol/L, although if > 10, or certainly > 20 nmol/L, there is a strong suggestion that ovulation has occurred but that the blood test was mistimed. It is essential to know when the test was performed in relation to both the preceding and subsequent menstrual period. If there is doubt the test should be repeated the following month and it is occasionally beneficial to measure the progesterone two or three times in the luteal phase. A combination of serum endocrinology with ultrasound monitoring of follicular growth and ovulation will of course provide the best picture of ovarian function.

Gonadotropins

Follicle stimulating hormone The best indicator of ovarian function is, at present, a measurement of the baseline serum FSH concentration. An elevated FSH level indicates reduced ovarian reserve and, generally, if greater than 10 i.u./L on more than one occasion the ovaries are unlikely to be ovulating regularly and will also be resistant to exogenous stimulation. When the serum concentration of FSH is above 15 i.u./L the chance of ovarian activity is slim and levels greater than 25 i.u./L are suggestive of the menopause or premature ovarian failure (Table 4.4).

Table 4.4 Diagnoses suggested by levels of FSH and LH

FSH	LH	Diagnosis
Normal	Elevated	PCOS
Normal	Low	Weight-related amenorrhea
Low	Low	Hypogonadotropic hypogonadism, functional or organic
Elevated	Elevated	If oligo-/amenorrheic: ovarian failure
Elevated	Elevated	If mid-cycle think of mid-cycle surge

FSH, follicle stimulating hormone; LH, luteinizing hormone; PCOS, polycystic ovarian syndrome.

Inhibin is thought to be the ovarian hormone which has the greatest influence on pituitary secretion of FSH. Assays for inhibin can detect the dimeric peptide hormone and do not crossreact with free subunits (which was the problem with earlier assays). It is thought that serum concentrations of inhibin B might provide better quantification of ovarian reserve than serum FSH concentrations and data are being accumulated to test this hypothesis.

Luteinizing hormone An elevated serum concentration of LH suggests that the patient has PCOS – usually associated with a level greater than 10 i.u./L in the early to mid-follicular phase of the cycle. In a series of over 1700 women with PCOS we found that approximately 40% of patients had an elevated serum concentration of LH, which was associated with a significantly higher risk of infertility than those with normal LH levels.[5] Other causes of an elevated LH are the mid-cycle surge and ovarian failure.

The association of amenorrhea with very low levels of FSH and LH (usually < 2 i.u./L or below the range of the assay) suggests pituitary failure or hypogonadotropic hypogonadism. Gonadotropin measurements are best interpreted together with the findings of a pelvic ultrasound scan as the combination of ovarian morphology, endometrial thickness, and serum gonadotropin levels will provide the diagnosis in most cases (Table 4.4).

Androgens

The normal female range for total serum testosterone (T) is 0.5–3.5 nmol/L. The most usual cause of an elevated serum testosterone is PCOS. Most women with PCOS, however, have a normal total serum testosterone concentration (about 70% in our experience). Measurement of the sex hormone binding globulin (SHBG) concentration (normal range 16–119 nmol/L) will permit the calculation of the "free androgen index" (FAI) [(T × 100)/SHBG], which should be less than 5. Women who are obese have high circulating levels of insulin which reduce synthesis of SHBG by the liver so that the FAI is often elevated when the total T is in the normal range.

If the T is greater than 5 nmol/L it is necessary to exclude other causes of hyperandrogenemia: late onset CAH, Cushing's syndrome, and androgen-secreting tumors. Women with the most common form of CAH (21-hydroxylase deficiency) will have an elevated serum 17-hydroxyprogesterone concentration (17-OHP > 20 nmol/L) and an exagerated response to an intramuscular or subcutaneous bolus of adrenocorticotropic hormone (ACTH: 250 mcg of tetracosactrin will cause a normal elevation of 17-OHP, usually between 50 and 60 nmol/L).

In Cushing's syndrome the 24-hour urinary free cortisol is elevated (> 400 nmol/24 h). The normal serum concentration of cortisol is 140–700 nmol/L at 8a.m. and less than 140 nmol/L at midnight. In normal people a low dose dexamethasone suppression test (0.5 mg 6-hourly for 48 h) will cause a suppression of serum cortisol by 48 hours. A simpler screening test is an overnight suppression test, using a single midnight dose of dexamethasone (1 mg, or 2 mg if obese) and measuring the serum cortisol concentration at 8a.m. when it should be less than 140 nmol/L. If Cushing's syndrome is confirmed a high dose dexamethasone suppression test (2 mg 6-hourly for 48 h) should suppress serum cortisol by 48 hours if there is a pituitary ACTH-secreting adenoma (Cushing's disease). Failure of suppression suggests an adrenal tumor or ectopic secretion of ACTH; further tests and detailed imaging will then be required and the opinion of an endocrinologist is essential.

The measurement of other serum androgen levels can be helpful. Dehydroepiandrosterone sulfate (DHEAS) is primarily a product of the adrenal androgen pathway (normal range < 10 μmol/L). If the serum androgen concentrations are greatly elevated the possibility of an ovarian or adrenal tumor should be excluded by ultrasound scan or computed tomography (CT). A serum T concentration of greater than 5 nmol/L associated with a normal DHEAS suggests an ovarian source, while if combined with an elevated DHEAS, the source is likely to be adrenal.

Thyroid function

Thyroid disease is common in women, affecting about 5% of reproductive years, and subtle disturbances of thyroid function may have a profound effect on fertility. While the RCOG guidelines[6] on the investigation of infertility suggest that routine assessment of thyroid function is not necessary, we found that 5% of women attending our infertility clinic had thyroid dysfunction – often in the absence of symptoms – and so we still recommend what is a cheap and simple screening test.[7] A measurement of thyroid stimulating hormone (TSH, range 0.5–5.0 U/L) is the most sensitive test of thyroid function, an elevation suggesting hypothyroidism; the additional measurement of free thyroxine (T_4: 9–22 pmol/L) may be helpful. If hyperthyroidism is suspected a suppressed TSH and elevated free T_4 will usually reveal the diagnosis; if the free T_4 is normal, then measure free triiodothyronine (T_3: 4.3–8.6 pmol/L). The measurement of total T_4 (60–160 nmol/L) and T_3 (1.2–3.1 nmol/L) rarely provides additional information. Thyroid autoantibodies should be measured because of the risk of their transplacental passage. Hypothyroidism is sometimes associated with a mild elevation in serum prolactin levels. It is essential that thyroid disease is treated and thyroid function stabilized prior to conception. Hypothyroidism in particular is very bad for the baby (see Ch. 3).

Prolactin

Mild elevations in serum prolactin concentration are associated with stress and may occur simply as a result of having blood taken. Prolactin measurements vary day to day and if elevated to more than 1000 mU/L should be repeated before imaging of the pituitary gland is arranged (see Ch. 6). About 15% of women with PCOS have hyperprolactinemia, and about 50% of these have a microadenoma. It used to be thought that, as stress can lead to a slight elevation in serum prolactin concentration, this might itself cause subfertility. However, the treatment of ovulatory women who have mild hyperprolactinemia with dopamine agonists such as bromocriptine does not enhance fertility.

Estrogen

This is of little value in pretreatment evaluation of infertile women. Sometimes an early follicular phase measurement of estradiol can be useful as, in the normal cycle, FSH remains fairly constant from days 1–3 while estradiol starts to rise on day 3 with follicular growth. It has been suggested that a relationship between serum FSH and estradiol concentrations can be used in order to enhance the prediction of "ovarian reserve," although this has not become generally adopted in clinical practice.

Glucose tolerance

Women who are obese, and also many slim women with PCOS, will have insulin resistance and elevated serum concentrations of insulin (usually < 30 mU/L fasting). We suggest that a 75 g oral glucose tolerance test (GTT) be performed in women with PCOS and a body mass index (BMI) > 30 kg/m^2, with an assessment of the fasting and 2 hour glucose concentration (Table 4.5). It has been suggested that South Asian women should have an assessment of glucose tolerance if their BMI is greater than 25 kg/m^2 because of the greater risk of insulin resistance at a lower BMI than seen in the Caucasian population.

Table 4.5 Definitions of glucose tolerance after a 75 g glucose tolerance test (GTT)

	Diabetes mellitus	Impaired glucose tolerance (IGT)	Impaired fasting glycemia
Fasting glucose (mmol/l)	≥ 7.0	< 7.0	≥ 6.1 and < 7.0
2 hour glucose (mmol/l)	≥ 11.1	≥ 7.8	< 7.8
Action	Refer to diabetic clinic	Dietary advice; check fasting glucose annually	Dietary advice; check fasting glucose annually

Chromosomal analysis

It is sensible to study the chromosomes of women with infertility and any dysmorphic features, and also of women with recurrent miscarriages (and their partners) (see Ch. 20) and those with premature ovarian failure (see Ch. 8). Men with severe oligospermia (< 5 million/ml) should also have a chromosomal analysis (see Ch. 11).

Autoantibodies

Women with premature ovarian failure sometimes have ovarian autoantibodies or signs of other autoimmune disease (thyroid pernicious anemia, diabetes mellitus, SLE) (see Ch. 8). The presence of autoantibodies alerts the clinician to the risk that these conditions may become manifest.

Anticardiolipin syndrome

Women with recurrent miscarriage might have elevated levels of lupus anticoagulant and anticardiolipin antibodies and may benefit from a full thrombophilia screen (see Ch. 20).

Pelvic Ultrasound

When first scanning the pelvis, many radiographers and radiologists suggest performing a transabdominal scan to obtain first an overview of the pelvic organs, and also to assess the kidneys and renal tract if indicated. Subsequently a transvaginal ultrasound examination (Fig. 4.8) of the pelvic organs is preferred to the transabdominal approach as it not only obviates the need for a full bladder, with its associated discomfort, but also allows high frequency probes (5–7.5 Mhz) to be used so that higher resolution and greater precision in measurements of the pelvic structures, follicular diameters, and endometrial thickness can be achieved. It is especially advantageous in patients who are undergoing assisted conception as they commonly have lower abdominal scars, which impair the penetration of ultrasound and, furthermore, periadnexal adhesions may tether the ovaries deep in the pelvis and limit the elevation of these structures that normally occurs when the bladder is filled for a transabdominal scan. A study comparing transabdominal with transvaginal scanning demonstrated that the margins of the follicles were more sharply defined in 90% of cases when the transvaginal approach was used compared with only 41% with a transabdominal approach.[8] The same study found that the numbers and sizes of the dominant follicles correlated better with the serum estradiol concentrations when transvaginal scanning was used.

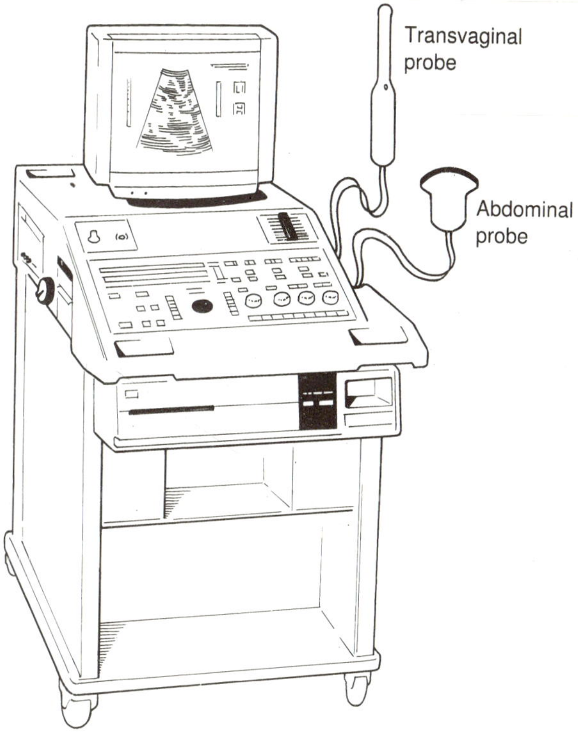

Figure 4.8 Ultrasound machine with transabdominal and transvaginal probes.

An ultrasound assessment of ovarian volume and antral follicle count in the early follicular phase has been used as a predictor for ovarian response prior to IVF treatment, with small volume ovaries indicating reduced ovarian reserve.[9] Indeed, a recent study correlated antral follicle count, ovarian volume, and day 3 levels of FSH, estradiol, and inhibin B and found that it was the follicle count that best correlated with subsequent ovarian response and pregnancy rates with IVF.[10]

Ovarian morphology

We recognize in the ovary three distinct morphological appearances: normal (Fig. 4.9), polycystic (Fig. 4.10), and multicystic (Fig. 4.11).[11] Multicystic ovaries are characteristically observed in pubertal girls and women recovering from weight loss-related amenorrhea. These multicystic (or multifollicular) ovaries are normal in size or slightly enlarged and contain six or more cysts that are 4–10 mm in diameter;[12] in contrast to women with polycystic ovaries (PCO), the stroma is not increased. The multicystic ovary appears to develop as a consequence

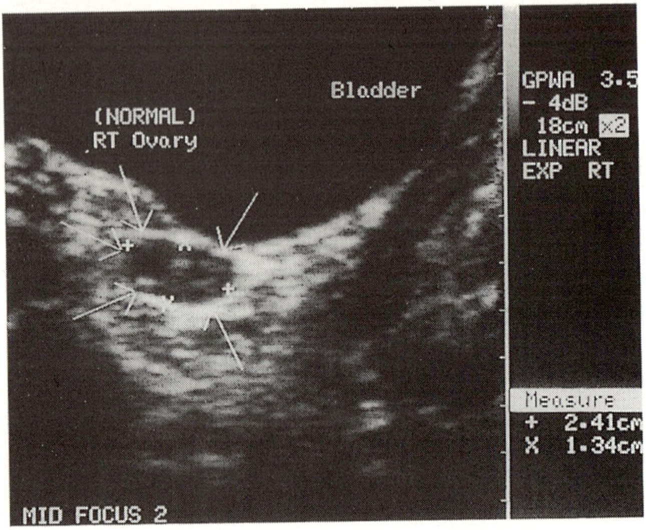

Figure 4.9 Transabdominal ultrasound scan of a normal ovary.

of reduced hypothalamic secretion of gonadotropin-releasing hormone (GnRH) which results in subnormal stimulation of the ovaries by the gonadotropins.[11] The multicystic ovary has a normal response to exogenous stimulation, by either pulsatile GnRH or gonadotropins, and the ultrasound appearance of the ovary usually reverts to normal.

Polycystic ovaries are a separate entity and have a distinct response to induction of ovulation and ovarian stimulation for IVF. The association of enlarged, sclerocystic ovaries with amenorrhea, infertility, and hirsutism was first described by Stein and Leventhal in 1935,[13] and is now known as the polycystic ovary syndrome (PCOS). Since then, it has become apparent that PCO may be present in women who are non-hirsute and who have regular menstrual cycles.[14] Thus, a clinical spectrum exists between the typical Stein–Leventhal picture on the one hand (PCOS) and the symptomless on the other (PCO). Even patients described as having the PCOS exhibit considerable heterogeneity (see Ch. 7).

Differentiating between PCO and PCOS

It is important to differentiate between PCO and the PCOS. The former describes the morphological appearance of the ovary whereas the latter term is only appropriate when PCO are found in association with a menstrual disturbance (amenorrhea or, more commonly, oligomenorrhea), the complications of hyperandrogenization (seborrhea, acne, and hirsutism) and obesity. The PCOS is also associated with

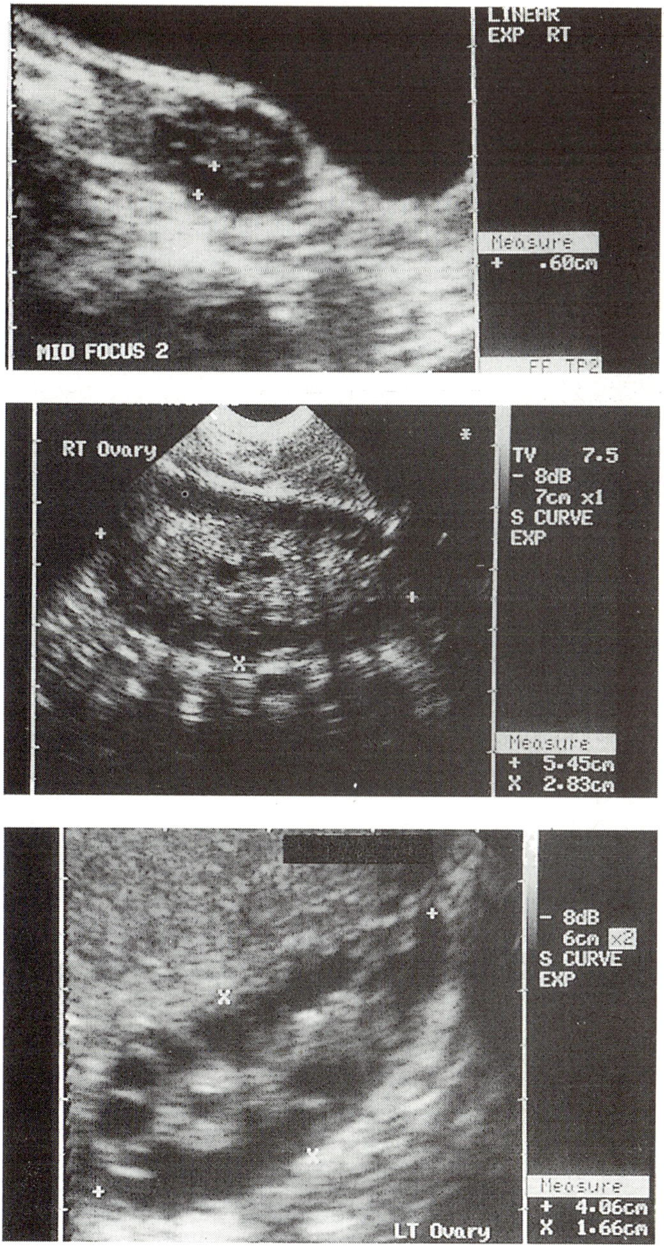

a

b

c

Figure 4.10a,b,c (**a**) Transabdominal ultrasound scan of a polycystic ovary. (**b**&**c**) Transvaginal ultrasound scans of a polycystic ovary.

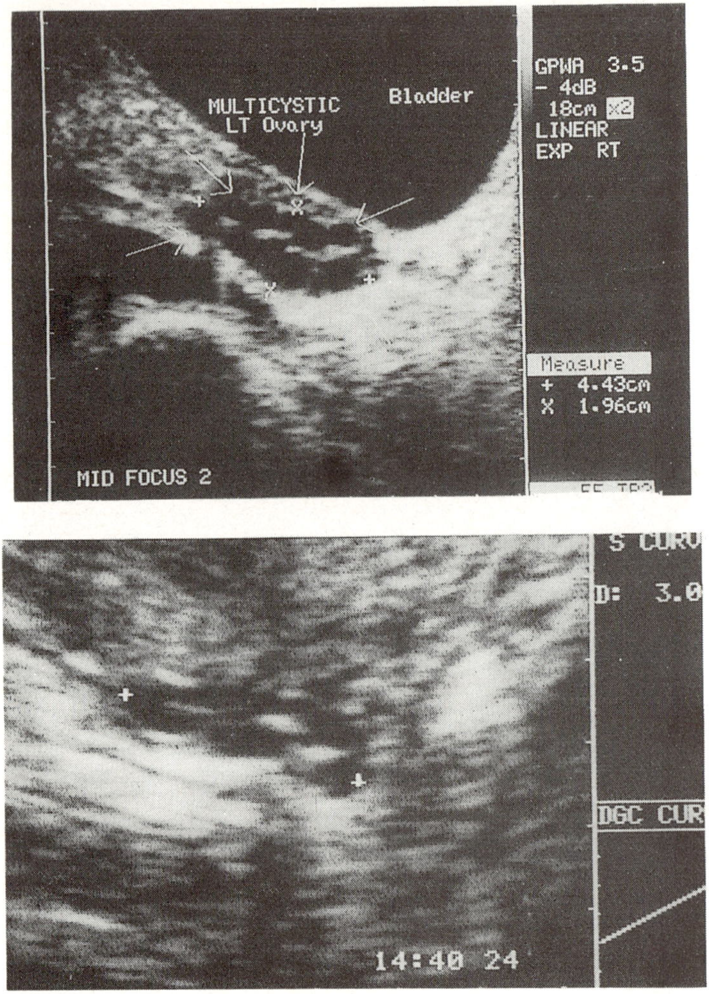

a

b

Figure 4.11a,b (**a**) Transabdominal scan of a multicystic ovary. (**b**) Transvaginal ultrasound scan of a multicystic ovary.

endocrinological abnormalities and in particular with elevated serum concentrations of LH, prolactin, estrogens, and androgens. As with the clinical picture, these changes are variable and patients with PCOS may have normal endocrine concentrations (see further discussion in Ch. 7).

The diagnosis of PCO is therefore best made not on the clinical presentation, but rather on the ovarian morphology (Figs 4.12 and 4.13). With the advent of high-resolution ultrasound, identification of

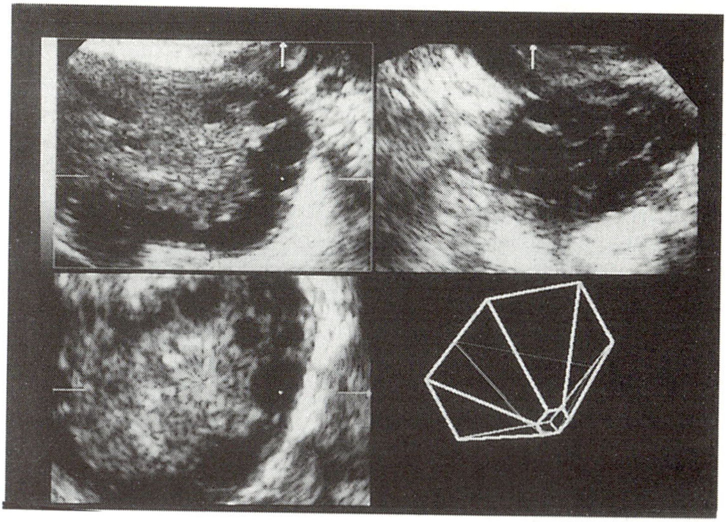

Figure 4.12 Three-dimensional transvaginal ultrasound scan of a polycystic ovary. (Courtesy of Dr A. Kyei-Mensah.)

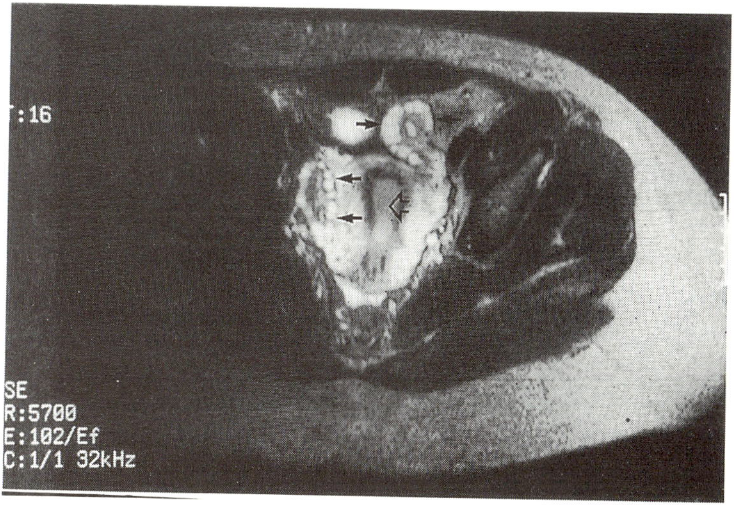

Figure 4.13 Magnetic resonance imaging (MRI) of a pelvis, demonstrating two polycystic ovaries (closed arrows) and a hyperplastic endometrium (open arrow).

PCO is simple, rendering ovarian biopsy – which is invasive and possibly damaging to future fertility because it can cause adhesions – unnecessary. Ovaries were described by transabdominal ultrasonography as being polycystic if there were 10 or more cysts, 2–8 mm in diameter, arranged around a dense stroma or scattered throughout an increased amount of stroma.[11] Some authors are attempting to redefine the morphological appearance of the PCO using transvaginal ultrasonography, three-dimensional transvaginal ultrasonography, and magnetic resonance imaging. Ovarian stromal volume has been correlated with serum testosterone concentrations and may provide more useful information than the volume of the cysts. There is, unfortunately, little standardization in the ultrasound diagnosis of PCO with virtually every department of radiology using its own, often subjective, definition. Most authorities now accept that the diagnosis of PCO is made when at least 10 cysts are seen using a transabdominal ultrasound, or 15–20 cysts with transvaginal ultrasound. Ovarian volume is usually greater than 10 ml, compared with normal ovarian volume of 5 ml.

Prevalence The prevalence of PCO in women with ovulatory disorders has been well documented. Using high-resolution ultrasound, it has been shown that as many as 87% of patients with oligomenorrhea and 26% with amenorrhea have PCO.[8] We have also identified PCO in women with hypogonadotropic hypogonadism who attended our ovulation induction clinic and, while these patients had no endogenous production of gonadotropins, they responded to stimulation in a characteristically "polycystic" fashion with a sudden growth of multiple follicles.[14,15] Polson *et al.*[16] found the prevalence of PCO to be 22% of a volunteer "normal" population, while Michelmore *et al.*[17] found PCO in 33% of "normal" young women (see Ch. 7 for more details). The prevalence in patients referred for IVF is not well known. We studied over 500 patients who underwent IVF and found 34% to have ultrasound detected PCO.[18]

Summary PCO with or without clinical symptoms are a common finding in patients referred for ovulation induction or IVF. Indeed, the patient's primary diagnosis is often not PCOS but rather another cause of subfertility that necessitates assisted conception therapy. It is of the utmost importance to make a careful assessment of the morphological appearance of the ovary prior to commencing ovarian stimulation as the presence of PCO should alert one to the risks and complications that might occur (see Ch. 17).

Ovarian cysts

Besides making a careful assessment of ovarian morphology, it is necessary to perform a baseline ultrasound scan of the ovaries before commencing ovarian stimulation in order to detect the presence of ovarian cysts (Figs 4.14–4.16). There remains controversy as to the effect of ovarian cysts on the treatment cycle (see Ch. 13). It is obviously necessary to record the presence of any cystic structures prior to commencing ovarian stimulation in order to monitor accurately

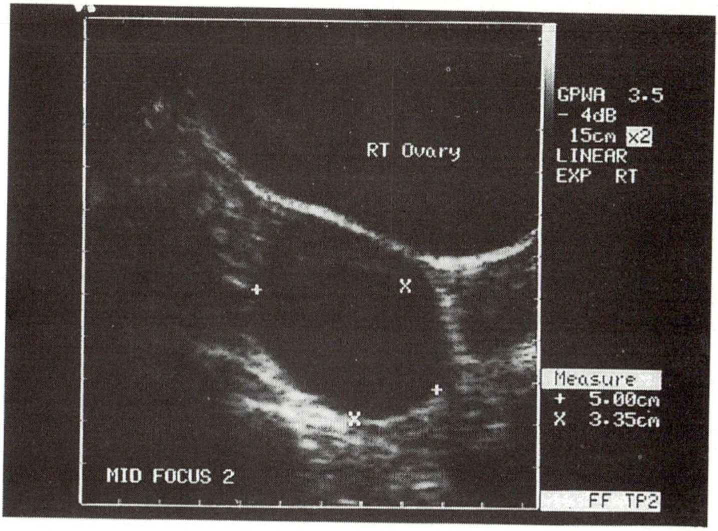

Figure 4.14 Transabdominal ultrasound scan of a "simple," functional cyst.

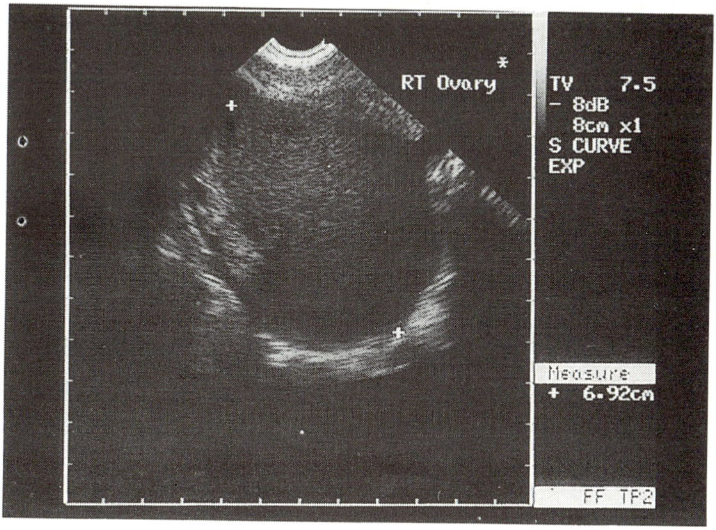

Figure 4.15 Transvaginal ultrasound scan of a mucinous cystadenoma.

the development of new follicles. Although it has been suggested that the presence of ovarian cysts reduces the success of the subsequent IVF cycle,[19,20] other studies have failed to confirm this.[21,22] It is also necessary to distinguish between cysts that are present before the administration of hormonal agents and those which might arise as a

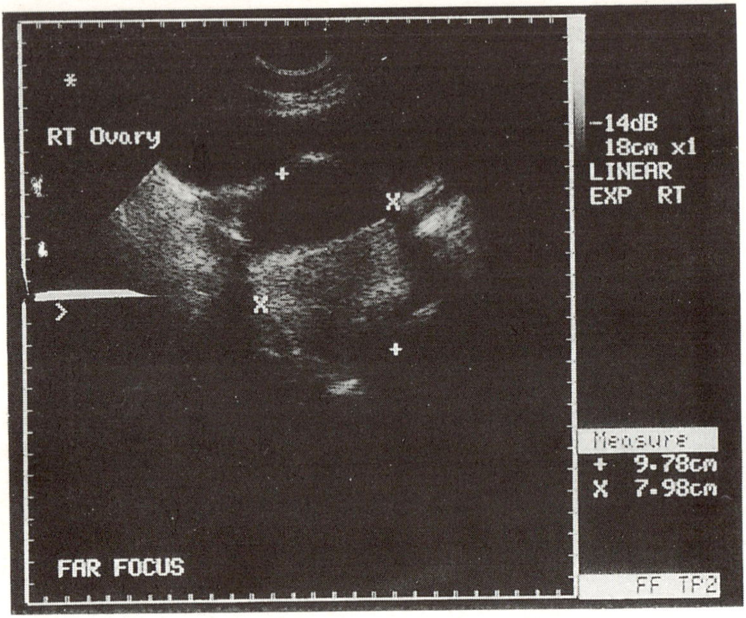

Figure 4.16 Transvaginal ultrasound scan of a benign cystic teratoma (dermoid cyst).

result of hormonal stimulation because of the exaggerated release of the gonadotropins that occurs when GnRH agonist therapy is commenced (pretreatment with the combined oral contraceptive pill reduces the occurrence of such GnRH agonist-stimulated cysts).

The situation is slightly different in patients who are undergoing ovulation induction for anovulatory infertility. In such patients cysts are usually functional and secrete estrogens or progesterone. If a cyst is detected on a baseline ultrasound scan, the usual policy is to commence ovarian stimulation only after the patient has had a spontaneous menstrual bleed, which indicates that the endogenous secretion of ovarian hormones has returned to baseline levels. Further confirmation of this is provided by a thin endometrium (less than 5 mm). Simple ovarian cysts that are less than 5 cm in diameter rarely require surgical intervention.

If the patient is known to have endometriosis it is important to avoid aspirating the cyst, either before ovarian stimulation is commenced or during the oocyte retrieval procedure itself, because of the risk of infection (see Ch. 13). An endometrioma has the characteristic hazy, echodense appearance of blood in a cyst. Inadvertent, or unavoidable, aspiration of an endometrioma necessitates full antibiotic cover. Dermoid cysts are sometimes seen in women of reproductive age and may be difficult to distinguish from endometriomas, as both may be bilateral with a hazy, homogeneously echodense appearance of lipid matter in dermoids and blood in endometriomas. Dermoids can sometimes be differentiated by brightly echogenic areas caused by the presence of solid components.

All but obviously simple cysts should be treated with caution as ovarian malignancy may occur in young women. Therapeutic stimulation of the ovaries should not be performed until complex ovarian cysts have resolved, either spontaneously or surgically.

The baseline ultrasound scan also permits inspection of the other pelvic structures and might reveal the presence of hydrosalpinges, fibroids (Fig. 4.17) (submucous fibroids are of particular importance), or even an elusive intrauterine contraceptive device – which on removal should cure the patient's subfertility![23] A patient with hydrosalpinges visible on ultrasound should be counseled to consider salpingectomy in order to improve the outcome of IVF (see Ch. 10).

The resolution of transvaginal and transabdominal scans is 2–3 mm and 3–5 mm, respectively, and so small follicles can be visualized easily as echo-free structures, which are usually toward the periphery of the more echogenic ovarian tissue.[24] The internal diameter of the follicle should be measured in three planes and the mean value calculated.[25] In one study the intraobserver standard deviation of transabdominal follicular measurement was reported to be 0.6 mm and the interobserver standard deviation 1.2 mm, irrespective of the follicular diameter.[26]

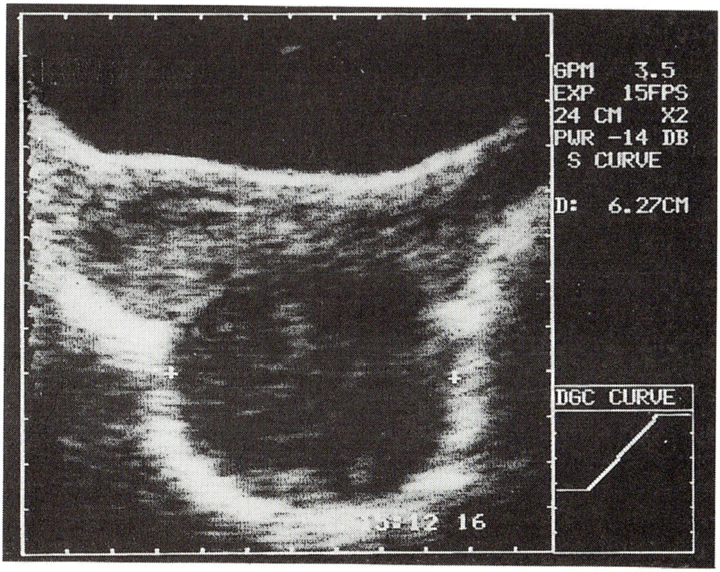

Figure 4.17 Transabdominal ultrasound scan of a serous fibroid.

The 95% confidence limits for any particular measurement would therefore be ±2.4 mm. One would expect transvaginal measurements to confer greater precision. In spontaneous cycles, therefore, the small follicles can generally be visualized about 10 days before the day of ovulation (day 4). By day 5 there is usually a dominant follicle which then grows at a rate of approximately 2–3 mm daily until the day of ovulation. (For illustration of ultrasound scans of follicular growth, see p. 171.)[27,28]

Plasma estradiol concentrations correlate well with follicular diameter in natural cycles, but not in superovulated cycles (when there is not only great variation but also differential effects of the different drug regimens that may be used).[29] The increase in circulating estrogen levels results in an increase in the overall uterine size and a thickening of the endometrium, which serves as a useful bioassay for estrogen production.

It is important to perform an ultrasound scan in the mid-luteal phase in both natural and stimulated cycles for IVF. The corpus luteum may have a number of appearances, being either ovoid or irregular in outline with a cystic, echo-free interior, or it may have a hazy, echodense appearance because of the presence of cellular debris and blood (see Ch. 6). The combination of a corpus luteum seen on ultrasound and an elevated serum progesterone concentration provides the best possible evidence of ovulation, although only a pregnancy will confirm that an oocyte was released from the follicle. Occasionally there is no follicular rupture and a cystic structure persists in the luteal phase of the cycle associated with an elevated serum progesterone concentration. This is referred to as "luteinized unruptured follicle" (LUF).[30] There is some debate about the incidence of the LUF syndrome. LUF occurs in less than 5% of cycles of patients undergoing ovulation induction therapy and does not tend to be a recurrent phenomenon.[31]

Endometrial assessment

Endometrial changes can be seen clearly using pelvic ultrasound (Figs 4.18 and 4.19). In the early follicular phase, when the endometrium is thin, there is a single hypoechogenic line produced by the opposed walls of the endometrial cavity. In the periovulatory phase the estrogenized endometrium takes on a characteristic "triple line" appearance. In the luteal phase the functional layer becomes hyperechogenic because of stromal edema.[32,33] The endometrial thickness in the early follicular phase is 4–6 mm, by the time of ovulation it is about 8–10 mm, and in the mid-luteal phase it reaches 14 mm. It has been suggested that there is a reduced chance of pregnancy if the triple line appearance is absent or if the preovulatory endometrial thickness is less than 7 mm.[34,35]

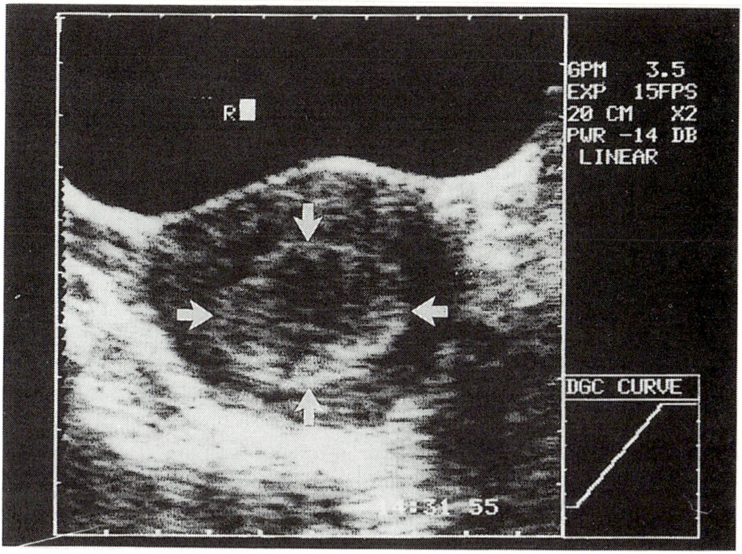

Figure 4.18 Transabdominal ultrasound scan demonstrating endometrial hyperplasia (30 mm diameter) in an amenorrheic woman with polycystic ovary syndrome.

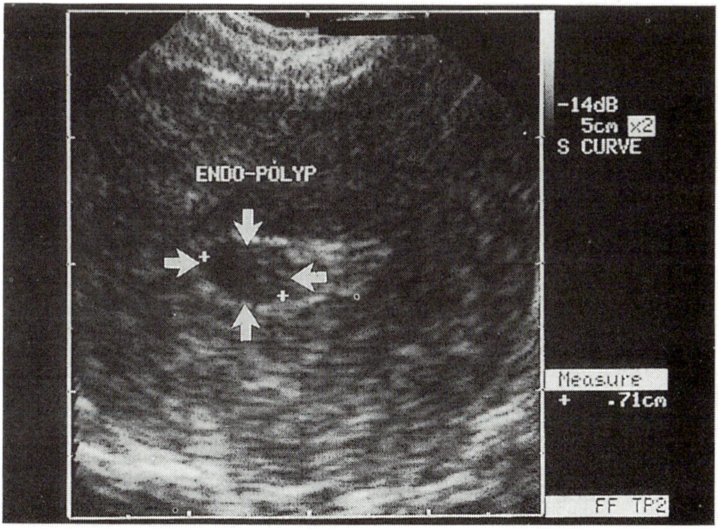

Figure 4.19 Transvaginal ultrasound scan demonstrating an endometrial polyp.

Doppler ultrasound in assisted conception

The combination of transvaginal ultrasound with color Doppler measurements is beginning to provide a detailed picture of follicular events around the time of ovulation and it allows assessment of the uterine blood flow to predict endometrial receptivity. The precise uterine requirements for successful implantation have yet to be elucidated fully. The probability of a pregnancy occurring during assisted conception procedures depends on embryo quality and uterine receptivity. In order to improve the chance of conception it has become customary to transfer two, three, or four pre-embryos and in some centers even more. In the UK it is now illegal to transfer more than three pre-embryos in any one cycle and the current recommendation is for the routine transfer of two pre-embryos, particularly in women under the age of 40 years who have a higher chance of a multiple pregnancy and a reduced rate of miscarriage. Methods to improve our ability to assess endometrial receptivity for implantation might help prevent the transfer of precious pre-embryos in cycles that are virtually doomed to failure. The embryos could then be frozen and transferred later, in a cycle that is judged to be optimal for implantation, perhaps following hormonal manipulation of the endometrial response. Until recently, the only way to assess endometrial receptivity was by endometrial biopsy. Doppler ultrasound is proving to be a valuable, non-invasive method which provides an instantaneous picture of uterine blood flow.[36]

Blood flow through the uterine and ovarian arteries has been extensively investigated in spontaneous and stimulated cycles.[37] Doppler studies of the ovarian circulation are still at the research stage. It was reported in one study of natural cycles that resistance to arterial flow was lower on the side bearing the dominant follicle. In gonadotropin-stimulated cycles it was reported that ovarian impedance was inversely proportional to the number of follicles greater than 15 mm in diameter.[38] It has also been reported that, in IVF cycles, there was a lower ovarian impedance 3 days after embryo transfer in those patients who conceived compared with those who did not.[39] In the future, it might be possible to time the administration of hCG to coincide with optimal ovarian blood flow for either the release or collection of the highest quality oocytes.[40]

Assessment of Tubal Patency and the Uterine Cavity

Hysterosalpingography

Tubal infertility is diagnosed in between 15% and 50% of couples presenting with subfertility. X-ray hysterosalpingography (HSG) (Figs 4.20–4.25) provides a delineation of both the uterine cavity and the Fallopian tubes. An HSG is the simplest preliminary test for the

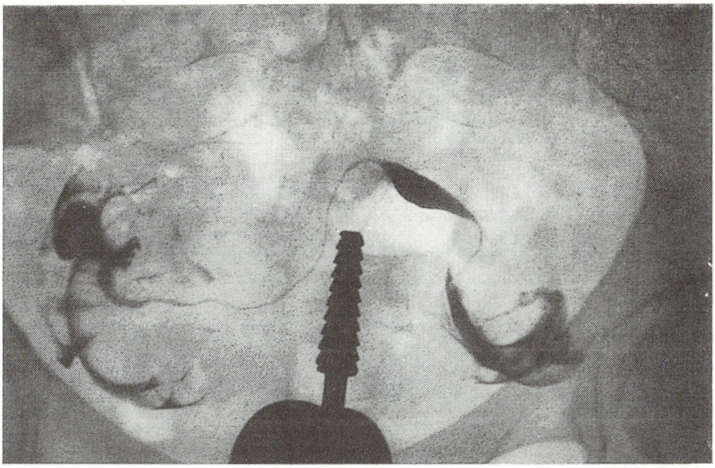

Figure 4.20 X-ray hysterosalpingogram (HSG) performed using a digital system. The iodine-based X-ray contrast medium appears black. In this picture free spill into the peritoneal cavity can be seen flowing from each Fallopian tube. In this procedure a metal cannula was used.

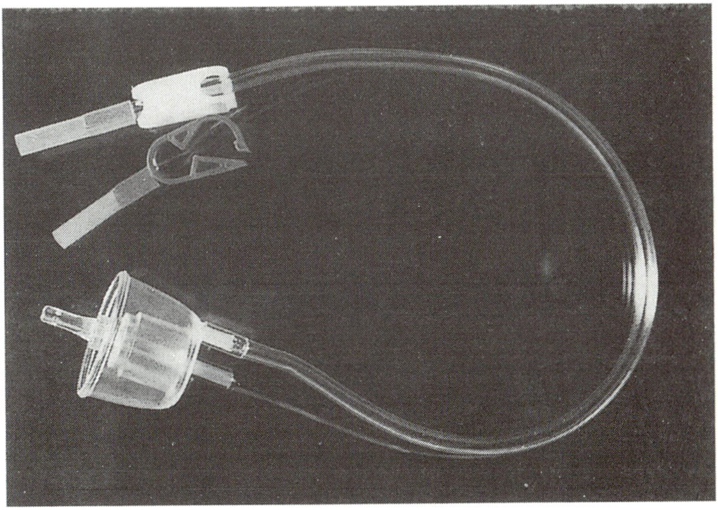

Figure 4.21 Plastic Malmstrom–Westerman vacuum suction cup. The cup fits over the cervix and negative pressure is applied by a hand-driven pump. Once the cup fits snugly over the cervix, contrast medium is injected through the central channel (see text).

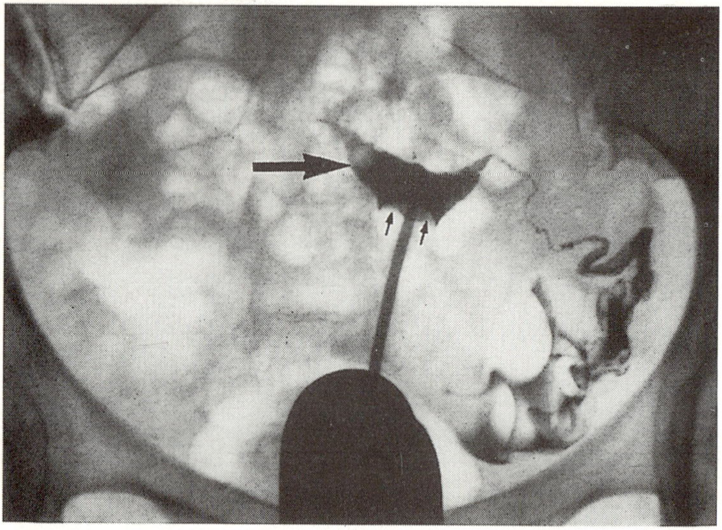

Figure 4.22 X-ray HSG demonstrating free spill from the left Fallopian tube but obstruction of flow through the right tube by an intrauterine lesion that was later found to be an endometrial polyp (large arrow). For this procedure, a balloon catheter (Fig. 4.23) was used and the inflated balloon can be seen occupying the lower portion of the uterus (small arrows).

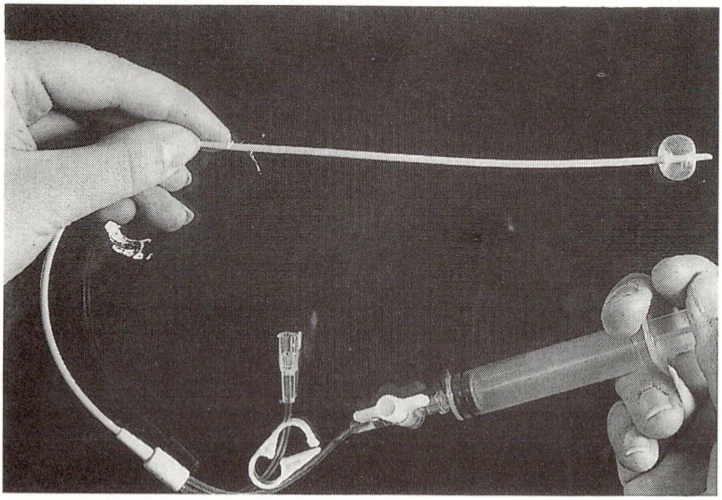

Figure 4.23 Balloon catheter. The catheter is inserted gently through the cervix and the balloon inflated within the uterine cavity. Gentle traction is applied to prevent backward flow of contrast medium.

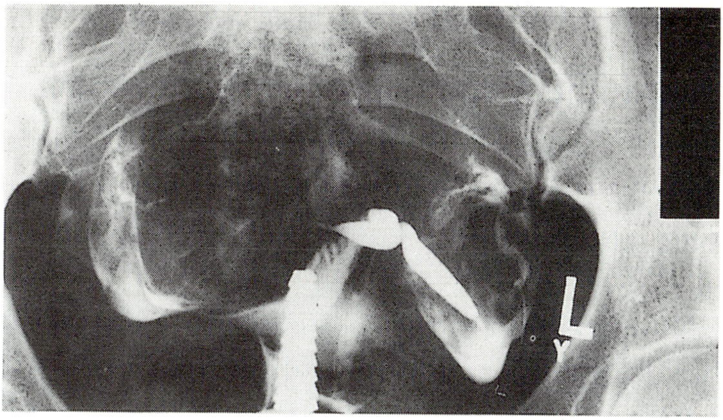

Figure 4.24 X-ray HSG of a uterus didelphys, which is acutely anteflexed. An older style metal Leisch–Wilkinson cannula has been used and a conventional X-ray system, in which the contrast medium appears white.

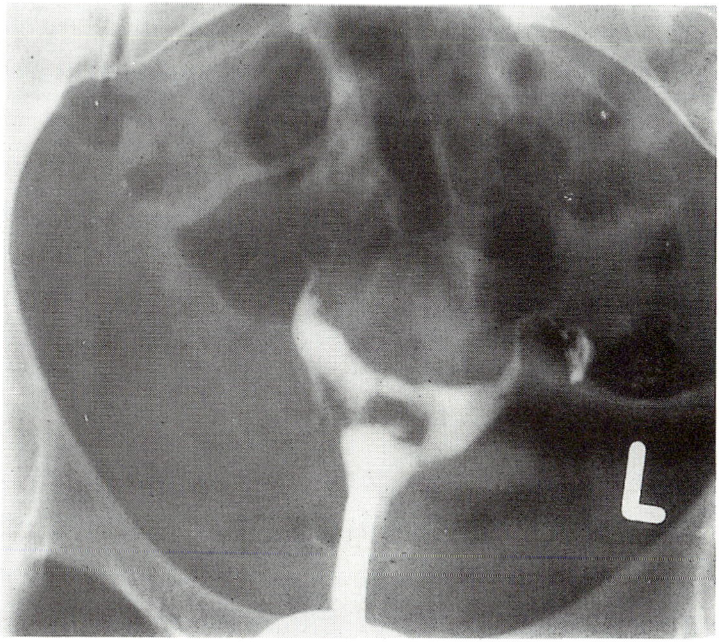

Figure 4.25 Conventional X-ray HSG demonstrating Ashermann's syndrome, with intrauterine synechiae. There is no flow of contrast medium through the right tube, although thickening of the cornual end of the tube suggests the possibility of tubal spasm. There is flow to the end of the left Fallopian tube, but no free spill into the peritoneal cavity. This raises the possibility of sacculated adhesions around the fimbrial end of the tube.

delineation of the uterine cavity and Fallopian tubes and has few complications.[1]

It is important that the procedure is performed by an experienced radiologist who is able both to position the cannula over or into the cervical canal and gently to inject the contrast medium while imaging the pelvis to get a dynamic view of the passage of dye. There are a number of different cannulae ranging from the old-style metal Leisch–Wilkinson or Green–Armytage cannula, which may have to be virtually screwed into the cervix, to the more modern plastic Malmstrom–Westerman vacuum suction cup that fits over the cervix, or balloon catheters that either fit into the endocervical canal or are passed into the uterine cavity itself. We prefer to use the last two techniques.

A water-soluble contrast medium is usually used and will be absorbed after an hour. While there is reported to be up to a 90% concordance between HSG and laparoscopic findings, a false-positive diagnosis of unilateral tubal blockage has also been reported in up to two-thirds of cases of apparently blocked tubes using either method. In a meta-analysis of 20 studies comparing HSG and laparoscopy it was found that for tubal patency, the sensitivity of HSG was 0.65 and the specificity 0.83.[41] HSG has generally been found to be unreliable for the detection of peritubular adhesions. Sometimes the cause of an apparent blockage is a mucus plug, which might be flushed through the tube by the contrast medium. Thus there are reports of an increased chance of pregnancy in the 2 or 3 months that follow either an HSG or laparoscopic insufflation of the tubes.

Oil-based contrast media are more irritant than water-soluble media and have gone out of favor because of the risk of venous intravasation of contrast agent and subsequent embolism in the immediate post-menstrual phase of the cycle. Fluoroscopic control of the procedure should ensure that this serious complication does not happen. Oil-based media are absorbed slowly and can cause granuloma formation when trapped within a hydrosalpinx. Interestingly, oil-based media are thought to "unblock" more tubes than water-based media. Indeed a meta-analysis of ten studies[42] indicated that spontaneous pregnancy rates were significantly higher after oil-based contrast media were used than after the use of water-soluble agents. This benefit was greatest for patients with unexplained infertility, suggesting the possibility of tubal "plugs" as a cause. We have also recently reported a therapeutic benefit in a randomized controlled trial in couples with unexplained infertility.[43] A similar beneficial effect has been reported after falloposcopic flushing of the tube or transcervical Fallopian tube catheterization. Despite these findings, it is unclear if oil-based media will return to favor as not only is their use more painful, but the high viscosity leads to a prolonged injection time and the need, in some cases, for an image to be taken 24 hours after the procedure.

Timing An HSG should be performed optimally within 10 days of a menstrual period when there should be no risk of a pregnancy. It should not be performed when the patient is bleeding. We advise that contraceptive precautions should be used during the cycle in which the HSG is performed. If a woman is oligo-/amenorrheic we induce a withdrawal bleed with a progestogen after a negative pregnancy test. If there is erratic bleeding or any doubt about the possibility of an early pregnancy, the procedure should be delayed and a pregnancy test should be performed.

The HSG can be uncomfortable, especially if there is either tubal spasm or a tubal obstruction. We advise patients to take an analgesic (e.g., mefenamic acid, naproxen, or diclofenac) 30–45 minutes before the procedure. Preparation for the HSG takes about 5 minutes and the average length of time spent screening for the flow of contrast is 40 seconds. Tubal spasm can occur and antispasmodics have been employed (glucagon, diazepam, hyoscine) with varying success. Probably the best way to avoid tubal spasm, however, is by slow injection of contrast.

Antibiotic prophylaxis If there has been a history of pelvic inflammatory disease antibiotic prophylaxis should be given (either a 3- or 5-day course of doxycycline and metronidazole or Augmentin), although patients with a history of pelvic infection are probably better assessed by laparoscopy than HSG. While the HSG will have been performed in aseptic conditions, patients should be warned to report immediately severe pelvic pain or pyrexia in the 24–48 hours after the procedure, as admission to hospital is then required in order to administer intravenous antibiotics. Because of "silent" pelvic infection, in particular *Chlamydia*, some advocate routine antibiotic prophylaxis for all procedures that involve instrumentation of the cervix (see Ch. 2).

Characteristic findings Small filling defects can be caused by air bubbles and small polyps (which can represent normal endometrium in the premenstrual phase of the cycle). The cavity of the body of the uterus is usually triangular, sometimes with a concave or convex fundus. The diameter of the cornual portion of the uterus is approximately 35 mm. The Fallopian tubes are 56 cm long and free spill of contrast medium into the peritoneal cavity should be seen. Hydrosalpinges appear as large sacculated structures that are often either convoluted or retort shaped. One of the criticisms of the HSG is that it is not possible to detect peritubal adhesions, which can interfere with oocyte pick-up by the fimbrial end of the tube. A convoluted distal tube may, however, suggest the presence of peritubular adhesions and the contrast medium tends to be immobile at the end of the tube rather than continue to spill freely into the peritoneal cavity.

If there is tubal blockage the commonest histological finding after surgical excision of the occluded portion of the tube is obliterative fibrosis, followed by salpingitis isthmica nodosa (Figs 4.26 and 4.27), chronic inflammation, and intramucosal endometriosis. Salpingitis isthmica nodosa is seen on an HSG as multiple small (2 mm diameter) diverticula of the proximal 2 cm of the Fallopian tubes; the condition is bilateral and the tubes are often blocked. The appearance of tubal damage after tuberculous salpingitis differs in that there is a ragged outline, often with multiple strictures and a beaded appearance; occasionally the tube is rigid, with a "pipe stem" appearance. Pelvic TB may lead to calcification, which can be seen on an X-ray.

A proximal tubal occlusion may be cannulated by selective salpingography, using guide wires, balloons, and catheters under fluoroscopic control in an attempt to unblock the obstruction (see p. 263).

Asherman's syndrome is a condition in which intrauterine adhesions prevent normal growth of the endometrium. This may be the result of a too vigorous endometrial curettage affecting the basalis layer of the endometrium or adhesions may follow an episode of endometritis. Estrogen deficiency may increase the risk of adhesion formation in breastfeeding women who require a curettage for retained placental tissue. Typically amenorrhea is not absolute, and it may be possible to induce a withdrawal bleed using a combined estrogen/progestogen preparation. Intrauterine adhesions may be seen on an HSG. Alternatively,

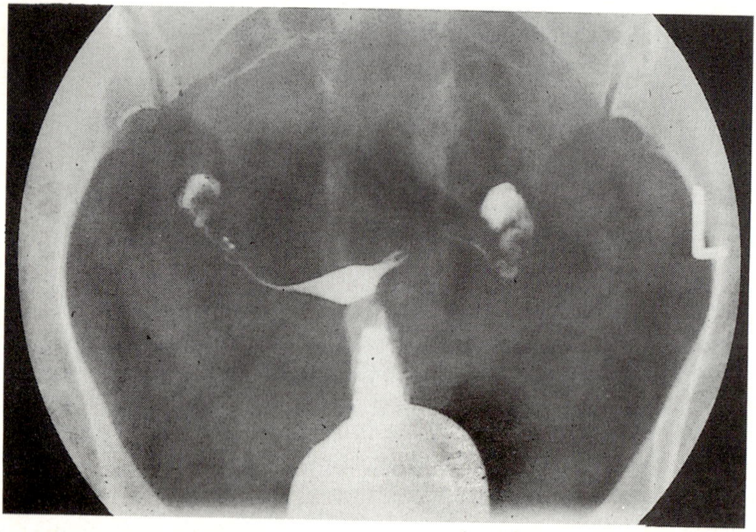

Figure 4.26 HSG of salpingitis isthmica nodosa (SIN) (please refer to plate section for color figure).

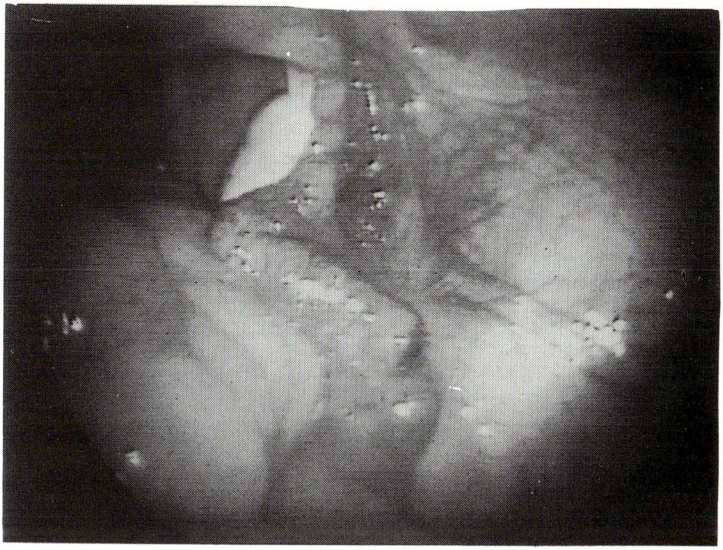

Figure 4.27 Salpingitis isthmica nodosa (SIN) seen at laparoscopy with blue dye appearing in the herniation through the serosal layer of the tube (please refer to plate section for color figure).

hysteroscopic inspection of the uterine cavity will confirm the diagnosis and enable treatment by adhesiolysis. Following surgery, a 3-month course of cyclical progesterone/estrogen should be given. The insertion of an intrauterine contraceptive device for 2–3 months may prevent the recurrence of adhesions.

Ultrasound contrast hysterosalpingography (or hysterosalpingo-contrast sonography, HyCoSy) (Figs 4.28–4.32)

It is now possible to perform an HSG using ultrasonography and an ultrasound contrast medium which contains galactose microparticles[29] (Echovist®) and is therefore free of the possible risks of radiation.[44] The procedure should be conducted in a similar fashion and at a similar time in the cycle as conventional HSG. Not only can tubal patency be assessed but before the contrast agent is injected, ultrasound enables the visualization of ovarian morphology and soft tissue abnormalities, such as fibroids or congenital anomalies of the uterus and cervix. Fibroids are not seen on X-ray HSG unless they are calcified or the uterine cavity is distorted and then the cause will not usually be apparent. Submucosal fibroids can cause tubal obstruction (usually at the cornual end) and can sometimes disrupt implantation and be associated with recurrent miscarriage. It is debatable whether myomectomy improves matters, in the absence of a tubal blockage

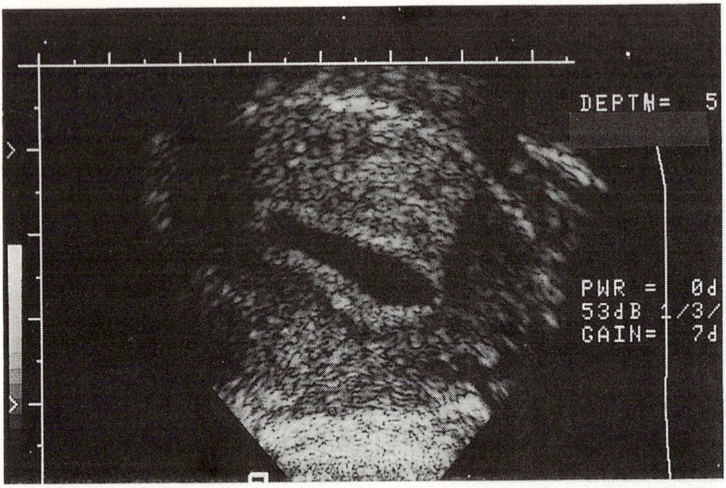

Figure 4.28 Ultrasound HSG (or hysterocontrast salpingography – HyCoSy). Transvaginal ultrasound scan showing negative contrast (saline) outlining a smooth endometrial cavity.

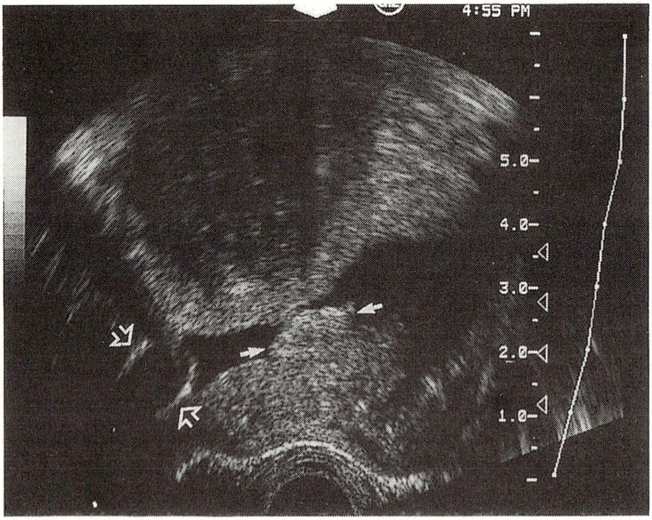

Figure 4.29 Transvaginal ultrasound HSG with saline demonstrating an endometrial polyp (small arrows). Note the transcervical balloon catheter (open arrows).

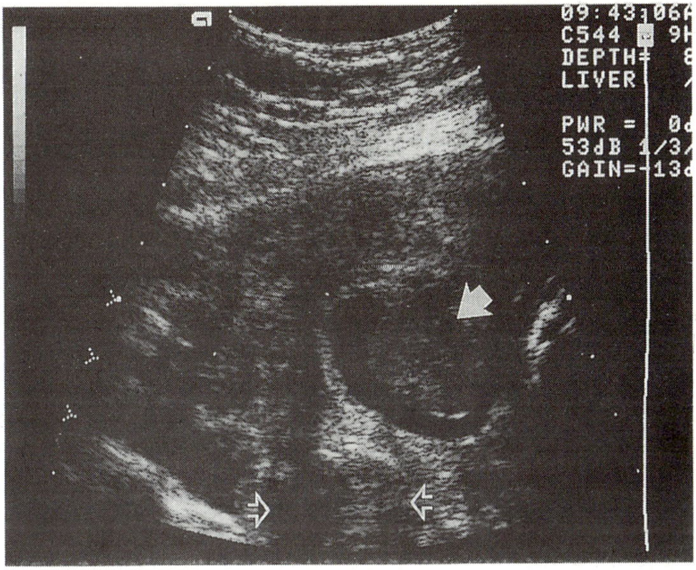

Figure 4.30 Transabdominal ultrasound HSG showing a submucosal fibroid (large arrow). There is also an intramural fibroid (open arrows). (See also Fig. 10.11, p. 267.)

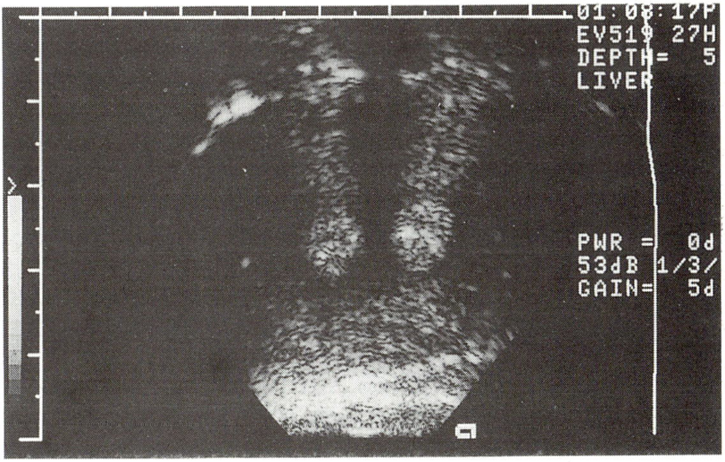

Figure 4.31 Transvaginal ultrasound HSG, using positive contrast medium (Echovist®) which has increased echogenicity on ultrasound. The two cavities of a uterus didelphys are seen (same patient as Fig. 4.24).

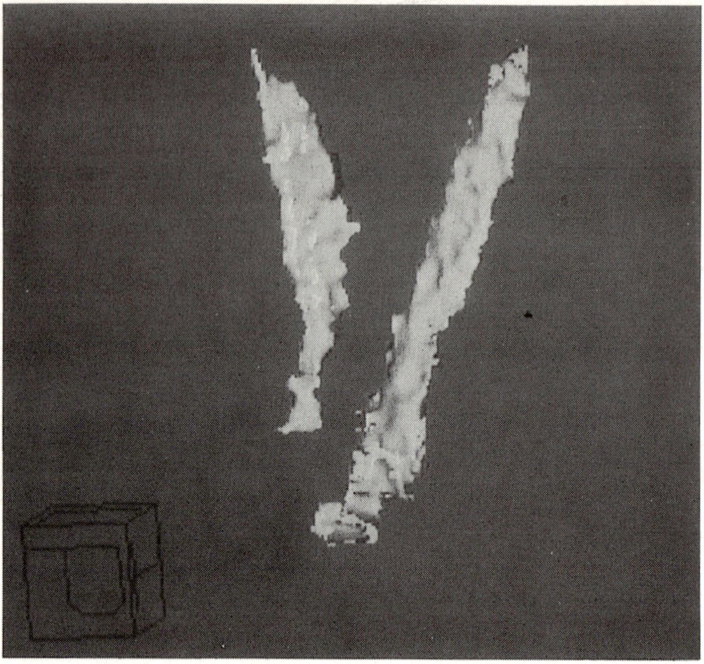

Figure 4.32 Three-dimensional reconstruction of the image obtained in Figure 4.31 of the uterus didelphys to show the relationship between the two cavities.

(see Ch. 10).[45] There is increasing evidence that intramural fibroids affect implantation, even when there is no deformation of the uterine cavity.[46] A recent study found that the presence of fibroids of less than 5 cm diameter reduced ongoing pregnancy rates by half following assisted conception.[47] Myomectomy is a major procedure with potential risks to the integrity and viability of the uterus. There has yet to be a randomized controlled study of myomectomy prior to assisted conception. Less invasive procedures are being evaluated for the management of fibroids, including uterine artery embolization and magnetic resonance imaging (MRI)-guided laser coagulative necrosis or high intensity focused ultrasound for the destruction of fibroids. The place of these techniques in the management of infertility is still being evaluated.

Advantages Hycosy provides a good alternative to conventional X-ray HSG and appears to have an 80–90% concordance with laparoscopy and dye insufflation. Some have used saline as an alternative ultrasound contrast medium, with similar success rates, particularly if a Doppler gate is placed over the Fallopian tube to

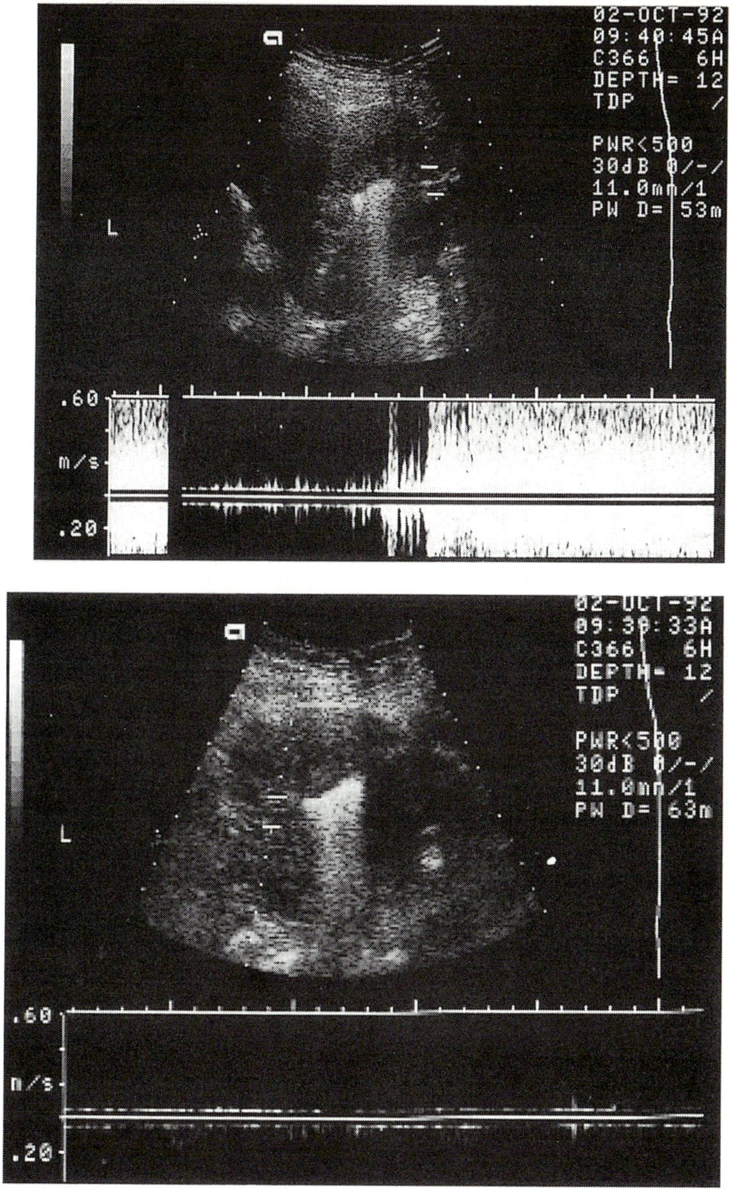

a

b

Figure 4.33a,b Transabdominal ultrasound HSG using Echovist®. The fundus of the uterus is visualized with a Doppler gate over the intramural portion of the Fallopian tube.. Flow is readily detected on the left when the intrauterine contrast medium is injected, while there is no flow on the right.

observe forward flow of the medium (Fig. 4.33). Furthermore, the uterine cavity can be reconstructed using three-dimensional imaging techniques to facilitate the diagnosis of uterine anomalies and differentiate between septate and bicornuate uteri (Fig. 4.31).[48]

Disadvantages Disadvantages of the HyCoSy procedure are that it takes longer than a conventional HSG (10–15 min) because of the additional time spent performing the transvaginal assessment of the pelvis, both the ultrasound transducer and catheter are in the vagina at the same time, and only one Fallopian tube can be visualized at a time. A HyCoSy requires trained personnel and we are not convinced that it will become adopted widely. We are certainly advocates of ultrasound assessment of ovarian and uterine morphology and consider that it should be performed by a skilled ultrasonographer. Then, if indicated, a conventional X-ray HSG should be performed separately by a radiologist.

Selective salpingography and falloposcopy

Transcervical cannulation of the tube can be performed using ultrasound guidance – selective salpingography – or with a falloposcope (Fig. 4.34). Selective salpingography might allow passage of the catheter through a stenotic region of the tube or permit flushing of inspissated mucus or fibrinous deposits.[49–51] Balloon tuboplasty can be achieved under fluoroscopic guidance. Falloposcopy, on the other hand, allows visualization

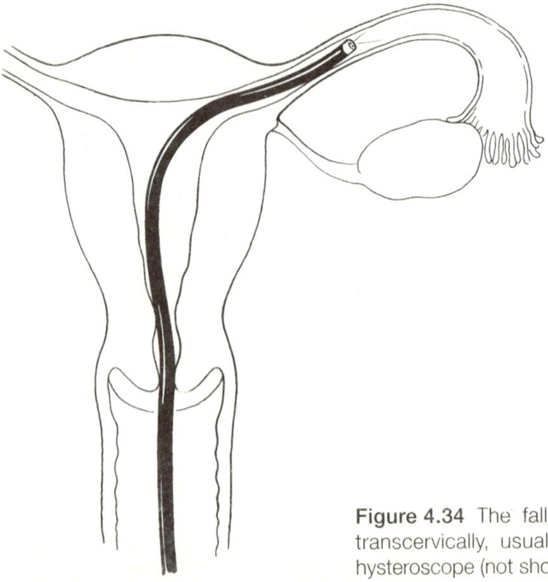

Figure 4.34 The falloposcope is inserted transcervically, usually via a channel in a hysteroscope (not shown).

of the tubal lumen (Fig. 4.35) and enables tuboplasty to be performed. The linear everting falloposcope eliminates the need for a hysteroscope and appears to be less traumatic to the tube.[52] The visualization of mucosal abnormalities might lead one to guide the patient to IVF sooner than if the architecture of the recannulated tube appeared normal. The salpingoscope, inserted laparoscopically,[53] provides clear visualization of the ampullary segment of the tube, which should normally have three to five major folds (4 mm in height) and several minor folds (1 mm in height).[54] These anatomical folds are not easily seen during salpingography and so salpingoscopy may enable a more appropriate decision to be made about whether to proceed with tubal surgery or IVF. While these are attractive techniques they have yet to be adopted in routine practice, largely because the optical systems have considerable limitations – particularly for falloposcopy, which is now no longer being performed.

Laparoscopy and Hysteroscopy (Figs 4.36–4.38)

It is our current practice to include a hysteroscopic evaluation of the uterine cavity whenever we perform a laparoscopy in the investigation of a woman with infertility. While it is uncommon to detect significant uterine anomalies, the procedure is simple and safe. The hysteroscopy can be performed while carbon dioxide is being instilled into the peritoneal cavity for the laparoscopy and need not lengthen the procedure if two gynecologists are available. While carbon dioxide can be used to distend the uterine cavity, we prefer to use saline. It is important to visualize both tubal ostia, make note of any intrauterine adhesions, which can usually be divided quite easily, and remove polyps (although we accept that the effect of endometrial polyps on fertility is uncertain). Congenital anomalies of uterine development occur in about 4% of women; although rarely affecting fertility they may sometimes predispose to an increased risk of second trimester miscarriage. It is not our routine practice to perform an endometrial biopsy unless the endometrium appears abnormal, as endometrial dating is of little diagnostic value.

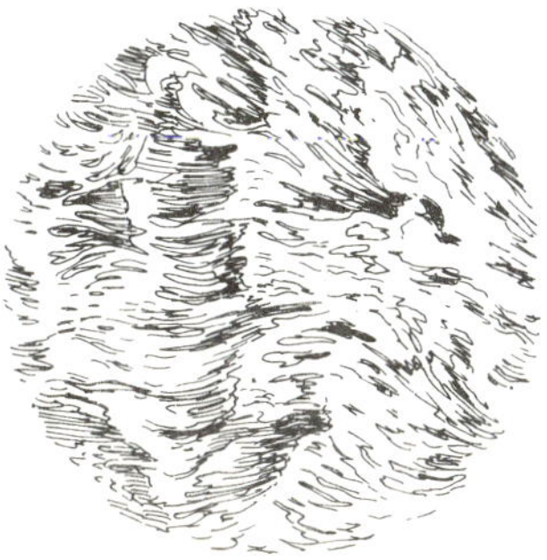

Figure 4.35 Schematic diagram of normal ciliated mucosa of the Fallopian tube.

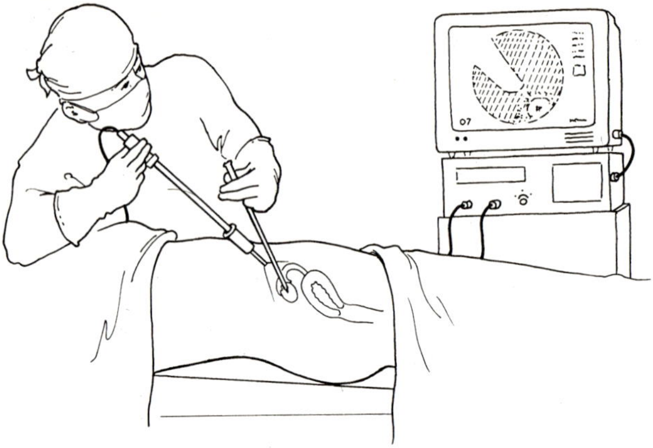

Figure 4.36 Diagnostic videolaparoscopy.

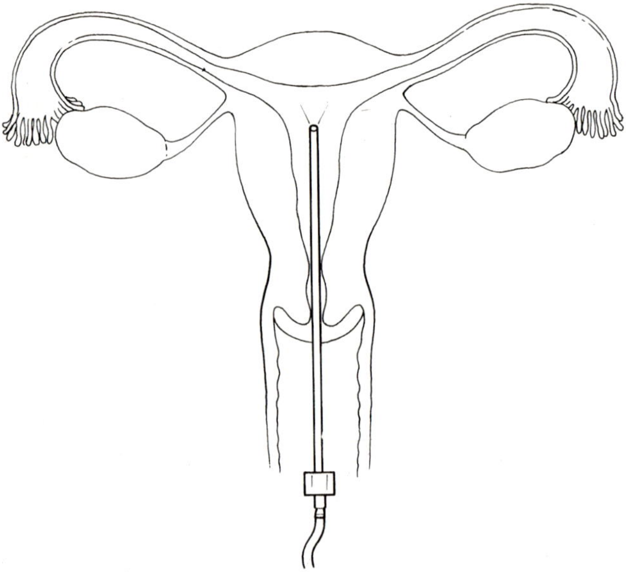

Figure 4.37 Hysteroscopy can be performed with rigid or flexible instruments and is often possible as an outpatient procedure with minimal analgesia.

Just as with HSG assessment of tubal patency, it is important to ensure that there is no risk of the patient being pregnant before undertaking the procedure. Laparoscopic assessment of the pelvis should include careful inspection of the peritoneal surface of the uterus, bladder and bowel. The area around the appendix should be visualized to check for occult inflammation and the subdiaphragmatic

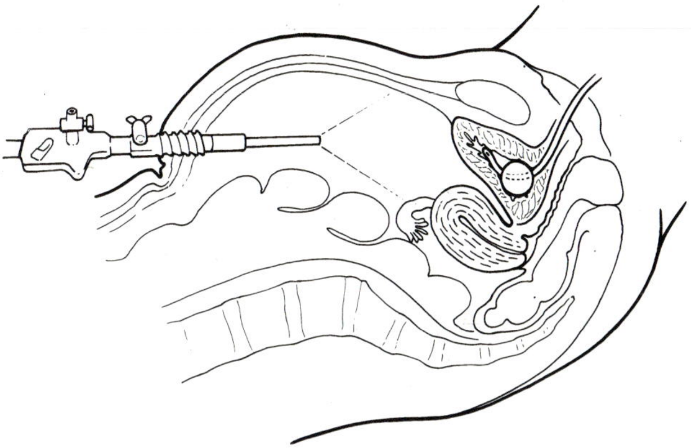

Figure 4.38 Laparoscopic view of pelvis.

surface of the liver inspected for adhesions, which might indicate chlamydial or gonococcal pelvic inflammatory disease in the past (the Fitz-Hugh Curtis syndrome) (Fig. 4.39).

The ovaries should be inspected for signs of follicular activity and ovulation, abnormal morphology, and endometriosis, which often occurs on the undersurface of the ovary or in the ovarian fossa. Endometriosis elsewhere in the pelvis should be noted carefully. Endometriosis can take on a number of appearances (see Ch. 9) and the pelvis should be inspected in a careful and systematic way (Fig. 4.38). There is evidence that even mild endometriosis may adversely affect fertility and so ablation, with diathermy or laser, can be performed during the initial diagnostic procedure. Thus it is our practice to obtain consent for treatment of mild endometriosis or adhesiolysis from all patients undergoing diagnostic laparoscopy; this should not prolong the procedure by more than 15–20 minutes.

It helps to make drawings of the laparoscopic findings and also to take still photographs which can be placed in the patient's notes. Video recordings of endoscopic procedures require careful cataloging and it is our experience that they are rarely viewed and so are of less practical value than still photographs – unless being used for demonstrations and teaching purposes. None the less, we do keep a record of operative procedures on cd both as a personal record and for medico-legal purposes.

Methylthioninium chloride (methylene blue) dye is injected transcervically and the fimbrial ends of the Fallopian tubes observed for spill (Fig. 4.40). If there is unilateral spill the isthmic part of the patent tube can be compressed gently in order to encourage the flow of dye through the contralateral tube. Fine periovarian and peritubal adhesions can often be broken down at the time of the initial laparoscopy.

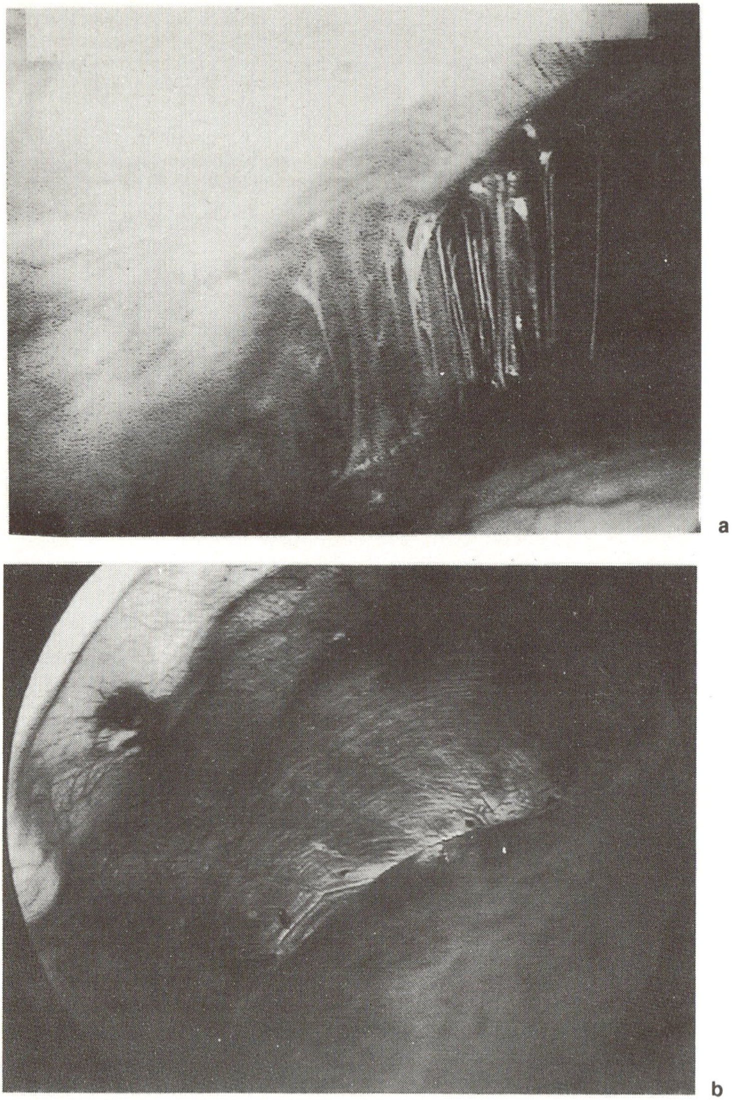

Figure 4.39a&b The laparoscopic views of the liver and undersurface of the diaphragm to illustrate the importance of assessing this area. (a) Fitz-Hugh Curtis syndrome, (b) endometriosis (please refer to plate section for color figures).

If, however, a more complicated adhesiolysis or tubal surgery is required it is our practice to inform the patient and plan an elective procedure, unless there is a high index of suspicion because of a past history of pelvic inflammatory disease, for example, in which case we would schedule a longer time for the diagnostic procedure.

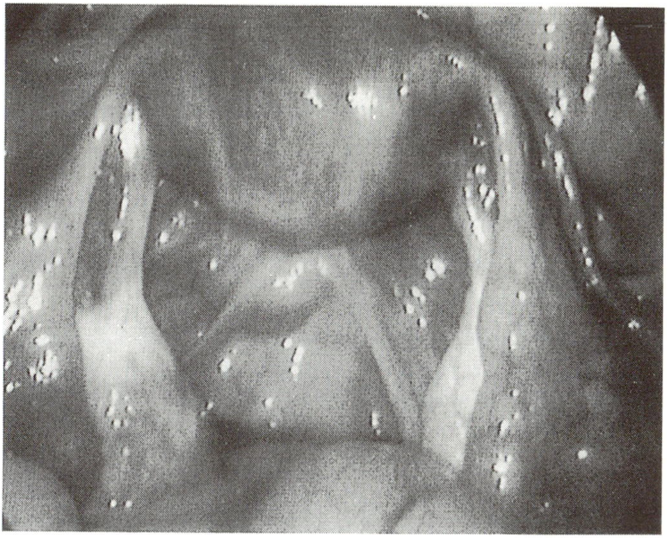

Figure 4.40 Laparoscopy with intubation of methylene blue dye. There is bilateral cornual obstruction to flow and on the right the dye can be seen suffusing the myometrium and vessels of the broad ligament. Externally the pelvic structures appear normal (please refer to plate section for color figure).

Ovarian cysts should have been detected by preoperative ultrasonography. Simple cysts can be aspirated while endometriotic or complicated cysts should be removed carefully. If there is doubt about the diagnosis a laparotomy should be performed together with either a careful cystectomy or even an oophorectomy if there is a strong suspicion of malignancy (usually after a positive biopsy). These possibilities must be discussed in detail with the patient prior to surgery and appropriate consent obtained.

Every patient should be warned that there is a possibility of a laparotomy because of the risks of perforation of viscera or accidental intraperitoneal hemorrhage. It should be remembered that diagnostic laparoscopy carries a mortality of 1:12 000 and so the less invasive diagnostic methods (see above) should be considered first.

Transvaginal Hydroculdoscopy/Hydrolaparoscopy/ Salpingoscopy

Transvaginal salpingoscopy is a technique that has been recently developed to visualize pelvic anatomy and tubal architecture.[55] The procedure can be performed with the patient awake. A small incision is made high in the vagina in the posterior cul de sac and the pouch of Douglas filled with warm Hartmann's solution. A fine 4 mm scope may then be inserted to inspect the underside of the ovaries and the fimbrial ends of the Fallopian tubes, which are beautifully demonstrated by hydroflotation. Tubal patency is assessed, salpingoscopy can be undertaken, and minor operative procedures also performed (e.g., adhesiolysis and ovarian diathermy for PCOS). Transvaginal salpingoscopy is not commonly performed in the UK.

MRI/CT Scans

MRI of the pituitary fossa is indicated in cases of persistent hyperprolactinemia, in patients with hypogonadotropic hypogonadism and Cushing's disease (see Ch. 6). Imaging of the adrenal glands might additionally be required if Cushing's syndrome or androgen-secreting tumors are suspected. MRI or CT of the pelvis is useful when there is doubt about the development of the internal genitalia and ultrasonography has been uninformative (for example when there are complex uterine anomalies or to look for testes in women with androgen insensitivity syndromes). MRI will provide beautiful images of the ovaries although it is rarely required for routine practice (see Fig. 4.13).

Investigating the Male Partner

Examination (Figs 4.41 and 4.42)

The general examination should include an assessment of body mass index (see p. 28) blood pressure, secondary sexual characteristics, the abdomen, and genitalia (Table 4.6). Some chest diseases are associated with infertility (congenital absence of the vas, spermatic duct obstruction – see Ch. 11 – and Kartagener's syndrome with dextrocardia) and might be elicited at the time of the examination. An absent or deficient sense of smell in patients with hypogonadotropic hypogonadism gives the diagnosis of Kallman's syndrome – and saves lots of further tests.

Men with androgen deficiency of prepubertal origin will have a high pitched voice, small soft testes and a small penis, lack of adult hair, and decreased muscle mass. They are often tall with a large arm span that exceeds their height. If hypogonadism develops after puberty the skin becomes fine and body hair and beard growth diminish. There may be gynecomastia, as in Klinefelter's syndrome. Gynecomastia may also occur with hyperthyroidism, liver disease, estrogen or hCG-producing tumors or with some drugs (most notably antiandrogens such as cimetidine, spironolactone, digitalis). Transient gynecomastia is normal during puberty. Other signs of endocrine disease (Cushing's syndrome, thyroid disease, pituitary tumor) should also become evident on the general examination. A full neurological examination is required when there are problems with sexual function.

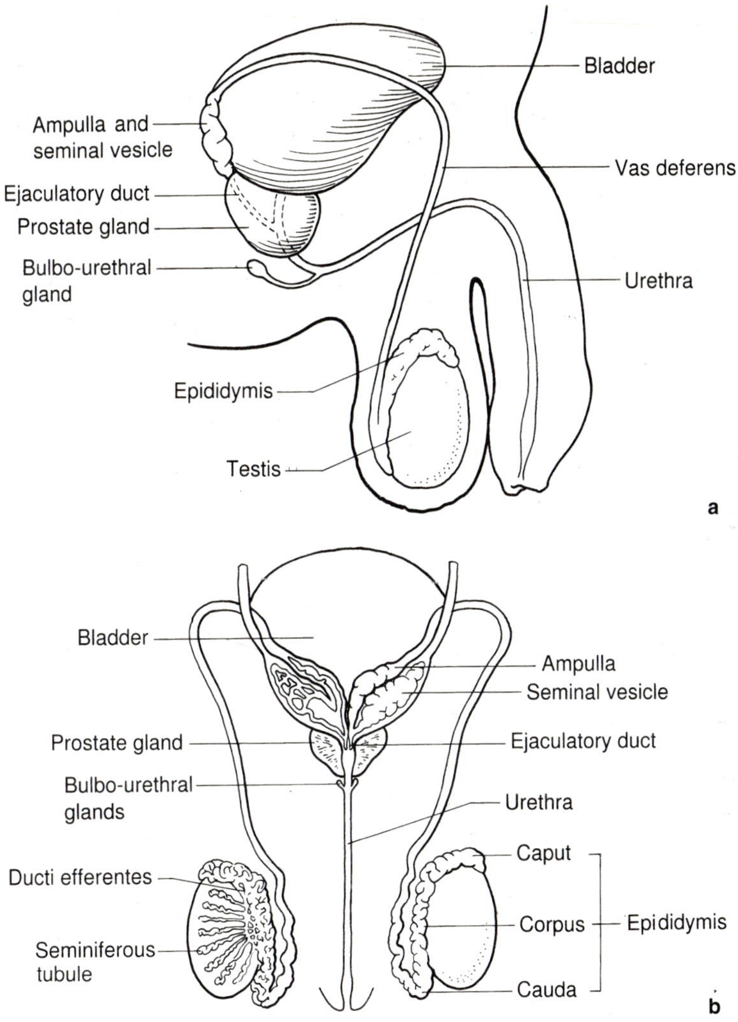

Figure 4.41a&b Male reproductive tract.

Abdominal examination

Abdominal examination should reveal the presence of abnormal masses and herniae. Scars from herniorrhaphy in childhood should be sought as often the history is either forgotten or unknown and damage to the vas deferens or testicular blood supply may follow surgery. Similarly a history of orchidopexy in childhood may not be revealed and has important implications for future fertility.

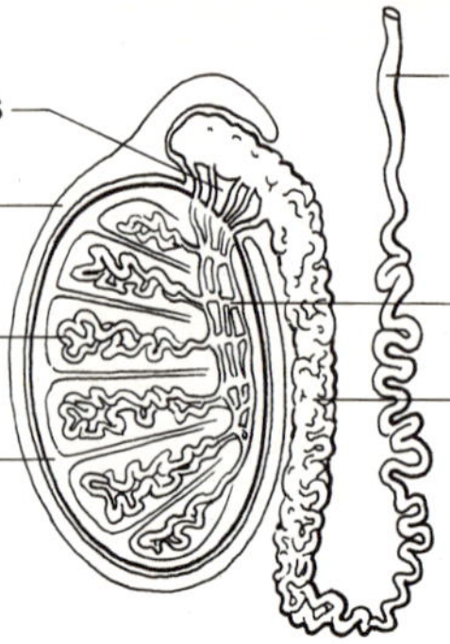

Figure 4.42 The testis and vas deferens.

Table 4.6 Examination of the male

General: weight, BP, urinalysis	
Secondary sexual characteristics	
Muscle bulk	
Signs of endocrine disease (see text)	
Gynecomastia	
Abdominal examination: masses, liver, scars, herniae	
Genital examination:	urethral meatus
	testicular volume, masses
	epididymis
	varicocele
Rectal examination of prostate	

Genital examination

The penis should be inspected for the location of the urethral opening and the foreskin retracted if possible. Congenital deformities of the penis or hypo-/epispadias may cause problems with semen deposition. Testicular size should be assessed using an orchidometer and is normal if over 15 ml. Small testes that are soft are usually associated with gonadotropin deficiency, as in hypopituitarism or Kallman's syndrome. Small testes that are firm (implying fibrosis) are usually associated with severe and permanent destruction of germinal epithelium (as in Klinefelter's syndrome) and androgenization may be normal. The plane of the testis has no bearing on fertility, but testes that lie in a horizontal plane are more likely to tort than those that lie more vertically. Testicular masses or asymmetry warrant further investigation by ultrasound in the first instance. Scrotal swellings are best palpated with the patient standing. It is then easier to palpate the epididymis and vas deferens and ascertain the presence of cysts, thickening, and tenderness, which are all associated with infection.

A varicocele may be palpated with the patient standing in the upright position because the valves are incompetent and the varicocele fills with venous blood due to increased intra-abdominal pressure. Varicoceles are more common on the left, because of the differential venous drainage between left and right, and can be graded depending whether they (1) fill only during a Valsalva maneuver, (2) are detectable by palpation, or (3) are clearly visible.[56]

Rectal examination of prostate

The prostate should be palpated by rectal examination. Undue tenderness indicates infection. Prostatic massage may produce a urethral secretion that should be sent for microscopy and culture; a urine specimen should also be sent after prostatic massage. Some men are aware of changes of seminal color or smell in association with infection of the epididymis, prostate, or seminal vesicles and the semen should be sent for microscopy and culture.

The Semen Analysis

The specimen of semen should be produced by masturbation into a clean, dry container and delivered to the laboratory within 30 minutes of its production. There should have been a period of abstinence of 3 days. A fixed period of abstinence not only improves the standardization of the test but more than 5 days' abstinence is associated with a decrease in motility despite an increase in sperm number. There are large swings in semen parameters in healthy, fertile sperm donors and so the results of a single semen analysis should be viewed with caution and repeated on two or more occasions, 3 months apart.[57] The results of four samples should provide average values that are within one standard deviation of the mean, although in most cases two semen analyses will suffice. There may be regional differences in semen quality dependent both on ambient temperature (with counts being higher in winter months) and environmental exposures or lifestyle differences.[58] Sperm production by the testis takes 10–12 weeks (Figs 4.43 and 4.44) and so an abnormal semen specimen is a reflection of testicular function 3 months previously. Thus, when assessing the effects of therapy, it is necessary not to be too hasty before repeating the analysis.

The conventional semen analysis provides poor prognostic information about male fertility and the criteria defined by the World Health Organization[59] have been dismissed by some authorities as providing minimal values that are well into the fertile range[60] (Table 4.7). There is also considerable intra- and interobserver variation of semen assessment, both within and between laboratories.

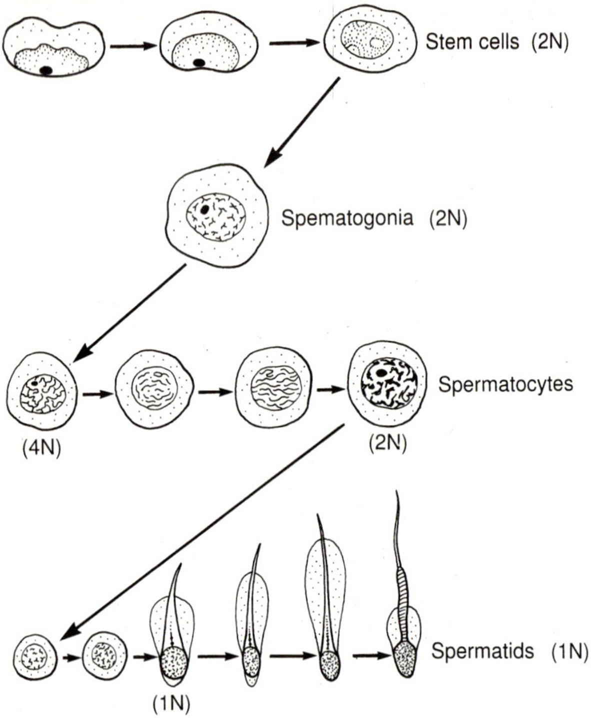

Figure 4.43 Spermatogenesis. The stem cells proliferate to become spermatogonia. The DNA is then replicated to produce the first spermatocytes, after which two meiotic reduction divisions produce the spermatids. These undergo spermiogenesis to produce mature spermatozoa.

Reduced sperm concentration (oligozoospermia)

The chance of natural conception falls significantly when the sperm concentration is less than 5×10^6/ml. When the total count is low there is often a corresponding reduction in motility.[61]

Impaired sperm morphology (teratozoospermia)

It has been suggested that sperm morphology is one of the better prognosticators for fertility and that the percentage of normal forms should be adjusted downwards to 14% when the "strict" criteria, developed by Kruger, are employed.[62,63] By this definition a normal spermatozoon is oval, with a smooth contour, an acrosome comprising 40–70% of the distal part of the head, a normal neck, mid-piece, and tail and no large cytoplasmic droplets (Fig. 4.45). The normal size of the sperm head is 5–6 µm × 2.5–3.5 µm. Using strict criteria for morphology, fertilization rates during IVF are in the region of 37–47%

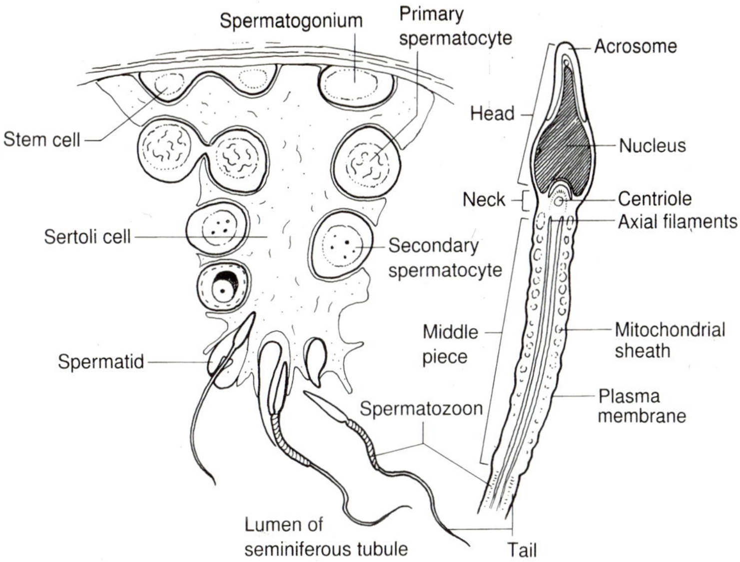

Figure 4.44 Spermatogenesis within the seminiferous tubule.

Table 4.7 Normal semen parameters (WHO 1999)[59]

Standard tests	
Volume	= 2.0 ml
pH	= 7.2–8.0
Sperm concentration	= 20 × 10^6/ml
Total sperm count	= 40 × 10^6/ejaculate
Motility (within 60 min of ejaculation)	= 25% with rapid progression (category 'a') = 50% with forward progression (categories 'a' and 'b')
Vitality	= 75% live (categories 'a', 'b,' and 'c') = 25% dead (category 'd')
Morphology	= 30% normal forms (morphology is still being defined in ongoing studies)
White blood cells	< 1 × 10^6/ml
Immunobead test	< 50%
Mixed antiglobulin reaction	< 50%
Additional tests	
Fructose	= 13 μmol/ejaculate
Acid phosphatase	= 200 U/ejaculate
α-Glucosidase	= 20 mU/ejaculate
Zinc	= 2.4 μmol/ejaculate
Citric acid	= 52 μmol/ejaculate

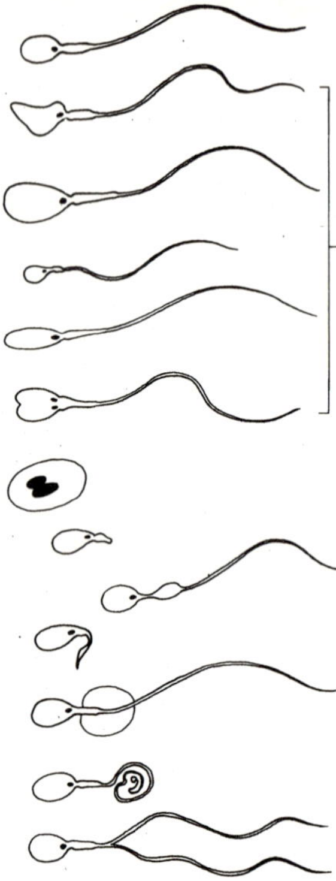

Figure 4.45 Sperm morphology.

when the percentage of normal sperm is < 14% and 85–88% when the percentage is greater; a percentage of less than 4% indicates a poor chance of fertilization.[64,65] Thus assessment of sperm morphology, while not strictly a "sperm function test," provides a good reflection of sperm function.[63] The lack of objectivity in the morphological assessment of sperm has led to the development of automated computer morphology analyzers, which are still in their infancy.[63]

Globozoospermia ("roundheaded" spermatozoa) is often missed and requires a skilled andrology technician to make the diagnosis. There is no acrosome on these spermatozoa and so fertilization cannot occur. IVF intracytoplasmic sperm injection (ICSI) might be a possibility for these patients although very few cases have been successful.

Reduced sperm motility (asthenozoospermia)

If most of the sperm are immotile the method of collection should be scrutinized and the sample should be repeated ensuring that there is no delay between production and arrival at the laboratory and that sperm have been delivered directly into a pot and not into a condom, which might contain lubricating or spermicidal agents. It is important that the man does not use lubricating jelly, soap, or water, all of which can cause sperm death. Good hygiene when producing the specimen also prevents contamination and so the patient should be advised to wash his hands and penis first. If the man has difficulties producing a specimen, there are inert silicon condoms that can be used to collect sperm during vaginal intercourse – in these situations it is sensible to consider cryopreservation of sperm as a back-up for use in future assisted conception cycles in case there is a complete inability to produce a sample on the day that it is required for treatment.

True immotility can be caused by infection, superoxide production by leukocytes, antisperm antibodies or defects in the microtubules and dynein arms of the sperm tail.[66] Sperm agglutination is often due to infection rather than antisperm antibodies and the appropriate tests should be performed (see below).

A precise analysis of sperm motility can be obtained using a computerized image analysis system which tracks motile sperm and provides data on several parameters, including forward velocity, curvilinear velocity, and amplitude of lateral head displacement. Not only is forward movement required for sperm to reach their target, but there must also be adequate lateral head displacement for penetration of the cervical mucus. Hyperactivation can also be observed. This is the process of increasing beat amplitude that occurs with capacitation of the sperm in the female reproductive tract as the sperm prepares to penetrate the zona pellucida. Computerized assessment of sperm motility and action correlate well with its IVF ability and these techniques are now used by most large centers that can afford the equipment.

Cause of sperm dysfunction

Sperm function can be impaired by lipid peroxidation in the sperm plasma membrane. Oxidative stress correlates with reduced motility and a decreased capacity for oocyte fusion. Reactive oxygen species (ROS) initiate lipid peroxidation and are produced either within the dysfunctional spermatozoa or by leukocytes. An end-product of lipid peroxidation is malondialdehyde, which can be measured to give an index of oxidative stress. Luminometry employs expensive equipment to measure ROS and differentiates between those released from sperm and leukocytes. Hydrogen peroxide appears to be the most important cytotoxic oxygen metabolite. Seminal plasma contains a rich concentration of antioxidants and removal of sperm from seminal plasma during preparative procedures for assisted conception can expose the sperm to damaging ROS. Current research is aimed at the study of antioxidants in IVF culture media.

A matter of some concern is the notion that ROS are well-known mutagens and sperm-derived genetic damage to embryos might occur through chromosomal breakage (while oocyte-derived damage occurs through chromosomal rearrangement).[67] It has been suggested that spermatozoa that have been exposed to ROS are at increased risk of carrying chromosomal breakages; at present this is speculative but clearly has to be investigated further.

Sperm activation and the acrosome reaction are dependent upon the influx of calcium before the sperm fuses with the oocyte. Progesterone appears to play a role in this process, although progesterone receptors have been found on only 10% of spermatozoa. The significance of this is unknown. It is difficult to assess the acrosome reaction *in vitro* as it cannot be visualized by light microscopy and so the acrosome has to be labeled with fluorescent monoclonal antibodies or lectins which attach to the acrosome membrane. The acrosome reaction occurs spontaneously in only about 5–10% of sperm *in vitro* and so the normal range is very low. All sperm that have bound to the zona are acrosome reacted. The acrosome reaction has been stimulated artificially using the calcium ionophore A23187 as a bioassay for sperm responsiveness. The so-called "acrosome reaction ionophore challenge" (ARIC) test has not lived up to its initial promise so the search is continuing for new tests of sperm functional capacity.

Leukospermia

It is difficult to distinguish leukocytes from immature germ cells by microscopy and semen culture rarely yields a positive result even in the presence of a significant concentration of leukocytes.[68] Sometimes bacteria are visualized by direct microscopy or grown in culture. Bacteria are most often thought to arise from contamination at the time of sperm production as repeat analysis usually fails to reveal an underlying infection.[69] If a lower genital tract infection is suspected a Stamey–Meares test should be performed. This involves collecting three small samples of urine in succession. The first indicates urethral infection, the second (a mid-stream specimen) urinary infection and the third, collected after prostatic massage, prostatic infection. The samples are then sent out for microscopy and culture.

More Detailed Tests of Sperm Function

The following two tests are included for completeness but we do not as a rule either use them or recommend their routine use.

Zona-free hamster egg sperm penetration assay (SPA)

This is a bioassay of the ability of human spermatozoa to penetrate hamster eggs that have been stripped of their zona pellucida. The semen sample must be suitably prepared (by incubation in TEST-yolk buffer, follicular fluid, or with the calcium ionophore A23187) to enable the sperm to undergo capacitation and the acrosome reaction prior to incubation with the hamster ova. The SPA is not used widely because of the high incidence of false-negative results, although this might be a reflection of too short an incubation time.[70] Many authors feel that the SPA might be a good test of sperm function providing standardization is improved.

The hemizona assay (HZA)

In contrast to the SPA, the HZA tests the ability of human sperm to bind to the human zona pellucida, where sperm activation occurs prior to the acrosome reaction. Dead human oocytes can be used for this assay, as the integrity of the ZP3 protein component of the zona pellucida survives indefinitely and this is the binding site for the spermatozoon. The oocyte is first divided microscopically, with one half being incubated with fertile donor sperm and the other half with the patient's sperm. The test requires a considerable degree of technical expertise and the use of human eggs but does appear to correlate well with subsequent IVF.[71,72]

Cervical Mucus Penetration and the Postcoital Test

The parameters of sperm movement correlate well with its ability to penetrate cervical mucus. The postcoital test (PCT) has been traditionally employed to assess sperm survival in cervical mucus. A PCT should be performed mid-cycle, when the estrogenized cervical mucus is most receptive to sperm. The couple should be asked to have intercourse the night before the test and the woman should refrain from washing inside the vagina afterwards. A sample of cervical mucus is aspirated from the cervical os and placed on a microscope slide for examination under high power. The characteristics of the cervical mucus should be recorded, including its: cellularity, viscosity, Spinnbarkeit, and ferning pattern when allowed to dry on the slide (Fig. 4.46). A cervical score can be obtained by quantifying each of these characteristics from 0 to 3, a score of less than 5 indicating cervical hostility, greater than 10 being satisfactory, and 15 maximal. A score of 3 is obtained if the volume is at least 0.3 ml, there is no cellularity (i.e., no white cells), normal viscosity, Spinnbarkeit of at least 9 cm and a ferning pattern with tertiary and quaternary stems (Table 4.8).

The methodology of performing the PCT varies enormously between centers. Indeed, a recent European survey indicated that while over 92% of 200 centers used the PCT there were wide variations in the timing of the test in relation to intercourse,[73] the magnification used, and the cut-off level for normality in terms of motile sperms per high power field (which ranged from 1 to 50). It has been suggested that

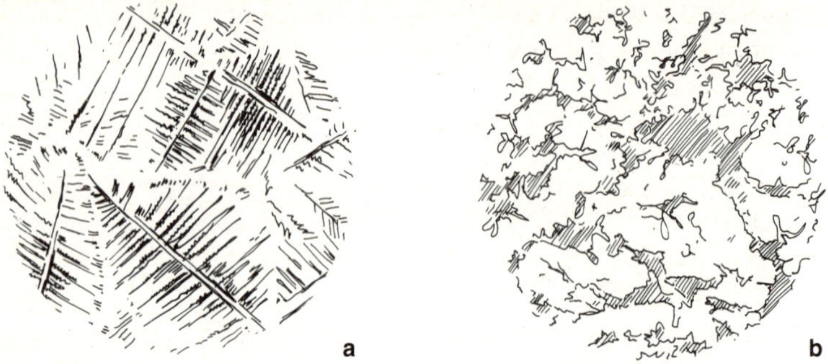

Figure 4.46 Ferning pattern of (**a**) ovulatory (estrogenized) cervical mucus which has dried on a microscope slide, contrasted with (**b**) non-ovulatory mucus.

Table 4.8 Cervical score

	0	1	2	3
Quantity (ml)	0	0.1	0.2	= 0.3
Viscocity	Thick	Intermediate	Mildly viscous	Normal
Cellularity	= 11 cells/HPF	6–10 cells/HPF	1–5 cells/HPF	0 cells/HPF
Ferning	No crystallization	Atypical pattern	1° and 2° stems	3° and 4° stems
Spinnbarkeit	< 1 cm	1–4 cm	5–8 cm	= 9 cm

HPF = high power field

the only useful parameter is the presence of a single sperm, as any number above this does not correlate better with fertility. The World Health Organization has recommended that the optimal time interval is 9–24 hours after intercourse and that at a magnification of 400× there should be more than 20 motile sperm per high power field.

The PCT can help to identify the presence of antisperm IgA antibodies which, if present on the sperm surface, bind to mucin chains in the mucus and cause the sperm to display a characteristic shaking movement.

Couples often find the PCT very stressful and precise timing at midcycle is often difficult to achieve. It is seen to be an invasion of their privacy by focusing on the most intimate part of their relationship, which is under close enough scrutiny in any case when attending the fertility clinic. Additionally, it is necessary to have the facility to perform the test on every weekday. And while the finding of motile sperm is reassuring, their absence does not necessarily indicate a problem providing intercourse has taken place. There is also little consensus among clinicians and scientists on the interpretation of test results. It is not our current practice to perform a PCT as part of a couple's investigation.

Advocates of the PCT have suggested that, in the absence of a clear explanation for a couple's infertility, the PCT is an effective predictor of conception if there is less than 3 years' infertility, with 68% of couples conceiving within 2 years after a positive test compared with 17% when the test is negative.[74] With more than 3 years' infertility, the corresponding rates are similar at 14% and 11%. The PCT may also be helpful in selected cases, for example in the work-up for intrauterine insemination (IUI). A crossed hostility test, using the couple's sperm and mucus with donor sperm and donated or artificial mucus, will indicate whether the problem lies with the sperm or the mucus. If the latter, then IUI might be beneficial, while if the problem is with the sperm, IVF ± ICSI is appropriate (see also p. 314).

An alternative to the PCT is the observation of the distance traveled by sperm over a period of time through hyaluronic acid polymers, which serve as an artificial substitute for cervical mucus. The results correlate very well with those observed in aspirated cervical mucus but can be better controlled and quantified. Furthermore, the test is not dependent on the stage of the woman's cycle. It has been suggested that this assay, combined with a measurement of antisperm antibodies, should replace the PCT. We concur with this opinion.

Antisperm Antibodies

IgG antisperm antibodies (ASABs) are found in the serum while those in the cervical mucus are IgA, and both classes of antibody are found in the seminal fluid. There are a number of different assays for the measurement of ASABs and the cut-off levels for a significant concentration of antibody vary depending on the assay and the laboratory's normal range.[56,57,60,75] We recently performed a survey in the UK and found that there is still tremendous variation, and confusion, about appropriate tests for ASABs and their interpretation.[76]

- *Sperm agglutination tests* (tray agglutination test): sperm agglutinate if bound to bivalent antibodies; agglutination can occur due to non-immune causes; based on serum antibodies; quantitative; poor specificity and poor correlation with fertility.
- *Mixed agglutination reaction* (MAR test): sperm agglutinates with sensitized rhesus-positive red cells in the presence of anti-IgG antiserum; detects antibodies bound to sperm in semen; measures IgG and IgA only; good specificity, non-quantitative.
- *Sperm immobilization test*: antibody binding activates complement to immobilize sperm; good specificity for complement fixing antibodies, poor sensitivity.
- *ELISA*: enzyme linked antibody reacts with ASAB; quantitative; requires fixation or homogenization and exposes internal antigens

so irrelevant antigens might be detected; good specificity, poor sensitivity.
- *Indirect immunofluorescence*: fluorescent labeled antibody reacts with antisperm antibody; both IgA and IgG detected; high false-positives, good sensitivity.
- *Radiolabeled antiglobulin assay*: radiolabeled antibody reacts with ASAB; both IgA and IgG detected; quantitative; good specificity and sensitivity.
- *Immunobead binding test (IBT)*: polyacrylamide beads with bound antibody react with ASAB; both IgA and IgG detected; good specificity and sensitivity.

The IBT appears to be the best test as it also detects the binding loci (i.e., head, mid-piece, or tail) on living sperm, which can be viewed by light microsocopy. This is important as head-bound ASABs have the most serious impact on fertility. The levels of ASABs are considered to be significant when more than 50–80% of the motile sperm are affected (depending on the assay).

Serum Endocrinology in the Male

An endocrine profile should be performed in men with oligospermia (counts less than 10×10^6/ml) or if there are signs or symptoms suggestive of either androgen deficiency or endocrine disease.

Testosterone

Serum testosterone levels undergo diurnal variation, with the highest levels in the morning. The time of the test – and its comparison with measurements performed on other days – may be important if the result is borderline. The normal range is 10–35 nmol/L.

FSH and LH

Normal serum concentrations of both gonadotropins are less than 10 i.u./L (although it is important to know the normal range for the individual laboratory).

The combination of azoospermia with normal sized testes and normal levels of testosterone, FSH, and LH indicates a mechanical obstruction to the passage of sperm. An elevated serum concentration of FSH indicates germinal cell insufficiency or primary testicular failure if combined with an elevated serum LH concentration; and the serum testosterone level will be low. The combination of azoospermia and an elevated serum FSH concentration has, until recently, been taken as an indication of no spermatogenesis. However, cases have been reported of a few spermatozoa being found during testicular aspiration/biopsy which have then been used to perform IVF/ICSI. Thus, unless the testes are absolutely tiny (e.g., less than 2 ml), some andrologists now suggest that all men with an elevated serum FSH concentration should be offered a testicular biopsy – with an option for cryopreservation of any retrieved spermatozoa at the same time.

Low serum concentrations of all three hormones indicate hypothalamic or pituitary insufficiency, which may be amenable to hormonal therapy.

Inhibin

Serum inhibin concentrations have not shown any correlation with spermatogenic activity and have no role in the current investigation of the infertile male.

Prolactin and thyroid function

These hormones should be measured to provide a complete endocrine profile when serum testosterone levels are low or when there is gynecomastia or thyroid disease.

Pituitary imaging and further investigation by an endocrinologist may be required if there are abnormalities of the hypothalamic–pituitary–gonadal axis.

Chromosomal analysis

Both men and women with primary gonadal failure should undergo karyotyping to aid diagnosis and enable the provision of appropriate genetic counseling in cases when gonadal failure is not absolute since there might be the possibility of extracting a few spermatozoa for IVF/ICSI. A karyotype is indicated in azoospermia and for men with severely impaired semen parameters, because of an increased risk of structural chromosomal anomalies and sex chromosomal anomalies (e.g., Klinefelter's syndrome, 47XXY). Furthermore, microdeletions on the long arm of the Y chromosome have been causally linked to anomalies in spermatogenesis and may be passed on to the male offspring of men who undergo IVF/ICSI. These microdeletions are often at the azoospermia factor (AZF) locus at q11.23 of the Y chromosome and may be found in 7% of infertile men and 2% of normal men[77] (see Chs 11, 13, and 16). Congenital bilateral absence of the vas deferens (CBAVD) is associated with mutations in the cystic fibrosis gene and so when CBAVD is detected both partners should be screened.

Imaging in Male Infertility

Varicoceles can be investigated by a combination of ultrasonography (± Doppler flow studies), nuclear scintigraphy, thermography, or venography.[78–80] The patient can be asked to perform a Valsalva maneuver to accentuate the varicocele. As the diagnostic significance of a varicocele is debatable its classification by these methods is imprecise, particularly as the size of varicocele does not correlate with the degree of impairment of spermatogenesis (see Fig. 11.1).

A vasogram can be performed if an obstruction is suspected. Sometimes this is done in the operating theater at the time of testicular exploration (see Fig. 11.2).

Testicular Exploration and Biopsy

Testicular exploration is indicated if the sperm densitiy is less than 5×10^6/ml and the serum FSH concentration is normal. If an obstruction is found it may be bypassed during the same procedure (see Ch. 11). Facilities should be available for sperm cryopreservation whenever surgery is performed on the testis and collecting system and sperm stored in case the procedure is unsuccessful (see Ch. 11).

A testicular biopsy will aid in the diagnosis of severe oligospermia or azoospermia. If there is obstructive azoospermia spermatogenesis is normal but there may be sloughing of the superficial layers of the seminiferous epithelium. Absent spermatogenesis suggests the diagnosis of the Sertoli-cell-only (Del Castillo) syndrome while after orchitis there might be hyalinization and tubular atrophy.

The degree of spermatogenesis can be scored using the mean Johnsen score (Table 4.9), which is obtained after the examination of a number of tubules. A score of 8–10 is normal, a score of 2 indicates the Sertoli-cell-only syndrome, and intermediate scores suggest varying degrees of disordered spermatogenic or maturation arrest. When cells of increasing maturity are seen all of the preceding stages will also be seen in the biopsy.

Table 4.10 summarizes the tables for the investigation and treatment of infertility, with suggestions for tests that can be initiated by the GP.

Table 4.9. The Johnsen score

1	No cells in the tubule
2	Sertoli cells only
3	Spermatogonia only
4	Few spermatocytes
5	Only spermatocytes
6	Few spermatids
7	Only spermatids
8	Few spermatozoa
9	Many spermatozoa, central sloughing, no lumen
10	Many spermatozoa with central lumen

Table 4.10 Summary tables for the investigation and treatment of infertility

Scheme for the investigation of infertility	
GP:	Semen analysis – twice if first abnormal
	Rubella status
	Baseline endocrine profile (FSH, LH, TSH, ± prolactin, testosterone)
	Luteal phase progesterone
	Hysterosalpingogram
Infertility clinic:	Baseline pelvic ultrasound scan
	Laparoscopy and dye/hysteroscopy
	More detailed endocrinology if indicated
	Further investigation of endocrine disorders
	More detailed sperm function tests
	Postcoital test?
Scheme for the treatment of infertility	
GP:	General health and sexual advice
	Folic acid
	Cervical smear
	Rubella immunization
	Referral for preconceptional counseling if other health concerns, drug therapy, older age group, family history of genetic disease
Infertility clinic:	All ovulation-inducing agents (including clomiphene citrate) with appropriate monitoring
	Laparoscopic surgery
	Assisted conception
	Male treatments
	Collaborative clinics with endocrinologist, urologist, pyschosexual counselor
	General counseling

References

1. ESHRE Capri Workshop Group (2000) Optimal use of infertility diagnostic tests and treatments. *Hum Reprod* **15**: 723–732.
2. Templeton A (ed) (1996) Recommendations arising from the 31st RCOG Study Group. The prevention of pelvic infection. In: *The prevention of pelvic infection.* RCOG Press, London.
3. Wilcox AJ, Dunson D & Baird DD (2000) The timing of the "fertile window" in the menstrual cycle: day specific estimates from a prospective study. *BMJ* **321**: 1259–1262.
4. Wilcox AJ, Weinberg CR & Baird DD (1995) Timing of sexual intercourse in relation to ovulation. *N Engl J Med* **333**: 1517–1521.
5. Balen AH, Conway GS, Kaltsas G *et al.* (1995) Polycystic ovary syndrome: the spectrum of the disorder in 1741 patients. *Hum Reprod* **10**: 2107–2111.
6. RCOG (1998) *Evidence-based clinical guidelines. The initial investigation and management of the infertile couple.* RCOG Press, London.
7. Stratford GA, Barth JH, Rutherford AJ & Balen AH (2000) The value of thyroid function tests in women in the routine investigation of uncomplicated infertility. *Hum Fertil* **3**: 203–206.

8. Gonzalez CJ, Curson R & Parsons J (1988) Transabdominal versus transvaginal ultrasound screening of ovarian follicles: are they comparable? *Fertil Steril* **50**: 657.
9. Lass A, Skull J, McVeigh E *et al.* (1997) Measurement of ovarian volume by transvaginal sonography before human menopausal gonadotropin superovulation for *in vitro* fertilization can predict poor response. *Hum Reprod* **12**: 294–297.
10. Bancsi LFJMM, Broekmans FJM, Eijkemans MJC, de Jong FH, Habbema JDF & te Velde ER (2002) Predictors of poor ovarian response in *in vitro* fertilization: a prospective study comparing basal markers of ovarian reserve. *Fertil Steril* **77**: 328–336.
11. Adams J, Polson DW, Abdulwahid N *et al* (1985) Multifollicular ovaries: clinical and endocrine features and response to pulsatile gonadotropin releasing hormone. *Lancet* **ii**: 1375–1378.
12. Adams J, Polson DW & Franks S (1986) Prevalence of polycystic ovaries in women with anovulation and idiopathic hirsutism. *Br Med J* **293**: 355–358.
13. Stein IF, Leventhal ML (1935) Amenorrhea associated with bilateral polycystic ovaries. *Am J Obstet Gynecol* **29**: 181–191.
14. Shoham Z, Conway GS, Patel A & Jacobs HS (1992) Polycystic ovaries in patients with hypogonadotropic hypogonadism: similarity of ovarian response to gonadotropin stimulation in patients with polycystic ovary syndrome. *Fertil Steril* **58**: 37–45.
15. Schachter M, Balen AH, Patel A & Jacobs HS (1996) Hypogonadotropic patients with ultrasonographically diagnosed polycystic ovaries have aberrant gonadotropin secretion when treated with pulsatile gonadotropin releasing hormone – a new insight into the pathophysiology of polycystic ovary syndrome. *Gynecol Endocrinol* **10**: 327–334.
16. Polson DW, Wadsworth J, Adams J & Franks S (1988) Polycystic ovaries: a common finding in normal women. *Lancet* **ii**: 870–872.
17. Michelmore KF, Balen AH, Dunger DB & Vessey MP (1999) Polycystic ovaries and associated clinical and biochemical features in young women. *Clin Endocrinol* **51**: 779–786.
18. Balen AH, Tan SL, MacDougal J & Jacobs HS (1993) Miscarriage rates following *in vitro* fertilisation are increased in women with polycystic ovaries and reduced by pituitary desensitisation with buserelin. *Hum Reprod* **8**: 959–964.
19. Hornstein MD, Barbieri RL, Ravnikar VA & McShane PM (1989) The effects of baseline ovarian cysts on the clinical response to controlled ovarian stimulation in an in-vitro fertilisation program. *Fertil Steril* **52**: 437–440.
20. Thatcher SS, Jones E & DeCherney AH (1989) Ovarian cysts decrease the success of controlled ovarian stimulation and in-vitro fertilisation. *Fertil Steril* **52**: 812–816.
21. Karande VC, Scott RT, Jones GS & Muasher SJ (1990) Non-functional ovarian cysts do not affect ipsilateral or contralateral ovarian performance during in-vitro fertilisation. *Hum Reprod* **5**: 431–433.
22. Rizk B, Tan SL, Kingsland C, Steer C, Mason BA & Campbell S (1990) Ovarian cysts aspiration and the outcome of in-vitro fertilisation. *Fertil Steril* **54**: 661–664.
23. Ayida G, Balen FG & Balen AH (1996) The usefulness of ultrasound in fertility management. *Contemp Rev Obstet Gynaecol* **8**: 32–38.
24. Yee B, Barnes RB, Vargyas JM & Marrs RP (1987) Correlation of transabdominal and transvaginal ultrasound measurements of follicle size and number with laparoscopic findings for in-vitro fertilisation. *Fertil Steril* **47**: 828–832.
25. Andreotti RF, Thompson GH, Janowitz W, Shapiro AG & Zusmer NR (1989) Endovaginal and transabdominal sonography of ovarian follicles. *J Ultrasound Med* **8**: 555–560.
26. Eissa MK, Hudson K, Docker MF, Sawers RS & Newton JR (1985) Ultrasound follicle diameter measurement: an assessment of interobserver and intraobserver variation. *Fertil Steril* **44**: 751–754.

27. Ritchie WGM (1985) Ultrasound in the evaluation of normal and induced ovulation. *Fertil Steril* **43**: 167.
28. Hackeloer BJ, Fleming R, Robinson HP, Adam AH & Coutts JRT (1979) Correlation of ultrasonic and endocrinologic assessment of human follicular development. *Am J Obstet Gynecol* **135**: 122–128.
29. Balen FG, Allen CM, Gardener JE, Siddle NC & Lees WR (1993) Three-dimensional reconstruction of ultrasound images of the uterine cavity. *Br J Radiol* **66**: 588–591.
30. Daly DC, Soto-Albors C, Walters C *et al.* (1985) Ultrasonographic assessment of luteinized unruptured follicle syndrome in unexplained infertility. *Fertil Steril* **43**: 62.
31. Marik J & Hulka J (1978) Luteinized unruptured follicle syndrome: a subtle cause of infertility. *Fertil Steril* **29**: 270.
32. Deichert U, Hackelöer BJ & Daume E (1986) The sonographic and endocrinologic evaluation of the endometrium in the luteal phase. *Hum Reprod* **1**: 219.
33. Grunfeld L, Walker B, Bergh P, Sandler B, Hofman G & Navot D (1991) High resolution endovaginal ultrasonography of the endometrium: a noninvasive test for endometrial adequacy. *Obstet Gynecol* **78**: 200–204.
34. Gonen Y, Casper RF, Jacobson W & Blankier J (1989) Endometrial thickness and growth during controlled ovarian stimualation: a possible predictor for implantation in *in vitro* fertilisation. *Fertil Steril* **52**: 446–450.
35. Ueno J, Oehninger S, Brzyski RG, Acosta AA, Philput CB & Muasher SJ (1991) Ultrasonographic appearance of the endometrium in natural and stimulated *in vitro* fertilisation cycles and its correlation with outcome. *Hum Reprod* **6**: 901–904.
36. Scholtes MCW, Wladimiroff JW, van Rijen HJM *et al.* (1989) Uterine and ovarian flow velocity waveforms in the normal menstrual cycle: a transvaginal Doppler study. *Fertil Steril* **52**: 981–985.
37. Bourne TH (1991) Transvaginal color Doppler in gynecology. *Ultrasound Obstet Gynecol* **1**: 359–373.
38. Bourne TH, Jurkovic D, Waterstone J, Campbell S & Collins WP (1991) Intrafollicular blood flow during human ovulation. *Ultrasound Obstet Gynecol* **1**: 53–59.
39. Steer C, Campbell S, Pampiglione J, Kingsland C, Mason BA & Collins W (1990) Transvaginal colour flow imaging of the uterine arteries during ovarian and menstrual cycles. *Hum Reprod* **5**: 391–395.
40. de Ziegler D, de Quay N & Fanchin R (2000) Combined Doppler and hormonal studies of uterine receptivity . In: Kupesic S, de Ziegler D (eds) *Ultrasound and infertility*. Parthenon Publishing, Carnforth, England, pp 195–204.
41. Swart P, Mol BW, van der Veen F, van Beurden M, Redekop WK & Bossut PM (1995) The accuracy of hysterosalpingography in the diagnosis of tubal pathology: a meta-analysis. *Fertil Steril* **64**: 486–491.
42. Watson A, Vanderkerckhove P, Lilford R, Vail A, Brosens I & Hughes E (1994) A meta-analysis of the therapeutic role of oil soluble contrast media at hysterosalpingography: a surpising result? *Fertil Steril* **61**: 470–477.
43. Nugent D,.Watson AJ, Killick SR, Balen AH & Rutherford AJ (2002) A randomized controlled trial of tubal flushing with lipiodol for unexplained infertility. *Fertil Steril* **77**: 173–176.
44. Schlief R & Deichert U (1991) Hysterosalpingo-contrast sonography of the uterus and Fallopian tubes: results of a clinical trial of a new contrast medium in 120 patients. *Radiology* **178**: 213–215.
45. Pellerito JS, McCarthy SM, Doyle MB, Glickman MG & de Cherney AH (1992) Diagnosis of uterine anomalies: relative accuracy of MR imaging, endovaginal sonography and hysterosalpingography. *Radiology* **183**: 795–800.
46. Eldar-Geva T, Meagher S, Healy DL, MacLachlan V, Breheny S & Wood C (1998) Effect of intramural, subserosal and submucosal uterine fibroids on the outcome of assisted reproductive technology treatment. *Fertil Steril* **70**: 687–691.

47. Hart R, Khalaf Y, Yeong C-T, Seed P, Taylor A & Braude P (2001) A prospective controlled study of the effect of intramural uterine fibroids on the outcome of assisted conception. *Hum Reprod* **16**: 2411–2417.
48. Balen FG, Allen CM, Siddle NC & Lees WR (1993) Ultrasound contrast hysterosalpingography – evaluation as an outpatient procedure. *Br J Radiol* **66**: 592–599.
49. Capitanio GL, Ferraiolo A, Groce S, Gazzo R, Anserini P & de Cecco L (1991) Transcervical selective salpingography: a diagnostic and therapeutic approach to cases of proximal tubal injection failure. *Fertil Steril* **55**: 1045–1050.
50. Kerin JF, Surrey ES, Williams DB, Daykhovsky L & Grundfest WS (1992) Falloposcopic observations of endotubal isthmic plugs as a cause of reversible tubal obstruction. *J Laparoendoscop Surg* **1**: 103–110.
51. Lederer KJ (1993) Transcervical tubal cannulation and salpingoscopy in the treatment of tubal infertility. *Curr Opin Obstet Gynecol* **5**: 240–244.
52. Kerin JF, Williams DB, San Romano GA, Pearlstone AC, Grundfest WS & Surrey ES (1992) Falloposcopic classification and treatment of Fallopian tube lumen disease. *Fertil Steril* **57**: 731–741.
53. Hershlag DB, Deiter DB, Carcangiu ML, Patton DL, Diamond MP & de Cherney AH (1991) Salpingoscopy: light microsocpic and electron microscopic designations. *Obstet Gynecol* **77**: 399–405.
54. Fortier KJ & Haney AF (1985) The pathological spectrum of uterotubal junction obstruction. *Fertil Steril* **65**: 93–98.
55. Gordts S, Campo R, Rombauts L & Brosens I (1998) Transvaginal salpingoscopy: an office procedure for infertility investigation. *Fertil Steril* **70**: 523–526.
56. Hirsh A (1999) The investigation and therapeutic options for infertile men presenting in assisted conception clinics. In: Brinsden PR (ed) *A textbook of in vitro fertilisation and assisted reproduction.* Parthenon Publishing, Carnforth, Lancashire, pp 27–52.
57. Glezerman M & Lunenfeld B (1993) Diagnosis of male infertility. In: Insler V & Lunenfeld B (eds) *Infertility: male and female.* Churchill Livingstone, Edinburgh, pp 317–334.
58. Jorgensen N, Andersen A-G, Eustache F, Irvine DS *et al.* (2001) Regional differences in semen quality in Europe. *Hum Reprod* **16**: 1012–1019.
59. World Health Organization (1999) WHO *Laboratory manual for the examination of human semen and sperm-cervical mucus interaction*, 4th edn. Cambridge University Press, Cambridge.
60. Aitken RJ (1992) Diagnosis of male infertility. In: Templeton AA, Drife JO (eds) *Infertility.* RCOG Springer-Verlag, London, pp 81–100.
61. Glezerman M & Bartoov B (1993) Semen analysis. In: Insler V, Lunenfeld B (eds) *Infertility: male and female.* Churchill Livingstone, Edinburgh, pp 285–316.
62. Kruger TF, Acosta AA, Simmons KF, Swanson RJ, Matta JF & Veeck LL (1987) New method of evaluating sperm morphology with predictive value for human *in vitro* fertilisation. *Urology* **30**: 248.
63. Kruger TF & Coetzee K (1999) The role of sperm morphology in assisted reproduction. *Hum Reprod Update* **5**: 172–178.
64. Grow DR, Swanson RJ, Oehninger S *et al.* (1994) Sperm morphology as diagnosed by strict criteria: probing the impact of teratozoospermia on fertilisation rate and pregnancy outcome in a large *in vitro* fertilisation population. *Fertil Steril* **62**: 559–567.
65. Kruger TF, Acosta AA, Simmons KF, Swanson RJ, Matta JF & Oehninger S (1988) Predictive value of abnormal sperm morphology in *in vitro* fertilisation. *Fertil Steril* **49**: 112–117.
66. Aitken RJ (1994) Pathophysiology of human spermatozoa. *Curr Opin Obstet Gynecol* **6**: 128–135.
67. Aitken RJ, Clarkson JS & Fishel S (1989) Generation of reactive oxygen species, lipid peroxidation and human sperm function. *Biol Reprod* **40**: 183–197.

68. Eggert-Kruse W, Bellman A, Rohr G, Tilgen W & Runnebaum B (1992) Differentiation of round cells in semen by means of monoclonal antibodies and relationship with male infertility. *Fertil Steril* **58**: 1046–1055.
69. Wolf H & Anderson DJ (1988) Immunohistologic characterisation and quantitation of leucocyte subpopulations in human semen. *Fertil Steril* **49**: 497–504.
70. Aitken RJ (1994) On the future of the hamster oocyte penetration assay. *Fertil Steril* **62**: 172–175.
71. Bamzu R, Lessing J, Yogev L, Homonnai ZT, Amit A & Yavetz H (1994) The hemizona assay is of good prognostic value for the ability of sperm to fertilise oocytes *in vitro*. *Fertil Steril* **62**:1056–1059.
72. Burkman LJ, Coddington CC, Fraken DR, Kruger TF, Rosenwalks Z & Hodgen GD (1988) The hemizona assay: development of a diagnostic test for the binding of human spermatozoa to the human hemizona pellucida to predict fertilisation potential. *Fertil Steril* **49**: 688–697.
73. Oei SG, Keirse MJNC, Bloemenkamp KWM & Helmerhorst FM (1995) European postcoital tests: opinions and practice. *Br J Obstet Gynaecol* **102**: 621–624.
74. Glazener CMA, Ford WCL & Hull MGR (2000) The prognostic power of the poistcoital test for natural conception depends on duration of infertility. *Hum Reprod* **15**: 1953–1957.
75. Sokol RZ (1995) The diagnosis and treatment of male infertility. *Curr Opin Obstet Gynecol* **7**: 177–181.
76. Krapez J, Hayden C, Rutherford A & Balen AH (1998) Survey of the diagnosis and management of antisperm antibodies. *Hum Reprod* **13**: 3363–3367.
77. Pryor JL, Kent-First M, Muallem A *et al.* (1997) Microdeletions in the Y chromosome of infertile men. *N Engl J Med* **336**: 534–539.
78. Geatti O, Gasparini D & Shapiro B (1991) A comparison of scintigraphy, thermography, ultrasound and phlebography in grading of clinical varicocele. *J Nucl Med* **32**: 2092–2097.
79. Horstmann W, Middleton W, Melson G & Siegel B (1991) Color Doppler US of the scrotum. *Radiographics* **11**: 941–957.
80. Petros J, Andriole G, Middleton W & Picus D (1991) Correlation of testicular color Doppler ultrasonography, physical examination and venography in the detection of left varicoceles in men with infertility. *J Urol* **145**: 785–788.

Further Reading

ESHRE Capri Workshop (1996) *Prevalence, diagnosis, treatment and management of infertility. Excerpts on human reproduction No. 4*. Oxford University Press, Oxford.

Kupesic S & de Ziegler D (eds) (2000) *Ultrasound and infertility*. Parthenon Publishing, Carnforth, England.

RCOG (1998) *Evidence-based clinical guidelines: the initial investigation and management of the infertile couple*. RCOG Press, London.

Templeton AA, Cooke I & O'Brien PMS (eds) (1998) *Evidence based fertility treatment*. RCOG Press, London.

Chapter 5

Counseling

Introduction

The counselor in a fertility clinic should be versatile both in dealing with the psychological stresses of couples with subfertility and with the special ethical and social dilemmas that need to be confronted when certain treatments are contemplated. The counselor therefore has to be compassionate in understanding the particular emotional strains of subfertility and have knowledge of the various treatments and the law as it applies to them.

Infertility

Many couples feel that they are infertile rather than subfertile. They do not see an end to their problem or believe that a pregnancy can ever occur. The woman's menstrual period is a monthly reminder that pregnancy has not occurred and this can compound what is already a low point of the month psychologically. Infertility treatments have attained a high profile since the advent of IVF. This can aggravate the stresses felt by couples who are undergoing the early stages of investigation and treatment because they sometimes perceive that they are embarking on a long track before they are offered "high-tech" and, supposedly, higher success therapies. It is important to try and place a couple's investigations in the context of their expected chance of conception over the next 6–12 months and to provide a proposed plan of management so that they can see how their treatment is envisaged by the clinician.

Society expects young couples to start a family – and many do. The couple with subfertility see relatives and friends expanding their families while their own pregnancy seems never to happen. Their working lives take over and they become more involved in work, both to fill time otherwise spent with a family and as an excuse to others for not starting a family. This process can sometimes result in tremendous isolation, especially if the couple also avoid contact with others who have a young family. Sometimes, particularly with professional couples, child-rearing is not a consideration until the female partner is in her mid to late thirties, when the natural and assisted chance of conception declines quite rapidly. It has been suggested that, in the future, we might be able to freeze ovarian biopsies from young professional women and either reimplant the ovarian tissue or culture the follicles *in vitro*, at a time when the couple wants to start a family. In the meantime these women require support and not blame for "leaving things too late."

Usually one partner is more affected psychologically than the other. This might be because they are going through the process of grieving at different times. Thus it is common for the male to be denying that there is a problem while the woman is feeling angry and distressed. Sometimes there is a feeling of guilt, exacerbated if there has been a history of pregnancies in other relationships which might have resulted either in abortion or in the birth of a child or children that are now with an ex-partner or that have been adopted. It is common for women, but not usually men, to disclose information about previous pregnancies to the clinic but to wish to keep this information from their partner. If the woman has had pelvic infection leading to tubal damage, or if the man has had a sexually transmitted disease that has impaired his fertility, these issues might not have been discussed previously and may come to light for the first time in the clinic. Guilt has also been described in subfertile couples in relation to normal activities such as premarital sex and masturbation.

While infertility is not thought to cause psychiatric illness, there is no doubt that psychological distress and psychosexual problems are commonly found in couples attending fertility clinics. This does not mean that couples with infertility are more prone to personality disorders or anxiety than the fertile population, as this has generally not been found to be so. In fact patients with subfertility appear to have a lower incidence of serious psychiatric disorders than the rest of the population. There is no difference in the overall rates of psychological problems and those in the general population, which might be because subfertile individuals tend to be in an older age group and usually in stable relationships. This is not to say that infertility does not cause psychological morbidity. Indeed, as some couples with unexplained infertility conceive after they have adopted a baby, it has been suggested that stress might have accounted for their infertility. While this might sometimes be true; the rates of conception are low (between 2% and 4% overall) and no higher than in couples with unexplained infertility who do not adopt.

Couples with infertility have a tendency to become increasingly isolated and avoid family gatherings and friends who have young families. Leisure time becomes focused on activities that do not involve children – and this can sometimes cause problems when the long-awaited child is born.

Some psychological disorders are relatively more common in young women, such as disordered eating habits. Bulimia, for example, is associated with polycystic ovary syndrome and may be diffficult to detect, particularly if the patient is of normal body weight – as is often the case. Chronic stress can lead to alcohol and drug abuse and this has important implications not only for ovarian and testicular function but also teratogenesis.

Women appear to differ from men in the ways in which they are affected by infertility, and the gap tends to widen as treatment progresses. Many women absorb infertility as a part of their identity, as opposed to men, who see infertility as a problem to be dealt with. Women become very preoccupied with their problem and often talk only with their partners. A study from Nottingham found that only 75% of women had told their mothers by the end of a year of attending the clinic and by this time 47% had given up their jobs. Particular treatments bring their own stresses, for example the humiliation that can sometimes be caused by having a postcoital test or the use of donor gametes. Fertility drugs such as clomifene, the gonadotropins and gonadotropin releasing hormone (GnRH) agonists can also have profound effects on a patient's psychological well-being.

After the failure of one IVF treatment cycle, as many as 25% of women are thought to have clinical depression and this rate rises with repeated failures. Men, on the other hand, tend to have more clinical anxiety (38% compared with 10% in the community) although the rate does not worsen with repeated treatment cycles – and may sometimes improve. As time goes on women begin to feel frustrated and more reliant on their partner; they become guilty, feel greater responsibility, and have a need to talk. Men, on the other hand, become fed up with the constant focus on their wife's ovarian function and throw themselves into other activities as a distraction; they become more introverted and less able to talk with their partners about their infertility and other personal issues.

Psychosexual Problems

Couples who are trying for a pregnancy tend to make love less frequently than those who have no concerns about fertility. The reasons for this include the mistaken notion that long periods of abstinence improve the sperm and that the days around ovulation are the only time when intercourse should take place. Women become very aware of their cycle and sometimes become obsessive about recording dates of menstruation and keeping temperature charts or testing urine for luteinizing hormone (LH) surges. Their partners often feel that they are having to "perform to order" rather than make love for pleasure and affection, so excuses are made, intercourse does not take place, and tensions increase. Furthermore, the couple know that when they are next seen in the clinic they will be asked about frequency of intercourse, or requested to have a postcoital test, or told to make love on a particular day during an ovulation induction cycle.

Major psychosexual problems and impotence account for less than 5% of cases of subfertility but require careful counseling and expert advice. Most couples with subfertility, however, have varying degrees of stress placed upon their sex lives and it is necessary to be sensitive to these issues and to try to de-medicalize this most personal part of a couple's relationship. A careful explanation about the optimum frequency of intercourse will help a couple to appreciate that it is not necessary to have long periods of abstinence before the day of ovulation and that intercourse every 2–3 days in the follicular phase of the cycle will result in satisfactory numbers of motile sperm in the Fallopian tube on the day of ovulation (see Ch. 4). This should diffuse the pressure associated with a monthly focus on the middle part of the cycle. Indeed it has been reported that up to 10% of men having fertility treatment have sexual difficulties mid-cycle and 35% of couples have sexual problems during fertility treatment. A negative postcoital test might suggest azoospermia but might also have resulted from unreported impotence or failure of ejaculation. Whether a negative result indicates a recurrent problem is uncertain, however, as the postcoital test is the most invasive of tests when it comes to examining a couple's sexual relationship. One of the few benefits of keeping a temperature chart for a few months is the record of the frequency of intercourse, which can be noted by the physician.

In caring for couples with subfertility it is essential not to over-medicalize sexual performance so that the loving and enjoyable aspects of love-making are not lost. It is also important to talk about these issues openly with an acknowledgement of the problems in order to break the "chain of silence."

How to Deal With Work

A major source of stress for women is the logistical difficulties of fitting repeated visits to the clinic into the working week. While many employers are cooperative and understanding, fertility treatment is aiming to get the woman pregnant and therefore results in maternity leave and maternity pay. It is not surprising that many women try to hide their reasons for repeated absences from work. The clinic can help by trying to perform scans early in the morning, at lunch time, and after work, although this has implications for the staffing of the unit.

Another factor is the attention paid to a couple undergoing fertility treatment by their friends and family. The couple feel under pressure to succeed, even though success is really out of their hands. They are confronted by continual requests for progress reports and this makes the lack of a pregnancy all the harder to bear. Couples should be advised to discuss their treatment only with those who they know will be discreet so as not to increase the pressures already on them. This necessity to be selective about whom to talk to does, unfortunately, perpetuate the mystique of fertility treatments and the ability of those who are affected to talk openly about the need for an improved service. In other words, the topic remains relatively taboo on an individual level despite the publicity that surrounds the scientific breakthroughs.

The Special Needs of the Male Partner

The male partner should certainly be encouraged to become involved in the investigations and treatments. His role in fertility therapy is relatively easy, irrespective of whether there are male factors in the couple's subfertility. As treatment centres largely around the female partner the man can sometimes feel left out and guilty, particularly if there is nothing specifically wrong with his partner and she is undergoing stressful treatment with potentially dangerous side-effects. While couples should be encouraged to confront feelings of guilt and emotional difficulties in order to help each other cope better with fertility treatment, many feel unable to communicate either with a counselor or, more importantly, with each other. Furthermore, research that has been conducted in this area is limited because of not being able to include those who do not attend the clinic or those who will not see a counselor. We can also only guess at the number of couples who never attend for investigation because they are unable to address their infertility and couples who actually make it to the clinic might be those better able to cope with the stresses of infertility and its management.

Adjustment to Parenthood

Couples who have experienced infertility can have difficulties adjusting to parenthood. They may have been together as a couple for a long time and the intrusion of a baby can disrupt their daily regime. The female partner may have to give up work after many years of building up a career. She may resent her baby and at the same time feel guilty about such feelings. There is an increased rate of postnatal depression among women who have experienced subfertility, which rises with the duration of marriage.

Prior to conception there is a tremendous focus on conceiving, yet after the birth of the baby life has to assume "normal" dimensions, although interestingly women still see themselves as being infertile. Multiple births bring with them additional stresses and difficulties with parenting. Not only do the parents find it difficult to relate to each of the babies, they often avoid close affection in order to prevent favoritism. Furthermore, pre-existing children are at risk of being excluded because so much time has to be spent with the babies.

How to Tell Children of Donated Gametes

All couples who undergo donor insemination (DI) or oocyte donation (OD) have to undergo counseling both as an essential part of the treatment and as a prerequisite of the Human Fertilisation and Embryology Authority (HFEA). They need to understand how the donors are selected, how they are screened and the limitations of accurate matching. The counselor should also describe the law with respect to the legal position of the child and the parents to it and also the rules governing confidentiality and anonymity. At present, sperm donors are invariably anonymous. Oocyte donors, however, are often provided by the recipient couple, sometimes by the sister of the patient. If the donor is known to the recipient couple it is virtually impossible to prevent the child from knowing his/her genetic origins. In the case of DI, the choice lies with the parents, who need not tell anyone if they do not wish to. The parents' names go on the child's birth certificate and so no one need ever know that donated gametes were used. If the parents choose to tell their child then they will need guidance about when and how. It is suggested that they tell the child in stages, initially with a simple explanation of how medical help was needed for conception, gradually expanding over the years and always emphasizing that the child was very much wanted and all the more so because of his/her special beginning. If the couple decide not tell their child it is important that they are advised not to tell anyone else, as the worst scenario is for the child to find out as the result of an accidental slip of the tongue.

More recipients of donated eggs are thought to tell their children than those who conceive through DI, with only 20% in the UK and 30% in the rest of Europe informing their children of their origins.[1] There is a move toward greater openness although this can potentially bring with it another set of problems, as many children who discover that they were conceived using donated gametes then wish to discover more about the gamete donor. In the UK, at the time of writing, only non-identifying information is available and so for those who are keen to find out more about their origins the lack of information may lead to great frustration, anger, and misery.

Surrogacy

Surrogacy involves a host mother carrying a pregnancy for a couple in which the woman is unable to go through a pregnancy, usually because she does not have a uterus or because she has a serious medical condition that makes it unwise for her to conceive. "Natural" surrogacy involves the host donating her egg as well as lending her uterus and is achieved by artificial insemination with the recipient father's sperm or intercourse with the recipient father. These forms of surrogacy are performed by private arrangement and not usually by fertility clinics. IVF surrogacy, on the other hand, involves the host receiving embryos that have been conceived *in vitro* using the recipient parents' gametes and is offered by a few assisted conception clinics in the UK. The ethical aspects of surrogacy are considerable and the host, her family, and the recipient couple require extensive counseling before embarking upon treatment.

Problems of Different Cultural Groups in the UK

Some cultures associate infertility with impotence and, for example, some African men will only marry a woman once she has borne his child. If a conception fails to occur, the woman might still be blamed for the couple's infertility, even if the man is found to be azoospermic.

We give here a simplified account of the teachings of the major religions – the reader involved in these transcultural problems is encouraged to consult priests and teachers of the religions concerned.

The Christian Church

The Anglican Church has a fairly open mind about fertility treatment, as does Buddhism. The Roman Catholic Church considers that infertility is predestined and has suggested that infertile couples should spend their energies usefully by adopting or helping other families, or helping poor or handicapped children. Furthermore, the Catholic Church considers life to begin at the time of fertilization. This can pose a dilemma for couples who decide to undergo IVF, as they may only permit two or three eggs to be exposed to sperm and so, if more than three oocytes are collected, they have to be disposed of, rather than allow the possibility of the disposal of pre-embryos. This prevents the selection of the best quality pre-embryos for transfer and might cause problems if there is poor fertilization. In some South American, predominantly Catholic, countries all embryos that are generated during IVF have to be frozen, irrespective of their quality; if they are not transferred in a subsequent cycle at a time when a conception could occur they have to be placed in the uterus during the luteal phase, thus "returning the embryo to the site of its origin" even though a conception could not occur. Catholics do not favor the use of donated sperm, eggs, or embryos which all run contrary to the concept of the unity of marriage and the child's right to be born in marriage.

The Jewish Faith

The Jewish faith varies depending on the degree of orthodoxy, with the most orthodox groups forbidding masturbation and hence any treatment that requires the production of sperm outside the woman's body. This is because there should be no destruction of germ cells. For this reason laparoscopic ovarian diathermy is also forbidden. A semen analysis can usually be obtained by ejaculation into a condom (free of spermicides) during intercourse, or alternatively a postcoital test can be performed. Contraception is banned and intercourse permitted during the most fertile time of the cycle so the size of Jewish families tends to be large. The couple without children therefore feels immense pressure and distress in such a procreation-oriented society. It is, however, our experience that most couples who are intent upon seeking treatment seem to be able to find a Rabbi who will give them a special exemption and bless their treatment.

It has been suggested by Hirsh[2] that sperm could be retrieved postcoitally from the wife of an orthodox Jew and then prepared for either conventional IVF if the number of sperm is sufficient, or for IVF-intracytoplasmic sperm injection (ICSI) if only a few sperm are retrieved. This would require the couple to have intercourse prior to oocyte retrieval at a time when the stimulated ovaries are enlarged and possibly tender. Postcoital assisted conception (PC-IVF or PC-ICSI) provides the possibility of fertility without the need for masturbation, semen collection devices, or coitus interruptus.

The use of donated spermatozoa is forbidden by Jewish law, which does not permit the insemination of a married woman with spermatozoa that are not her husband's. The main issue is that of incest, as the father of the child is an unknown sperm donor, although some have got round this by using the sperm from a non-Jewish donor. If donated sperm has been used, the owner of the sperm is considered to be the legal father of the child.

Muslims and Hindus

Many Muslims and Hindus tend to live in close-knit family-oriented communities and so subfertility brings with it particular stresses. In the UK many families are first generation immigrants and the women often have a poor grasp of English and so become isolated within their community. They also have difficulty in knowing where to go for help. While the men are often better integrated because they are usually employed, they too have difficulty in accessing help and relationships can become highly stressed. Islamic law prohibits the use of donated gametes and states that infertility should be accepted rather than engaging in "adulterous" treatments. The Hindu faith, on the other hand, will permit DI using spermatozoa from a close relative of the husband, provided all other treatments have failed. Buddhism allows relative freedom.

Emotional Support for Clinic Staff

Dealing with stress is stressful in itself and it is important for nurses, doctors, embryologists, and administrative staff to be able to meet and defuse tensions that have been absorbed during the course of difficult consultations and encounters. Some patients latch on to an individual member of staff, who might not be the appropriate person to deal with their medical problems or able to cope with the constant demands made upon them. For example, a particular nurse or doctor might be requested always to perform a couple's insemination treatment or embryo transfer after a successful attempt resulted in a pregnancy that then miscarried. The couple might have an unrealistic belief that that nurse/doctor is the only member of the clinic who can help them to achieve a pregnancy, yet with each failed attempt the pressure on the nurse/doctor increases to an unreasonable level. Some consultations can be extremely tense and emotions can run so high as to make communication impossible. Tensions are transmitted to the staff and it is sometimes necessary to ask another member of staff to take over either for the present or, sometimes, in all future consultations.

It is important that there is a forum to discuss all consultations at the end of the clinic or at the end of the week, not only as an educational forum but also so that concerns about the emotional problems of the patients can be aired. Each member of staff should also be able to talk in confidence to a colleague about personal concerns and difficulties and even the counselor sometimes needs a counselor!

It is inevitable that some members of the clinic staff will themselves experience infertility or miscarriage and may even require treatment on the unit where they work. This may create immense tensions, with a combination of factors including lack of privacy and a feeling of being in the spotlight during treatment. If therapy can be offered elsewhere the situation might be made easier, although geographical constraints often render this option impractical.

The Infertility Counselor

The HFEA requires that each assisted reproduction clinic has access to a counselor. Furthermore, an infertility clinic can barely survive without a suitably trained counselor who is able to help couples deal with the emotional and ethical issues of modern fertility treatment. The clinic nurse has traditionally fulfilled the role of counselor but it is now recognized that patients should be able to communicate in confidence with the counselor and the counselor should not be involved with the patients' treatment. There are now a number of courses for counselors with an interest in infertility and a British Infertility Counsellors' Association (BICA), which has now unified training and accreditation for fertility counseling. Counselors in the clinic should be trained and should also receive regular supervision from a senior colleague, who might not necessarily work in the fertility unit.

The counselor has to support couples through the acceptance of their fertility problem(s) and in making the right decisions for themselves as an individual couple about whether to have treatment. The couple should be aware that in any one cycle of treatment, whether by DI, ovulation induction, or IVF, the greater chance is that they will not be pregnant and they may need support through several attempts. Some months there will be pitfalls in the treatment, for example lack of ovarian response to stimulation, or a canceled cycle because of ovarian overstimulation. The counselor therefore needs to have a detailed understanding of the clinic's protocols and should be able to help to clarify the expectations of the couple. If a pregnancy occurs there is still the possibility of miscarriage, ectopic pregnancy, and problems later in pregnancy, particularly if a multiple pregnancy has occurred. Whatever the outcome of the treatment, counseling aims to help the couple to accept their situation and feel comfortable with their emotions.

The counselor may work in a variety of ways but must be familiar with the likely procedures and patterns of experience that present in a fertility clinic and the dilemmas, griefs, and joys that these bring. She/he should be able to detect major depression and other severe psychiatric disorders and be able to recognize when the couple's difficulties are beyond her expertise. She/he should be familiar with the psychological processes of adjustment, the process of grief, the resilience of the mind, and its defenses.

Counselors can also help to educate the rest of the team about psychological issues and communication skills. Some counselors work very closely with their nursing and clinical colleagues, while others keep the entire contents of their sessions confidential. We believe that patients should of course have the right to complete confidentiality if they wish but that it is helpful for there to be a summary of the counseling sessions in the clinical notes. The detailed content of counseling is not usually required by the gynecologist but where misunderstandings or grief have been engendered, further upset can be avoided by the sensitive involvement of the gynecologist in the relevant psychological concerns. A well-informed team works best all round and if good communication does not occur between the counselor and clinical staff, patients may find themselves splitting the staff and directing woe or anger against individuals.

Counselors need to be able to accept non-judgmentally the decisions that couples make about treatment and should be aware how their own psychological dilemmas interact with those of the patient and gynecologist. It is our experience that counselors contribute enormously to the successful operation of a clinic and those that we have met are able to empathize with the patients and take a genuine interest in their concerns.

Counseling – key points

- Counseling is an integral part of the management of infertility
- Subfertile men and women have different needs and approach their problems in different ways
- It is important to be conscious of the needs of different religious and cultural societies
- Working in a fertility clinic can be mentally and emotionally exhausting – special consideration should be made of the needs of the staff
- Counselors should be properly trained and selected
- Counseling subfertile patients requires different skills and knowledge to general counseling

References

1. Golombok S, Brewaeys A, Cook R *et al.* (1996) The European study of assisted reproduction families: family functioning and child development. *Hum Reprod* **10**: 2324–2331.
2. Hirsh A (1996) Post-coital sperm retrieval could lead to the wider approval of assisted conception by some religions. *Hum Reprod* **11**: 101–103.

Further Reading

Appleton T (1994) *Surrogacy – a guide for patients*. Infertility Support Counselling Presentations, Cambridge.

Appleton T (1994) *The pain of childlessness*. Infertility Support Counselling Presentations, Cambridge.

Demyttenaere K (1998) Coping with infertility. In: Templeton AA, Cooke I, O'Brien PMS (eds) *Evidence based fertility treatment*. RCOG Press, London, pp 345–353.

Friedman T (1989) Infertility and assisted reproduction. In: Psychological aspects of obstetrics and gynaecology. *Baillière's Clinical Obstetrics and Gynaecology* **3**: 751–768.

Houghton D & Houghton P (1987) *Coping with childlessness*. Unwin Paperbacks, London.

Snowden R & Snowden E (1984) *The gift of a child* (about donor insemination). George Allan & Unwin, London.

SECTION 2

Management – diagnosis and treatment

Introduction – Cost-effectiveness of Therapy

When determining appropriate treatment for the management of infertility, there may be one clear treatment or a number of potential options. Furthermore there are often a variety of drugs to choose between and several potential treatment protocols. It is important to consider not only efficacy of treatment but also cost-effectiveness based on a combination of scientific evidence and health economics. There has been a trend recently for cost-effectiveness analyses to be sponsored by the pharmaceutical industry. While much research could not take place without industry support, it is important to be cautious when interpreting such data.[1] Reproductive medicine is evolving continually – and often rapidly – therefore guidelines for management and its funding require regular revision. Statements on cost-effectiveness often make reference to eligibility criteria without providing a balanced view on "fairness." For example, a woman aged 28 with two children and tubal infertility will have a much better chance of conceiving with IVF than a woman aged 35 with no children and tubal infertility – yet who deserves the treatment more? In the UK the National Institute for Clinical Excellence (NICE) is currently deliberating on guidelines for the National Health Service funding of fertility treatment and we await the outcome with great interest. We have tried to provide an up-to-date, practical guide to the management of infertility and have made reference to issues of cost-effectiveness where appropriate.

Reference

1. Barlow D (2001) Cost effectiveness modelling. *Hum Reprod* **16**: 2479–2480.

Further Reading

AEGISS Report (2000) Department of Health, Scotland.

Cochrane Database of Systematic Reviews. Cochrane Collaboration, Oxford.

EHC (1992) *The Management of Subfertility*. Effective Health Care Bulletin Number 3. School of Public Health, University of Leeds.

Gleicher N (2000) Cost effective fertility care. *Hum Reprod Update* **6**: 190–199.

Hull MGR (1996) Managed care of infertility. *Curr Opin Obstet Gynecol* 8: 302–313.

Philips Z, Barraza-Llorens M & Posnett J (2000) Evaluation of the relative cost-effectiveness of treatments for infertility in the UK. *Hum Reprod* **15**: 95–106.

RCOG Guidelines (1998–2000) *The initial investigation and management of the infertile couple* (1998); *The management of infertility in secondary care* (1998); *The management of infertility in tertiary care* (2000). RCOG Press, London.

Chapter 6

Anovulatory infertility and ovulation induction

Introduction

The principles of the management of anovulatory infertility are: first, to correct any underlying disorder (e.g., nutritional deficiency in hypogonadotropic patients who are underweight); second, to optimize health before commencing therapy (e.g., women with polycystic ovary syndrome (PCOS) who are overweight); and third, to induce regular unifollicular ovulation.

A semen analysis should be performed before ovulation induction therapy is commenced. Tubal patency should be assessed by either hysterosalpinography (HSG) or laparoscopy before embarking upon gonadotropin therapy. If there are no firm indications (e.g., past history of pelvic infection, pelvic pain) our policy has been to delay a test of tubal patency until there have been up to three or six ovulatory cycles. In order to minimize the risks of therapy (see Ch. 17), and also to ensure a cost-effective approach to treatment, we should perhaps now be thinking about performing an assessment of tubal patency in every woman before choosing the appropriate therapy for her.

Before considering the management of specific disorders of anovulation we present a classification of primary and secondary amenorrhea. Of course not all women with anovulatory infertility are amenorrheic – some have oligomenorrhea, particularly those with PCOS. The classification still holds and the diagnosis is made by following the steps described in Chapter 4.

Pituitary and Hypothalamic Causes of Anovulation

The causes of primary and secondary amenorrhea are listed in Tables 6.1 and 6.2. Pituitary and hypothalamic etiologies occur after surgery for pituitary tumors, pituitary ablation in addition to Kallmann's syndrome, and idiopathic hypogonadotropic hypogonadism (Tables 6.3 and 6.4). Initial clues to the presence of a pituitary tumor can be seen on a skull X-ray (Figs 6.1–6.2) although magnetic resonance imaging (MRI) and computed tomography (CT) are preferred (see below).

Table 6.1 Classification of primary amenorrhea

Uterine causes	Mullerian agenesis (e.g., Rokitansky syndrome)
Ovarian causes	Polycystic ovary syndrome Premature ovarian failure (usually genetic, e.g., Turner's syndrome)
Hypothalamic causes (hypogonadotropic hypogonadism)	Weight loss Intense exercise (e.g., track athletes, ballerinas) Genetic (e.g. Kallmann's syndrome) Idiopathic
Delayed puberty	Constitutional delay or secondary (see text)
Pituitary causes	Hyperprolactinemia Hypopituitarism
Causes of hypothalamic/pituitary damage *(hypogonadism)*	Tumors (craniopharyngiomas, gliomas, germinomas, dermoid cysts) Cranial irradiation, head injuries (rare in young girls)
Systemic causes	Chronic debilitating illness Weight loss Endocrine disorders (thyroid disease, Cushing's syndrome, etc.)

Table 6.2 Classification of secondary amenorrhea

Uterine causes	Asherman's syndrome
Cervical stenosis	Ovarian causes: Polycystic ovary syndrome Premature ovarian failure (genetic, autoimmune, infective, radio/chemotherapy)
Hypothalamic causes *(hypogonadotropic hypogonadism)*	Weight loss Exercise Chronic illness Psychological distress Idiopathic
Pituitary causes	Hyperprolactinemia Hypopituitarism Sheehan's syndrome
Causes of hypothalamic/ pituitary damage *(hypogonadism)*	Tumors (e.g., craniopharyngiomas) Cranial irradiation Head injuries Sarcoidosis Tuberculosis
Systemic causes	Chronic debilitating illness Weight loss Endocrine disorders (thyroid disease, Cushing's syndrome, etc.)

Table 6.3 Etiology of primary amenorrhea in 90 consecutive patients attending the endocrine clinic at the Middlesex Hospital, London

Premature (primary) ovarian failure	36%
Hypogonadotropic hypogonadism	34%
Polycystic ovary syndrome	17%
Hypopituitarism	4%
Hyperprolactinemia	3%
Weight-related amenorrhea	2%
Congenital abnormalities	4%

Table 6.4 Etiology of secondary amenorrhea in 570 patients attending the endocrine clinic at the Middlesex Hospital, London

Polycystic ovary syndrome	36.9%
Premature ovarian failure	23.6%
Hyperprolactinemia	16.9%
Weight-related amenorrhea	9.8%
Hypogonadotropic hypogonadism	5.9%
Hypopituitarism	4.4%
Exercise-related amenorrhea	2.5%

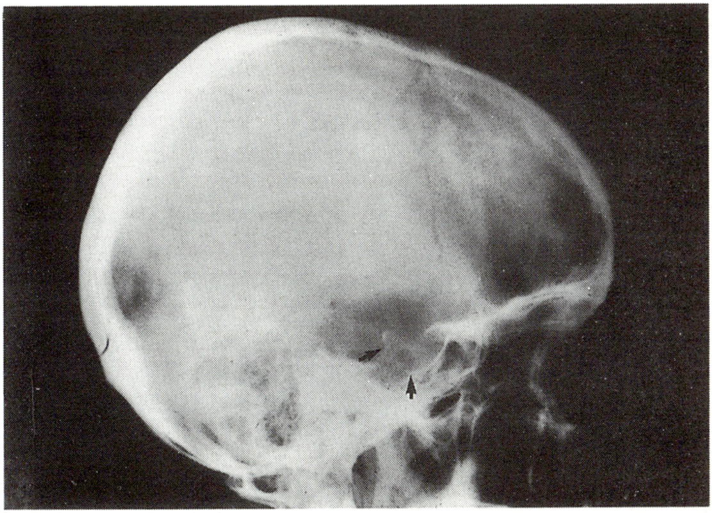

Figure 6.1 Lateral skull X-ray of a patient with a pituitary macroadenoma. The pituitary fossa is enlarged and the floor of the sella turcica is eroded (black arrows).

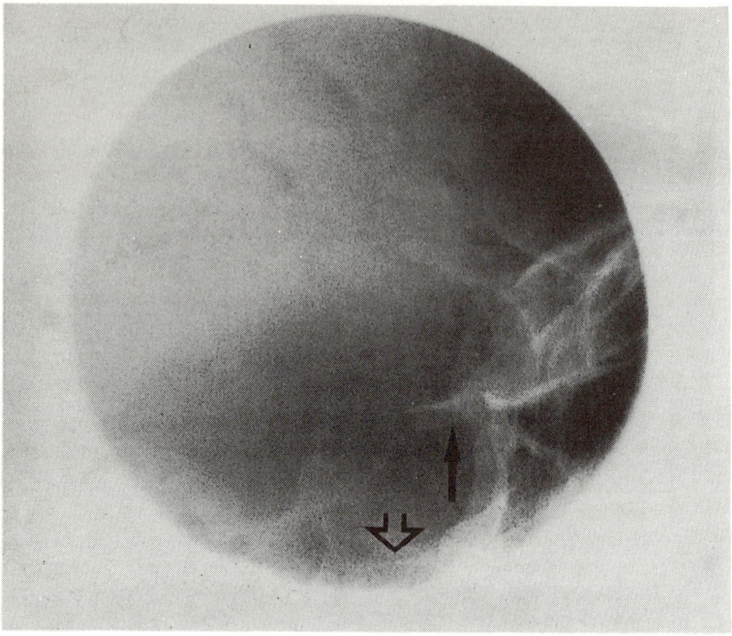

Figure 6.2 Magnified view of the pituitary fossa, in a different patient with a macroadenoma, showing an eroded floor of the sella with asymmetrical ballooning (open arrow). The anterior clinoid processes are eroded from beneath and appear pointed (closed arrow).

Hypogonadotropic Hypogonadism

One should suspect hypogonadotropic hypogonadism if the gonadotropin concentrations are subnormal (less than 5 i.u./L), in the presence of estrogen deficiency. The cause may be at the level of the pituitary or hypothalamus. Stimulation with gonadotropin releasing hormone (GnRH) does not help in distinguishing between a hypothalamic and pituitary etiology, as there is great heterogeneity in the response to a single 100 μg dose of GnRH. We therefore no longer perform the GnRH test.[1] The diagnosis of Kallmann's syndrome is made if the patient has hyposmia or anosmia associated with hypogonadotropic hypogonadism. Radiology of the hypothalamus and pituitary is otherwise indicated and abnormalities on a skull X-ray (nowadays rarely performed) should be investigated with CT or MRI.

Pulsatile LHRH or GnRH (Fig. 6.3)

Ovulation is optimally induced in women with intact pituitary function by application of pulsatile luteinizing hormone releasing hormone (LHRH or GnRH), administered subcutaneously or intravenously by a

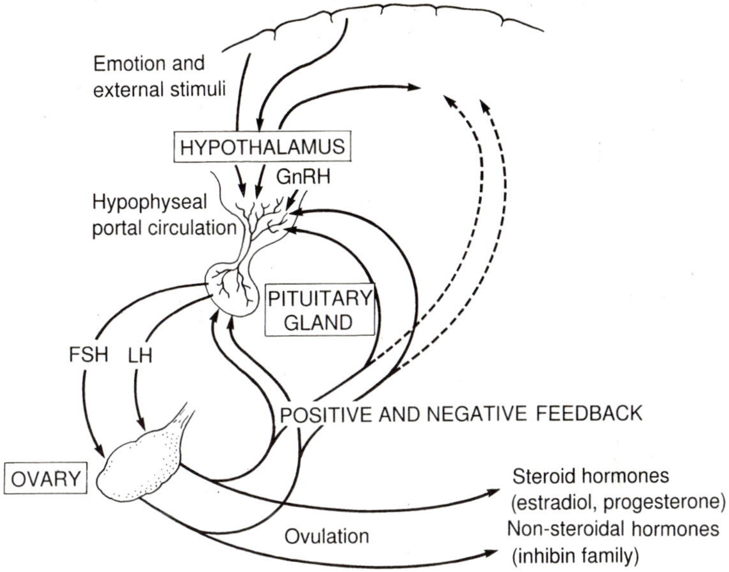

Figure 6.3 The hypothalamic–pituitary–ovarian axis.

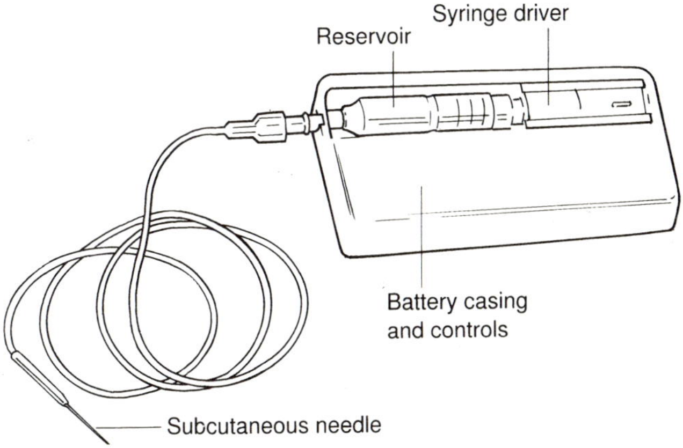

Figure 6.4 Mini-infusion GnRH (LHRH) pump.

miniaturized infusion pump (Fig. 6.4). The injections are given at intervals of 90 minutes at a dose of either 15 micrograms subcutaneously or 5–10 micrograms intravenously.[2–4] This therapy provides the most physiological correction of the primary disturbance with little risk of multiple pregnancy or ovarian hyperstimulation. Ultrasound monitoring can be kept to a minimum and cumulative conception and live birth rates equal those expected of normal ovulating women (see

Fig. 6.8).[5–7] Some women with hypogonadotropic hypogonadism also have polycystic ovaries, which are "suppressed" because they have not been exposed to cyclical stimulation by gonadotropins. These small polycystic ovaries are usually larger than normal ovaries in patients with hypogonadotropic hypogonadism and can be identified prior to stimulation – transabdominally (Fig. 6.5) or transvaginally (Fig. 6.6). Sometimes, however, they are first recognized after stimulation (Fig. 6.7). If overstimulated, these ovaries behave in a typically "polycystic" fashion. It is also interesting to note that when stimulated with pulsatile GnRH, these patients often develop abnormally elevated serum LH concentrations.

If pulsatile GnRH cannot be used (if the patient is unhappy with the equipment or if a pump is not available) then women with hypogonadotropic hypogonadism, of whatever cause, respond better to human menopausal gonadotropin (hMG) than to purified follicle stimulating hormone (FSH), because the former contains the LH which is necessary to stimulate androgen steroidogenesis – the substrate for estrogen biosynthesis.[8] Gonadotropin therapy is described on p. 165.

Adjuvant therapy

Adjuvant therapy with recombinantly derived human growth hormone has been shown to be of benefit to some women with hypogonadotropic hypogonadism who respond poorly to gonadotropin therapy.[9] The optimum dose has not been clearly defined. We would give alternate day injections of 12 i.u. over 2 weeks. Growth hormone appears to be of particular benefit to women with prolonged estrogen deficiency or pituitary failure. Growth hormone deficiency can be diagnosed by a negative response of growth hormone to clonidine, which stimulates growth hormone-releasing hormone secretion and thus assesses the growth hormone-secreting capacity of the pituitary. Baseline measurements of growth hormone are less useful. Growth hormone has been used in combination with a number of treatment regimens and does not appear to be of benefit to women with PCOS or hypergonadotropic ovarian failure; it has also been used in IVF regimens with little benefit.

Weight-related Amenorrhea (Fig. 6.8)

A body mass index (BMI) of less than 20 kg/m^2 is subnormal. It is also necessary to achieve a BMI of more than 19 kg/m^2 prior to the menarche for puberty to progress normally. Fat seems to be the critical component and it has been estimated that for the maintenance of ovulatory cycles fat should comprise at least 22% of body weight. The gonadotropin deficiency seen with weight loss is greater for LH than FSH, as is the diminished response to stimulation with exogenous GnRH. Subnormal secretion of gonadotropins, particularly an impairment

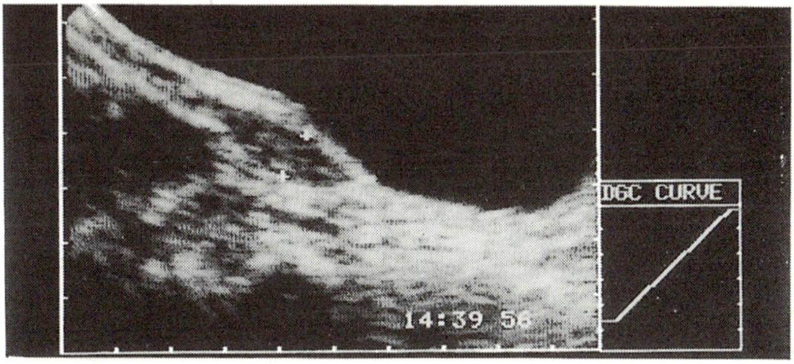

Figure 6.5

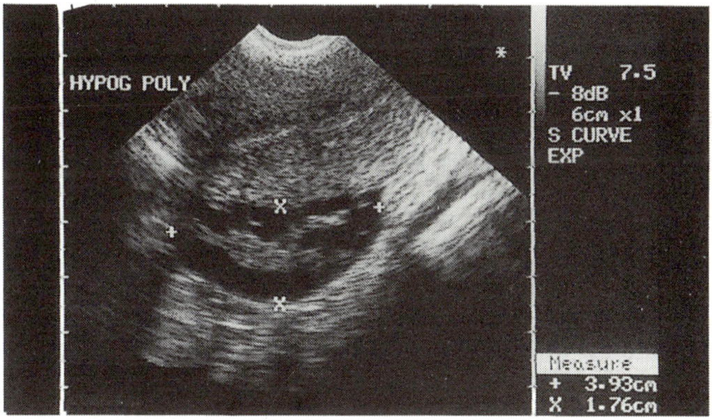

Figure 6.6

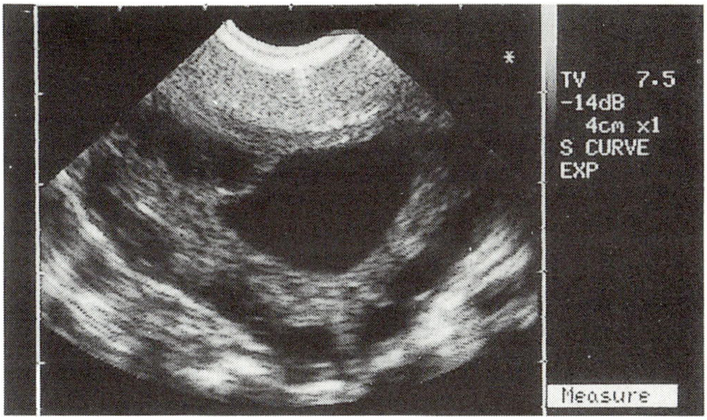

Figure 6.7

Figures 6.5–6.7 Transabdominal (**6.5**) and transvaginal (**6.6**) ultrasound scans of suppressed polycystic ovaries in patients with hypogonadotropic hypogonadism before and after (**6.7**) stimulation.

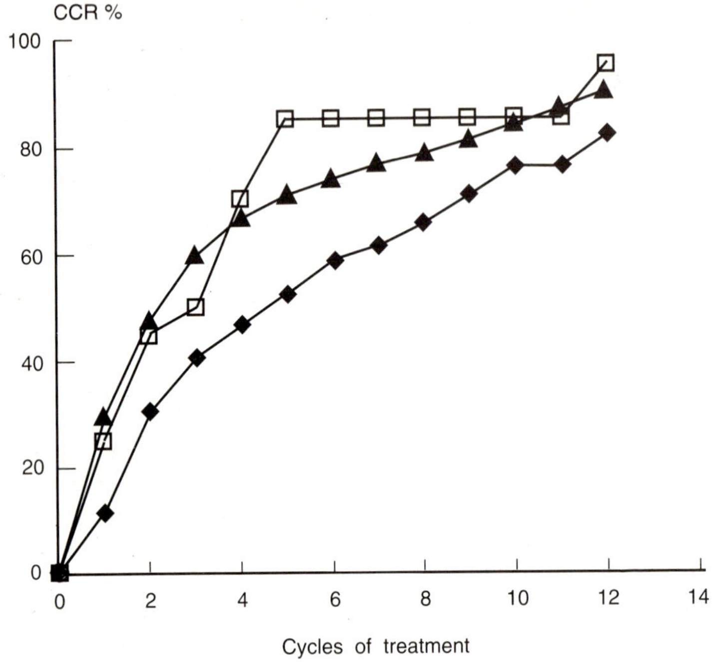

Figure 6.8 Cumulative conception rates (CCR) over successive cycles in normal women (triangle) and 20 patients with weight-related amenorrhea (square) and 77 with hypogonadotropic hypogonadism (diamond) who have undergone ovulation induction. (From Balen *et al.* (1994) *Hum Reprod* **9**: 1563.)[5]

of the pulsatility of gonadotropin secretion, may result in a "multicystic" pattern in the ovary,[10] as demonstrated by ultrasonography. This ovarian appearance is characteristic of normal puberty (see p. 69–70). The endocrine link between nutrition and reproduction has recently been described: white fat cells secrete a hormone (leptin) which is thought to signal satiety by suppressing the activity of the central neurotransmitter neuropeptide Y (NPY). NPY, as well as stimulating appetite and eating behavior, controls GnRH activity (and therefore reproduction) as well as adrenocorticotropic hormone (ACTH) and thyroid stimulating hormone (TSH) secretion (so modifying metabolism and the response to stress). Leptin levels are low in starvation, resulting in heightened NPY activity, a voracious appetite, with elevated ACTH and cortisol concentrations and low TSH and thyroxine concentrations – as typically seen in patients with severe anorexia nervosa. As weight is regained, leptin secretion resumes, NPY activity falls, and GnRH secretion resumes, thus permitting the return of fertility as nutrition returns to normal. It is thought that leptin plays an important role in the initiation of puberty.

Not all women who attain a normal BMI resume regular menstruation. In some cases this is dependent on levels of exercise, in which case the serum LH concentration may still be low. Approximately 20% of women have PCOS (see also Chs 4 and 7), which is also associated with an increased rate of eating disorders. Women with PCOS will be prone to oligomenorrhea or amenorrhea irrespective of their BMI.

Anorexia nervosa accounts for between 15% and 35% of patients with amenorrhea. It is now recognized that there is a spectrum of psychosomatic dysfunction from anorexia nervosa to bulimia, and menstrual disturbances are invariably associated. While the extreme forms of dietary abuse are more readily recognized now than in the past, there are many women with weight-related amenorrhea who have an appropriate body image perception and a lesser degree of weight loss than that seen in classic anorexia nervosa. It should be appreciated that these groups may form part of a continuum, with the possibility of an apparently innocent dieting pattern leading eventually to true anorexia. Many of these women will have presented with either amenorrhea or infertility without perceiving that they have a problem related to weight. It is essential to encourage weight gain as the main therapy and a careful explanation of the cause of their amenorrhea will help in this aim. Women with anorexia nervosa should be managed in collaboration with a psychiatrist and those with less severe dieting problems usually benefit from counseling or psychotherapy.

The prescription of an oral contraceptive, while inducing an artificial cycle, masks the underlying problem by allowing the denial of weight loss as the etiological factor. On the other hand, the degree of osteopenia caused by estrogen deficiency may be so great that the benefits of estrogen replacement therapy outweigh any putative psychiatric risks. Estrogen and leptin deficiency, reduced calcium and protein intake, reduced levels of vitamin D, and elevated cortisol levels can all contribute to osteoporosis and so estrogen therapy alone does not always rectify the problem. The age of onset of anorexia nervosa is also important, as prolonged amenorrhea before the normal age at which peak bone mass is obtained (approximately 25 years) increases the likelihood of severe osteoporosis. Pregnancy and lactation make significant demands on the skeleton's calcium reserves and so conception when significantly osteoporotic carries additional risks.

While ovulation may be readily induced with either GnRH or exogenous gonadotropins, treatment of infertility in the underweight patient is not necessarily in the baby's best interests as embarking upon a pregnancy when severely underweight results in a significant risk of intrauterine growth retardation and neonatal problems. In our experience few women have difficulty in perceiving and accepting that being underweight poses an avoidable risk to the unborn child and that consequently weight gain is an essential prelude to conceiving.[11]

Furthermore, since three-quarters of the cell divisions that occur during pregnancy take place during the first trimester, it is essential that nutritional status is optimized before conception. In an increasing number of studies low birth weight is also being related to an increased risk of cardiovascular disease, obstructive lung disease, and other illnesses in adult life.[12] Thus it seems that fetal nutritional status determines the pattern of adult disease. It is therefore the duty of the fertility specialist to provide a holistic approach to the patient and her desire for a family, with appropriate involvement of other health care professionals (dietician, nutritionalist, counselor, psychiatrist) in providing support both before and after pregnancy.

World-wide, involuntary starvation is the commonest cause of reduced reproductive ability, resulting in delayed pubertal growth and menarche in adolescents and infertility in adults. Acute malnutrition, as seen in famine conditions and during and after the Second World War, has profound effects on fertility and fecundity. Ovulatory function usually returns quickly on restoration of adequate nutrition. The chronic malnutrition common in developing countries has less profound effects on fertility, but is associated with small and premature babies.

Systemic disorders causing secondary amenorrhea and anovulation

Chronic disease may result in menstrual disorders as a consequence of the general disease state, weight loss or by the effect of the disease process on the hypothalamic–pituitary axis. Furthermore, a chronic disease that leads to immobility, such as chronic obstructive airways disease, may increase the risk of amenorrhea-associated osteoporosis.

In addition, certain diseases affect gonadal function directly. Women with chronic renal failure have a discordantly elevated LH, possibly as a consequence of impaired clearance. Prolactin is also elevated in these women, due to failure of the normal dopamine inhibition. Diabetes mellitus may result in functional hypothalamic–pituitary amenorrhea and be associated with an increased risk of PCOS. Liver disease affects the level of circulating sex hormone binding globulin, and thus circulating free hormone levels, thereby disrupting normal feedback mechanisms. Metabolism of various hormones, including testosterone, is also liver dependent; both menstruation and fertility return after liver transplantation. Endocrine disorders such as thyrotoxicosis and Cushing's syndrome are commonly associated with gonadal dysfunction. Management of these patients should concentrate on the underlying systemic problem and on preventing complications of estrogen deficiency. If fertility is required, it is desirable to achieve maximal health and where possible to discontinue teratogenic drugs.

Studies have failed to demonstrate a link between stressful life events and amenorrhea of longer than 2 months. However, stress may lead to physical debility such as weight loss which may then cause menstrual disturbance.

Exercise related amenorrhea Menstrual disturbance is common in athletes undergoing intensive training. Between 10% and 20% have oligomenorrhea or amenorrhea, compared with 5% in the general population. Amenorrhea is more common in athletes under 30 years of age and is particularly common in women involved in the endurance events (such as long distance running). Up to 50% of competitive runners training 80 miles per week may be amenorrheic.[13] Studies of women who train for competitive sport have reported rates of oligo-/amenorrhea of 16–79% in dancers, 47% in gymnasts, 24–50% in runners, and 12% in swimmers and cyclists.[14,15] The main etiological factors are low weight and percentage body fat content, but other factors have also been postulated. Physiological changes are consistent with those associated with starvation and chronic illness. In order to conserve energy, there may be a fall in TSH, a reduction in triiodothryonine (T_3) and an elevation of the inactive reverse-T_3. Exercise also leads to a fall in circulating insulin and insulin like growth factor 1 (IGF1), and therefore decreases their stimulation of the pituitary and ovary. Amenorrhea occurs when percentage body fat falls below a threshold of 17% and when serum LH concentrations are less than 5 i.u./L.

Female ballet dancers provide an interesting, and much studied, subgroup of sportswomen, because their training begins at an early age. They have been found to have a significant delay in menarche (15.4 compared to 12.5 years) and a retardation in pubertal development which parallels the intensity of their training. Menstrual irregularities are common and up to 44% have secondary amenorrhea.[16] In a survey of 75 dancers, 61% were found to have stress fractures and 24% had scoliosis; the risk of these pathological features was increased if menarche was delayed or if there were prolonged periods of amenorrhea. These findings may be explained by delayed pubertal maturation resulting in attainment of a greater than expected height and a predisposition to scoliosis, as estrogen is required for epiphyseal closure.

Exercise-induced amenorrhea has the potential to cause severe long-term morbidity, particularly with regard to osteoporosis. Studies on young ballet dancers have shown that the amount of exercise undertaken by these dancers does not compensate for these osteoporotic changes. Estrogen is also important in the formation of collagen and soft tissue injuries are also common in dancers.

Whereas moderate exercise has been found to reduce the incidence of postmenopausal osteoporosis, young athletes may be placing themselves at risk at an age when the attainment of peak bone mass is important for long-term skeletal strength.

It is sometimes difficult to unravel the interaction between desire to exercise and an eating disorder, as "undereating and over-exercising are mutually reinforcing and self-perpetuating behaviors".[17] The psyche of the young athlete is affected not only by pressure to compete against peers but also by parents and coaches. Stresses – mental as well as physical – may be immense and some athletes are found to be abusing performance enhancing drugs at a young age. Appropriate advice should be given, particularly regarding improving diet, vitamin, calcium, and iron supplements and the use of a cyclical estrogen/progestogen preparation should be considered. If possible the amount of exercise itself should be reduced – for which the support of parents and coaches is essential. Unfortunately the long-term health of the young girl is often overridden by the ambitions of those around her.

Hyperprolactinemia

There are many causes of a mildly elevated serum prolactin concentration, including stress and a recent physical or breast examination. If the prolactin concentration is greater than 1000 mu/L then the test should be repeated and if still elevated, it is necessary to image the pituitary fossa (usually by MRI).[18] Hyperprolactinemia may result from a prolactin-secreting pituitary adenoma or from a large non-functioning "disconnection" tumor in the region of the hypothalamus or pituitary, which disrupts the inhibitory influence of dopamine on prolactin secretion. Large non-functioning tumors are usually associated with serum prolactin concentrations of less than 3000 mu/L (Fig. 6.9), while prolactin-secreting macroadenomas usually result in concentrations of 4000 mu/L or more and the figures may rise to 50 000 mu/L or so. Other causes of mild hyperprolactinemia include hypothyroidism, PCOS (occurs in 15%, up to 2500 mu/L) and several drugs (e.g., the dopaminergic antagonist phenothiazines, selective serotonin reuptake inhibitors (SSRIs), domperidone and metoclopramide). In fact the SSRIs are now the most common cause of drug-induced hyperprolactinemia (Table 6.5).[19]

In women with hyperprolactinemic amenorrhea the main symptoms are usually those of estrogen deficiency (vaginal dryness, dyspareunia) and libido is usually reduced, irrespective of estrogen status. Prolonged estrogen deficiency may result in osteoporosis and while in many cases there will be an improvement of trabecular bone mineral density with resumption of regular menses, full recovery is not seen in all patients. In contrast, when hyperprolactinemia is associated with PCOS, the syndrome is characterized by adequate estrogenization, polycystic ovaries on ultrasound scan, and a withdrawal bleed following a progestogen challenge; the bone mineral density is usually normal. Galactorrhea may be found in up to a third of hyperprolactinemic patients, although its appearance is not correlated with prolactin levels or with the presence of a tumor.[18] About 5% present with visual field defects.

A prolactin-secreting pituitary microadenoma (Fig. 6.10) is usually associated with a moderately elevated prolactin (1500–4000 mu/L) and is unlikely to result in abnormalities on a lateral skull X-ray. On the other hand, a macroadenoma (Fig. 6.11), associated with a prolactin typically greater than 4000–8000 mu/L, and by definition greater than 1 cm in diameter, may cause typical radiological changes – that is,

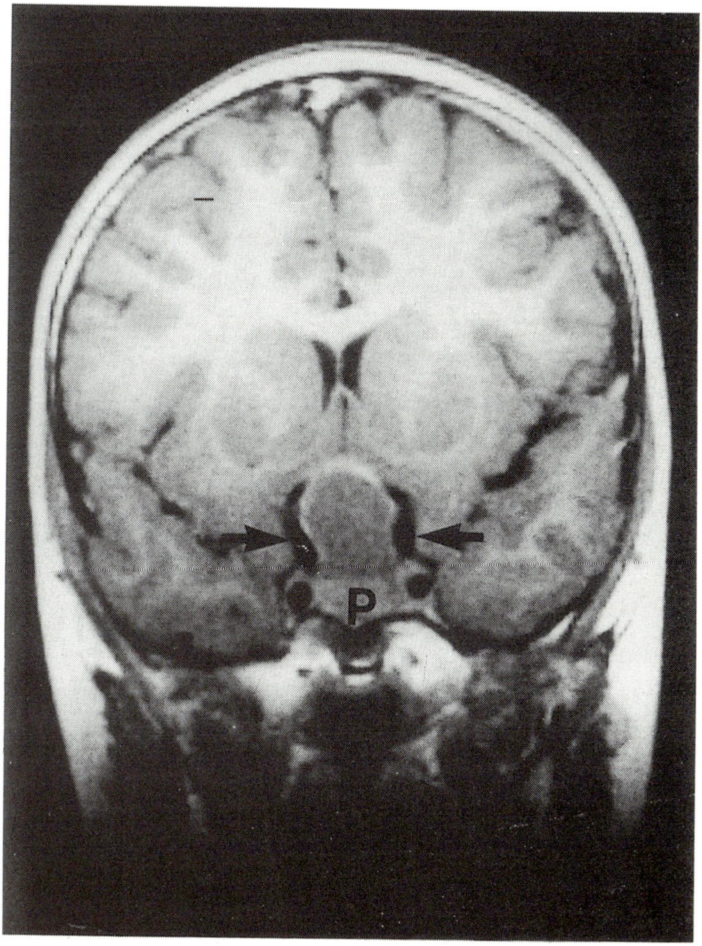

a

Figure 6.9

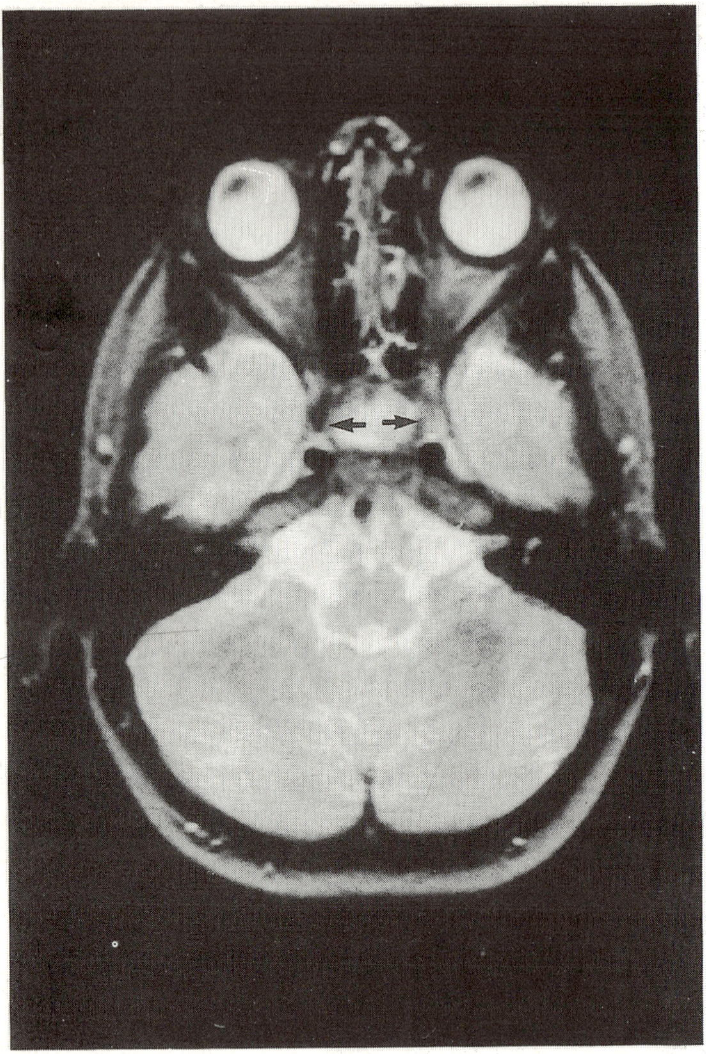

b

Figure 6.9a&b Craniopharyngioma. Cranial MRI: (**a**) coronal T1-weighted section after gadolinium enhancement. (The tumor signal intensity is reduced on the T1 image and only part of the periphery of the tumor enhances.) The carotid arteries have a low signal intensity (black arrows) due to the rapid flow within them and are deviated laterally and superiorly by the mass, which arises out of the pituitary fossa (P). (**b**) Axial T2-weighted section, without enhancement, made just above the level of the pituitary gland and through the chiasmatic cistern. There is a high signal in the suprasellar extension of the tumor (arrowed).

Table 6.5 Causes of hyperprolactinemia

Physiological	Pregnancy, lactation, neonatal period, stress
Hypothalamic	Tumors, transection pituitary stalk, cranial irradiation
Pituitary	Adenoma, acromegaly, Cushing's disease, tumors compressing pituitary stalk, empty sella syndrome
Miscellaneous	Primary hypothyroidism, PCOS, chronic renal failure, cirrhosis, ectopic prolactin secretion (bronchogenic carcinoma, hypernephroma), seizures. Hypersecretion of biologically less active isoforms of prolactin (e.g. "big prolactin")
Drugs[19]	Selective serotonin reuptake inhibitors (SSRIs): citalopram, fluoxetine, fluvoxamine, paroxetine, sertraline Classic neuroleptics: perphenazine, fluphenazine, flupentixol, thioridazine, promazine, haloperidol, loxapine, chlorpromazine, sulpiride Atypical neuroleptics: amisulpride, sertindole, risperidone Antiemetics: metoclopramide, domperidone Cardiovascular drugs: verapamil, reserpine, methyldopa Estrogens: high dose oral contraceptives Opiates Miscellaneous: bezafibrate, omeprazole, trimethoprim, histamine H_2 antagonists

Table 6.6 Drug therapy for hyperprolactinemia

Bromocriptine	2.5–20 mg daily, divided doses	Maintenance usually 5–7.5 mg/day
Cabergoline	0.25–1 mg twice weekly	Maintenance usually 1 mg/week
Quinagolide	25–150 µg daily, divided doses	Maintenance usually 75 µg/day

an asymmetrically enlarged pituitary fossa, with a double contour to its floor and erosion of the clinoid processes. CT and MRI now allow detailed examination of the extent of the tumor and, in particular, identification of suprasellar extension and compression of the optic chiasma or invasion of the cavernous sinuses. Prolactin is an excellent tumor marker and so the higher the serum concentration, the larger the size of the tumor expected on the MRI scan. In contrast, a large tumor on the scan with only a moderately elevated serum prolactin concentration (2000–3000 mu/L) suggests a non-functioning tumor compressing the pituitary stalk with "disconnection" from the hypothalamus.

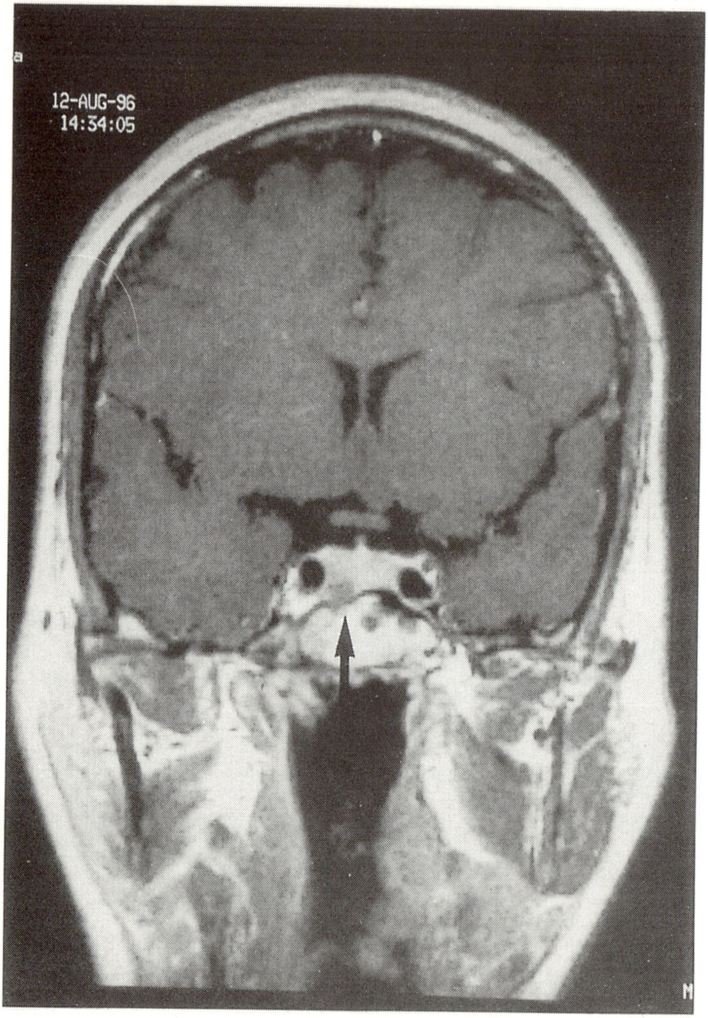

Figure 6.10 Pituitary microadenoma. Cranial MRI. A coronal section T1-weighted spin echo sequence after i.v. gadolinium. The normal pituitary gland is hyperintense (bright) while the tumor is seen as a 4 mm area of non-enhancement (gray) in the right lobe of the pituitary, encroaching up to the right cavernous sinus. It is eroding the right side of the sella floor.

Management (Table 6.6)

The management of hyperprolactinemia centers around the use of a dopamine agonist. Bromocriptine is still the most widely used preparation despite cabergoline being today's drug of choice (see below). Of course, if the hyperprolactinemia is drug induced, the relevant preparation should be discontinued. However, this may not be appropriate if the cause is a psychotropic medication, for example a phenothiazine being used to treat schizophrenia. In these cases it is reasonable to continue the drug and, after imaging the pituitary fossa, prescribe a low-dose combined oral contraceptive in order to counteract the symptoms of estrogen deficiency. Serum prolactin concentrations must then be carefully monitored to ensure that they do not rise further. Sometimes it is possible to change to an alternative drug, such as an atypical neuroleptic. The use of a dopamine agonist combined with an antipsychotic may lower serum prolactin concentrations but may also antagonize the therapeutic effects of the antipsychotic agent. Furthermore, dopaminergic drugs can occasionally induce or worsen psychotic symptoms (probably more so with bromocriptine than the longer-acting cabergoline) and so should only be used with great caution in patients with pre-existing psychotic illness and in conjunction with input from a psychiatrist.[19]

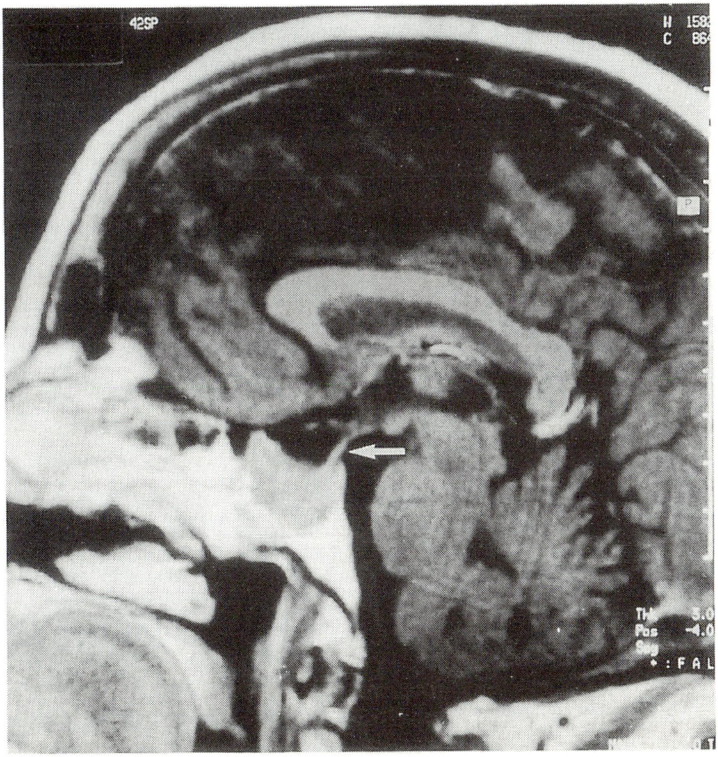

a

Figure 6.11

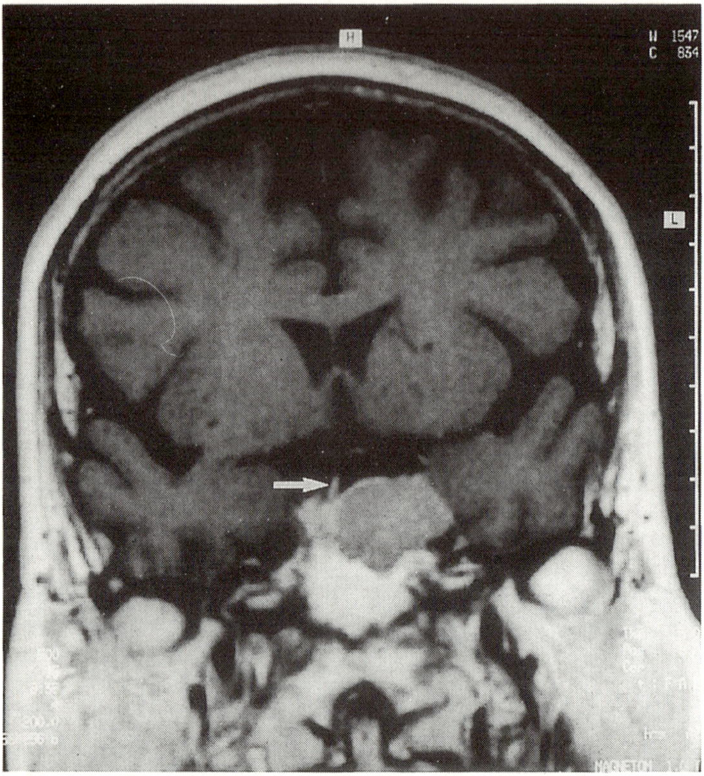

b

Figure 6.11a&b Pituitary macroadenoma. Cranial MRI. T1-weighted sections made after gadolinium enhancement. (**a**) Mid-line sagittal section and (**b**) coronal section at the level of the pituitary stalk (white arrows). There is a macroadenoma which enhances to a considerably lesser degree than the normal pituitary substance within and expanding from the left lobe of the pituitary gland into the left cavernous sinus. The tumor bulges the pituitary diaphragms superiorly and deviates the pituitary stalk towards the right side.

Most patients show a fall in prolactin levels within a few days of commencing dopamine agonist therapy and a reduction of tumor volume within 6 weeks (Figs 6.12–6.14).

Bromocriptine

Bromocriptine should be commenced at a dose of half a tablet at night (1.25 mg) and increased gradually every 3–5 days to 2.5 mg at night and then 1.25 mg in the morning with 2.5 mg at night until the daily dose is 7.5 mg (in two or three divided doses). The maintenance dose should be the lowest that works and is often lower than that needed at first to initiate a response. Side-effects can be troublesome (nausea, vomiting, headache, postural hypotension) and are minimized by commencing the therapy at night for the first 3 days of treatment and taking the tablets in the middle of a mouthful of food. Longer-term side-effects include Raynaud's syndrome, constipation, and psychiatric changes – especially aggression, which can occur at the start of treatment.[18]

Quinagolide and cabergoline

Longer acting preparations (e.g., quinagolide or twice-weekly cabergoline) may be prescribed to those patients who develop unacceptable side-effects. Cabergoline generally appears to be better tolerated and more efficacious than bromocriptine and is now the drug of choice for hyperprolactinemia. A monthly intramuscular depot bromocriptine preparation is not yet available in the UK but has distinct advantages in that it results in a very rapid fall in serum prolactin concentration and adverse effects rarely persist after the first 24 hours. Both quinagolide and cabergoline are highly effective in suppressing prolactin

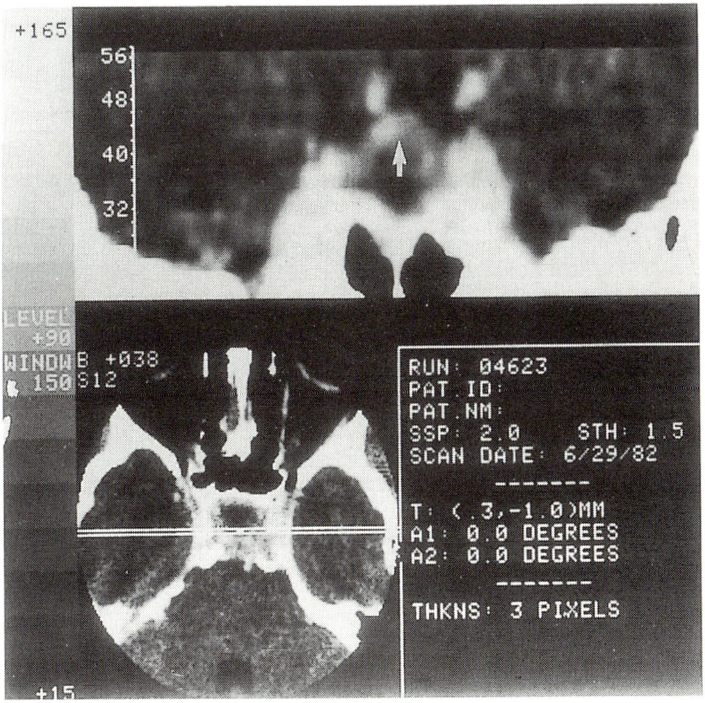

a

Figure 6.12a Pituitary macroadenoma. CT scan of the pituitary fossa with coronal reconstructions. A 1.3 mm slice taken after contrast enhancement showing a mixed density tumor (arrow) with suprasellar extension.

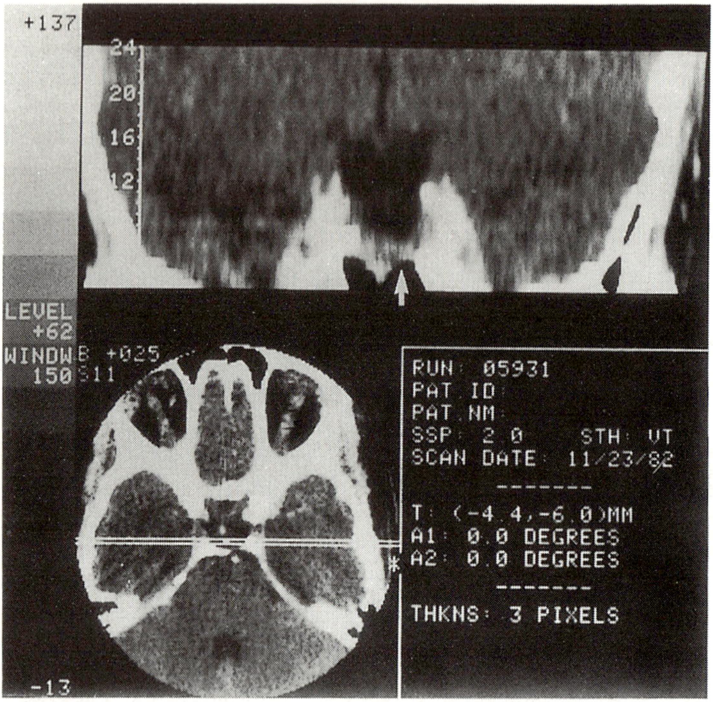

b

Figure 6.12b The same patient after treatment with bromocriptine showing considerable shrinkage of the tumor, with no suprasellar component but evidence on this section of erosion of the floor of the sella into the sphenoid sinus (arrow).

secretion although the latter appears more effective in reducing tumour volume.[20]

Dopamine agonist therapy may be discontinued for a trial period after a variable period of time, usually 1–5 years; approximately 25% of patients will remain normoprolactinemic.[20]

Surgery

Surgery, in the form of a trans-sphenoidal adenectomy, is reserved for cases of drug resistance and failure to shrink a macroadenoma or if there are intolerable side-effects from the drugs (the most common indication). Non-functioning tumors should be removed surgically and are usually detected by a combination of imaging and a serum prolactin concentration of less than 3000 mu/L. These tumors may expand with invasion of the cavernous sinus or compression of the optic chiasma (with impairment of vision). Occasionally such tumours are subject to hemorrhage (pituitary apoplexy). When the prolactin level is between

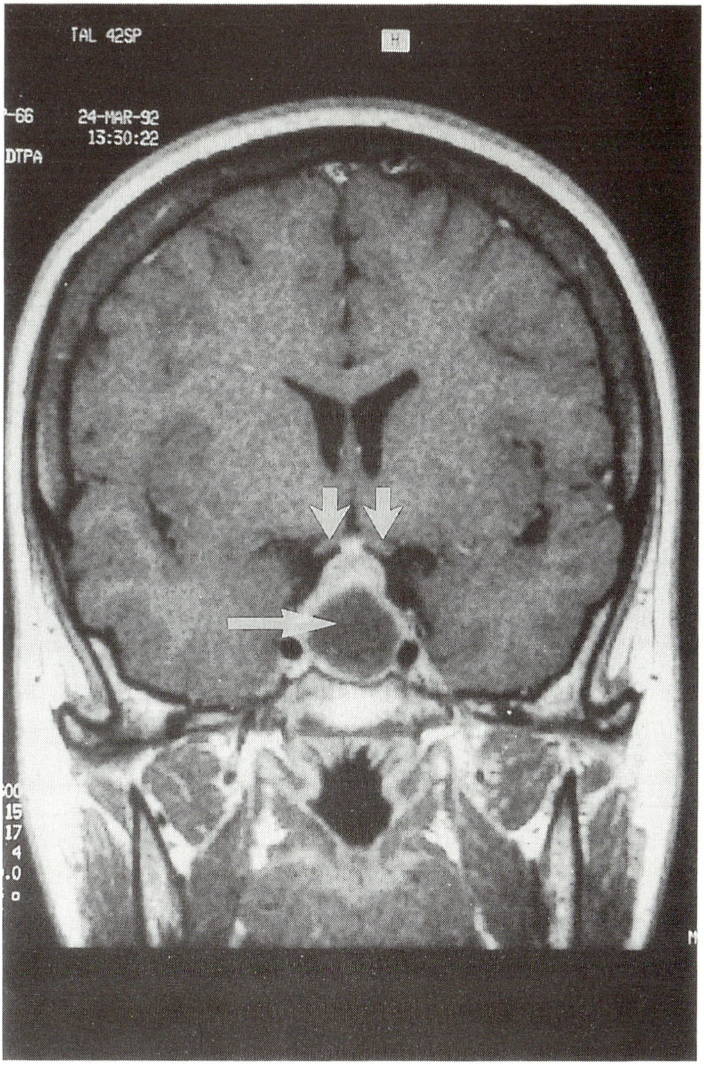

Figure 6.13 MRI scan of a pituitary macroadenoma before bromocriptine therapy. T1-weighted image after gadolinium enhancement demonstrating a macroadenoma with a large central cystic component (large arrow) There is suprasellar extension with compression of the optic chiasm (small arrows).

3000 and 8000 mu/L a trial of bromocriptine is warranted and if the prolactin level falls it can be assumed that the tumor is a prolactin-secreting macroadenoma. Operative treatment is also required if there is suprasellar extension of the tumor that has not regressed during treatment with bromocriptine and a pregnancy is desired. With the

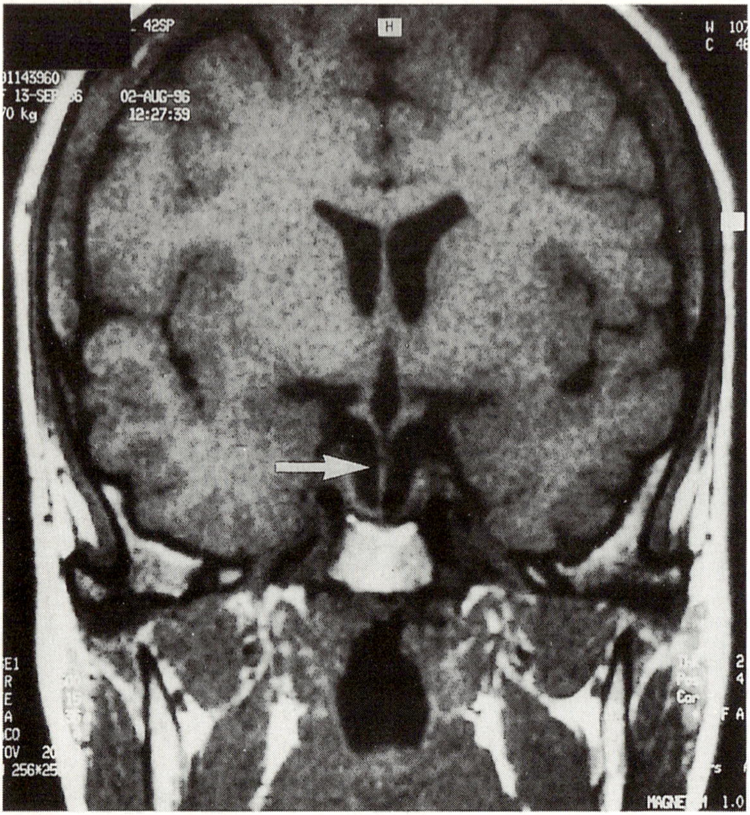

Figure 6.14 MRI scan of a pituitary macroadenoma after bromocriptine therapy. The tumor has almost completely resolved and there is tethering of the optic chiasm (arrow) to the floor of the sella.

current skills of neurosurgeons in trans-sphenoidal surgery, it is seldom necessary to resort to pituitary irradiation, which offers no advantages. Furthermore, long-term surveillance is required after irradiation to detect the inevitable hypopituitarism, which is immediately apparent if it occurs after surgery.

Women with a microprolactinoma who wish to conceive should be prescribed bromocriptine, as there are no safety data for the use of cabergoline in pregnancy. Bromocriptine may be discontinued when pregnancy is diagnosed and no further monitoring is required, as the likelihood of significant tumor expansion is very small (less than 2%). On the other hand, if a patient with a macroprolactinoma is not treated with bromocriptine the tumor has a 25% risk of expanding during pregnancy. This risk is probably also present if the tumor has been treated but has not shrunk, as assessed by CT or MRI scan.

The first-line approach to treatment of macroprolactinomas is therefore with cabergoline combined with barrier methods of contraception. In cases with suprasellar expansion, follow-up CT (or MRI) scan should be performed after 3 months of treatment to ensure tumor regression before it is safe to embark upon pregnancy. The patient should be switched to bromocriptine if she is trying to conceive; this can be discontinued during pregnancy, although if symptoms suggestive of tumor re-expansion occur an MRI scan should be performed and if there is continuing suprasellar expansion it is necessary to recommence bromocriptine therapy. These patients also require expert assessment of their visual fields during pregnancy.

If the serum prolactin is found to be elevated and the patient has a regular menstrual cycle, no treatment is necessary unless the cycle is anovulatory and fertility is desired. Amenorrhea is the "bioassay" of prolactin excess and should be corrected for its sequelae, rather than for the serum level of prolactin.

Polycystic Ovary Syndrome (Fig. 7.1)

PCOS (see Ch. 7 for a more general account of PCOS) is defined by the detection of polycystic ovaries by ultrasound scan (enlarged ovaries with more than 10 cysts 2–8 mm in diameter, scattered either around or through an echodense, thickened central stroma) in a patient with symptoms of oligoamenorrhea, obesity, and/or hyperandrogenism (acne, hirsutism).[10] A detailed description of the definition of PCOS, its pathophysiology, and long term sequelae is given in Chapter 7. Here we deal with PCOS in the context of anovulatory infertility, of which, in the developed world, it is the commonest cause. Various factors influence ovarian function and fertility is adversely affected by an individual being overweight or having elevated serum concentrations of LH (Fig. 6.15). Strategies to induce ovulation include weight loss, oral antiestrogens (principally clomiphene citrate), parenteral gonadotropin therapy and laparoscopic ovarian surgery. There have been no adequately powered randomized studies to determine which of these therapies provides the best overall chance of an ongoing pregnancy. Women with PCOS are at risk of ovarian hyperstimulation syndrome (OHSS) and so ovulation induction has to be carefully monitored with serial ultrasound scans. The realization of an association between hyperinsulinemia and PCOS has resulted in the use of insulin sensitizing agents, such as metformin, which appear to ameliorate the biochemical profile and improve reproductive function.

PCOS accounts for approximately 80% of women with anovulatory infertility. There are a number of interlinking factors that affect expression of PCOS.[21] A gain in weight is associated with a worsening

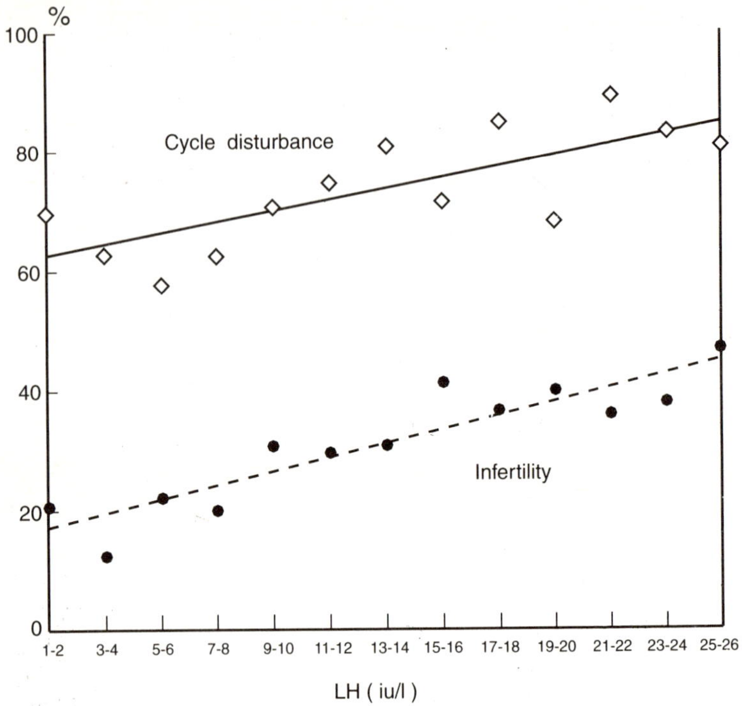

Figure 6.15 Relationship of serum LH concentration to rate of infertility and cycle disturbance.

of symptoms while weight loss will ameliorate the endocrine and metabolic profile and symptomatology.[22] Feedback from the polycystic ovary to both the pituitary and hypothalamus appears to be disturbed due to abnormalities in the secretion of ovarian steroid hormones and – probably more important – of non-steroidal hormones, for example inhibin and related proteins.[23,24] Normal ovarian function relies upon the selection of a follicle, which responds to an appropriate signal (FSH) in order to grow, become "dominant" and ovulate. This mechanism is disturbed in women with PCOS, resulting in multiple small cysts, most of which contain potentially viable oocytes but within dysfunctional follicles.

Hypersecretion of LH is found in 40% of women with PCOS and is associated with a reduced chance of conception and an increased risk of miscarriage, possibly through an adverse effect of LH on oocyte maturation.[23] Genetic studies to date have demonstrated abnormalities in both the steroidogenic pathway for androgen biosynthesis and the regulation of expression of the insulin gene. Elevated serum concentrations of insulin are more common in both lean and obese women

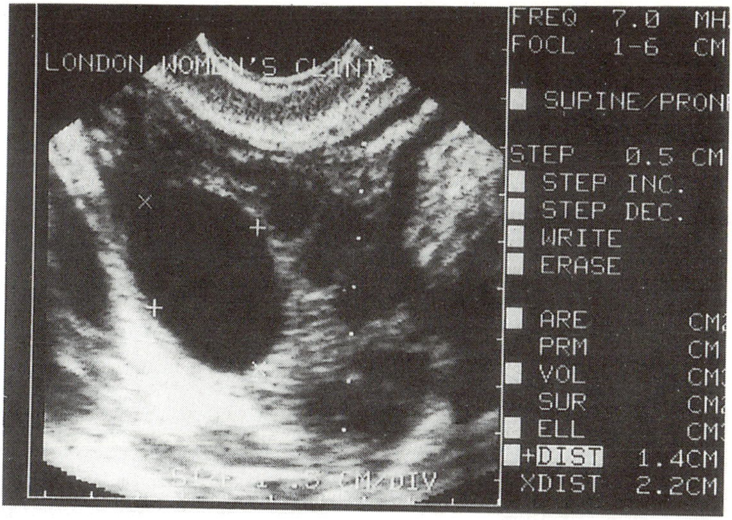

Figure 6.16 Stimulation of a single mature follicle in a polycystic ovary (transvaginal ultrasound scan).

with PCOS than weight-matched controls. Indeed it is hyperinsulinemia that many feel is the key to the pathogenesis of the syndrome as insulin stimulates androgen secretion by the ovarian stroma and appears to affect the normal development of ovarian follicles, both by the adverse effects of androgens on follicular growth and possibly also by suppressing apoptosis and permitting the survival of follicles otherwise destined to disappear (see Ch. 7).

The management of the PCOS is symptom-oriented. While obesity worsens the symptoms, the metabolic scenario conspires against weight loss. Initial reports of the use of insulin-sensitizing agents (e.g., metformin, D-*chiro*-inositol)[25,26] have been encouraging and suggest an improvement in biochemistry, symptoms and an increase in fertility. Ovulation induction has traditionally involved the use of clomiphene citrate and then gonadotropin therapy or laparoscopic ovarian surgery in those who are clomiphene resistant. The principles of management of anovulatory infertility are firstly to optimize health before commencing therapy, for example weight loss for those who are overweight, and then induce regular unifollicular ovulation, while minimizing the risks of OHSS and multiple pregnancy.

Endocrine and Metabolic Factors in Anovulation

Hypersecretion of LH is particularly associated with menstrual disturbances and infertility (Table 6.7 and Fig. 6.16). Indeed, it is this endocrine feature that appears to result in reduced conception rates

Table 6.7 Serum LH concentrations (i.u./L) with respect to fertility status[21]	
Proven fertility	7.2 ± 2.1
Untested fertility	7.4 ± 2.2
Primary infertility	11.0 ± 2.2[a]
Secondary infertility	9.0 ± 2.0[b]

[a] Different from proven fertile and secondary infertile groups.
[b] Different from proven fertile group.

and increased rates of miscarriage in both natural and assisted conception.[23] The finding of a persistently elevated early to mid-follicular phase LH concentration in a woman who is trying to conceive suggests the need to suppress LH levels by either pituitary desensitization, with a gonadotropin-releasing hormone agonist, or laparoscopic ovarian diathermy. There are, however, no large prospectively randomized trials that demonstrate a therapeutic benefit from a reduction in serum LH concentrations during ovulation induction protocols.

The patient's BMI correlates with both an increased rate of cycle disturbance and infertility,[21,27] secondary to disturbances in insulin metabolism.[28] Even moderate obesity (BMI > 27 kg/m^2) is associated with a reduced chance of ovulation[29] and a body fat distribution leading to an increased waist:hip ratio appears to have a more important effect than body weight alone.[30] Obese women (BMI > 30 kg/m^2) should be encouraged to lose weight. A study by Clark *et al.*[22] looked at the effects of a weight loss and exercise program on women with anovulatory infertility, clomiphene resistance, and a BMI > 30 kg/m^2. The emphasis of the study was a realistic exercise schedule combined with positive reinforcement of a suitable eating program over a 6-month period. Thirteen out of the 18 women enrolled completed the study. Weight loss had a significant effect on endocrine function, ovulation, and subsequent pregnancy. Fasting insulin and serum testosterone concentrations fell and 12 of the 13 subjects resumed ovulation; 11 became pregnant (five naturally). Thus, with appropriate support, patients may ovulate spontaneously without medical therapy. An extension of this study, in women with a variety of diagnoses, demonstrated that in 60 out of 67 subjects weight loss resulted in spontaneous ovulation with lower than anticipated rates of miscarriage and a significant saving in the cost of treatment.[31]

Weight loss should also be encouraged prior to ovulation induction treatments, as they appear to be less effective when the BMI is greater than 28–30 kg/m^2.[32] It has been shown that insulin sensitizing agents such as metformin ameliorate hyperandrogenism and abnormalities of gonadotropin secretion in women with PCOS[33,34] and can restore menstrual cyclicity and fertility.[35]

Insulin Sensitizing Agents

Not all authors agree that metformin is beneficial,[36] particularly if there is no weight loss with metformin therapy.[37] The insulin-sensitizing agent troglitazone also appeared significantly to improve the metabolic and reproductive abnormalities in PCOS[38] although this product has been withdrawn because of reports of fatal liver damage. The new generation of thiazolidinediones (rosiglitazone and pioglitazone) may be of benefit to the older woman with PCOS but should not be prescribed to women wishing to conceive because of an uncertain safety profile in pregnancy. Newer insulin sensitizing agents are currently being evaluated, as is the phosphoglycan containing drug D-*chiro*-inositol.[26]

Metformin is the most promising and safe sensitizer to insulin available in the UK. The major concern with biguanides has been the risk of lactic acidosis. This is a very rare and serious metabolic complication of metformin therapy, occurring mainly in women with renal impairment and does not appear to be a problem for otherwise fit women with PCOS who are not frankly diabetic and who have normal renal and liver function. The most commonly reported minor side effects of metformin include bloating, nausea, vomiting, flatulence and diarrhoea. These symptoms appear to be dose-dependent and may be substantially minimised by taking the tablet with meals. It is likely that an incremental dosage protocol (500 mg up to 850 mg initially once and then twice daily) will be helpful to acclimatise patients and minimise undesirable gastrointestinal complaints.

In the last few years a number of mostly uncontrolled short-term studies have assessed the effects of metformin on insulin sensitivity and endocrine profile in women with PCOS. Velazquez *et al* 1994[25] demonstrated that an improvement in insulin sensitivity induced by 1500 gm of metformin a day for 8 weeks leads to a favourable change in serum concentrations of androgens, SHBG and gonadotropins. Metformin resulted in a rapid fall in insulin and the insulin to glucose ratio with a concurrent significant decrease in serum concentrations of testosterone (T), free T, DHEAS and androstenedione.[25] A significant increase in the concentration of SHBG was also noted. As far as gonadotropin concentrations were concerned there was a significant decrease in LH concentrations, an increase in FSH and a normalisation of the LH:FSH ratio.

However, not all the data has been so encouraging. Two trials with essentially identical recruitment criteria and using slightly higher doses of metformin (850 mg twice and three times a day) over similar lengths of time, showed little or no benefit with respect to insulin metabolism, hormone concentrations or lipid variables in a study that was designed to balance dietary intake and sustain body weight, found that hyperinsulinaemia and androgen excess in obese non diabetic women with PCOS were not improved by the administration of high dose metformin.[37,38] The reasons for these disagreements are unclear but could be due to different methods used to assess insulin action and large BMI differences (29 versus 39 Kg/m^2) between the study groups. In fact, it has been claimed that the ability of metformin to alter insulin sensitivity in individuals with major obesity (BMI of 40 Kg/m^2 and above) is limited.[39]

Metformin, by reducing fasting insulin and insulin response to glucose in hyperinsulinaemic PCOS patients, reduces the hyperinsulinemia-driven hyperandrogenism and can reverse the endocrinopathy, often enough to allow regular menstrual cycles, reversal of infertility and spontaneous pregnancy. The achievement of normal menstrual cycles may also reduce the risk of endometrial hyperplasia and adenocarcinoma associated with PCOS.

Evidence supporting ovarian responsiveness to metformin has accumulated from several institutions through small studies published during the past decade. For example, among 22 PCOS patients receiving metformin for 6 months, Velazquez *et al*[35] demonstrated a restoration of menstrual cyclicity in 96% of oligo/amenorrhoeic women. This menstrual regularisation was accompanied by an ovulatory response in 87% of patients with regular menses and of pregnancy rates of 19%. All patients who had normalisation of menstrual irregularities showed a metformin-induced reduction in insulin levels at baseline and after a glucose load that was associated with a substantial decrease in serum-free T concentrations and the LH/FSH ratio.

Similarly, an extensive two-year investigation of 43 amenorrhoeic, hyperinsulinaemic PCOS patients treated with metformin demonstrated the return of normal menses in more than 90% of women.[40] Many other studies have shown, to varying degrees, improvements in both spontaneous and drug-induced ovulatory function, development of normal menses and restoration of fertility, independent of changes in body weight. Indeed a significant decline in serum concentrations of testosterone and LH occurred within one week in a small group of patients indicating a rapid effect of metformin on ovarian function.[41] The reasons for the striking differences in clinical response to metformin might reflect the heterogeneity in the pathogenesis of the syndrome and different patient populations.

Metformin is not an ovulation induction agent. Indeed, unlike gonadotropins or CC, metformin does not accelerate ovarian follicular recruitment or growth. Rather, the physiologic aim of metformin therapy in PCOS is the resumption of normal, monofollicular gonadal function. Metformin has no known direct stimulant effect on the ovarian stromal or germ-cell compartment. Therefore, there is no associated increased risk for multiple gestation when metformin is used to enhance fertility in PCOS. While many women with PCOS may benefit from treatment with insulin-lowering agents, the ideal candidates for such therapy are probably those who are overweight with elevated serum androgen concentrations and/or fasting insulin levels ≥ 10mU/l.

Metformin can increase the frequency of induced ovulation in previously CC resistant patients. Administration of metformin to 11 CC resistant women with a mean BMI of 38 kg/m^2 was shown to increase the number of ovulatory cycles induced with CC by almost three fold and increase the pregnancy rate by almost eight fold compared with a control group given a placebo.[42] In addition a conception rate of 21% after ovulation, similar to normal cycle fecundity, was observed suggesting that combined metformin and CC use have no adverse effects on postovulatory reproductive events.

A study by Nestler *et al*,[43] involved the prescription of metformin (500 mg t.d.s.) or placebo to 61 women with a mean BMI of 32 kg/m^2 for 35 days, by which time 12 of the 35 who received metformin had ovulated (34%) compared with only 1 of the 26 given placebo (4%, $p < 0.001$). On day 35 of the study all those who had yet to ovulate were given clomiphene citrate (50 mg for 5 days) and progesterone measured after 11 and 19 days, when the study was stopped. Of the 21 who received metformin and CC, 19 had ovulated (90%) compared with only 2 of the 25 given placebo and CC (8%, $p < 0.001$). This study provided striking results in the absence of a change in BMI, yet criticisms have been made about the study design (with assessment finishing 19 days after CC administration) and the surprisingly low rate of ovulation in the CC/placebo group.

The largest prospective RCT to date is that of Fleming and colleagues[44] who randomized 94 patients to receive either metformin 850 mg bd or placebo. Interestingly, significantly more patients withdrew in the metformin arm due to side effects (15 versus 5, $p < 0.05$). The patients treated with metformin were found to have an increased rate of ovulation (23% vs 13%, $p < 0.01$) and a quicker first time to ovulation (24 vs 42 days, $p < 0.05$). Significant weight loss was reported in the treated group, whilst the placebo group gained weight ($p < 0.05$) over the 14 weeks of therapy, although glucose tolerance was not improved in either group. The study also a reported an inverse relationship between body mass and efficacy of metformin.

Improvements in ovulatory function in women given metformin plus CC or FSH may be due to a decrease in the direct effects of insulin on ovary, to the normalisation of clomiphene-induced gonadotropin secretion or to a direct tissue-sensitizing effect of the drug at the ovarian level. Differences in the reported studies may be due to variations in patient populations, definitions of PCOS, degrees of obesity and insulin resistance and the definition of clomiphene citrate resistance (that is failure of response or failure of conception).

Clomiphene Citrate Therapy (Table 6.8 and Fig. 6.17)

Antiestrogen therapy with clomiphene citrate or tamoxifen has traditionally been used as first line therapy for anovulatory PCOS. Clomiphene citrate has been available for many years and its use has tended not to have been closely monitored. There have been no prospective, randomized studies comparing the efficacy of clomiphene citrate with other therapies[45] and it may be time to rethink our approach to the initial mangement of anovulation.

Antiestrogen therapy should be commenced on day 2 of the cycle and given for 5 days. If the patient has oligo/amenorrhea it is necessary to exclude pregnancy and then induce a withdrawal bleed with a 5-day course of medroxyprogesterone acetate 10–20 mg (or norethisterone 5 mg). The starting dose of clomiphene is 50 mg. If the patient has not menstruated by day 35 and she is not pregnant, a withdrawal bleed should be induced. The dose should only be increased if there is no response after three cycles as, of those women who will respond to 50 mg, only two-thirds will do so in the first cycle. Doses of 150 mg or more confer no benefit and only worsen the side-effects, particularly of a more tenacious cervical mucus. If there is an exuberant response to 50 mg, as in some women with PCOS, the dose can be decreased to 25 mg. Antiestrogen therapy should be discontinued if the patient is anovulatory after the dose has been increased up to 100 mg for clomiphene citrate or from 20 mg to 40 mg for tamoxifen. If the patient

Table 6.8 Protocol for clomiphene citrate therapy

Pre-treatment investigations: semen analysis, assessment of tubal patency	
If BMI > 30 kg/m^2 advise weight loss and consider metformin therapy	
Monitoring of therapy:	serial ultrasound scans until response is confirmed gold standard would be ultrasound monitoring for each cycle luteal phase progesterone each cycle mid-follicular phase (day 8) LH in first cycle of a new dose consider postcoital test if not pregnant after three cycles
Dose: start with 50 mg, increase to 100 mg if no response and drop to 25 mg if over-response	

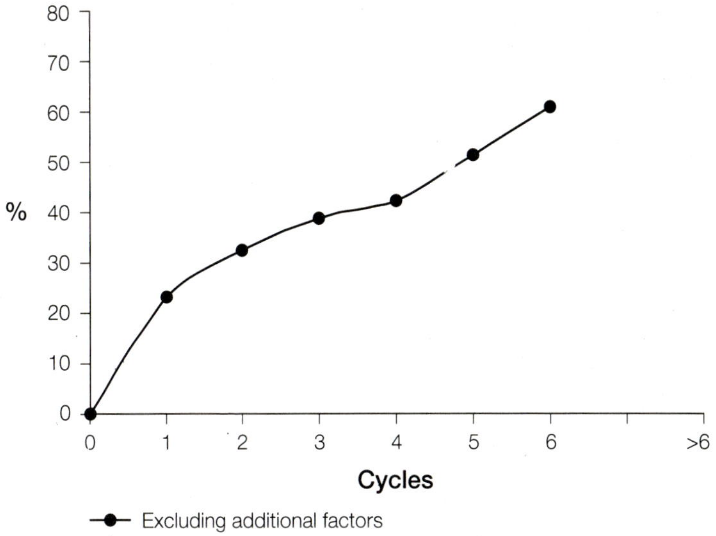

Figure 6.17 Use of clomiphene citrate in induction of ovulation. (From Kousta *et al.* (1997) *Hum Reprod Update* **3**: 359.)[49]

is ovulating, it is not necessary to increase the dose if conception does not occur and conception is expected to occur at a rate determined by factors such as the patient's age. Clomiphene can cause thickening of the cervical mucus and this can impede passage of sperm through the cervix. A postcoital test may be a good idea if a pregnancy hasn't occurred after 3 cycles of treatment.[46]

Monitoring

All women who are prescribed clomiphene should be carefully monitored with a combination of endocrine and ultrasonographic assessment of follicular growth and ovulation because of the risk of multiple pregnancy (see Fig. 6.15). Clomiphene therapy should therefore be prescribed and managed by specialists in reproductive medicine, or, in some cases, by GPs who have access to ultrasound monitoring.

An ovulatory trigger in the form of human chorionic gonadotropin (hCG) is very rarely required and should only be given if there has been repeated evidence of an unruptured follicle, by ultrasound and serum progesterone monitoring. When an ovulatory dose is reached it is useful to confirm that a correctly timed postcoital test is normal or alternatively assess the cervical mucus at the time of ovulation. Women with PCOS should have a measurement of LH on day 8 in a cycle that follows an ovulatory cycle; if the LH is > 10 i.u./L the chance of conception is reduced and risk of miscarriage is elevated. In this case the options include laparoscopic ovarian diathermy or gonadotropin therapy (see below). Side-effects of clomiphene include visual disturbances (stop drug immediately), multiple pregnancy (in about 10%), abdominal distension, ovarian cysts, hot flushes, breast tenderness, dizziness, nausea. Some women who experience troublesome side-effects with clomiphene benefit from tamoxifen (20–40 mg, days 2–6). Monitoring should be the same as for clomiphene.

Results of clomiphene citrate therapy

Clomiphene citrate induces ovulation in approximately 70–85% of patients although only 40–50% conceive.[47] It has been suggested that the most important reason for reduced overall pregnancy rates with clomiphene citrate therapy is discontinuation of therapy and that cumulative conception rates approach 100% after 10 cycles, when corrected for those who discontinue therapy (which might be considered to be a rather biased way of analyzing data).[47] None the less, there is no doubt that the majority of cycles of clomiphene citrate treatment go unmonitored and it is recommended that at least the first cycle of treatment, if not all cycles, should be monitored with a combination of serial ultrasound scans and serum endocrinology.[48] Kousta *et al.*[49] reported treatment of 167 patients with clomiphene citrate in whom there was a cumulative conception rate of 67% over 6 months in those who had no other subfertility factors, which continued to rise up to 12 cycles of therapy (see Fig. 6.17). They reported a multiple pregnancy rate of 11%, similar to that described in other series, and a miscarriage rate of 23.6%, with those who miscarried tending to have a higher serum LH concentration immediately after clomiphene administration. Reviews about the safety of clomiphene citrate with respect to congenital anomalies indicate that there is no increased risk.[50,51]

Shoham and colleagues[52] studied the hormonal profiles in a series of 41 women treated with clomiphene citrate, of whom 28 ovulated. In those who ovulated, 17 exhibited normal patterns of hormone secretion and five conceived, while 11 exhibited an abnormal response, characterized by significantly elevated serum concentrations of LH from day 9 until the LH surge, together with premature luteinization and higher estradiol levels throughout the cycle (none of the patients with this abnormal response conceived). This strengthens the argument for careful monitoring of therapy and discontinuation if the response is abnormal. A useful approach for clomiphene-resistant patients is the administration of progesterone prior to clomiphene citrate treatment,[53] which at an intramuscular dose of 50 mg over 5 days caused a suppression of FSH and LH secretion. LH levels fell in seven out of 10 women treated with progesterone, all became responsive to clomiphene (those whose LH levels were not suppressed remained unresponsive), and three conceived in the first cycle of treatment.

Clomiphene is currently licenced for only 6 months' use in the UK as the initial application for the license was only made for 6 months. It has been suggested that there is an association between clomiphene and ovarian cancer with more than 12 months' therapy, although in most cases of prolonged use the indication was unexplained infertility rather than anovulation.[54] It would seem reasonable that patients should be counseled about the possible risks if treatment is to continue beyond 6 months. If pregnancy has not occurred after 10–12 normal ovulatory cycles it is then appropriate to offer the couple assisted conception.

The therapeutic options for patients with anovulatory infertility who are resistant to antiestrogens are either parenteral gonadotropin therapy or laparoscopic ovarian diathermy. The role of metformin therapy is still being evaluated (see above). The term clomiphene resistance should be applied to mean failure to ovulate (i.e., no response) rather than failure to conceive despite ovulation, which should be termed clomiphene failure.

Gonadotropin Therapy

Gonadotropin therapy is indicated for women with anovulatory PCOS who have been treated with antiestrogens if they have failed to ovulate or if they have a response to clomiphene that is likely to reduce their chance of conception (e.g., persistent hypersecretion of LH, or antiestrogenic effect on cervical mucus).

In order to prevent the risks of overstimulation and multiple pregnancy, the traditional standard step-up regimens (when 75–150 i.u. are increased by 75 i.u. every 3–5 days[55] have been replaced by either low-dose step-up regimens[56,57] or step-down regimens (Fig. 6.18).[58] The low-dose step-up regimen employs a starting dose of 25–50 i.u., which is only increased after 14 days if there is no response and then by only half an ampoule every 7 days.[57] Treatment cycles using this approach can be quite long – up to 28–35 days – but the risk of multiple follicular growth is lower than with conventional step-up regimens. With the step-down protocol, follicular recruitment is achieved using 150–225 i.u. daily for 3 or 4 days before decreasing the dose to 50–75 i.u. to maintain follicular development.[58,59] Experimental studies have indicated that initiation of follicular growth requires a 10–30% increment in the dose of exogenous FSH and the threshold changes with follicular growth, due to an increased number of FSH receptors, so that the concentration of FSH required to maintain growth is less than that required to initiate it.[60] More recently, a sequential step-up, step-down protocol has been employed, in which the FSH threshold dose is reduced by half when the leading follicle has reached 14 mm.[61] This approach also appears to reduce the number of lead follicles when compared with a classic step-up protocol.[61] In all the above-mentioned ovulation induction regimens, gonadotropins are used alone, without a background of pituitary desensitization, which does not confer any advantage. Furthermore the different gonadotropin preparations appear to work equally well.

It can be extremely difficult to predict the response to stimulation of a woman with polycystic ovaries – indeed this is the greatest therapeutic challenge in all ovulation induction therapies. The polycystic ovary is characteristically quiescent, at least when viewed by ultrasound (Fig. 6.19), before often exhibiting an exuberant and explosive response to stimulation. It can be very challenging to stimulate the development of a single dominant follicle, and while attempts have been made to predict a multifollicular response by looking at mid-follicular endocrine profiles and numbers of small follicles, it is harder to do so prior to commencing ovarian stimulation and hence determine the required starting dose of gonadotropin.[62] In order to prevent OHSS and multiple pregnancy, however, the strategy of cancelling cycles on day 8 of stimulation if there are more than seven follicles (≥ 8 mm) seems to be reasonable.[62]

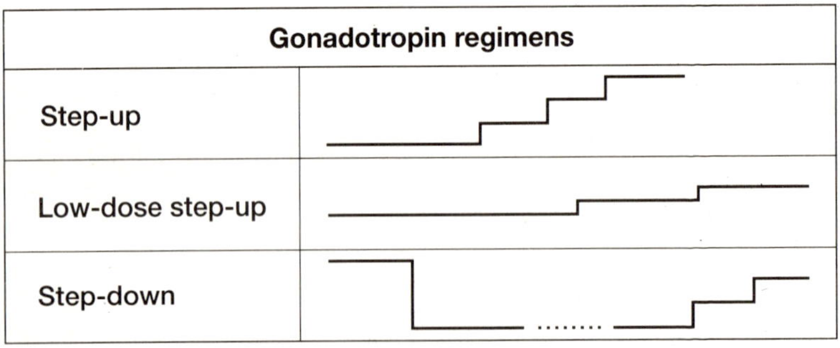

a

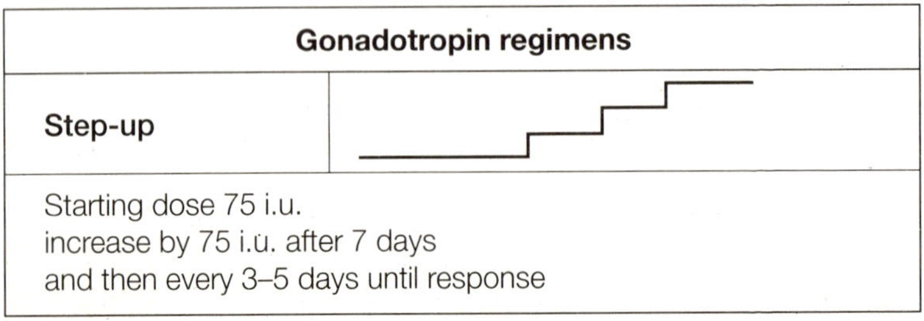

b

Figure 6.18a–b

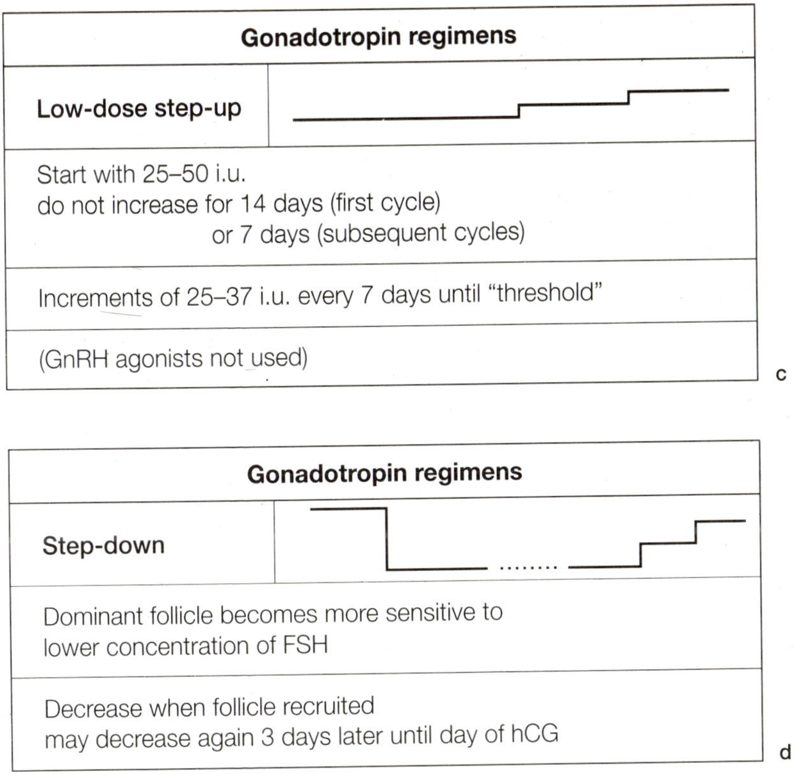

Figure 6.18c–d Gonadotropin step-up and step-down regimens.

White and colleagues[63] reported their extensive experience of the low-dose regimen in 225 women over 934 cycles of treatment resulting in 109 pregnancies in 102 women (45%). Of the cycles, 72% were ovulatory (fewer than 5% of patients failed to ovulate) and 77% of these were uniovulatory. The multiple pregnancy rate was 6%. Despite using a low-dose protocol, 18% of cycles were abandoned because more than three large follicles developed – a further reminder of the sensitivity of the polycystic ovary even when attempts are made to reduce the response. At the start of their series the initial starting dose was 75 i.u. but this was reduced to 0.7 of an ampoule (i.e. 52.5 i.u.) for the last 429 cycles of treatment in order to reduce further the rate of multiple follicle development (84% of cycles with the lower starting dose were uniovulatory). Interestingly, their previously reported miscarriage rate of 35% when the higher starting dose was used fell to 20% when they used the 52.5 i.u. starting dose.[63] Once again it was noted that the only factor that influenced the outcome significantly was the patient's BMI. Those with a BMI > 25 kg/m^2 had a higher rate

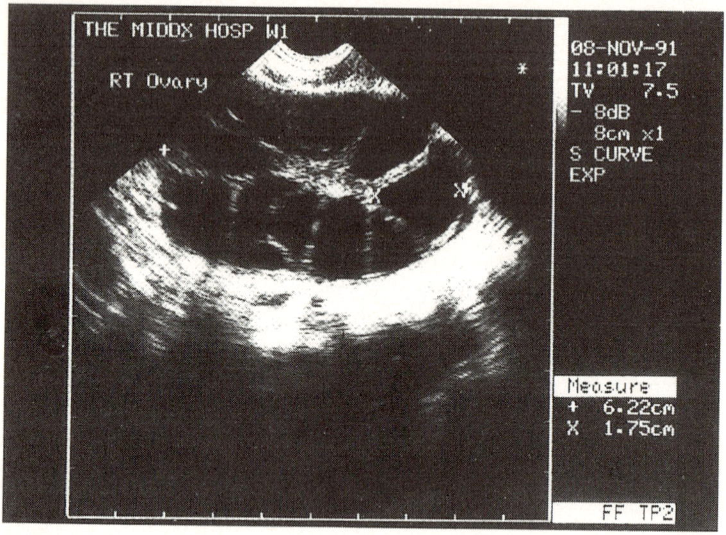

Figure 6.19 . Transvaginal ultrasound scan of an overstimulated polycystic ovary. Both ovaries are likely to have this appearance and the treatment must be discontinued to minimize the risk of multiple pregnancy and ovarian hyperstimulation syndrome.

of abandoned cycles (31% vs 15% in those of normal weight) and a lower cumulative conception rate over six cycles (46.8% vs 57% for the whole group) and a miscarriage rate of 31%. We reported the cumulative conception and live birth rates in 103 women with clomiphene citrate-resitant PCOS (Fig. 6.20).[5] While the cumulative conception and live birth rates after 6 months were 62% and 54%, respectively, and after 12 months 73% and 62%, respectively, the rate of multiple pregnancy was 19% and there were three cases of moderate to severe OHSS. We found that the rate of multiple pregnancy fell to 4% after the introduction of real-time transvaginal ultrasound monitoring of follicular development. This emphasizes the central role of effective surveillance in programs of ovulation induction.[5]

Dosage (Fig. 6.21)

Because of the sensitivity of the polycystic ovary to stimulation by hormones, it is important to start with low doses of gonadotropins and very carefully monitor follicular development by ultrasound scans. Close monitoring should enable treatment to be suspended if three or more follicles develop, as the risk of multiple pregnancy obviously increases.[64] We suggest the algorithm for gonadotropin therapy shown in Figure 6.21.

Treatment with gonadotropins should be commenced within the first 5 days of a natural or induced menstrual bleed, when a pelvic

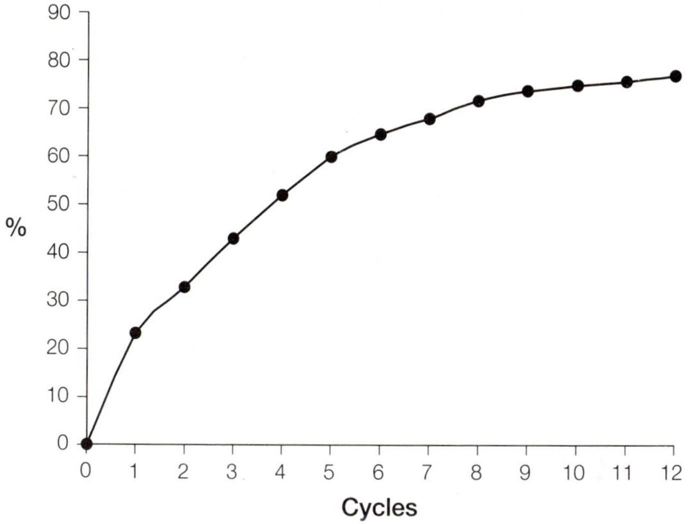

Figure 6.20 Gonadotropin therapy in 103 women with PCOS. (From Balen *et al.* (1994) *Hum Reprod* **9**: 1563.)[5]

ultrasound examination indicates that the endometrium is thin (less than 6 mm in depth) and that there are no ovarian cysts. The initial dose, usually 50 i.u. of FSH, is increased by 25 i.u. per day after 14 days in the first cycle of treatment (and 7 days in subsequent cycles) if there is an inadequate response, as assessed by ultrasound scan. There is no value in increasing the initial dose before the fifth day (at the earliest) as recruitment of follicles takes between 5 and 15 days. Further increases are made at 4–7-day intervals. In subsequent cycles the starting dose is determined by the patient's previous response and can be reduced in some cases to 25 i.u. and increased in others to 100 i.u. or even 150 i.u. per day.

A number of pre-stimulation protocols have been used in order to suppress endogenous pituitary gonadotropin secretion and ovarian activity before commencing gonadotropin therapy. These include treatment for 2–3 months with the combined oral contraceptive pill or with a GnRH agonist for 6–8 weeks. In our view this approach simply prolongs the treatment cycle, resulting in fewer ovulations and hence chances of conception in a given period of time without conferring a significant benefit on the pregnancy rates. The use of GnRH agonists also increases the requirement for FSH. A role for GnRH antagonists in ovulation induction has yet to be found.

Ovulation is triggered with a single injection of human chorionic gonadotropin (hCG) 5000 units (i.m. or s.c.). The inclusion criterion for hCG administration should be the development of at least one follicle of at least 17 mm in its largest diameter. In order to reduce

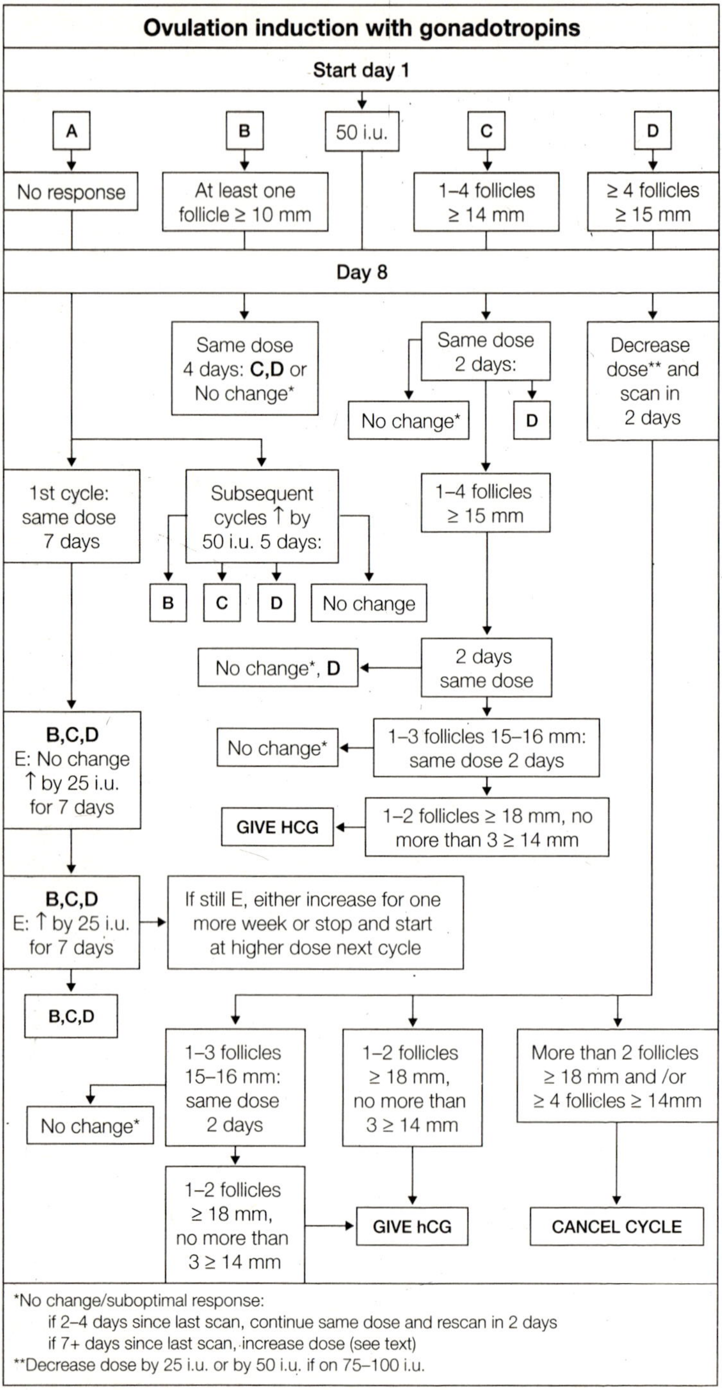

Figure 6.21 Ovulation induction protocol.

the risks of multiple pregnancy and OHSS, the exclusion criteria for hCG administration are the development of a total of three or more follicles larger than 14 mm in diameter. In overstimulated cycles hCG is withheld, and the patient counseled about the risks and advised to refrain from sexual intercourse (Figs 6.22–6.24).

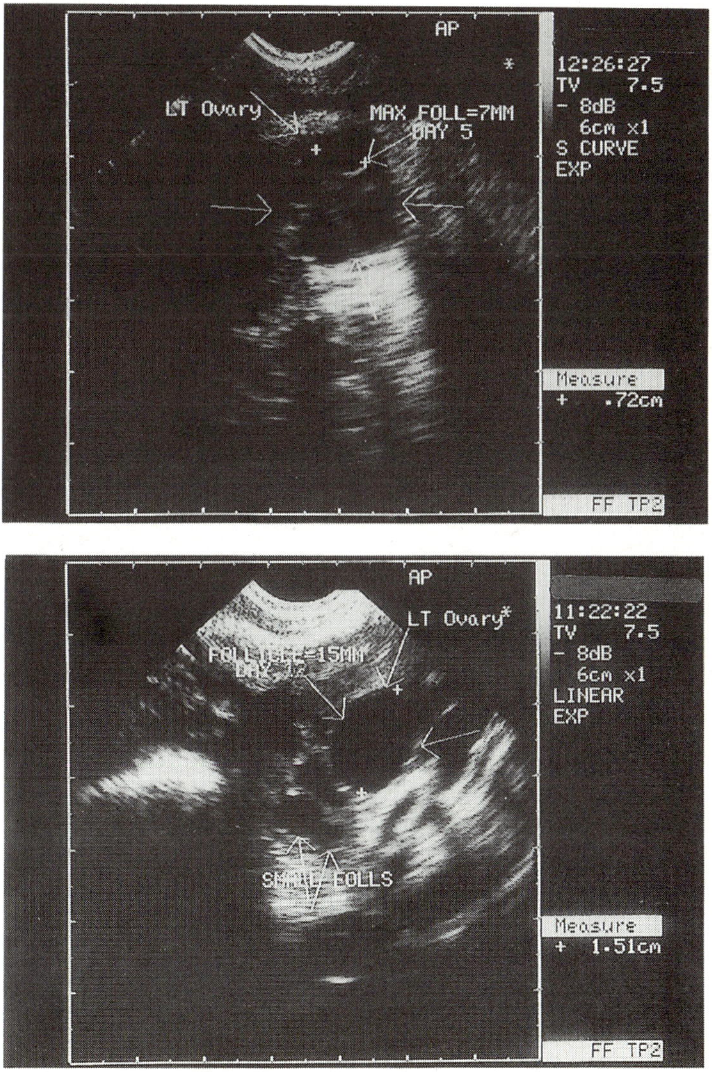

a

b

Figure 6.22a–b Ovulation induction in a polycystic ovary, transvaginal ultrasound monitoring. (**a**) On day 5 the largest follicle has a diameter of 7 mm; (**b**) by day 12 it is 15 mm in diameter.

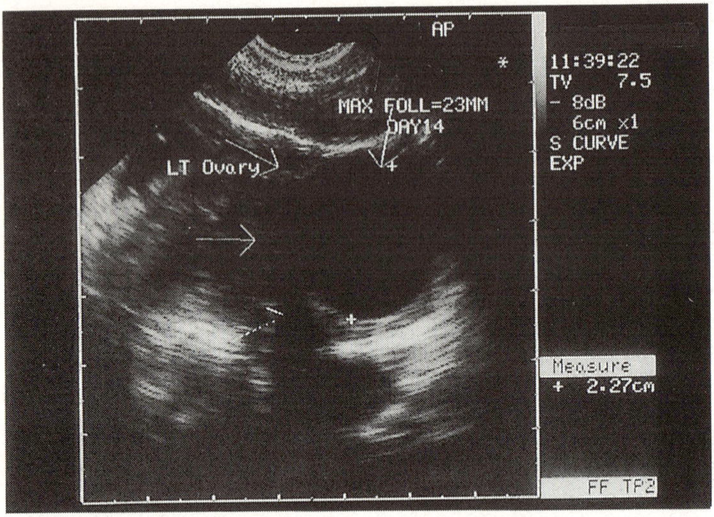

c

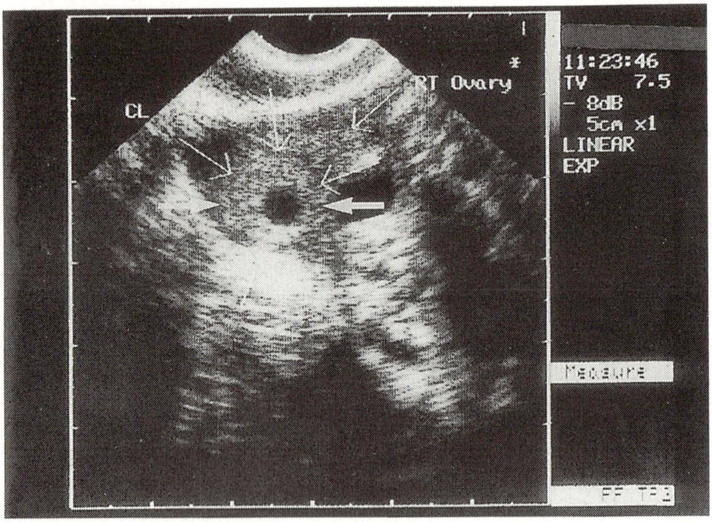

d

Figure 6.22c–d Ovulation induction in a polycystic ovary, transvaginal ultrasound monitoring. (**c**) Two days later the diameter is 23 mm and ovulation can be triggered using hCG 5000–10 000 units. (**d**) Seven days later a corpus luteum should be visualized (between arrows).

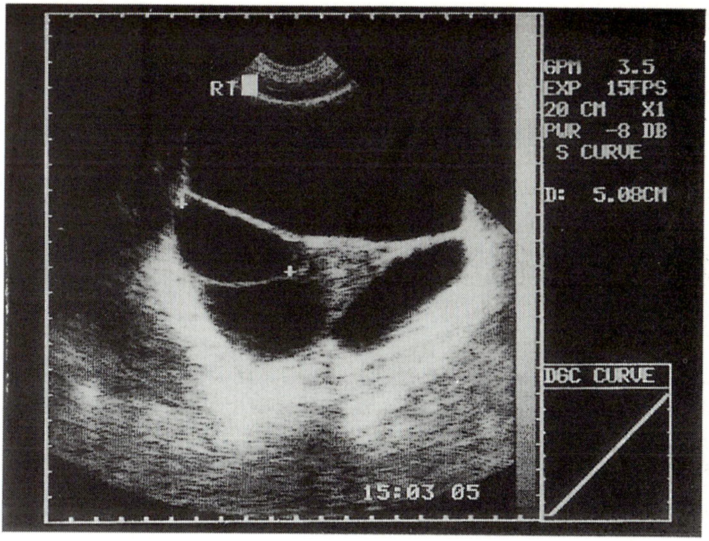

Figure 6.23 Transvaginal ultrasound scan of "luteinized unruptured follicles" (LUF) – in this case four large cysts are seen 7 days after hCG administration. While it is often assumed that cysts represent failure of ovulation, the only actual proof of ovulation is the subsequent fertilization of the egg. An oocyte can be released from a follicle that becomes cystic subsequently.

If conception has failed to occur after six ovulatory cycles in a woman younger than 25 years or after 12 ovulatory cycles in women older than 25, then it can be assumed that anovulation is unlikely to be the cause of the couple's infertility (Fig. 6.25). The couple should have been comprehensively investigated by this stage with a laparoscopy ± hysteroscopy or hysterosalpingography and sperm function tests. If no other explanation has been found for their infertility assisted conception (usually IVF) is now indicated.

Complications of ovulation induction (see also Ch. 17)

Women with PCOS are at an increased risk of developing OHSS.[65] This occurs if many follicles are stimulated, leading to ascites, pleural and, sometimes, pericardial effusions with the symptoms of abdominal distension, discomfort, nausea, vomiting, and difficult breathing. Hospitalization is sometimes necessary in order for intravenous fluids (colloids preferable to crystalloids) and heparin to be given to prevent dehydration and thromboembolism. Although this condition is rare it is a potentially fatal complication and should be avoidable with appropriate monitoring of treatment (see Fig. 6.19) (see also Ch. 17).

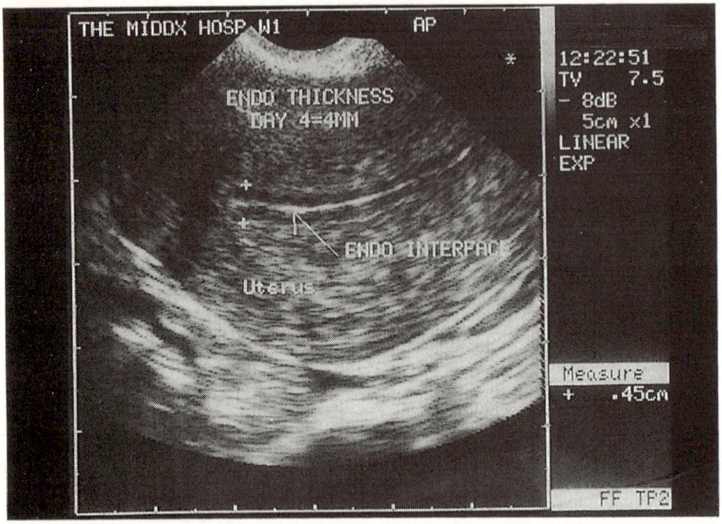

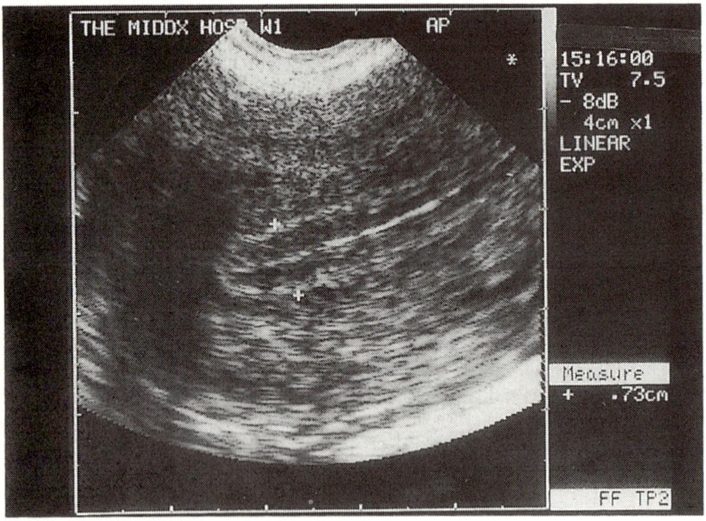

b

Figure 6.24a–b

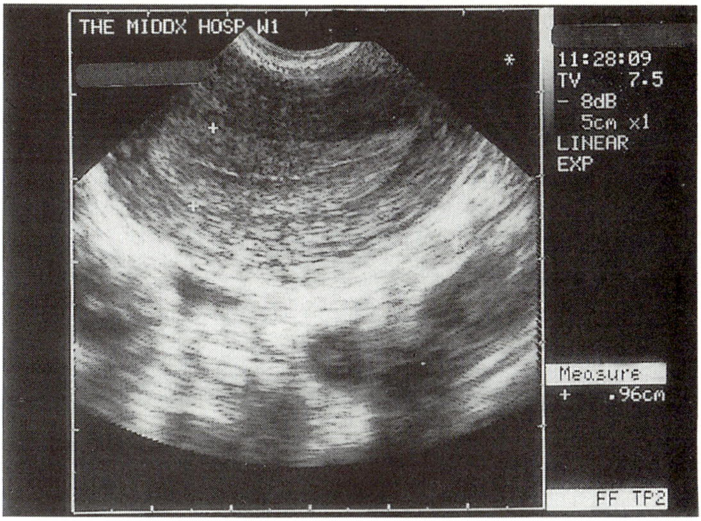

c

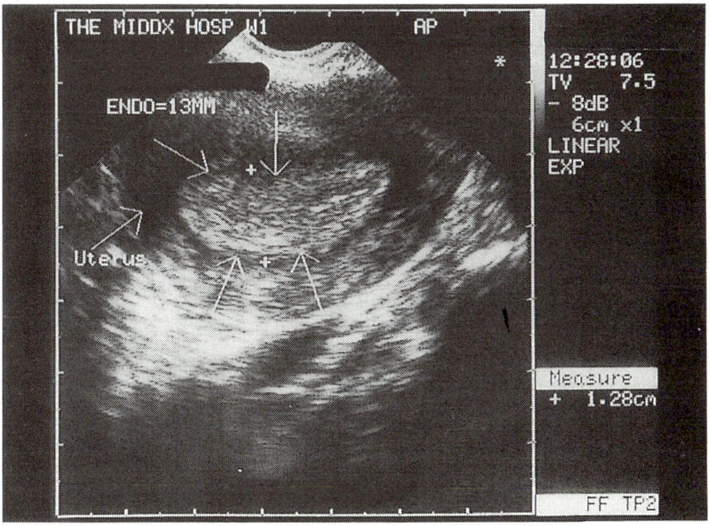

d

Figure 6.24a–d Monitoring of endometrial development during ovulation induction (transvaginal ultrasound): (**a**) Early follicular, thin endometrium (4.5 mm); (**b**) mid-follicular (7 mm); (**c**) preovulatory (9.6 mm); (**d**) mid-luteal, postovulation (13 mm).

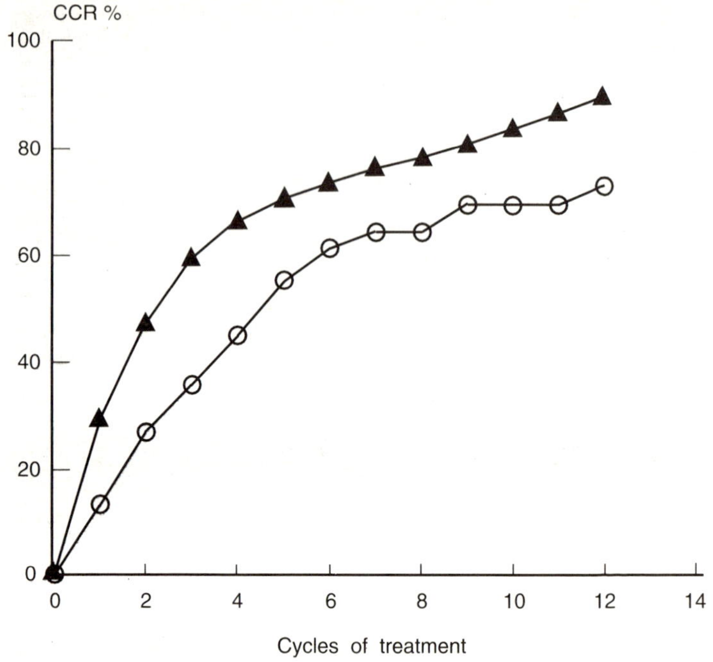

Figure 6.25 Cumulative conception rates over successive cycles in normal women (triangles) and 103 patients with anovulatory PCOS (circles) who have undergone ovulation induction. (From Balen *et al.* (1994), *Hum Reprod* **9**: 1563.)[5]

Multiple pregnancy is the other undesirable side-effect of fertility therapy, first because of the increased rates of perinatal morbidity and mortality and second because of the devastating effects on the family of caring for a large number of babies. In the UK the unmonitored use of oral antiestrogens accounts for more cases of triplets than gonadotropin therapy or assisted conception. High order multiple pregnancies (quadruplets or more) result almost exclusively from ovulation induction therapies.[64,66] Gonadotropins should be given in low doses to women with anovulatory infertility and strict criteria employed before the administration of the ovulatory trigger. Hull[67] reviewed the results of six studies of conventional dose gonadotropin therapy (111 patients) and compared them with six studies of low dose therapy (243 patients). The pregnancy rates per cycle (23%) and per ovulatory cycle (30%) were higher in the standard dose cycles than during low-dose therapy (11% and 15% respectively). The miscarriage rate was also lower in the standard dose cycles (17% versus 37%), resulting in an ongoing pregnancy rate per cycle of 20% compared with 7% in the low-dose cycles. The multiple pregnancy rate, however, was 23% in the standard dose cycles compared with 9% in the low-dose cycles. It is important to balance the benefits of a higher rate of pregnancy against the potential risks of multiple pregnancy and OHSS (see also Figs 6.26–6.28).

Source of gonadotropins

Gonadotropins are available in the form of urinary-derived hMG or FSH (Table 6.9). The gonadotropins are glycoprotein hormones. Biological activity is determined by the ability of the hormone to bind to its receptors (on granulosa cells) and its persistence in the circulation (its half-life). After the protein structure of the hormone is assembled

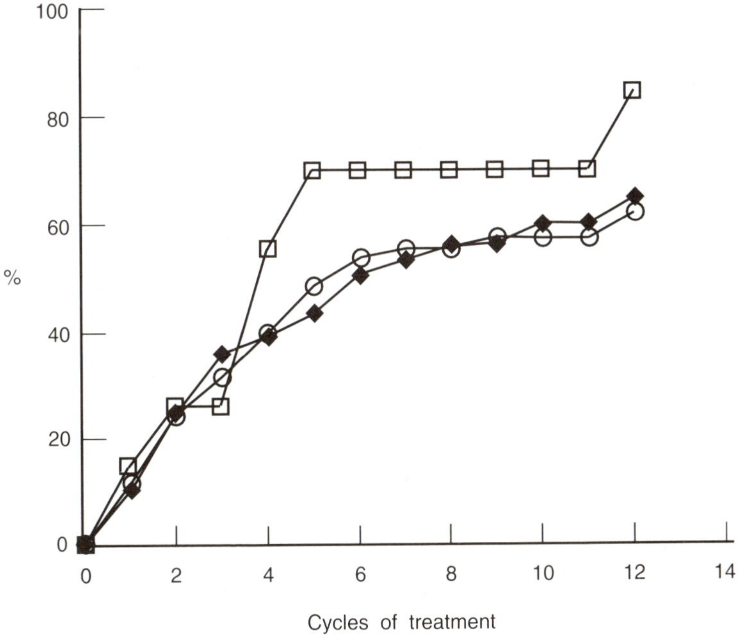

Figure 6.26 Cumulative live birth rate (CLBR): after one course of ovulation induction treatment for patients with PCOS (○, n = 103), hypogonadotropic hypogonadism (◆, n = 77), and weight-related amenorrhea (□, n = 20). (From Balen *et al.* (1994), *Hum Reprod* **9**: 1563, with permission).[5] The miscarriage rates were similar for patients with PCOS and hypogonadotropic hypogonadism, but higher in women with weight-related amenorrhea, leading to similar CLBRs for all three groups. Patients with weight-related amenorrhea should ideally be managed by encouraging weight gain rather than gonadotropin administration to correct their anovulatory infertility.

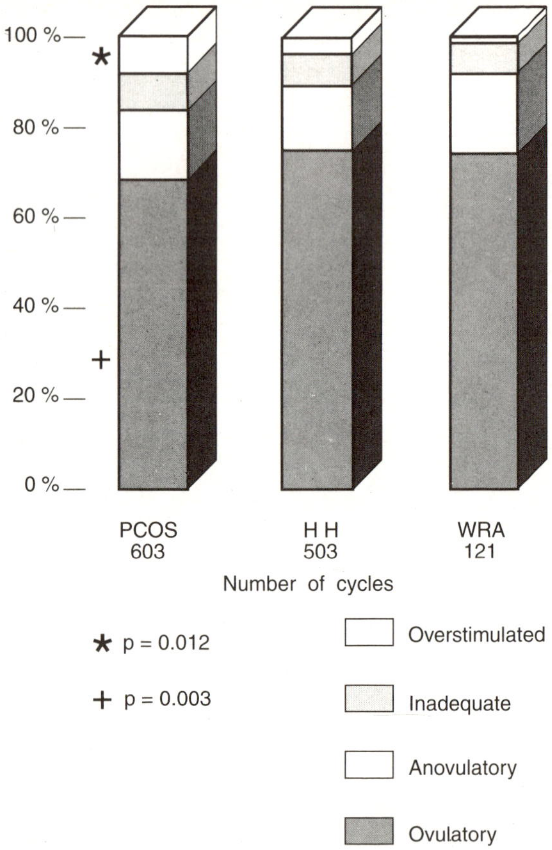

Figure 6.27 Response to treatment: Patients with polycystic ovary syndrome were less likely to have anovulatory cycles – the usual reason being the need to abandon the cycle because of an over exuberant response and the production of too many follicles. (From Balen *et al.* (1994) *Hum Reprod* **9**: 1563.)[5]

in the pituitary cell, the hormone is glycosylated (i.e., carbohydrate moieties are applied to the molecule). These carbohydrate components determine whether the molecule is positively or negatively charged. People in fact secrete a mixture of isoforms, i.e., molecules of the same peptide structure but different carbohydrate component and therefore different acidity and alkalinity. Preparations of gonadotropins which have a preponderance of alkaline isoforms bind well to the receptor but disappear rapidly from the circulation. Those with a low pH (acidic) persist in the circulation well and are thought to have a high total *in vivo* biopotency. The pituitary secretes a range of FSH and LH isoforms, the distribution of which depends on circulating estrogen

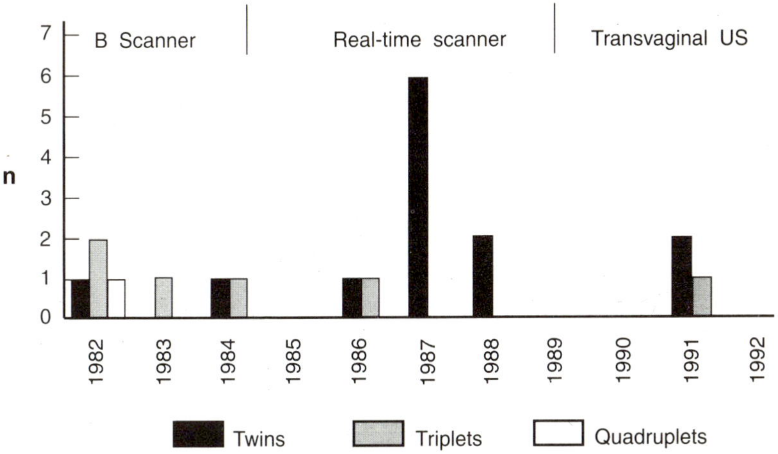

Figure 6.28 Distribution of multiple pregnancies. With the advent of real-time and then transvaginal ultrasonography (US), the rate of multiple pregnancy fell due to the increased accuracy of monitoring and detection of each follicle. (From Balen *et al.* (1994) *Hum Reprod* **9**: 1563.)[5]

Table 6.9 Gonadotropins available in the UK (2003)

Preparation	Trade names	Route	Urinary proteins
Human chorionic gonadotropin (hCG)	Chorogon, Pregnyl, Profasi	i.m./s.c.	++
Recombinant hCG: choriogonadotropin alpha (or α)	Ovitrelle	s.c.	0
Human menopausal gonadotropin (hMG) (FSH:LH = 1:1)	Menogon Menopur	i.m. s.c.	++ +
Urofollitropin (FSH)	Metrodin High Purity	s.c.	+
Recombinant FSH:			
follitropin alpha (or α)	Gonal-F	s.c.	0
follitropin beta (or β)	Puregon	s.c.	0
Recombinant LH: lutropin α	Luveris	s.c.	0

concentrations and other factors. Postmenopausal women secrete highly glycosylated gonadotropins with a long half-life and it is these that are purified from the urine of postmenopausal women to provide the preparations that are in current use. Because of the variation in bioactivity of the urinary-derived gonadotropins the allowable range in each ampoule is 20% either side of the mean – in other words between 60 and 94 units of activity in a 75-unit ampoule (a potential variation of up to 64% between ampoules from different batches). The original preparations of hMG were administered intramuscularly, while more purified preparations can now be given by subcutaneous injections, which can be self-administered and are tolerated better by the patient.

Recombinantly derived FSH, hCG, and LH are synthesized by transfecting the human gonadotropin genes into Chinese hamster ovary cell lines and are now widely available for therapeutic use. These preparations have far greater purity and homogeneity than the urinary-derived gonadotropins. There is heterogeneity between the different recombinantly derived preparations; in other words there is no single "physiological" preparation of FSH.

Hypersecretion of LH appears to have a significant effect on conception and miscarriage. Initial, non-randomized reports of GnRH agonist therapy in PCOS described encouraging rates of pregnancy but prospective randomized studies have indicated that using GnRH agonists during ovulation induction regimens provides no benefit over hMG therapy alone and, in particular, does not reduce the tendency of the polycystic ovary to multifollicular development, cyst formation, or OHSS. The "purified" and recombinant FSH preparations or those with a reduced LH content confer no therapeutic advantage over hMG as the LH content in hMG is trivial compared with the endogenous secretion of LH.

Surgical Ovulation Induction (Table 6.10 and Figs 6.29–6.31)

An alternative to gonadotropin therapy for clomiphene-resistant PCOS is laparoscopic ovarian surgery, which has replaced the more invasive and damaging technique of ovarian wedge resection. Laparoscopic ovarian surgery is free of the risks of multiple pregnancy and ovarian hyperstimulation and does not require intensive ultrasound

Table 6.10 Indications for LOD

Anovulatory PCOS:	Clomiphene citrate resistance Persistent hypersecretion of LH Repeated over-response to clomiphene citrate or gonadotropins Patients who find it difficult to travel for regular scans
No value for therapy of long-term effects of PCOS, e.g. hirsutism, obesity	

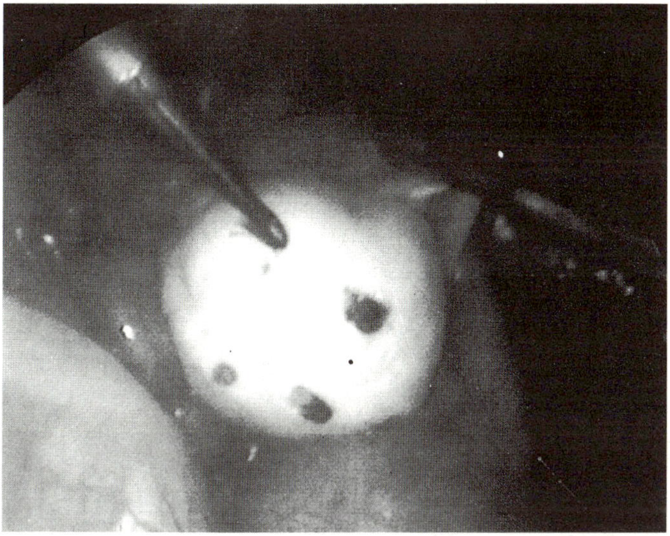

a

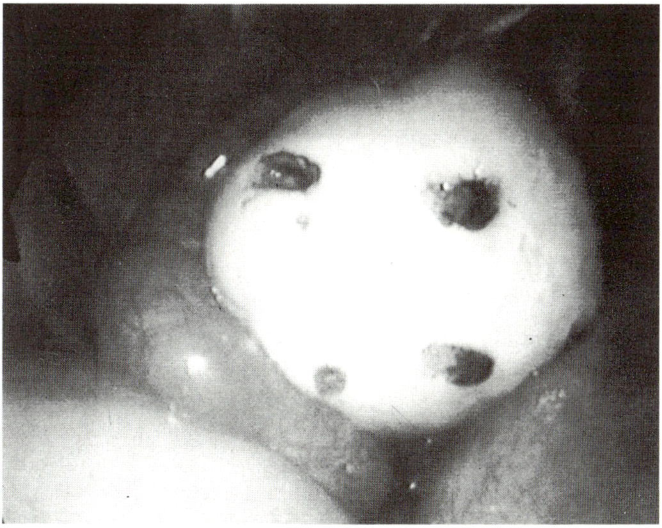

b

Figure 6.29a&b (**a**) Laparoscopic ovarian diathermy. The needle enters the ovarian capsule while the ovarian ligament is held steady, with the ovary supported on the front of the uterus. (**b**) At the end of the procedure the ovary has been diathermized at four sites (please refer to plate section for color figures).

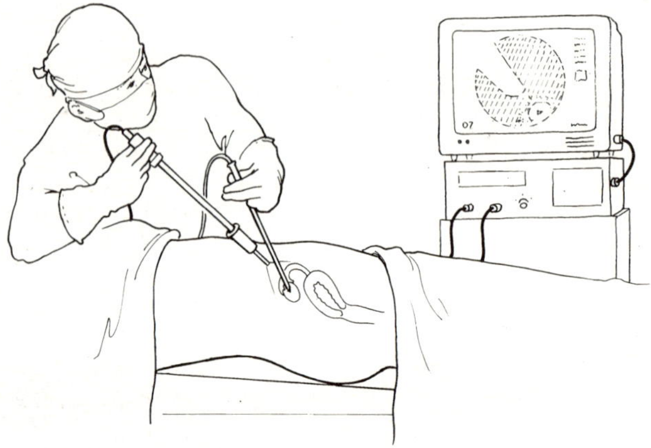

Figure 6.30 Laparoscopic ovarian diathermy.

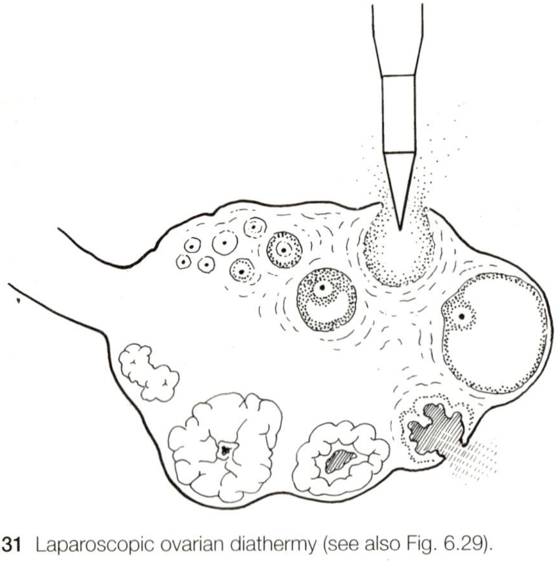

Figure 6.31 Laparoscopic ovarian diathermy (see also Fig. 6.29).

monitoring. Furthermore, ovarian diathermy appears to be as effective as routine gonadotropin therapy in the treatment of clomiphene-insensitive PCOS.[68,69] In addition, laparoscopic ovarian surgery is a useful therapy for anovulatory women with PCOS who fail to respond to clomiphene and who persistently hypersecrete LH, or need a laparoscopic assessment of their pelvis, or who live too far away from the hospital to be able to attend for the intensive monitoring required in gonadotropin therapy. Surgery does, of course, carry its own risks and must be performed only by fully trained laparoscopic surgeons.

After laparoscopic ovarian surgery, with restoration of ovarian activity serum concentrations of LH and testosterone fall.[70] A fall in serum LH concentrations both increases the chance of conception and reduces the risk of miscarriage, as demonstrated by Armar & Lachelin,[71] who observed a miscarriage rate of 14% in 58 pregnancies compared with the expected miscarriage rate of 30–40% seen in reports of hormonal induction of ovulation in women with PCOS.[72] Whether patients respond to laparoscopic ovarian diathermy (LOD) appears to depend on their pre-treatment characteristics, with patients with high basal LH concentrations having a better clinical and endocrine response.[73] Indeed neither the pre-treatment testosterone level, body mass index nor ovarian volume could be used to predict outcome[72]. We performed a small prospective study in which we randomized women to receiving either unilateral or bilateral LOD.[74] We found that unilateral diathermy restored bilateral ovarian activity, with the contralateral, untreated ovary often being the first to ovulate after the diathermy treatment. We also found that the only significant difference between the responders and non-responders was a post-diathermy fall in serum LH concentration.

While the mechanism of ovulation induction by LOD is uncertain, it appears that minimal damage to an unresponsive ovary either restores an ovulatory cycle or increases the sensitivity of the ovary to exogenous stimulation. Furthermore, the finding of an attenuated response of LH secretion to stimulation with GnRH[75] suggests an effect on ovarian–pituitary feedback and hence pituitary sensitivity to GnRH. Our study went one step further by demonstrating that unilateral diathermy leads to bilateral ovarian activity, suggesting that ovarian diathermy achieves its effect by correcting a perturbation of ovarian–pituitary feedback.[74] Our own hypothesis is that the response of the ovary to injury leads to a local cascade of growth factors and those such as IGF1, which interact with FSH, result in stimulation of follicular growth and the production of the hormone gonadotropin surge attenuating/inhibitory factor (GnSAF/GnSIF) which leads to a fall in serum LH concentrations.[76]

Commonly employed methods for laparoscopic surgery include monopolar electrocautery (diathermy)[77] and laser,[78] while multiple biopsy alone is less commonly used. In the first reported series, ovarian diathermy resulted in ovulation in 90% and conception in 70% of the 62 women treated.[77] A number of subsequent studies have produced similarly encouraging results, although the techniques used and degree of ovarian damage vary considerably. Gjonnaess[77] cauterized each ovary at five to eight points, for 5–6 seconds at each point with 300–400 watts. Naether *et al.*[79] treated five to 20 points per ovary, with 400 watts for approximately 1 second. They found that the rate of adhesions was 19.3% and 16.6% when peritoneal lavage with saline was used.[80] In an earlier study, Naether *et al.*[81] found that the post-diathermy fall in serum testosterone concentration was proportional to the degree of ovarian damage, with up to 40 cauterization sites being used in some patients. The greater the amount of damage to the surface of the ovary, the greater the risk of periovarian adhesion formation. This led Armar *et al.*[82] to develop a strategy of minimizing the number of diathermy points to four per ovary for 4 seconds at 40 watts; it is this last technique that we favor. The high pregnancy rate (86% of those with no other pelvic abnormality) reported by Armar & Lachelin[71] indicates that the small number of diathermy points used leads to a low rate of significant adhesion formation.

Wedge resection of the ovaries resulted in significant adhesions – in 100% of cases in some published series. The risk of adhesion formation is far less after laparoscopic ovarian diathermy (10–20% of cases) and the adhesions that do form are usually fine and of limited clinical significance. Our technique involves instilling 200 ml Hartmann's solution or Adept® into the pouch of Douglas, which, by cooling the ovaries, prevents heat injury to adjacent tissues and reduces the adhesion formation. The risk of periovarian adhesion formation may be further reduced by abdominal lavage and early second-look laparoscopy, with adhesiolysis if necessary.[83] We have also used liberal peritoneal lavage to good effect.[82] In another study 40 women undergoing laser photocoagulation of the ovaries using an Nd-YAG laser set at 50 W at 20–25 points per ovary were randomized to a second-look laparoscopy and adhesiolysis.[84] Of those who underwent a second-look laparoscopy, adhesions that were described as minimal or mild were found in 68% yet adhesiolysis did not appear to be necessary as the cumulative conception rate after 6 months was 47% compared with 55% in the expectantly managed group (not a statistically significant difference).

It is suggested that a minimum amount of ovarian destruction should be employed. Furthermore, a combined approach may be suitable for some women whereby low dose diathermy is followed by low dose ovarian stimulation. Ostrzenski,[86] for example, commenced all his patients on either clomiphene or FSH therapy immediately after laser wedge resection and Farhi *et al.*[81] also demonstrated an increased ovarian sensitivity to gonadotropin therapy after LOD. Now that we recognize the importance of insulin resistance in the pathophysiology of anovulation in PCOS, studies are needed of the use of metformin in patients who do not ovulate after LOD.

An additional concern is the possibility of ovarian destruction leading to ovarian failure, an obvious disaster in a woman wishing to conceive. Cases of ovarian failure have been reported after both wedge resection and laparoscopic surgery.[82] An unfortunate vogue has developed whereby women with polycystic ovaries who have over-responded to *superovulation* for IVF are subjected to ovarian diathermy as a way of reducing the likelihood of subsequent OHSS.[83] If one accepts that appropriately performed ovarian diathermy works by sensitizing the ovary to FSH then one could extrapolate that ovarian diathermy prior to superovulation for IVF should make the ovary *more* and not less likely to overstimulate. The amount of ovarian destruction that is required to reduce the chance of overstimulation is therefore likely to be considerable. We would urge great caution before proceeding with such an approach because of concerns about permanent ovarian atrophy.

Laser treatment seems to be as efficacious as diathermy and it has been suggested that it may result in less adhesion formation,[78,90] although the only study to compare the two techniques was non-randomized, reported similar ovulation and pregnancy rates, and did not examine adhesion formation.[90] Various types of laser have been used, from the CO_2 laser to the Nd:YAG and KTP lasers. As with the use of laser in other spheres of laparoscopic surgery, whether laser or diathermy is employed appears to depend upon the preference of the surgeon and the availability of the equipment.

It has been suggested that to demonstrate a 20% increase in pregnancy rate over 6 months from 50% to 70%, with an 80% power at least 235 patients would be required in each arm of a study to compare LOD with gonadotropin therapy.[91] The current meta-analysis in the Cochrane database includes a total of only 303 women.[91] The first prospective study to suggest that LOD appeared to be as effective as gonadotropin therapy in the treatment of clomiphene-insensitive PCOS prospectively randomised 88 patients,[68] who had failed to conceive after six CC cycles, to receiving either hMG, FSH or LOD. There were no differences in the rates of ovulation or pregnancy between the two groups, although those treated with LOD had fewer cycles with multiple follicular growth and a lower rate of miscarriage.[68] There have been few other prospective randomised studies since that have attempted to compare LOD with gonadotropin therapy. Farquhar *et al*,[92] randomised 50 patients and reported similar and somewhat disappointing cumulative pregnancy rates of 28% at six months for LOD and 33% after three cycles of gonadotropin therapy.

The ongoing pregnancy rate following ovarian drilling compared with gonadotropins differed according to the length of follow up. Overall, the pooled odds ration for all studies was not statistically significant (OR 1.27, 95% CI 0.77, 1.98).[91] Multiple pregnancy rates were reduced in the ovarian drilling arms of the four trials where there was a direct comparison with gonadotropin therapy (OR 0.16, 95%CI 0.03,0.98). There was no difference in miscarriage rates in the drilling group when compared with gonadotropin in these trials (OR 0.61, 955% 0.17, 2.16).[91]

The duration of follow-up varied amongst the studies that were included in the meta-analysis.[91] Furthermore it is difficult to produce a temporal comparison as not all women receiving gonadotropin therapy are treated in consecutive months and so it is therefore necessary to compare treatment cycles. The meta-analysis found that when comparing 6 months after ovarian drilling compared with 6 cycles of gonadotropin therapy the ongoing cumulative pregnancy rate was higher amongst women who received gonadotropins (OR 0.48, 95% CI 0.28, 0.81).[91] One large study (n=168) has only been published in abstract form and involved the administration of clomiphene citrate and then rFSH to those who were anovulatory after LOD.[93] They reported an improved cumulative ongoing pregnancy rate with six cycles of recombinant FSH (67%) compared with LOD six months after surgery (37%) (OR 0.28, 95% CI 0.15-0.52). And after 12 months the OR was 1.37 (95% CI 0.70, 2.69) for ovarian drilling (with the addition of rFSH for women who were anovulatory) compared with rFSH.[93]

Thus it was concluded that there is insufficient evidence of a difference in cumulative ongoing pregnancy rates between laparoscopic ovarian drilling after 6-12 months follow up and 3-6 cycles of ovulation induction with gonadotropins as a primary treatment for subfertile patients with anovulatory PCOS. The greatest advantage is that multiple pregnancy rates are considerably reduced.[91]

Summary (Table 6.11 and Fig. 6.32)

The underlying principle of all methods of ovulation induction for women with polycystic ovary syndrome must always be to use the lowest possible dose (of drug or surgery) to achieve unifollicular ovulation and thereby avoid the significant risks of multiple pregnancy and ovarian hyperstimulation syndrome. Clomiphene citrate remains the first line medical therapy for anovulatory PCOS. It may be time to

Table 6.11 Strategy for ovulation induction in anovulatory PCOS

Slim patient	Overweight patient – BMI > 30 kg/m^2
1. Clomiphene citrate therapy 2. LOD if LH elevated 3. Gonadotropin therapy if clomiphene citrate resistant 4. IVF	1. Lifestyle changes 2. Metformin therapy[a] 3. Clomiphene citrate therapy combined with metformin[a] 4. Gonadotropin therapy if clomiphene citrate resistant combined with metformin[a] 5. IVF combined with metformin[a]
In rare cases of insulin resistance treat as overweight patients	

[a] *The use of metformin is supposition until the results of large studies are available*

rethink current strategies, particularly with the promising early experience of metformin. Compared with medical ovulation induction with gonadotropins for the clomiphene-resistant patient, the advantage of laparoscopic diathermy is that it need only be performed once and intensive monitoring is not required as there is no danger of multiple ovulation or ovarian hyperstimulation. We are, however, still unsure of the right dose of diathermy to stimulate reliably the resumption of ovulatory cycles. Neither are we certain about the degree of permanent damage done to the ovary by different amounts (duration, power, number of sites) of treatment. Unifollicular ovulation induction requires a subtle approach, particularly in women with PCOS. Gonadotropin therapy adds appreciably to the cost of the treatment and for what appears to be an equivalent cumulative conception rate is more expensive than laparoscopic ovarian diathermy.

Gonadotropin therapy, however, is still the mainstay of most forms of fertility therapy and adds appreciably to the cost of assisted reproduction therapies; indeed, the costs of the preparations have risen fourfold over the last 5 years. Other costs have to be counted in terms of the successful outcome of treatment with a low rate of miscarriage and the birth of healthy, preferably singleton, babies, with no health risks to their mothers. Advances in recombinant-DNA technology have resulted in the development of long-acting FSH preparations, a single shot of which might be sufficient to induce unifollicular ovulation. We may also expect to see orally active agents. The results of current trials are awaited with interest.

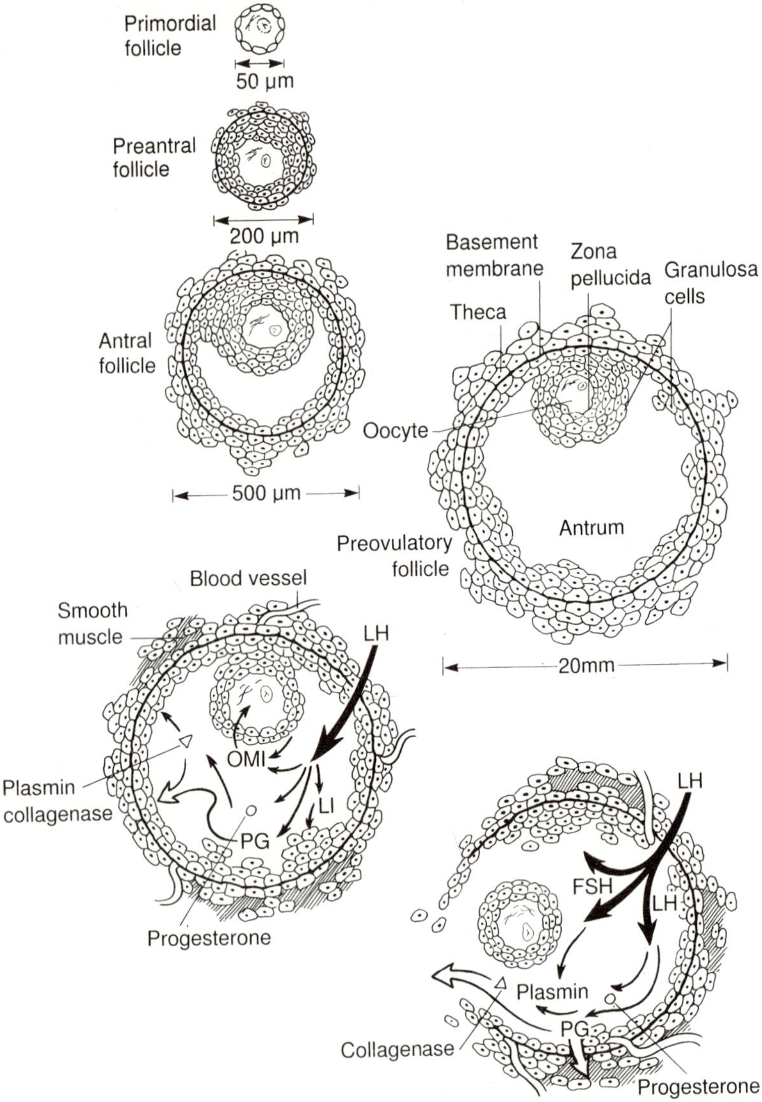

Figure 6.32 Schematic diagram to illustrate the principal steps in follicular development primordial follicle through to ovulation. Meiosis is arrested within the oocyte by maturation inhibitor (OMI) until the time of the LH surge (see text, page 63, and in greater detail on pages 157–158).

Ovulation induction – key points

- Correction of the cause of anovulatory infertility leads to cumulative conception rates that approach those expected for the female patient's age.
- It is important to optimize health, confirm tubal patency, and check the partner's semen analysis before commencing treatment.
- Hypogonadotropic hypogonadism is optimally treated with pulsatile GnRH (s.c.) but if gonadotropins are required use hMG rather than FSH.
- PCOS should be treated first with clomiphene citrate and if this fails, gonadotropin therapy and laparoscopic ovarian diathermy are equally efficacious.
- Insulin sensitizing agents, such as metformin, are still being evaluated in the management of PCOS.
- Clomiphene citrate therapy should be carefully monitored. Doses greater than 100 mg confer no benefit and if ovulation is occurring it is reasonable to continue for at least 6 but no more than 12 months.
- Gonadotropin therapy requires tight monitoring with serial ultrasound scans. The main risks are multiple pregnancy and OHSS.
- Laparoscopic ovarian diathermy is a single treatment which works well in selected patients; excellent results can be achieved using four-point diathermy on each ovary (4 seconds with 40 W).

References

1. Abdulwahid NA, Armar NA, Morris DV, Adams J & Jacobs HS (1985) Diagnostic tests with luteinising hormone releasing hormone should be abandoned. *Br Med J* **291**: 1471–1472.
2. Leyendecker G, Wildt L & Hansmann M (1980) Pregnancy following chronic intermittent (pulsatile) administration of LH-RH in women with hypothalamic and hyperprolactinaemic amenorrhea. *Arch Gynecol* **229**: 177–190.
3. Mason PW, Adams J, Morris DV *et al.* (1984) Induction of ovulation with pulsatile luteinising hormone-releasing hormone. *Br Med J* **288**: 181–185.
4. Schoemaker J, Simons AHM, van Osnabrugge GJC, Lugtenburg C & van Kessel H (1981) Pregnancy after prolonged pulsatile administration of luteinising hormone- releasing hormone in a patient with clomiphene-resistant secondary amenorrhoea. *J Clin Endocrinol Metab* **52**: 882.
5. Balen AH, Braat DDM, West C, Patel A & Jacobs HS (1994) Cumulative conception and live birth rates after the treatment of anovulatory infertility: an analysis of the safety and efficacy of ovulation induction in 200 patients. *Hum Reprod* **9**: 1563–1570.
6. Braat DDM, Schoemaker R & Schoemaker J (1991) Life table analysis of fecundity in intravenously treated gonadotropin-releasing hormone treated patients with normogonadotropic and hypogonadotropic amenorrhea. *Fertil Steril* **55**: 266–271.

7. Filicori M, Flamigni C, Dellai P *et al.* (1994) Treatment of anovulation with pulsatile GnRH: prognostic factors and clinical results in 600 cycles. *J Clin Endocrinol Metab* **79**: 1215–1220.
8. Shoham Z, Balen AH, Patel A & Jacobs HS (1991). Results of ovulation induction using human menopausal gonadotropins or purified follicle-stimulating hormone in hypogonadotropic hypogonadism patients. *Fertil Steril* **56**: 1048–1053.
9. European and Australian Multicenter Study (1995) Cotreatment with growth hormone and gonadotropin for ovulation induction in hypogonadotropic patients: a prospective, randomized, placebo-controlled, dose response study. *Fertil Steril* **64**: 917–923.
10. Adams J, Franks S, Polson DW *et al.* (1985) Multifollicular ovaries: clinical and endocrine features and response to pulsatile gonadotropin-releasing hormone. *Lancet* **ii**: 1375–1378.
11. Van der Spuy ZM, Steer PJ, McCusker M, Steele SJ & Jacobs HS (1988) Outcome of pregnancy in underweight women after spontaneous and induced ovulation. *Br Med J* **296**: 962–965.
12. Barker DJP (1990) The fetal and infant origins of adult disease. *Br Med J* **301**: 111.
13. Cumming DC & Rebar RW (1983) Exercise and reproductive function in women. *Am J Indust Med* **4**: 113–125.
14. Robinson TL, Snow-Harter C, Taaffe DR, Gillis D, Shaw J & Marcus R (1995) Gymnasts exhibit higher bone mass than runners despite similar prevalence of amenorrhoea and oligomenorrhoea. *J Bone Miner Res* **10**: 26–35.
15. To WW, Wong MW & Chan KM (1995) The effect of dance training on menstrual function in collegiate dancing students. *Aust NZ J Obstet Gynaecol* **35**: 304–309.
16. Warren MP, Brooks-Gunn J, Hamilton LH, Warren LF & Hamilton WG (1986) Scoliosis and fractures in young ballet dancers. *N Engl J Med* 314: 1348–1353.
17. Garner DM, Rosen LW & Barry D (1998) Eating disorders among athletes. *Sport Psychiatry* **4**: 839–857.
18. Soule SG & Jacobs HS (1995) Prolactinomas: present day management. *Br J Obstet Gynaecol* **102**: 178–181.
19. Korbonitis M & Grossman AB (2000) Drug-induced hyperprolactinaemia. *Prescribers' J* **40**: 157–164.
20. Webster J (2000) Cabergoline and quinagolide therapy for prolactinomas. *Clin Endocrinol* **53**: 549–550.
21. Balen AH, Conway GS, Kaltsas G *et al.* (1995) Polycystic ovary syndrome: the spectrum of the disorder in 1741 patients. *Hum Reprod* **10**: 2107–2111.
22. Clark AM, Ledger W, Galletly C *et al.* (1995) Weight loss results in significant improvement in pregnancy and ovulation rates in anovulatory obese women. *Hum Reprod* **10**: 2705–2712.
23. Balen AH, Tan SL & Jacobs HS (1993) Hypersecretion of luteinising hormone – a significant cause of subfertility and miscarriage. *Br J Obstet Gynaecol* **100**: 1082–1089.
24. Lockwood GM, Muttukrishna S, Groome NP, Matthews DR & Ledger WL (1998) Mid-follicular phase pulses of inhibin B are absent in polycystic ovary syndrome and are initiated by successful laparoscopic ovarian diathermy: a possible mechanism for the emergence of the dominant follicle. *J Clin Endocrinol Metab* **83**: 1730–1735.
25. Velazquez EM, Mendoza S, Hamer T, Sosa F & Glueck CJ (1994) Metformin therapy in polycystic ovary syndrome reduces hyperinsulinaemia, insulin resistance, hyperandrogenaemia and systolic blood pressure, while facilitating normal menses and pregnancy. *Metabolism* **43**: 647–654.
26. Nestler JE, Jakubowicz DJ, Reamer P, Gunn MS & Allan G (1999) Ovulatory and metabolic effects of D-*chiro*-inositol in the polycystic ovary syndrome. *N Engl J Med* **340**: 1314–1320.

27. Kiddy DS, Hamilton-Fairley D, Bush A, Anyaoku V, Reed MJ & Franks S (1992) Improvement in endocrine and ovarian function during dietary treatment of obese women with polycystic ovary syndrome. *Clin Endocrinol* **36**: 105–111.
28. Conway GS (1990) Insulin resistance and the polycystic ovary syndrome. *Contemp Rev Obstet Gynaecol* **2**: 34–39.
29. Grodstein F, Goldman MB & Cramer DW (1994) Body mass index and ovulatory infertility. *Epidemiology* **5**: 247–250.
30. Zaazdstra BM, Seidell JC, Van Noord PA *et al.* (1993) Fat and female fecundity: prospective study of effect of body fat distribution on conception rates. *Br Med J* **306**: 484–487.
31. Clark AM, Thornley B, Tomlinson L, Galletley C & Norman RJ (1998) Weight loss in obese infertile women results in improvement in reproductive outcome for all forms of fertility treatment. *Hum Reprod* **13**: 1502–1505.
32. Hamilton-Fairley D, Kiddy D, Watson H, Paterson C & Franks S (1992) Association of moderate obesity with poor pregnancy outcome in women with polycystic ovary syndrome treated with low dose gonadotropins. *Br J Obstet Gynaecol* **99**: 128–131.
33. Nestler JE & Jakubowicz DJ (1996) Decreases in ovarian cytochrome P450c17alpha activity and serum free testosterone after reduction of insulin secretion in polycystic ovary syndrome. *N Engl J Med* **335**: 617–623.
34. Velazquez EM, Mendoza SG, Wang P & Glueck CJ (1997) Metformin therapy is associated with a decrease in plasminogen activator inhibitor-1, lipoprotein(a) and immunoreactive insulin levels in patients with PCOS. *J Clin Endocrinol Metab* **82**: 524–530.
35. Velazquez EM, Acosta A & Mendoza SG (1997) Menstrual cyclicity after metformin therapy in PCOS. *Obstet Gynecol* **90**: 392–395.
36. Acbay O & Gundogdu S (1996) Can metformin reduce insulin resistance in polycystic ovary syndrome? *Fertil Steril* **65**: 946–949.
37. Ehrmann DA, Cavaghan MK, Imperial J, Sturis J, Rosenfield RL & Polonsky KS (1997) Effects of metformin on insulin secretion, insulin action and ovarian steroidogenesis in women with polycystic ovary syndrome. *J Clin Endocrinol Metab* **82**: 1241–1247.
38. Ehrmann DA, Schneider DJ, Sobel BE *et al.* (1997) Troglitazone improves defects in insulin action, insulin secretion, ovarian steroidogenesis and fibrinolysis in women with polycystic ovary syndrome. *J Clin Endocrinol Metab* **82**: 2108–2116.
39. Kahn SE, Prigeon RL, Mcculloch DK, Bayco EJ, Bergman RN *et al.* Quantification of the relationship between insulin sensivity and β cell function in human subjects. *Diabetes* 1993; **42**: 1663-1672.
40. Glueck CJ, Wang P, Fontaine R, Tracy T, Sieve-Smith L. Metformin-induced resumption of normal menses in 39 of 43 (91%) previously amenorrheic women with the polycystic ovary syndrome. *Metabolism* 1999; **48**: 511-519.
41. Pirwany IR, Yates RWS, Cameron IT, Fleming R. Effects of the insulin sensitizing drug metformin on ovarian function, follicular growth and ovulation rate in obese women with oligomenorrhoea. *Hum Reprod* 1999; **14**: 2963-2968.
42. Vandermolen D, Ratts V, Evans WS *et al.* Metformin increases the ovulatory rate and pregnancy rate from clomiphene citrate in patients with polycystic ovary syndrome who are resistant to clomiphene citrate alone. *Fertil Steril* 2001; **75**: 310-315.
43. Nestler JE , Jakubowicz DJ, Evans WS, Pasquali R. Effects of metformin on spontaneous and clomiphene-induced ovulation in the polycystic ovary syndrome. *N Engl J Med* 1998; **338**: 1876-80.
44. Fleming R, Hopkinson ZE, Wallace AM, Greer IA, Sattar N. Ovarian function and metablic factors in women with oligomenorrhoea treated with metformin in a randomised double-blind placebo controlled trial. JCEM 2002 (in press).
45. Hughes E, Collins J & Vandekerckhove P (2002) Clomiphene citrate for ovulation induction in women with oligo-amenorrhoea. Cochrane Database of Systematic Reviews, Issue 1.

46. Hammond MG, Halme JK & Talbert LM (1983) Factors affecting the pregnancy rate in clomiphene citrate induction of ovulation. *Obstet Gynecol* **62**: 196–202.
47. ESHRE (1997) Female infertility: treatment options for complicated cases. ESHRE Capri Workshop. *Hum Reprod* **12**: 1191–1196.
48. Balen AH (1997) Anovulatory infertility and ovulation induction: Recommendations for good clinical practice. *J Br Fertil Soc* **2**: 83–87.
49. Kousta E, White DM & Franks S (1997) Modern use of clomiphene citrate in induction of ovulation. *Hum Reprod Update* **3**: 359–365.
50. Shoham Z, Zosmer A & Insler V (1991) Early miscarriage and fetal malformations after induction of ovulation, *in vitro* fertilisation and gamete intrafallopian transfer. *Fertil Steril* **55**: 1–11.
51. Venn A & Lumley J (1994) Clomiphene citrate and pregnancy outcome. *Aust NZ J Obstet Gynaecol* **34**: 56–66.
52. Shoham Z, Borenstein R, Lunenfeld B & Pariente C (1990) Hormonal profiles following clomiphene citrate therapy in conception and nonconception cycles. *Clin Endocrinol* **33**: 271–278.
53. Homburg R, Weissglass L & Goldman J (1988) Improved treatment for anovulation in polycystic ovarian disease utilizing the effect of progesterone on the inappropriate gonadotropin release and clomiphene citrate response. *Hum Reprod* **3**: 285–288.
54. Rossing MA, Daling JR, Weiss NS *et al.* (1994) Ovarian tumors in a cohort of infertile women. *N Engl J Med* **331**: 771–776.
55. Lunenfeld B & Insler V (1974) Classifiaction of amenorrhoeic states and their treatment by ovulation induction. *Clin Endocrinol* **3**: 223–237.
56. Brown JB, Evans JH, Adey FD, Taft HP & Townsend L (1969) Factors involved in the induction of fertile ovulation with human gonadotropins. *J Obstet Gynaecol Br Comm* **76**: 289–307.
57. Hamilton-Fairley D, Kiddy D, Watson H, Sagle M & Franks S (1991) Low dose gonadotropin therapy for induction of ovulation in 100 women with polycystic ovary syndrome. *Hum Reprod* **6**: 1095–1099.
58. Fauser BC, Donderwinkel & Schoot DC (1993) The step-down principle in gonadotropin treatment and the role of GnRH analogues. *Baillières Clin Obstet Gynaecol* **7**: 309–330.
59. van Santbrink EJP, Donderwinkel PFJ, van Dessel TJHM & Fauser BCJM (1995) Gonadotropin induction of ovulation using a step-down dose regimen: single centre clinical experience in 82 patients. *Hum Reprod* **10**: 1048–1053.
60. Ben Rafael Z, Levy T & Schoemaker J (1995) Pharmacokinetics of follicle-stimulating hormone: clinical significance. *Fertil Steril* **63**: 689–700.
61. Hugues J-N, Cedrin-Durnerin I, Avril C, Bulwa S, Herve F & Uzan M (1996) Sequential step-up and step-down dose regimen: an alternative method for ovulation induction with FSH in polycystic ovary syndrome. *Hum Reprod* **11**: 2581–2584.
62. Farhi J & Jacobs HS (1997) Early prediction of ovarian multifollicular response during ovulation induction in patients with polycystic ovary syndrome. *Fertil Steril* **67**: 459–462.
63. White DM, Polson DW, Kiddy D *et al.* (1996) Induction of ovulation with low-dose gonadotropins in polycystic ovary syndrome: an analysis of 109 pregnancies in 225 women. *J Clin Endocrinol Metab* **81**: 3821–3824.
64. Levene MI, Wild J & Steer P (1992) Higher multiple births and the modern management of infertility in Britain. *Br J Obstet Gynaecol* **99**: 607–613.
65. Abdalla HI, Baber RJ, Kirkland A, Leonard T & Studd JWW (1989) Pregnancy in women with premature ovarian failure using tubal and intrauterine transfer of cryopreserved zygotes. *Br J Obstet Gynaecol* **96**: 1071–1075.
66. Botting BJ, Macfarlane AJ & Price FV (eds) (1990) *Three, four and more. a study of triplet and higher order births.* HMSO, London.
67. Hull MGR (1992) Gonadotropin therapy in anovulatory infertility. In: Howles CM (ed) *Gonadotropins, gonadotropin releasing hormone analogues and growth factors in infertility: future perspectives*. Medifax International, Sussex, pp 56–70.

68. Abdel Gadir A, Mowafi RS, Alnaser HMI, Alrashid AH, Alonezi OM & Shaw RW (1990) Ovarian electrocautery versus human menopausal gonadotropins and pure follicle stimulating hormone therapy in the treatment of patients with polycystic ovarian disease. *Clin Endocrinol (Oxf)* **33**: 585–592.
69. Donesky BW & Adashi EY (1995) Surgically induced ovulation in the polycystic ovary syndrome: wedge resection revisited in the age of laparoscopy. *Fertil Steril* **63**: 439–463.
70. Balen AH (1998) PCOS – medical or surgical treatment? In: Templeton A, Cooke I & O'Brien PMS (eds) *Evidence-based fertility treatment*. RCOG Study Group. RCOG Press, London, pp 157–177.
71. Armar NA & Lachelin GCL (1993) Laparoscopic ovarian diathermy: an effective treatment for anti-oestrogen resistant anovulatory infertility in women with polycystic ovaries. *Br J Obstet Gynaecol* **100**: 161–164.
72. Homburg R, Armar NA, Eshel A, Adams J & Jacobs HS (1988) Influence of serum luteinising hormone concentrations on ovulation, conception and early pregnancy loss in polycystic ovary syndrome. *Br Med J* **297**: 1024–1026.
73. Abdel Gadir A, Alnaser HMI, Mowafi RS & Shaw RW (1992) The response of patients with polycystic ovarian disease to human menopausal gonadotropin therapy after ovarian electrocautery or a luteinizing hormone-releasing hormone agonist. *Fertil Steril* **57**: 309–313.
74. Balen AH & Jacobs HS (1994) A prospective study comparing unilateral and bilateral laparoscopic ovarian diathermy in women with the polycystic ovary syndrome. *Fertil Steril* **62**: 921–925.
75. Rossmanith WG, Keckstein J, Spatzier K & Lauritzen C (1991) The impact of ovarian laser surgery on the gonadotropin secretion in women with polycystic ovarian disease. *Clin Endocrinol* **34**: 223–230.
76. Balen AH & Jacobs HS (1991) Gonadotropin surge attenuating factor – a missing link in the control of LH secretion? *Clin Endocrinol (Oxf)* **35**: 399–402.
77. Gjoannaess H (1984) Polycystic ovarian syndrome treated by ovarian electrocautery through the laparoscope. *Fertil Steril* **41**: 20–25.
78. Daniell JF & Miller N (1989) Polycystic ovaries treated by laparoscopic laser vaporization. *Fertil Steril* **51**: 232–236.
79. Naether OGJ, Fischer R, Weise HC, Geiger-Kotzler L, Delfs T & Rudolf K (1993) Laparoscopic electrocoagulation of the ovarian surface in infertile patients with polycystic ovarian disease. *Fertil Steril* **60**: 88–94.
80. Naether OGJ & Fischer R (1993) Adhesion formation after laparoscopic electrocoagulation of the ovarian surface in polycystic ovary patients. *Fertil Steril* **60**: 95–99.
81. Naether O, Weise HC & Fischer R (1991) Treatment with electrocautery in sterility patients with polycystic ovarian disease. *Geburtsh Frauenheilk* **51**: 920–924.
82. Armar NA, McGarrigle HHG, Honour JW, Holownia P, Jacobs HS & Lachelin GCL (1990) Laparoscopic ovarian diathermy in the management of anovulatory infertility in women with polycystic ovaries: endocrine changes and clinical outcome. *Fertil Steril* **53**: 45–49.
83. Naether OGJ (1995) Significant reduction of adnexal adhesions following laparoscopic electrocautery of the ovarian surface by lavage and artificial ascites. *Gynaecol Endoscopy* **4**: 17–19.
84. Gurgan T, Urman B *et al.* (1992) The effect of short internal laparoscopic lysis of adhesions in pregnancy rates following Nd:YAG laser photocoagulation of PCO. *Obstet Gynaecol* **80**: 45–47.
85. Ostrzenski A (1992) Endoscopic carbon dioxide laser ovarian wedge resection in resistant polycystic ovarian disease. *Int J Fertil* **37**: 295–299.
86. Farhi J, Soule S & Jacobs H (1995) Effect of laparoscopic ovarian electrocautery on ovarian response and outcome of treatment with gonadotropins in clomiphene citrate resistant patients with PCOS. *Fertil Steril* **64**: 930–935.
87. Cohen BM (1989) Laser laparoscopy for polycystic ovaries. *Fertil Steril* **52**: 167–168.

88. Rimmington MR, Walker SM & Shaw RW (1997) The use of laparoscopic ovarian electrocautery in preventing cancellation of in-vitro fertilization treatment cycles due to risk of ovarian hyperstimulation syndrome in women with polycystic ovaries. *Hum Reprod* 7: 1443–1447.
89. Keckstein G, Rossmanith W, Spatzier K, Schneider V, Borchers K & Steiner R (1990) The effect of laparoscopic treatment of polycystic ovarian disease by CO_2-laser or Nd:YAG laser. *Surg Endosc* 4: 103–107.
90. Heylen SM, Puttemans PJ & Brosens LH (1994) Polycystic ovarian disease treated by laparoscopic argon laser capsule drilling: comparison of vaporization versus perforation technique. *Hum Reprod* 9: 1038–1042.
91. Farquhar C, Vandekerckhove P, Lilford R. Laparoscopic "drilling" by diathermy or laser for ovulation induction in anovulatory polycystic ovary syndrome (Cochrane Review). In: *The Cochrane Library*, Issue 4, 2002. Oxford: Update Software.
92. Farquhar CM, Williamson K, Gudex G, Johnson NP, Garland J, Sadler L. A randomised controlled trial of laparoscopic ovarian diathermy versus gonadotropin therapy for women with clomiphene citrate-resistant polycystic ovary syndrome. *Fertil Steril* 2002; 78: 404-411.
93. Bayram N, Van Wely M, Bossuyt P, Van der Veen F. Randomised clinical trial of laparoscopic electrocoagulation of the ovaries versus recombinant FSH for ovulation induction in subfertility associated with polycystic ovary syndrome. Abstract 0-148 of the 17th Annual Meeting of the ESHRE, Lausanne, Switzerland. July 2001.

Further Reading

Filicori M & Flamigni C (eds) (1994) Ovulation induction. *Excerpta Medica*, Amsterdam, p 1046.

Evers JLH (ed) (1993) Ovulation induction: the difficult patient. *Baillière's Clinical Obstetrics and Gynaecology* 7: 2.

Shoham Z, Howles C & Jacobs HS (1999) *Female infertility therapy: current practice*. Martin Dunitz, London.

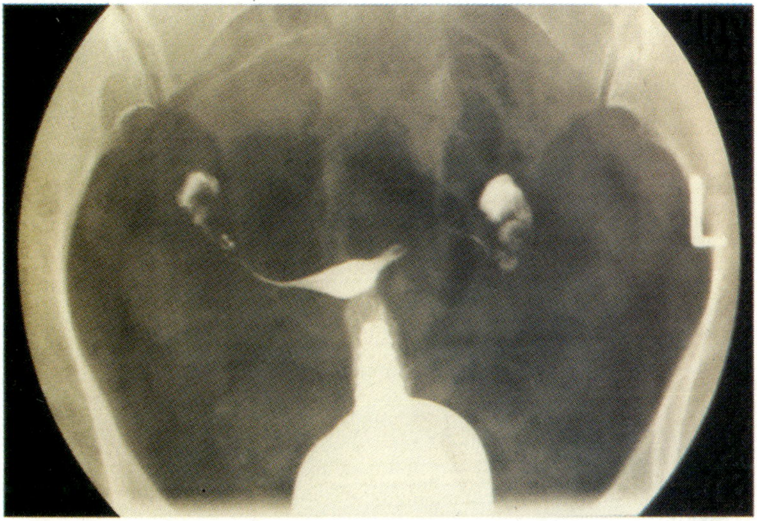

Figure 4.26 HSG of salpingitis isthmica nodosa (SIN).

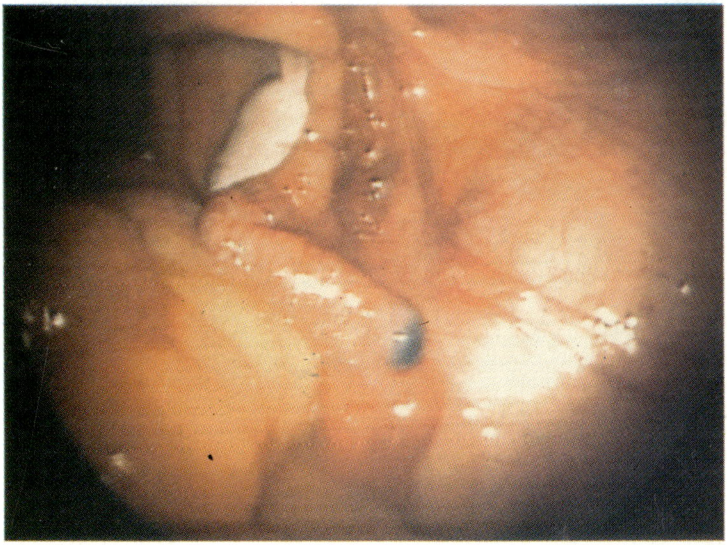

Figure 4.27 Salpingitis isthmica nodosa (SIN) seen at laparoscopy with blue dye appearing in the herniation through the serosal layer of the tube.

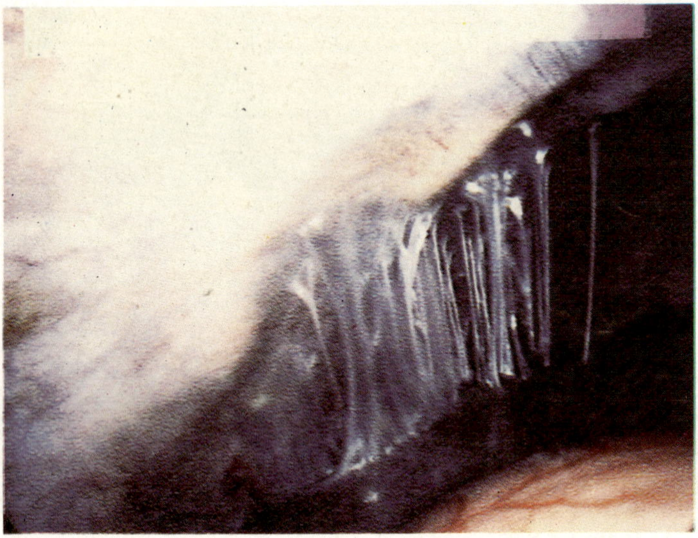

a

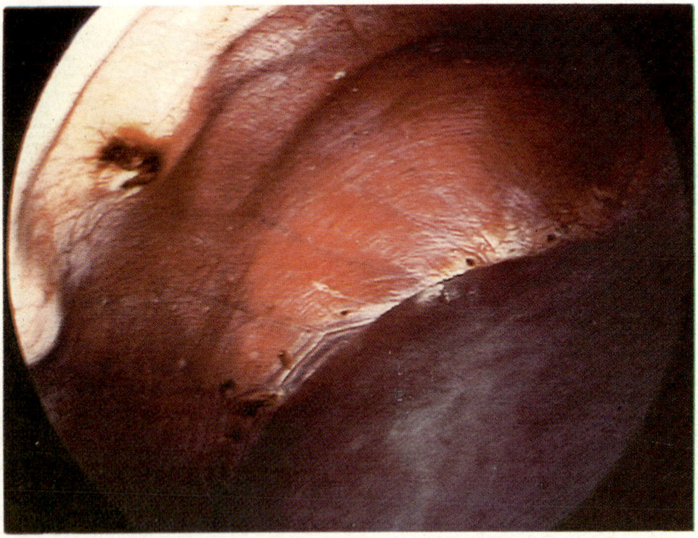

b

Figure 4.39 The laparoscopic views of the liver and undersurface of the diaphragm to illustrate the importance of assessing this area. (**a**) Fitz-Hugh Curtis syndrome, (**b**) endometriosis.

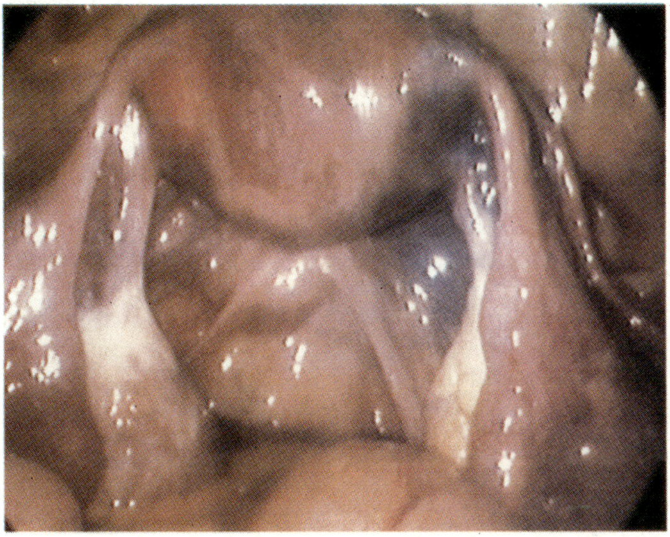

Figure 4.40 Laparoscopy with intubation of methylene blue dye. There is bilateral cornual obstruction to flow and on the right the dye can be seen suffusing the myometrium and vessels of the broad ligament. Externally the pelvic structures appear normal.

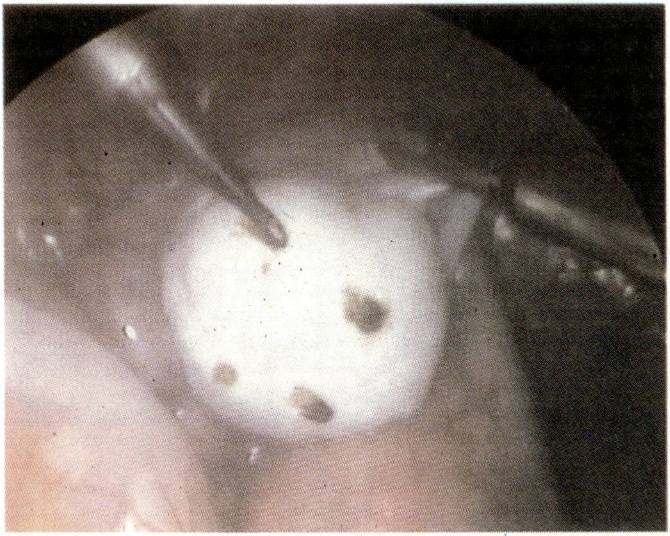

a

Figure 6.29 (**a**) Laparoscopic ovarian diathermy. The needle enters the ovarian capsule while the ovarian ligament is held steady, with the ovary supported on the front of the uterus.

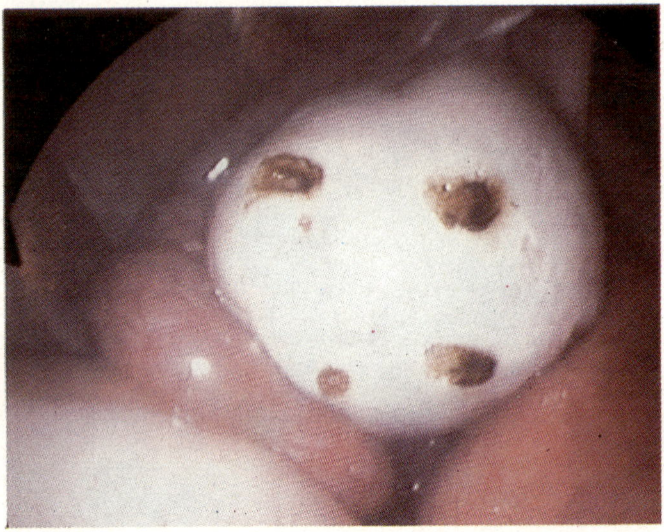

Figure 6.29 (**b**) At the end of the procedure the ovary has been diathermized at four sites.

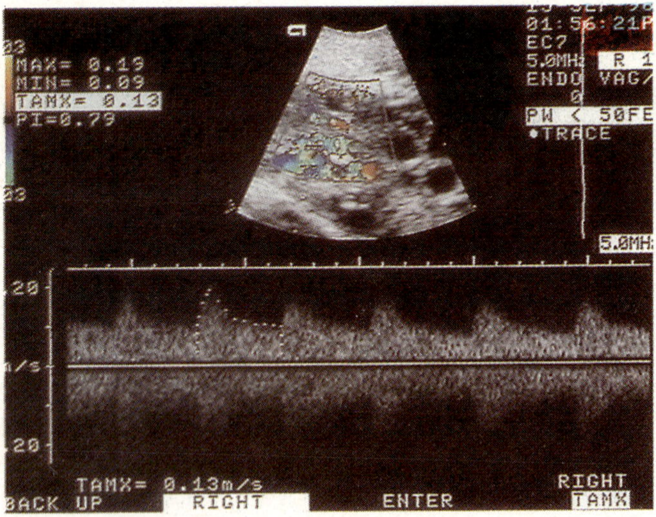

Figure 7.2 Color Doppler studies of a polycystic ovary. Transvaginal ultrasound (5 MHz) with superimposed pulsed Doppler demonstrating a typical ovarian stromal flow velocity waveform. In the early follicular phase the normal velocity is < 0.1 m/s (with thanks to Dr J. Zaidi).

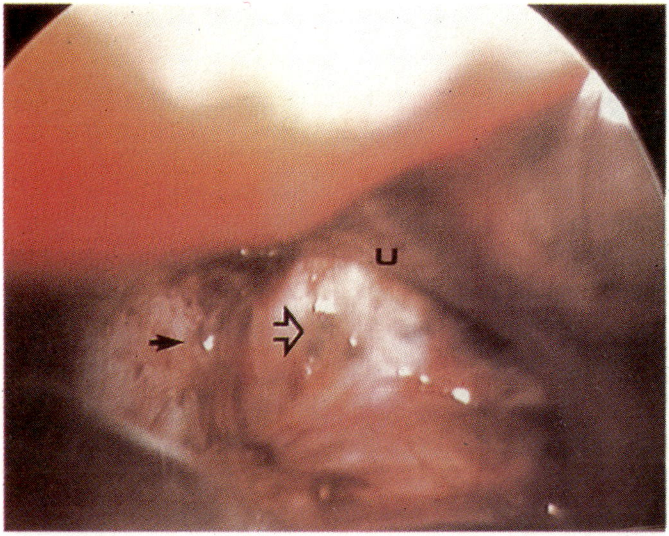

a

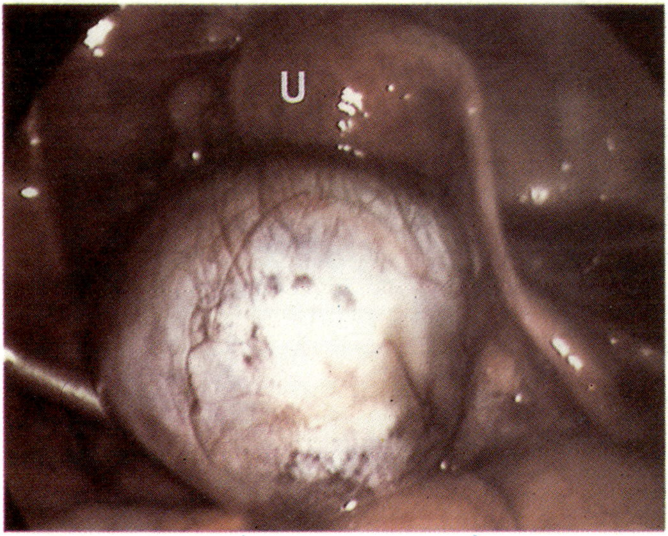

b

Figure 9.3 Endometriosis at laparoscopy. (**a**) Active spots of endometriosis are seen between the the uterosacral ligaments (u) and in the pouch of Douglas (open arrow) there is adjacent neovascularization and the new peritoneal formation (closed arrow). (**b**) The left ovary is supported behind the uterus (U) and is distended by a large endometriotic cyst.

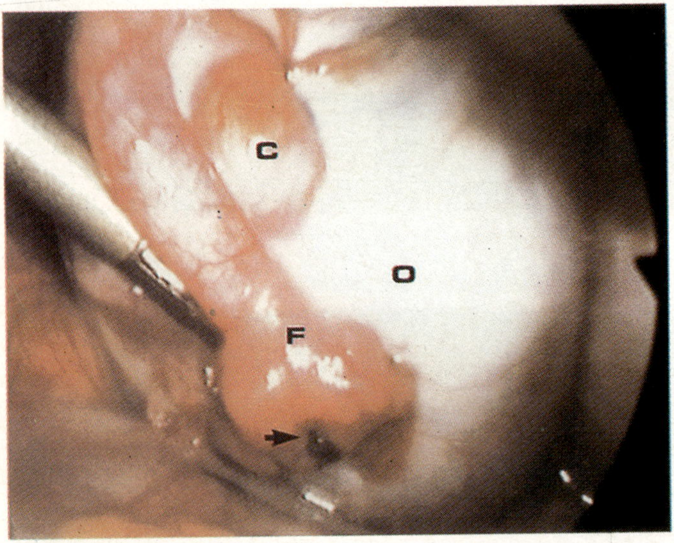

c

Figure 9.3 Endometriosis at laparoscopy: (**c**) Another view of the left ovary (O) indicates recent ovulation by virtue of a corpus luteum (C). The fimbrial end of the tube (F) appears reasonably healthy although there is an endometriotic deposit on its posterior margin (arrow).

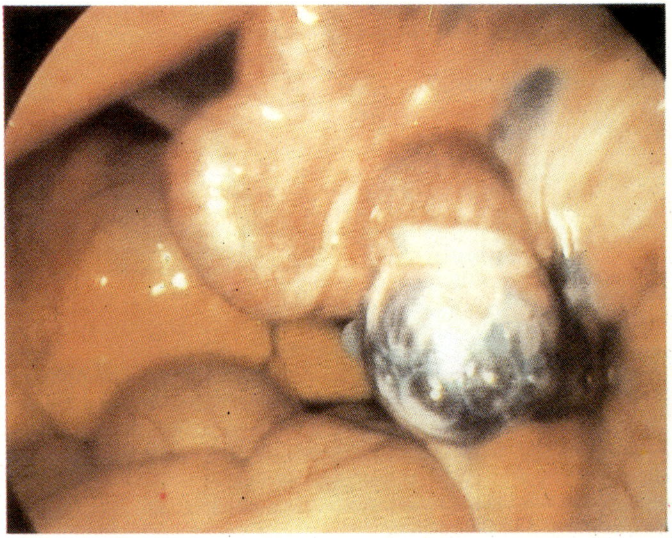

a

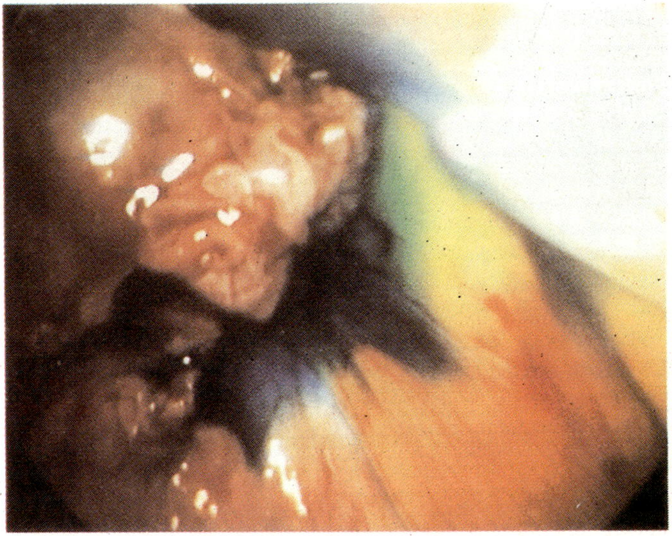

b

Figure 10.2 (**a**) Laparoscopy and dye: perifimbrial adhesions lead to loculation of the injected dye, yet there is some spill into the peritoneal cavity. In cases such as this an HSG examination can give the impression of normal tubal patency. (**b**) An adhesiolysis has been performed and the fimbrial end of the tube displayed to allow free flow of dye.

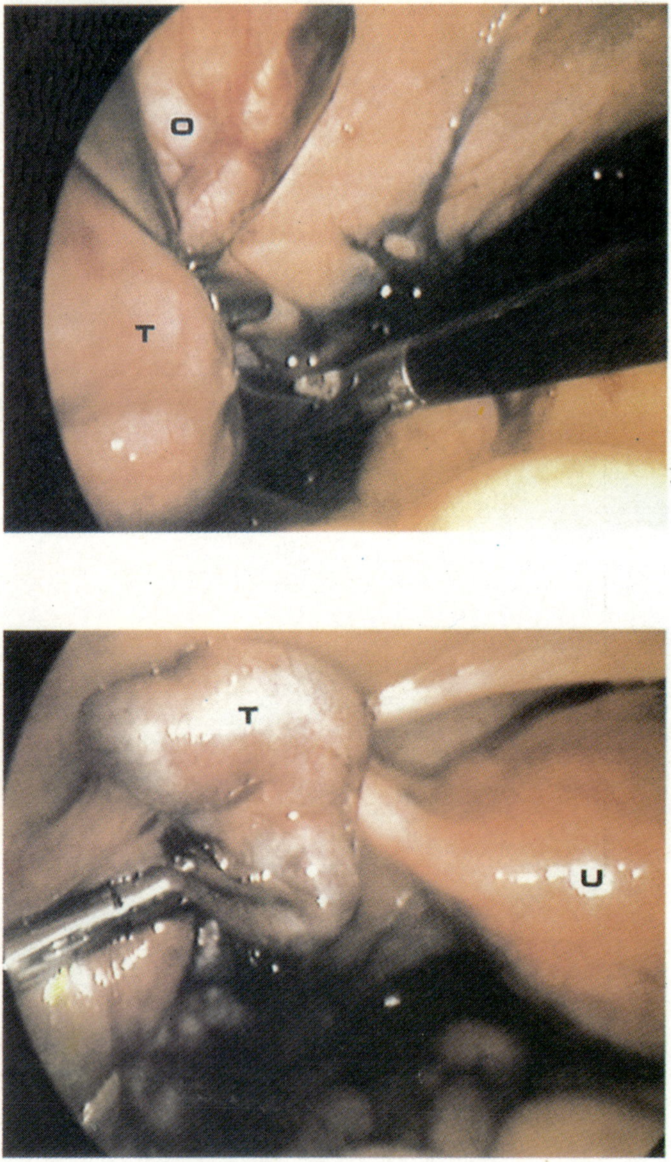

a

b

Figure 10.3 (**a**) Laparoscopy and dye: the left ovary (O) is tethered to the posterior leaf of the broad ligament and the tube (T) is adherent in the pouch of Douglas. Scissors are used to release the adhesions. (**b**) An adhesiolysis has been performed but the tube (T) is "retort" shaped, distended, and considerably damaged. The uterus (U) is seen to the right.

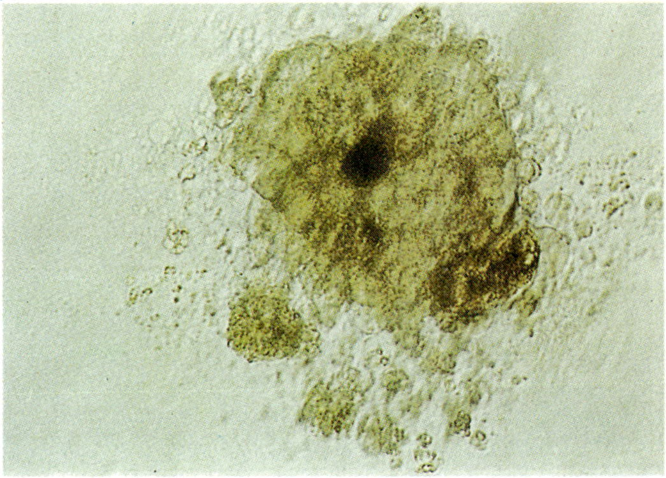

Figure 13.8 Oocyte immediately after follicular aspiration, covered in cumulus cells.

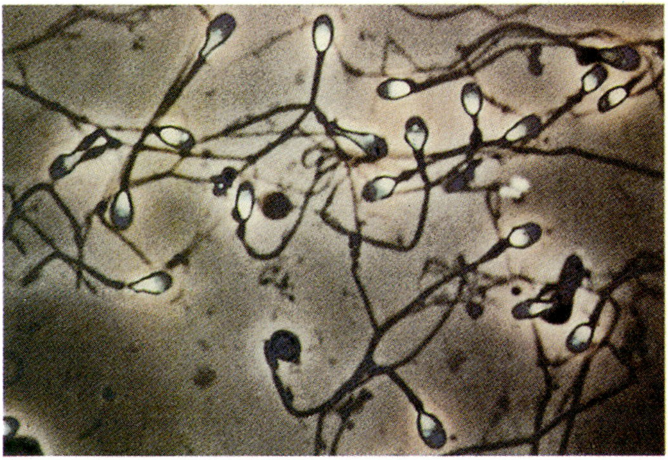

Figure 13.9 Phase contrast microscopy of normal spermatozoa.

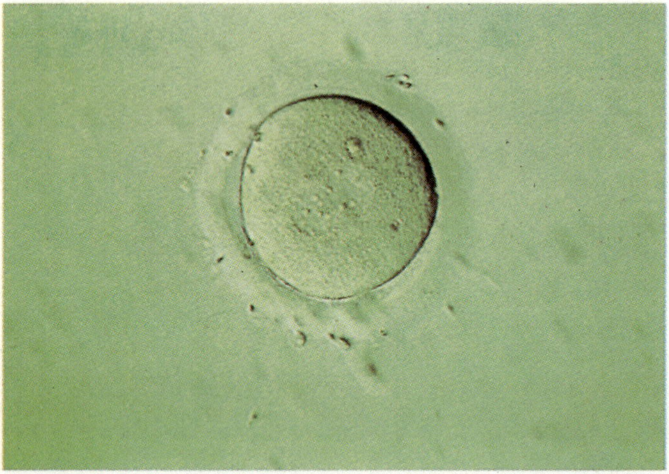

Figure 13.10 After fertlization two pronuclei can be seen clearly and spermatozoa can be seen attached to the outside of the zona pellucida.

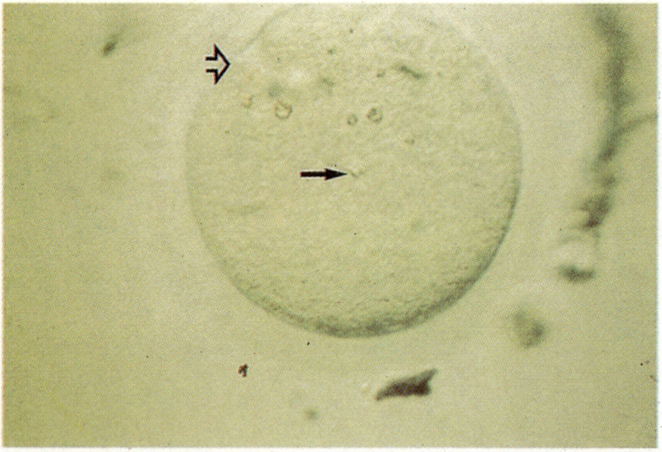

Figure 13.11 Oocyte immediately after ICSI has been performed. The site of the passage of the needle can be seen clearly (open arrow), as can the head of the spermatozoon.

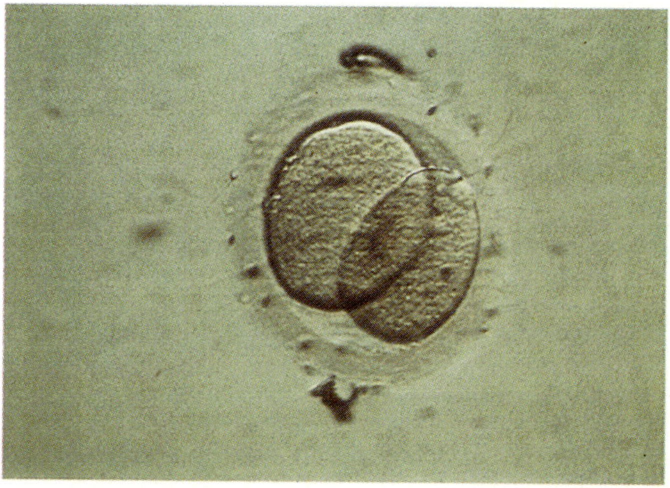

Figure 13.12 Two-cell pre-embryo.

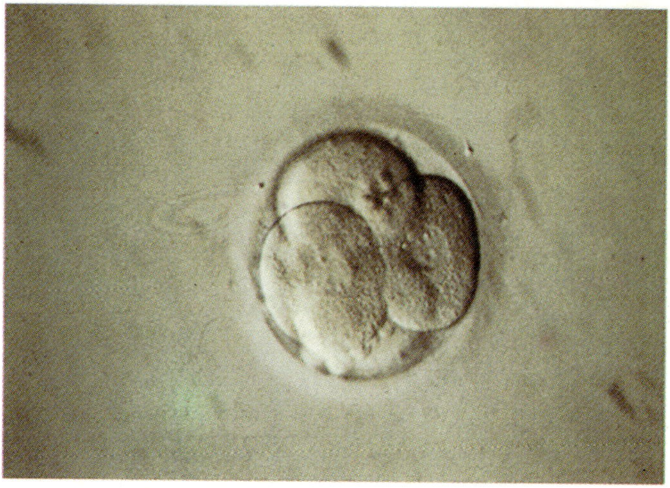

Figure 13.13 Four-cell pre-embryo.

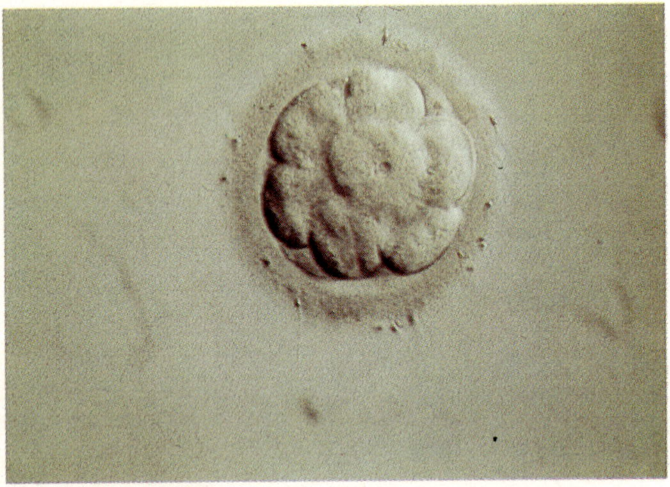

Figure 13.14 Morula stage.

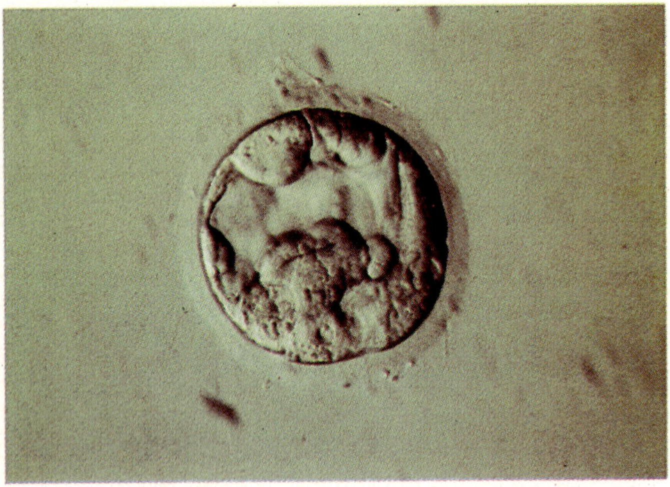

Figure 13.15 Blastocyst.

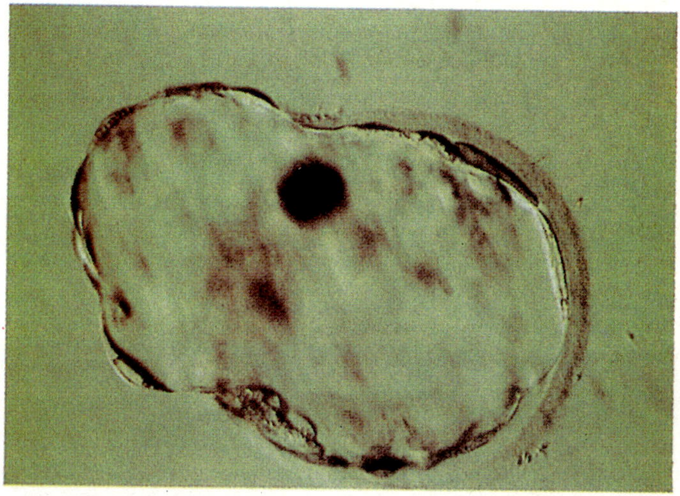

Figure 13.16 Blastocyst hatching.

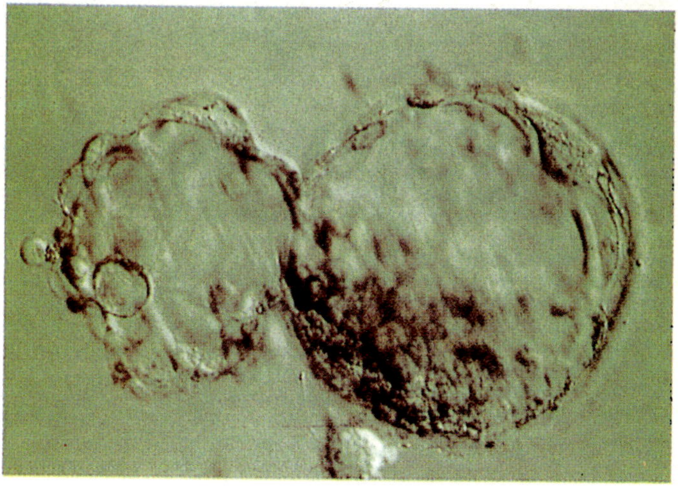

Figure 13.17 Hatched blastocyst (on right).

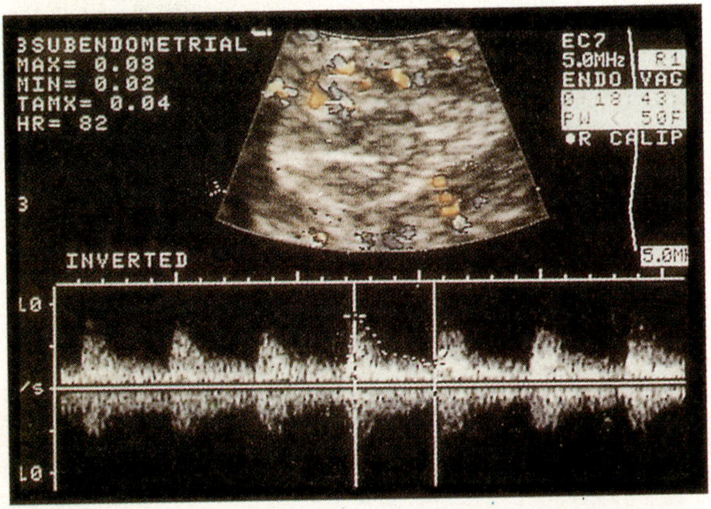

Figure 13.27 Color Doppler studies of the endometrium. Transvaginal ultrasound (5 MHz) with superimposed pulsed Doppler demonstrating flow through subendometrial vessels. Absent subendometrial or intraendometrial vascularization on the day of hCG administration during IVF appears to be a useful predictor of failure of implantation in IVF cycles, irrespective of the morphological appearance of the endometrium (with thanks to Dr J. Zaidi).

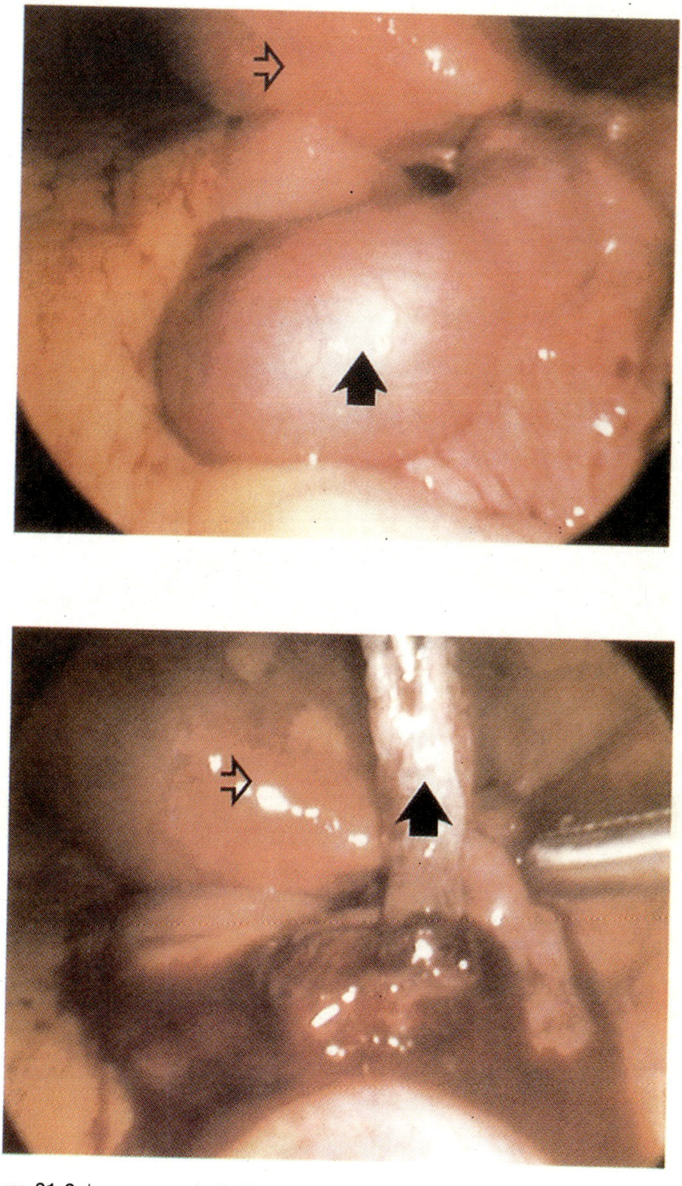

a

b

Figure 21.2 Laparoscopic findings of (**a**) an unruptured ectopic pregnancy (arrow) and (**b**) removal of the pregnancy through a linear salpingostomy. The uterus in (a) and (b) is denoted by an open arrow. (For the ultrasound findings of this case see Figure 21.1).

Chapter 7

Polycystic ovary syndrome

Introduction

The polycystic ovary syndrome (PCOS) is the commonest endocrine disturbance affecting women. However, there is no international consensus either on the definition of the syndrome or, indeed, on what constitutes a polycystic ovary. Terminology is important, and it is gratifying to see a shift away from the term "polycystic ovarian disease" to the more commonly accepted polycystic ovary *syndrome*. This confirms the notion of PCOS as a collection of signs, symptoms, and endocrine disturbances and reinforces the heterogeneous nature of the condition.[1]

We tend to take a pragmatic approach to the management of an individual's symptoms and needs, which may change over time. Hence an argument could be made that a precise definition of the condition does not help when providing therapy. Yet we feel that, while having practical relevance, this argument is flawed because it is necessary to evaluate scientifically the outcomes of treatment. It is then only possible to compare outcomes if the same starting points are employed. Furthermore, while PCOS is a familial condition, it is proving difficult to establish the genetic basis for the syndrome without a clear view of the phenotype – another reason to aim for a consensus in defining PCOS.

What is Polycystic Ovary Syndrome?

Polycystic ovaries are commonly detected by ultrasound or other forms of pelvic imaging, with estimates of the prevalence in the general population being in the order of 20–33%.[1–4] However, not all women with polycystic ovaries demonstrate the clinical and biochemical features which define the PCOS. These include menstrual cycle disturbances, obesity, hirsutism, acne, and abnormalities of biochemical profiles including elevated serum concentrations of luteinizing hormone (LH), testosterone, androstenedione, and insulin. Presentation of the syndrome is so varied that one, all, or any combination of the above features may be present in association with an ultrasound picture of polycystic ovaries – the defining features of PCOS in the UK and much of Europe (see Fig. 7.1).[5]

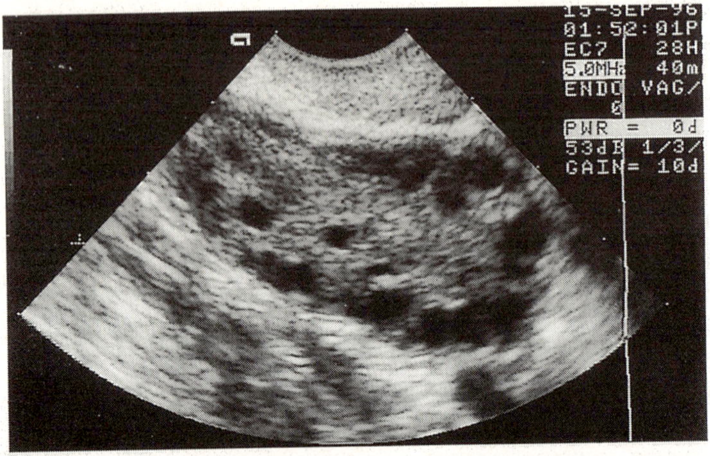

The spectrum of clinical manifestations of the polycystic ovary syndrome		
Symptoms	Serum endocrinology	Possible late sequelae
Obesity	↑ Androgens (testosterone and androstenedione)	Diabetes mellitus Dyslipidemia
Menstrual disturbance	↑ Luteinizing hormone	Hypertension
Infertility	↑ Fasting insulin ↑ Prolactin	Cardiovascular disease
Hyperandrogenism	↓ Sex hormone binding globulin	Endometrial carcinoma Breast cancer
Asymptomatic	↑ Estradiol, estrone	

Figure 7.1 Symptoms, signs, and endocrine disturbances in the PCOS can occur either together or separately but require the presence of polycystic ovarian morphology, as seen here by transvaginal ultrasound.

There is considerable heterogeneity of symptoms and signs among women with PCOS and for an individual these may change over time.[1] The PCOS is familial[6] and various aspects of the syndrome may be differentially inherited. Polycystic ovaries can exist without clinical signs of the syndrome, which may then become expressed over time. There are a number of interlinking factors that affect expression of PCOS. A gain in weight is associated with a worsening of symptoms while weight loss ameliorates the endocrine and metabolic profile and symptomatology.[7]

The pathogenesis of polycystic ovaries and the associated syndrome is still being elucidated, but the heterogeneity of presentation of PCOS suggests that a single cause is unlikely. Recent genetic studies have identified a link between PCOS and disordered insulin metabolism, and indicate that the syndrome may be the presentation of a complex genetic trait disorder.[8] The features of obesity, hyperinsulinemia, and hyperandrogenemia, which are commonly seen in PCOS, are also known to be factors which confer an increased risk of cardiovascular disease and non-insulin dependent diabetes mellitus (NIDDM) (see review by Rajkowha *et al.*[9]). There are studies which indicate that women with PCOS have an increased risk for these diseases which pose long-term risks for health, and this evidence has prompted debate as to the need to screen women for polycystic ovaries. There are also associations between the presence of PCOS and some cancers (see below). For studies of the long-term risks it is essential to have a clear view of definition.

Definitions

Historically the detection of the polycystic ovary required visualization of the ovaries at laparotomy with histological confirmation following biopsy.[10] As further studies identified the association of certain endocrine abnormalities in women with histological evidence of polycystic ovaries, biochemical criteria became the mainstay for diagnosis. Raised serum levels of LH, testosterone, and androstenedione, in association with low or normal levels of follicle stimulating hormone (FSH) and abnormalities of estrogen secretion, described an endocrine profile which many believed to be diagnostic of PCOS.[11] Well recognized clinical presentations included menstrual cycle disturbances (oligo-/amenorrhea), obesity, and hyperandrogenism manifesting as hirsutism, acne, or androgen-dependent alopecia. These definitions proved inconsistent, however, as clinical features were noted to vary considerably between women, and indeed some women with histological evidence of polycystic ovaries consistently failed to display any of the common symptoms. Likewise, the biochemical features associated with PCOS were not consistent in all women. Thus consensus on a single biochemical or clinical definition for PCOS was thwarted by the heterogeneity of presentation of the disorder.

The advent of high resolution ultrasound scanning provided a non-invasive technique for the assessment of ovarian size and morphology. Good correlation has since been shown between ultrasound diagnoses of polycystic morphology and the histopathological criteria for polycystic ovaries by studies examining ovarian tissue obtained at hysterectomy or after wedge resection.[12,13] The histopathological criteria have been defined as the observation of: increased numbers of follicles, hypertrophy and luteinization of the inner theca cell layer, and thickened ovarian tunica. Transabdominal and/or transvaginal ultrasound have since become the most commonly used diagnostic methods for the identification of polycystic ovaries. Although the ultrasound criteria for the diagnosis of polycystic ovaries have never been universally agreed, the characteristic features are accepted as being an increase in the number of follicles and the amount of stroma as compared with normal ovaries. The transabdominal ultrasound criteria of Adams *et al.*[14] defined a polycystic ovary as one which contains, in one plane, at least 10 follicles (usually between 2 and 8 mm in diameter) arranged peripherally around a dense core of ovarian stroma or scattered throughout an increased amount of stroma. These criteria have been adopted by many studies which have used ultrasound scanning to detect polycystic ovaries.[1,3,15–17]

It has been argued that transvaginal ultrasound is a more sensitive method for the detection of polycystic ovaries and that the transvaginal definition of a polycystic ovary should require the presence of at least 15 and usually more than 20 follicles (2–10 mm in diameter) in a single plane.[18] However, other authors examining transabdominal versus transvaginal scanning have not found significant differences in the detection rate of polycystic ovaries.[17] The innovation of three-dimensional ultrasound and the use of color and pulsed Doppler ultrasound are techniques which may further enhance the detection of polycystic ovaries and which may be more commonly employed in time (Fig. 7.2).[19,20] The use of magnetic resonance imaging (MRI) for the visualization of the structure of pelvic organs has been claimed to have even greater sensitivity than ultrasound for the detection

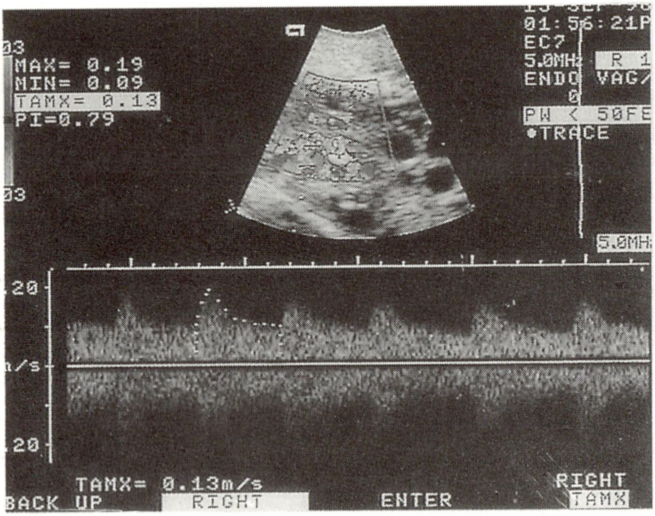

Figure 7.2 Color Doppler studies of a polycystic ovary. Transvaginal ultrasound (5 MHz) with superimposed pulsed Doppler demonstrating a typical ovarian stromal flow velocity waveform. In the early follicular phase the normal velocity is < 0.1 m/s (with thanks to Dr J. Zaidi) (please refer to plate section for color figure).

of polycystic ovaries.[21] However, the substantial cost and practical problems involved with this imaging technique limit its use.

The term "polycystic ovary" in some respects adds to the confusion that surrounds its diagnosis. The "cysts" are not cysts in the sense that they do contain oocytes. So truly it should be called a polyfollicular ovary, to reflect the finding that the "cysts" are actually follicles whose development has been arrested. Indeed the prerequisite of a certain number of cysts may be of less relevance than the volume of ovarian stroma, which has been shown to correlate closely with serum testosterone concentrations.[19] Furthermore, it has been suggested recently that an ultrasound assessment of the ratio of ovarian stromal area to total ovarian area gives the greatest sensitivity and specificity (both 100%) for the diagnosis of PCOS.[22] While this appears to be an attractive proposition, there are other studies that have examined various ultrasound parameters and found limited predictive value for abnormal hormone levels.[23]

While it is now clear that ultrasound provides an excellent technique for the detection of polycystic ovarian morphology, identification of polycystic ovaries by ultrasound does not automatically confer a diagnosis of PCOS. Controversy still exists over a precise definition of the syndrome and whether or not the diagnosis should require confirmation of polycystic ovarian morphology. Some authors suggest that the definition of PCOS should be based on biochemical evidence of ovarian hyperandrogenism rather than an ultrasound appearance, as hyperandrogenism may exist in women who have normal ovarian morphology as detected by ultrasound.[24] This viewpoint has been adopted in the USA, and the 1990 National Institute of Health conference on PCOS recommended that diagnostic criteria should include evidence of hyperandrogenism and ovulatory dysfunction, in the absence of non-classic adrenal hyperplasia, and that evidence of polycystic ovarian morphology is not essential.[25] This definition results in the mystifying condition of PCOS without polycystic ovaries! However, the more generally accepted theory in the UK and Europe is that a spectrum exists, ranging from women with polycystic ovarian morphology and no overt abnormality at one end, to those with polycystic ovaries associated with severe clinical and biochemical disorders at the other end. It is important also to appreciate that *in vitro* studies have demonstrated that theca cells from ovulatory women with polycystic ovaries produce increased androgens compared with normal ovaries, strengthening the argument for a fundamental dysfunction of ovarian steroidogenic activity.[26,27] Using a combination of clinical, ultrasonographic, and biochemical criteria, the diagnosis of PCOS is usually reserved for those women who exhibit an ultrasound picture of polycystic ovaries, and who display one or more of the clinical symptoms (menstrual cycle disturbances, hirsutism, obesity, hyperandrogenism), and/or one or more of the recognized biochemical disturbances (elevated LH, testosterone, androstenedione, or insulin).[1,23,28] This definition of PCOS requires the exclusion of specific underlying diseases of the adrenal or pituitary glands (e.g., hyperprolactinemia, acromegaly, and congenital adrenal hyperplasia) which could predispose to similar ultrasound and biochemical features.

We favor the following definitions:[5] first, the expression "polycystic ovaries" is used to describe the ultrasound appearance of polycystic morphology in the absence of overt symptoms of the syndrome. Second, the definition of "polycystic ovary syndrome" (PCOS1) is conferred in cases where polycystic ovaries have been identified ultrasonographically and where one or more of the clinical symptoms or biochemical features are present (i.e., oligo-/amenorrhea, hyperandrogenism, obesity, elevated serum tesosterone or LH concentrations). Thus, using this definition it is possible to have PCOS when polycystic ovaries are present together with obesity as the only other sign. It is, however, usually the case that more than one symptom, sign, or biochemical disturbance coexists with polycystic ovaries. Furthermore, the condition is dynamic and features in an individual may change over time. Third, the North American definition (PCOS2) requires evidence of hyperandrogenism and ovulatory dysfunction, in the absence of non-classic adrenal hyperplasia, without specific evidence of polycystic ovarian morphology. Nevertheless, it is widely recognized in the USA that positive ovarian findings predominate and there is considerable overlap between the European and US definitions (Table 7.1).

Heterogeneity of PCOS

A few years ago we reported a large series of women with polycystic ovaries detected by ultrasound scan.[1] All of the 1871 patients had at least one symptom of the PCOS, and the definition PCOS1 was employed (see Table 7.1). Thirty eight per cent of the women were overweight

Table 7.1 Definitions of PCOS

PCO	Polycystic ovarian morphology seen by ultrasound
PCOS 1 (favored in the UK)	Polycystic ovaries on ultrasound, plus: symptoms (obesity, hyperandrogenism, menstrual cycle disturbance) and/or: biochemical abnormalities (elevated serum concentrations of testosterone and/or LH)
PCOS 2 (favored in North America)	Hyperandrogenism and menstrual cycle disturbance

(body mass index (BMI) > 25 kg/m^2). Obesity was significantly associated with an increased risk of hirsutism, menstrual cycle disturbance, and an elevated serum testosterone concentration (Fig. 7.3). Obesity was also associated with an increased rate of infertility. Twenty six per cent of patients with primary infertility and 14% of patients with secondary infertility had a BMI of more than 30 kg/m^2. Approximately 30% of the patients had a regular menstrual cycle, 50% had oligomenorrhea, and 20% amenorrhea. In this study the classical endocrine features of raised serum LH and testosterone were found in only 39.8% and 28.9% of patients, respectively.[1]

Many other groups have similarly reported heterogeneity in their populations with PCOS. Franks's series, also from England,[29] related to 300 women recruited from a specialist endocrine clinic. Some years earlier Goldzieher.[30] compiled a comprehensive review of 1079 cases of surgically proven polycystic ovaries. The frequency of clinical symptoms and signs in these series was similar (Tables 7.2 and 7.3).

High serum LH concentrations were found to be associated with infertility or menstrual cycle disturbances in both of the studies. In the study by Balen *et al.*,[1] high serum testosterone levels were associated with an increased risk of hirsutism, infertility, and cycle disturbances.

Table 7.2 Clinical symptoms and signs in women with PCOS

	Percentage frequency of symptom or sign			
	Balen *et al.* (1995)[1] *n*=1741 %	Franks (1989)[29] *n*=300 %	Goldzieher (1981)[30] *n*=1079 %	(No. of cases[a])
Menstrual cycle disturbance:				
–oligomenorrhea	47	52	29[b]	(*n*=547)
–amenorrhea	19	28	51	(*n*=640)
Hirsutism	66	64	69	(*n*=819)
Obesity	38	35	41	(*n*=600)
Acne	34	27	–	–
Alopecia	6	3	–	–
Acanthosis nigricans	2	<1	–	–
Infertility (primary/secondary)	20	42	74	(*n*=596)

– Denotes feature not recorded.

[a] In the Goldzieher study clinical details were not available for all 1079 women, thus the number of cases which were used to determine the frequency of each symptom is stated.

[b] In this series, any abnormal pattern of uterine bleeding was included.

Table 7.3 Biochemical features of women with PCOS

	Percentage frequency	
	Balen *et al.* (1995)[1] *n*=1741 %	Franks (1989)[29] *n*=300 %
Elevated serum LH	39.8	51
Elevated serum testosterone	28.9	50
Elevated serum prolactin	11.8	7

Ovarian volume was significantly correlated with serum LH and with testosterone concentrations (see also Fig. 6.15 and text p. 157). Other authors have attempted to correlate predictors for the diagnostic criteria of women with PCOS. For example Fox *et al.*[18] found that a combination of the free androgen index (FAI) with serum LH concentration was the most accurate combination for making the diagnosis of PCOS in women with oligomenorrhea. This group also found that the progestogen challenge test – an assay of uterine estrogenization – was as good a predictor as the FAI and did not require the measurement of sex hormone binding globulin (SHBG) – an expensive and less commonly used test. In another series of women with oligomenorrhea, independent correlations with ovarian morphology were identified with LH concentrations and androgen levels.[31] Furthermore, markers of insulin resistance correlated with ovarian volume and stromal echogenicity, which in turn have been correlated with androgen production.[19,31,32]

Population-based Studies

Estimates of the prevalence of PCOS are greatly affected by the nature of the population which is being assessed. Populations of women who are selected on the basis of the presence of a symptom associated with the syndrome (e.g., hirsutism, acne, and menstrual cycle disturbances) would be expected to demonstrate a prevalence greater than that which exists in the general population.

In a study of 173 women presenting with anovulation or hirsutism, Adams *et al.*[14] found the prevalence of polycystic ovaries (using ultrasound criteria for diagnosis) to be 26% in women with amenorrhea, 87% in women with oligomenorrhea, and 92% in women with hirsutism and regular cycles. In another study of 389 women presenting with menstrual cycle disturbances, Gadir *et al.*[33] found the prevalence of polycystic ovaries to be 65%. In a third study of 350 women presenting with hirsutism and/or androgenic alopecia, O'Driscoll *et al.*[34] identified

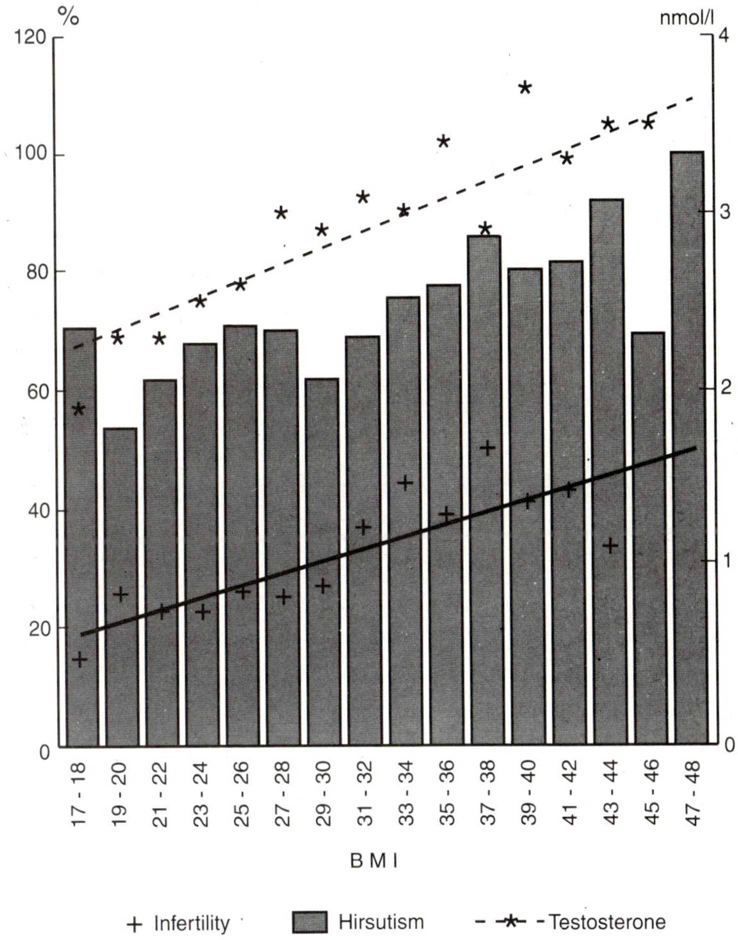

Figure 7.3 Relationship of body mass index (BMI) to the rate of hirsutism and testosterone concentration.[1]

polycystic ovaries in 60% of 282 women whose ovaries were successfully visualized by ultrasound. In a fourth study, examining 119 women with acne but no menstrual disorders, obesity, or hirsutism, Peserico *et al.*[35] found the prevalence to be 45% in this group. These results indicate that polycystic ovaries, and by definition PCOS, are very common in these specifically defined groups of women. However, the prevalence of PCOS in the general population has not been definitively determined. A cross-sectional study by Knochenhauer *et al.*[36] examined the prevalence of PCOS in a population of American women and determined a prevalence rate of 4%, but this study applied the US definition of PCOS and did not include polycystic ovarian morphology on ultrasound as part of the defining criteria.

Several studies have been performed to attempt to determine the prevalence of polycystic ovaries in the general population, as detected by ultrasound alone, and have found remarkably similar prevalence rates in the order of 17–22%. The study designs and results are summarized in Table 7.4. All of the studies used transabdominal ultrasound for the diagnosis of polycystic ovaries except for Cresswell *et al.*,[37] who converted to a transvaginal scan if the transabdominal picture was unclear.

The study populations recruited by Polson *et al.*,[2] Tayob *et al.*,[38] and by Botsis *et al.*[39] were subject to selection bias because they recruited women from hospital populations (although Polson's study recruited hospital workers and not patients) and not from the general population. The low response rates achieved in the community based studies by Clayton *et al.*[16] and Farquhar *et al.*[3] might reduce confidence in the validity of their estimates of prevalence, but reassuringly Cresswell *et al.*,[37] who achieved a much higher response rate in their sample, determined a very similar prevalence. In the absence of a large, cross-sectional population-based study, the prevalence rates detected above provide the best estimates of the occurrence of polycystic ovaries in the "normal" population. The pooled prevalence is 19%, indicating that polycystic ovaries (as defined by their ultrasound appearance) are extremely common.

The study by Tayob *et al.*[38] was primarily designed to identify women who were at risk of breakthrough ovulation while taking the combined oral contraceptive pill. Although the ovaries were assessed by trans-abdominal ultrasound, blood samples were not collected and clinical symptoms of PCOS are not recorded. In the other studies, clinical and biochemical features associated with PCOS were compared between women with and without polycystic ovaries. In all of the studies hirsutism was identified more commonly in women with polycystic ovaries. Menstrual cycle abnormalities were also found to be more common in the polycystic ovary groups, except in the study by Clayton *et al.*[16] which detected no significant difference in menstrual patterns when comparing women with polycystic vs those with normal ovaries. In the study by Polson *et al.*[2] a surprisingly low frequency of irregular menstrual cycles was detected in those women with normal ovaries. The explanation for this is not clear as the definition of "irregular cycles" is similar to that used in other studies, but may be related to the way in which menstrual histories were recorded from the participants. Botsis *et al.*[39] noted a greater tendency towards obesity in their group of women with polycystic ovaries, but significant differences in obesity were not identified in the other reports. All of these studies determined higher mean ovarian volumes in women with

Table 7.4 The prevalence of polycystic ovaries in the general population

	Polson *et al.* (1988)[2]	Tayob *et al.* (1990)[38]	Clayton *et al.* (1992)[16]	Farquhar *et al.* (1994)[3]	Botsis *et al.* (1995)[39]	Cresswell *et al.* (1997)[37]
Study population	Volunteers recruited from clinical and secretarial staff at St Mary's Hospital, London *n*=257	Volunteers using a low dose combined OCP, recruited from routine clinics at the Margaret Pyke Centre and the Royal Free Hospital, London *n*=120	Volunteers born between 1952 and 1969 recruited from a list of a group practice in Harrow, London, by random postal invitation *n*=190	Volunteers recruited from two electoral rolls in Auckland, NZ, by random postal invitation *n*=183	Volunteers recruited from women presenting to an outpatient clinic for routine Pap smear *n*=1078	Volunteers born between 1952 and 1953 recruited from records of the Jessop Hospital, Sheffield, by invitation and personal interview *n*=235
Response rate	Unknown	Unknown	18%	16%	Unknown	68%
Age range	18–36 years	18–30 years mean=24 years	18–36 years	18–45 years mean=33 years	17–40 years	40–42 years
Prevalence	22%	22%	22%	21%	17%	21%
95% CI	17–27%	14–30%	16–28%	14–27%	14–19%	16–26%

polycystic ovaries when compared with women with normal ovaries. The frequency of symptoms and signs identified in women with and without polycystic ovaries is summarized in Table 7.5. The inconsistencies between these studies may be due in part to differences in the definitions used for each symptom or sign which was recorded.

Comparison of hormone levels between women with and without polycystic ovaries was further complicated by the high proportion of women using the oral contraceptive pill (OCP) in these populations. This necessitated division of the "normal" and "polycystic ovary" groups of women into further subgroups dependent upon their oral contraceptive status. The women with polycystic ovaries tended to have disturbed biochemistry, with elevated serum testosterone concentrations and also sometimes elevated LH levels compared with those who had normal ovaries.

We studied 224 normal female volunteers between the ages of 18 and 25 years and identified polycystic ovaries using ultrasound in 33% of participants.[40] Fifty per cent of the participants were using some form of hormonal contraception, but the prevalence of polycystic ovaries in users and non-users of hormonal contraception was identical. Polycystic ovaries in the non-users of hormonal contraception were associated with irregular menstrual cycles and significantly higher serum testosterone concentrations when compared with women with normal ovaries; however, only a small proportion of women with polycystic ovaries (15%) had "elevated" serum testosterone concentrations outside the normal range. Interestingly there were no significant differences in acne, hirsutism, BMI, or body fat percentage between women with polycystic and normal ovaries and hyperinsulinism and reduced insulin sensitivity were not associated with polycystic ovaries in this group.

In our study, the prevalence of PCOS was as low as 8% using the USA definition for PCOS, or as high as 26% if the broader European criteria were applied. However, features included in the European criteria (menstrual irregularity, acne, hirsutism, BMI > 25 kg/m^2, raised serum testosterone, or raised LH) were found to occur frequently in women without polycystic ovaries, and 75% of women with normal ovaries had one or more of these attributes. Subgroup analyses of women according to the presence of normal ovaries, polycystic ovaries alone, or polycystic ovaries and features of PCOS revealed greater mean BMI in women with PCOS, but also indicated *lower* fasting insulin concentrations and *greater* insulin sensitivity in polycystic ovary and PCOS groups when compared with women with normal ovaries. This is in contrast to studies of older women.[25,41] These interesting findings were difficult to interpret in the light of current understanding of PCOS, but lead us to consider the possibility that this young, mainly non-overweight population might reflect women early in the natural

Table 7.5 Frequency of clinical symptoms and signs in women with and without polycystic ovaries

	Percentage frequency									
	Polson *et al.* (1988)[2]		Clayton *et al.* (1992)[16]		Farquhar *et al.* (1994)[17]		Botsis *et al.* (1995)[39]		Cresswell *et al.* (1997)[37]	
	PCO *n*=33[a.]	Normal *n*=116[a.]	PCO *n*=43	Normal *n*=165	PCO *n*=39	Normal *n*=144	PCO *n*=183	Normal *n*=823	PCO *n*=49	Normal *n*=186
Menstrual cycle disturbance	76%	1%	29%[a.b.]	27%	46%	20%	80%	–	41%	27%
Hirsutism	–	–	14%	2%	23%	4%	40%	10%	14%	2%
Obesity	–	–	33%	29%	23%	19%	41%	10%	35%	48%
Infertility[c.] primary/ secondary	–	–	12%	10%	26%	11%	–	–	16%	15%

– Denotes feature not recorded.
[a.] *Value includes only non-OCP users with PCO.*
[b.] *Percentage calculated for non-OCP users with PCO where n=34.*
[c.] *Includes only women who have tested their fertility.*

history of the development of PCOS, and that abnormalities of insulin metabolism might evolve following weight gain in later life.

In our study we were also able to determine genotype frequencies for the insulin gene minisatellite (*INS* VNTR) which has been linked to anovulatory PCOS.[42] Genotype frequency distributions were found to be similar in women with polycystic ovaries and those with normal ovaries. However, subdivision of those women with polycystic ovaries according to the "severity" of PCOS (classified using polycystic ovaries alone, polycystic ovaries and PCOS by European criteria, and polycystic ovaries and PCOS by USA criteria) revealed increasing frequency of the III/III genotype with increasing severity of the PCOS phenotype.[40] This could suggest that the *INS* VNTR locus may determine clinical severity of PCOS in women with polycystic ovaries. However, larger studies would be necessary to determine this conclusively.

National and racial differences in expression of PCOS

The highest reported prevalence of PCO has been 52% among South Asian immigrants in Britain, of whom 49% had menstrual irregularity.[43] Rodin *et al.*[43] demonstrated that South Asian women with polycystic ovaries, had a comparable degree of insulin resistance to controls with established type 2 diabetes mellitus. Generally, there has been a paucity of data of the prevalence of PCOS among women of South Asian origin, both among migrant and native groups. Type 2 diabetes and insulin resistance have a high prevalence among indigenous populations in South Asia, with a rising prevalence among women. Insulin resistance and hyperinsulinemia are common antecedents of type 2 diabetes, with a high prevalence in South Asians. Type 2 diabetes also has a familial basis, inherited as a complex genetic trait that interacts with environmental factors, chiefly nutrition, commencing from fetal life. We are currently exploring the hypothesis that ethnic variations in the overt features of PCOS (symptoms of hyperandrogenism, menstrual irregularity, and obesity) in women of South Asian descent are linked to the higher prevalence and degree of insulin resistance in South Asians. We have already found that South Asians with anovular PCOS[44a] have greater insulin resistance and more severe symptoms of the syndrome than anovular white Caucasians with PCOS. Furthermore, we have found that women from South Asia living in the UK appear to express symptoms at an earlier age than their white Caucasian British counterparts.[44a]

So is there evidence that the syndrome that we are discussing varies either in its prevalence or in its presentation around the world or in different racial groups within the same country? Michelmore *et al.*[4] demonstrated that 80% of those with polycystic ovaries (which was 26% of those from the community) had features of PCOS based on the UK/European definition of PCOS, in their post-menarchal years (i.e. ages 18–24). However, using the much more stringent USA criteria which do not utilize ovarian morphology, the prevalence rate for PCOS ranged from 4.5–11.2% from an unselected group of white Caucasian and blacks in a population-based study in Alabama,[36] to 9% in Greece[44] and 6.5% in Spain.[45] Generally, ethnic differences in the prevalence of PCOS have not been well explored. Dunaif and co-workers[46] reported an increased rate of PCOS among Caribbean Hispanic women. However, Knochenhauer *et al.*,[36] in a sample of 195 black women and 174 white women in the USA, found the prevalence of PCOS among black women to be comparable with that among white women (3.4% vs 4.7%). There may also be ethnic variation in overt features of PCOS when the prevalence of biochemical manifestations is similar across the races.[47] A study carried out comparing women with PCOS from the USA, Japan, and Italy reported less obesity in Japanese women, yet comparable rates of androgen excess and insulin resistance.[48] The question remains as to whether differences in expression of the syndrome are due to dietary and lifestyle factors or to genetic variations in hormone actions, such as polymorphisms in gonadotropin subunits or receptor function (affecting the expression of androgens, gonadotropins, or insulin). A full discussion of the genetics of PCOS is beyond the scope of this chapter and there are a number of candidate genes that have been proposed (see Franks *et al.*[8] for a recent review). It may be that some families or racial groups have genetic differences that affect the expression or presentation of PCOS.

Health Consequences of Polycystic Ovary Syndrome

Obesity and metabolic abnormalities are recognized risk factors for the development of ischemic heart disease (IHD) in the general population, and these are also recognized features of PCOS. IHD accounts for 18% of deaths in men and 14% of deaths in women in Europe. In men, the incidence of IHD increases after the age of 35 years, while in women an increased incidence is noted after the age of 55 years. The questions are whether women with PCOS are at an increased risk of IHD, and whether this will occur at an earlier age than women with normal ovaries. The basis for the idea that women with PCOS are at greater risk for cardiovascular disease is that these women are more insulin resistant than weight-matched controls and that the metabolic disturbances associated with insulin resistance are known to increase cardiovascular risk in other populations.

Insulin resistance is defined as a diminution in the biological responses to a given level of insulin (see glucose tolerance test, Ch. 4, p. 67). In the presence of an adequate pancreatic reserve, normal circulating glucose levels are maintained at higher serum insulin concentrations. In the general population cardiovascular risk factors include insulin resistance, obesity, glucose intolerance, hypertension, and dyslipidemia. A prospective population-based study of 1462 women aged between 38 and 60 years was undertaken in Gothenberg, to examine cardiovascular risk factors in women.[49] After a 12 year follow-up, they reported four independent risk factors for myocardial infarction in women; these were increased waist:hip ratio, raised serum triglyceride concentrations, diabetes, and hypertension. A further follow-up of the same cohort of women for a period of 20 years found that the two most important factors relating to cardiovascular mortality were central obesity and raised serum triglycerides. Central obesity was more important than obesity itself.

Two large American epidemiological studies on heart disease in women, the Framingham and Lipid Research Clinic Follow-up studies, demonstrated that mortality from cardiovascular disease was closely related to the lipid fractions, namely elevated serum triglycerides and reduced high-density lipoprotein (HDL) cholesterol levels. In 1988, Reaven[50] described syndrome X, or the insulin resistance syndrome, which is characterized by the presence of hyperinsulinemia, varying degrees of glucose intolerance, dyslipidemia, central obesity, and hypertension. It was suggested that the metabolic and hemodynamic abnormalities associated with syndrome X constitute a major role in the etiology/risk factors leading to coronary heart disease.

Burghen and colleagues[51] first suggested a relationship between the hyperandrogenism of PCOS and hyperinsulinemia. There was a significant correlation between basal insulin measurements and serum testosterone and androstenedione concentrations, and between insulin response during the oral glucose tolerance test and serum testosterone concentrations. Subsequently hyperinsulinemia has been demonstrated in non-obese PCOS subjects, demonstrating that a form of insulin resistance is specific to PCOS in addition to that caused by obesity. Since then there have been a large number of studies demonstrating the presence of insulin resistance and corresponding hyperinsulinemia in both obese and non-obese women with PCOS. Obese women with PCOS have consistently been shown to be more insulin resistant than weight-matched controls. It appears that obesity and PCOS have an additive effect on the degree and severity of the insulin resistance and subsequent hyperinsulinemia in this group of women.

Insulin sensitivity varies depending upon menstrual pattern. Women with PCOS who are oligomenorrheic are more likely to be insulin resistant than those with regular cycles – irrespective of their BMI. Women with PCOS have a defect in insulin signaling at the insulin receptor, which causes insulin resistance. The sex steroid induced increase of growth hormone that initiates the adolescent growth spurt also leads to insulin resistance and explains the timing of onset of symptoms in those prone to develop PCOS. The presence of obesity and/or type 2 diabetes worsens the degree of insulin resistance.

Insulin resistance is restricted to the extra-splanchnic actions of insulin on glucose dispersal. The liver is not affected (hence the fall in SHBG and HDL), neither is the ovary (hence the menstrual problems and hypersecretion of androgens) nor the skin, hence the development of acanthosis nigricans. The insulin resistance causes compensatory hypersecretion of insulin, particularly in response to glucose, so euglycemia is usually maintained at the expense of hyperinsulinemia.

Central obesity Simple obesity is associated with greater deposition of gluteo-femoral fat while central obesity involves greater truncal abdominal fat distribution. Obesity is observed in 35–60% of women with PCOS. Hyperandrogenism is associated with a preponderance of fat localized to truncal abdominal sites. Women with PCOS have a greater truncal abdominal fat distribution as demonstrated by a higher waist:hip ratio. The central distribution of fat is independent of BMI and associated with higher plasma insulin and triglyceride concentrations, and reduced HDL cholesterol concentrations.

Impaired glucose tolerance and diabetes Impaired glucose tolerance and diabetes are known risk factors for cardiovascular disease. It is reported that 18–20% of obese women with PCOS demonstrate impaired glucose tolerance. Dahlgren *et al.*[52] noted the prevalence of type 2 diabetes was 15% in women with PCOS compared with 2% in the controls. Most women with type 2 diabetes under the age of 45 years have PCOS. Insulin resistance combined with abdominal obesity is thought to account for the higher prevalence of type 2 diabetes in PCOS. There is a concomitant increased risk of gestational diabetes. We recommended a glucose tolerance test for white Caucasian women with PCOS and a BMI of > 30 kg/m^2 and for Asian women with PCOS if they have a BMI > 25 kg/m^2 (see p. 67). Women with PCOS are also at increased risk of developing gestational diabetes.

Hypertension The prevalence of treated hypertension is three times higher in women with PCOS between the ages of 40 and 59 years compared with controls.[52] In their series, Gjonnaess[53] reported the incidence of pre-eclampsia in obese women with PCOS conceiving after ovarian electrocautery to be 12.9% compared with 3.8% in the general pregnant population.

Dyslipidemia Women with PCOS have high concentrations of serum triglycerides and suppressed HDL levels, particularly a lower

HDL_2 subfraction. HDLs play an important role in lipid metabolism and are the most important lipid parameter in predicting cardiovascular risk in women. HDLs perform the task of "reverse cholesterol transport". That is, they remove excess lipids from the circulation and tissues to transport them to the liver for excretion, or transfer them to other lipoprotein particles. Cholesterol is only one component of HDL, a particle with constantly changing composition forming HDL_3 then HDL_2, as unesterified cholesterol is taken from tissue, esterified and exchanged for triglyceride with other lipoprotein species. Consequently, measurement of a single constituent in a particle involved in a dynamic process gives an incomplete picture.

In a detailed study of HDL composition it was found that obesity was the most important factor associated with elevated serum total triglyceride, cholesterol, and phospholipid concentrations in both PCOS subjects and controls.[54] In addition, obese women with PCOS had lower HDL cholesterol and phospholipid concentrations in all subfractions compared with obese controls. This was in the presence of normal quantities of the protein component of HDL – apolipoprotein-a_1. These findings imply that the number of HDL particles was the same in obese PCOS subjects compared with obese controls, but the HDL particles were lipid-depleted, hence less effective in function. The only factor which appeared to have an independent influence on the HDL composition was the presence of PCOS, rather than obesity or raised serum androgen or insulin concentrations.

Plasminogen activator inhibitor-I (PAI-1) is a potent inhibitor of fibrinolysis and has been found to be elevated in both obese women and non-obese women with PCOS. Plasma levels of PAI-1 correlate directly with serum insulin concentrations, and have been shown to be an important predictor of myocardial infarction.

Thus, in summary, examining the surrogate risk factors for cardiovascular disease, there is evidence that insulin resistance, central obesity, and hyperinsulinemia are features of PCOS and have an adverse effect on lipid metabolism. Women with PCOS have been shown to have dyslipidemia, with reduced HDL cholesterol and elevated serum triglyceride concentrations, along with elevated serum PAI-1 concentrations. The evidence is thus mounting that women with PCOS may have an increased risk of developing cardiovascular disease and diabetes later in life, which has important implications in their management.

PCOS in younger women At what stage do the risk factors for cardiovascular disease become apparent in women with PCOS? The majority of the studies which have identified the risk factors of obesity and insulin resistance in women with PCOS have investigated adult populations, commonly including women who have presented to specialist endocrine or reproductive medicine clinics. However, PCOS has been identified in much younger populations,[4] in which women with increasing symptoms of PCOS were found to be more insulin resistant. These data emphasize the need for long-term prospective studies of young women with PCOS in order to clarify the natural history, and to determine which women will be at risk of diabetes and cardiovascular disease later in life. A study of women with PCOS and a mean age of 39 years, followed over a period of 6 years, found that 9% of those with normal glucose tolerance developed impaired glucose tolerance (IGT) and 8% developed NIDDM,[55] while 54% of women with IGT at the start of the study had NIDDM at follow-up. The risks of disease progression, not surprisingly, were greatest in those who were overweight.

In 1992, Dahlgren and colleagues[52] extrapolated the findings of their earlier study to ascertain the relative risk of IHD in a group of 33 women diagnosed clinically and histologically to have PCOS between 1956 and 1965. By risk model analysis it was calculated that the women with PCOS had a 7.4-fold greater risk of myocardial infarction than age-matched controls. Compared with the control group, the women with PCOS aged 40 years or more showed a marked increase in the prevalence of central obesity and higher basal serum insulin concentrations, as well as a seven-fold higher prevalence of diabetes and three-fold higher prevalence of hypertension. However, in another study Pierpoint *et al.*[56] reported the mortality rate in 1028 women diagnosed as having PCOS between 1930 and 1979. All the women were older than 45 years and 770 women had been treated by wedge resection of the ovaries. A total of 786 women were traced; the mean age at diagnosis was 26.4 years and average duration of follow-up was 30 years. There were 59 deaths, of which 15 were from circulatory disease. Of these 15 deaths, 13 were from IHD. There were six deaths from diabetes as an underlying or contributory cause compared with the expected 1.7 deaths. The standard mortality rate both overall and for cardiovascular disease was not higher in the women with PCOS compared with the national mortality rates in women, although the observed proportion of women with diabetes as a contributory or underlying factor leading to death was significantly higher than expected (odds ratio 3.6, 95% CI 1.5–8.4). Thus, despite surrogate markers for cardiovascular disease, in this study no increased rate of death from cardiovascular disease could be demonstrated.

Endometrial Cancer

Endometrial adenocarcinoma is the second most common female genital malignancy but only 4% of cases occur in women less than 40 years of age. The risk of developing endometrial cancer has been shown to be adversely influenced by a number of factors including obesity, long-term use of unopposed estrogens, nulliparity, and infertility. The relative risk of endometrial cancer is 1.6 in women with a menarche before the age of 12 years and 2.4 in women who have their menopause after the age of 52 years.[57] Women with endometrial carcinoma have had fewer births compared with controls and it has also been demonstrated that infertility *per se* gives a relative risk of 2. Hypertension and type 2 diabetes mellitus have long been linked to endometrial cancer, with relative risks of 2.1 and 2.8 respectively[57] – conditions that are now known also to be associated with PCOS.

A study by Coulam *et al.*[58] examined the risk of developing endometrial carcinoma in a group of 1270 patients who were diagnosed as having "chronic anovulation syndrome." The defining characteristics of this group included pathological or macroscopic evidence of the Stein–Leventhal syndrome, or a clinical diagnosis of chronic anovulation. This study identified the excess risk of endometrial cancer to be 3.1 (95% CI, 1.1–7.3) and proposed that this might be due to abnormal levels of unopposed estrogen. The true risk of endometrial carcinoma in women with PCOS, however, is difficult to ascertain.

Endometrial hyperplasia may be a precursor to adenocarcinoma, with cystic glandular hyperplasia progressing in perhaps 0.4% of cases and adenomatous hyperplasia in up to 18% of cases over 2–10 years. Precise estimation of rate of progression is impossible to determine. Some authors have reported conservative management of endometrial adenocarcinoma in women with PCOS with a combination of curettage and high dose progestogens. The rationale is that cancer of the endometrium often presents at an early stage, is well differentiated, of low risk of metastasis, and therefore is not perceived as being life-threatening, while poorly differentiated adenocarcinoma in a young woman has a worse prognosis and warrants hysterectomy. In general, however, the literature on women with PCOS and endometrial hyperplasia or adenocarcinoma suggests that this group has a poor prognosis for fertility. This may be because of the factors that predisposed to the endometrial pathology – chronic anovulation combined often with severe obesity – or secondary to the endometrial pathology disrupting potential embryonic implantation. Thus a more traditional and radical surgical approach (i.e. hysterectomy) is suggested as the safest way to prevent progression of the cancer. Early stage disease may permit ovarian conservation and the possibility of pregnancy by surrogacy.

Although the degree of risk has not been clearly defined, it is generally accepted that for women with PCOS who experience amenorrhea, or oligomenorrhea, the induction of artificial withdrawal bleeds to prevent endometrial hyperplasia is prudent management. Indeed we consider it important that women with PCOS shed their endometrium at least every 3 months. For those women with oligo-/amenorrhea who do not wish to use cyclical hormone therapy, we recommend an ultrasound scan to measure endometrial thickness and morphology every 6–12 months (depending upon menstrual history). An endometrial thickness greater than 10 mm in an amenorrheic woman warrants an artificially induced bleed, which should be followed by a repeat ultrasound scan and endometrial biopsy if the endometrium has not been shed. Another option is consider a progestogen secreting intrauterine system, such as the Mirena.

Breast Cancer

Obesity, hyperandrogenism, and infertility occur frequently in PCOS, and are features known to be associated with the development of breast cancer. However, studies examining the relationship between PCOS and breast carcinoma have not always identified a significantly increased risk. The study by Coulam *et al.*[58] calculated a relative risk of 1.5 (95% CI 0.75–2.55) for breast cancer in their group of women with chronic anovulation, which was not statistically significant. After stratification by age, however, the relative risk was found to be 3.6 (95% CI 1.2–8.3) in the postmenopausal age group. More recently, Pierpoint *et al.*[56] reported a series of 786 women with PCOS in the UK who were traced from hospital records after histological diagnosis of polycystic ovaries between 1930 and 1979. Mortality was assessed from the national registry of deaths and standardized mortality rates (SMR) calculated for patients with PCOS compared with the normal population. The average follow-up period was 30 years. The SMR for all neoplasms was 0.91 (95% CI 0.60–1.32) and for breast cancer 1.48 (95% CI 0.79–2.54). In fact, breast cancer was the leading cause of death in this cohort.

Ovarian Cancer

In recent years there has been much debate about the risk of ovarian cancer in women with infertility, particularly in relation to the use of drugs to induce superovulation for assisted conception procedures. Inherently the risk of ovarian cancer appears to be increased in women who have multiple ovulations – that is, those who are nulliparous (possibly because of infertility) with an early menarche and late menopause. Thus it may be that inducing multiple ovulations in women with infertility will increase their risk (see Ch. 17) – a notion that is by no means proven. Women with PCOS who are oligo-/anovulatory might therefore be expected to be at low risk of developing ovarian cancer if it is lifetime number of ovulations rather than pregnancies that is critical. Ovulation induction to correct anovulatory infertility aims to induce unifollicular ovulation and so in theory should raise the risk of a woman with PCOS to that of a normal ovulating woman. The polycystic ovary, however, is notoriously sensitive to stimulation and it is only in recent years with the development of high resolution transvaginal ultrasonography that the rate of unifollicular ovulation has attained acceptable levels. The use of clomiphene citrate and gonadotropin therapy for ovulation induction in the 1960s, 1970s, and 1980s resulted in many more multiple ovulations (and indeed multiple pregnancies) than in recent times and might therefore present with an increased rate of ovarian cancer when these women reach their sixties – the age of greatest incidence.

There are a few studies which have addressed the possibility of an association between polycystic ovaries and ovarian cancer. The results are conflicting, and generalizability is limited due to problems with the study designs. In the large UK study of Pierpoint *et al.*[56] the standardized mortality rate for ovarian cancer was 0.39 (95% CI 0.01–2.17).

Management of Polycystic Ovary Syndrome

Investigations: for women with PCOS see Ch. 4, p. 63–74).

Obesity

The management of women with PCOS should be focused on the patient's particular problems. Obesity worsens both symptomatology and the endocrine profile and so obese women (BMI > 30 kg/m^2) should be encouraged to lose weight, by a combination of calorie restriction and exercise. Weight loss improves the endocrine profile, the likelihood of ovulation, and a healthy pregnancy.

Insulin sensitizing agents such as metformin are becoming increasingly popular in the management of PCOS (see also Ch. 6) as they act directly at the pathogenesis of the syndrome and help correct both metabolic and endocrine problems. Early studies suggest an improvement in reproductive function and menstrual cycle regulation and there may be benefits to health of long-term use, including deferring the onset of type 2 diabetes, although large prospective studies are required.

Menstrual Irregularity

The simplest way to control the menstrual cycle is the use of a low dose combined oral contraceptive preparation (COCP). This will result in an artificial cycle and regular shedding of the endometrium. It is also important once again to encourage weight loss. As women with PCOS are thought to be at increased risk of cardiovascular disease a "lipid friendly" combined contraceptive pill should be used. The third generation oral contraceptives are lipid friendly but present the potential disadvantage of venous thromboembolism, particularly in overweight women. Dianette® is a COCP that has antiandrogenic properties and will have additional benefits for women with hyperandrogenism and Yasmin® contains a newer antiandrogen, which is still being evaluated in women with PCOS (see below). Alternatives to the COCP include a progestogen, for example medroxyprogesterone acetate (Provera) or dydrogesterone (Duphaston), for 12 days every 1–3 months to induce a withdrawal bleed, or simply the insertion of a Mirena intrauterine system.

In women with anovulatory cycles the action of estradiol on the endometrium is unopposed because of the lack of cyclical progesterone secretion. This may result in episodes of irregular uterine bleeding, and in the long term endometrial hyperplasia and even endometrial cancer. An ultrasound assessment of endometrial thickness provides a bioassay for estradiol production by the ovaries and conversion of androgens in the peripheral fat. If the endometrium is thicker than 10 mm a withdrawal bleed should be induced and if the endometrium fails to shed then endometrial sampling is required to exclude endometrial hyperplasia or malignancy. The only young women to get endometrial carcinoma (< 35 years), which otherwise has a mean age of occurrence of 61 years in the UK, are those with anovulation secondary to PCOS or estrogen-secreting tumors (see above).

Infertility (see Ch. 6 for the management of anovulatory infertility in PCOS)

Hyperandrogenism and hirsutism

The bioavailability of testosterone is affected by the serum concentration of SHBG. High levels of insulin inhibit hepatic synthesis of SHBG and so increase the free fraction of androgen. Elevated serum androgen concentrations stimulate peripheral androgen receptors, resulting in an increase in 5α reductase activity, thereby increasing the conversion of testosterone to the more potent metabolite, dihydrotestosterone. Symptoms of hyperandrogenism include hirsutism, which is a distressing condition. Hirsutism is characterized by terminal hair growth in a male pattern of distribution, including chin, upper lip, chest, upper and lower back, upper and lower abdomen, upper arm, thigh, and buttocks. A standardized scoring system, such as the modified Ferriman and Gallwey score, should be used to evaluate the degree of hirsutism before and during treatments.

Optimally, treatment combines cosmetic and medical therapies. Medical regimens stop further progression of hirsuitism and slow the rate of hair growth. However, drug therapies may take 6–9 months or longer before any benefit is perceived and so physical treatments (see p. 53, Fig. 4.1) including laser, electrolysis, waxing, and bleaching may be helpful while waiting for medical treatments to work. Medical therapy is aimed at slowing the rate of hair growth while cosmetic treatments attempt to remove existing hair. Laser therapy works best in women with dark hair on fair skin, but is expensive and not usually permanent (despite claims to the contrary).

Symptoms of hyperandrogenism can be treated by a combination of an estrogen (such as ethinylestradiol, or a combined contraceptive pill), and the antiandrogen cyproterone acetate (50–100 mg). Estrogens lower circulating androgens by a combination of a slight inhibition of gonadotropin secretion and gonadotropin-sensitive ovarian steroid production and by an increase in hepatic production of SHBG resulting in lower free testosterone. The cyproterone is taken for the first 10 days of a cycle (the "reversed sequential" method) and the estrogen for the first 21 days. After a gap of exactly 7 days, during which menstruation usually occurs, the regimen is repeated. As an alternative, the preparation Dianette® contains ethinylestradiol in combination with cyproterone, although at a lower dose (2 mg). Cyproterone acetate acts as a competitive inhibitor at the androgen receptor. Cyproterone acetate can, rarely, cause liver damage and liver function should be checked after 6 months and then annually. Unfortunately this treatment increases insulin resistance.

Other antiandrogens such as ketoconazole, finasteride, and flutamide have been tried, but are not widely used in the UK due to their adverse side effects. Spironolactone, a potassium sparing diuretic, has antiandrogenic properties and is useful in women for whom the oral contraceptive pill is contraindicated (e.g., because of hypertension). Spironolactone, at a dose of 50–100 mg daily, may result in erratic menstrual bleeding and should be combined with reliable contraception. A new combined oral contraceptive preparation, Yasmin, contains a new progestogen, drosperinone, which is a derivative of spironolactone, with potential antiandrogenic properties and benefits for women with PCOS.

Conclusions

PCOS is one of the most common endocrine disorders. It may present, at one end of the spectrum, with the single finding of polycystic ovarian morphology as detected by pelvic ultrasound. At the other end of the spectrum, symptoms such as obesity, hyperandrogenism, menstrual cycle disturbance, and infertility may occur either singly or in combination. Women with PCOS are characterized by the presence of insulin resistance, central obesity, and dyslipidemia, which appears to place them at a higher risk of developing diabetes as well as cardiovascular disease. There are a number of environmental factors that may influence the expression of the syndrome, in particular a tendency to insulin resistant states induced by overeating and under-exercising. A plausible hypothesis for the survival of PCOS in the population is that of the "thrifty phenotype/genotype" whereby in times of famine, individuals who have a tendency to obesity preserve the population by maintaining fertility, while those of normal body weight fall below the threshold body weight for fertility. This might explain the greater prevalence of PCOS among South Asians in the UK, where there is relatively greater nutrition and thus the right environment to express PCOS. In addition the "thrifty phenotype" hypothesis suggests that *in utero* insulin resistance results as an adaptation to impaired nutrition and then persists through to adult life and is then amplified by over-nutrition (obesity).

PCOS is probably the same the world over, although without an agreed definition one cannot say for sure that this is the case. There may be factors that effect expression and presentation – whether because of racial differences in the color and distribution of hair (e.g., Japanese vs Mediterranean women) or variations in hormone production and receptor activity. Fundamentally, the underlying condition is likely to be the same. Management should be directed towards an individual's needs (whether cosmetic, reproductive, or metabolic) and attention given to potential long-term sequelae. In order to compare treatments and define the genotype we must be clear on the phenotype and so an international consensus is still required.

Women with PCOS are characterized by the presence of insulin resistance, central obesity, and dyslipidemia, which appears to place them at a higher risk of developing diabetes as well as cardiovascular disease. The retrospective long-term follow-up studies have confirmed the higher incidence of diabetes, though they have not shown a higher risk of mortality from ischemic heart disease. Cross-sectional studies have demonstrated a significant association between PCOS and IHD. Prospective longitudinal studies confirming this risk are still awaited. There does seem to be enough biochemical evidence regarding the potential for long-term risks of cardiovascular disease and diabetes, which need to be addressed when counseling women with PCOS. Therapeutic interventions in the form of metformin and other insulin sensitizing drugs appear to be potentially effective tools in ameliorating insulin resistance with improvement in clinical and hormonal parameters, and possible reduction in cardiovascular risk. But further evaluation is needed. Encouraging weight loss remains the most effective first line therapeutic intervention in these women, albeit hard to achieve. Further longitudinal studies need to be performed to investigate the natural history of PCOS and its sequelae for the health of women.

References

1. Balen AH, Conway GS, Kaltsas G *et al.* (1995) Polycystic ovary syndrome: the spectrum of the disorder in 1741 patients. *Hum Reprod* **10**: 2107–2111.
2. Polson DW, Adams J, Wadsworth J & Franks S (1988) Polycystic ovaries – a common finding in normal women. *Lancet* **1**: 870–872.
3. Farquhar CM, Birdsall M, Manning P, Mitchell JM & France JT (1994) The prevalence of polycystic ovaries on ultrasound scanning in a population of randomly selected women. *Aust N Z J Obstet Gynaecol* **34**: 67–72.
4. Michelmore KF, Balen AH, Dunger DB & Vessey MP (1999) Polycystic ovaries and associated clinical and biochemical features in young women. *Clin Endocrinol Oxf* **51**: 779–786.
5. Balen AH (1999) The pathogenesis of polycystic ovary syndrome: the enigma unravels. *Lancet* **354**: 966–967.
6. Franks et al 1997 [details to follow]
7. Clarke AM, Ledger W, Galletly C *et al.* (1995) Weight loss results in significant improvement in pregnancy and ovulation rates in anovulatory obese women. *Hum Reprod* **10**: 2705–2712.
8. Franks S, Gharani N & McCarthy M (2001) Candidate genes in polycystic ovary syndrome. *Human Reprod Update* **7**: 405–410.
9. Rajkowha M, Glass MR, Rutherford AJ, Michelmore K & Balen AH (2000) Polycystic ovary syndrome: a risk factor for cardiovascular disease? *Br J Obstet Gynaecol* **107**: 11–18.
10. Stein IF & Leventhal ML (1935) Amenorrhea associated with bilateral polycystic ovaries. *Am J Obstet Gynecol* **29**: 181–191.
11. Franks S (1995) Polycystic ovary syndrome. *N Engl J Med* **333**: 853–861.
12. Saxton DW, Farquhar CM, Rae T, Beard RW, Anderson MC & Wadsworth J (1990) Accuracy of ultrasound measurements of female pelvic organs. *Br J Obstet Gynaecol* **97**: 695–699.
13. Takahashi K, Eda Y, Abu Musa A, Okada S, Yoshino K & Kitao M (1994) Transvaginal ultrasound imaging, histopathology and endocrinopathy in patients with polycystic ovarian syndrome. *Hum Reprod* **9**: 1231–1236.
14. Adams J, Polson DW & Franks S (1986) Prevalence of polycystic ovaries in women with anovulation and idiopathic hirsutism. *Br Med J Clin Res Ed* **293**: 355–359.
15. Kiddy DS, Sharp PS, White DM *et al.* (1990) Differences in clinical and endocrine features between obese and non-obese subjects with polycystic ovary syndrome: an analysis of 263 consecutive cases. *Clin Endocrinol Oxf* **32**: 213–220.
16. Clayton RN, Ogden V, Hodgkinson J *et al.* (1992) How common are polycystic ovaries in normal women and what is their significance for the fertility of the population? [see comments] *Clin Endocrinol Oxf* **37**: 127–134.
17. Farquhar CM, Birdsall M, Manning P & Mitchell JM (1994) Transabdominal versus transvaginal ultrasound in the diagnosis of polycystic ovaries in a population of randomly selected women. *Ultrasound Obstet Gynecol* **4**: 54–59.
18. Fox R, Corrigan E, Thomas PA & Hull MG (1991) The diagnosis of polycystic ovaries in women with oligo-amenorrhea: predictive power of endocrine tests. *Clin Endocrinol Oxf* **34**: 127–131.
19. Kyei-Mensah A, Maconochie N, Zaidi J, Pittrof R, Campbell S & Tan SL (1996) Transvaginal three-dimensional ultrasound: reproducibility of ovarian and endometrial volume measurements. *Fertil Steril* **5**: 718–722.
20. Zaidi J, Campbell S, Pittrof R, Kyei-Mensah A, Jacobs HS & Tan SL (1995) Ovarian stromal blood flow in women with polycystic ovaries – a possible new marker for diagnosis? *Hum Reprod* **10**: 1992–1996.
21. Faure N, Prat X, Bastide A & Lemay A (1989) Assessment of ovaries by magnetic resonance imaging in patients presenting with polycystic ovarian syndrome. *Hum Reprod* **4**: 468–472.

22. Fulghesu AM, Ciampelli M, Belosi C, Apa R, Pavone V & Lanzone A (2001) A new ultrasound criterion for the diagnosis of polycystic ovary syndrome: the ovarian stroma/total area ratio. *Fertile Steril* **76**: 326–331.
23. van Santbrink EJP, Hop WC & Fauser BCJM (1997) Classification of normogonadotropic infertility: polycystic ovaries diagnosed by ultrasound versus endocrine characteristics of polycystic ovary syndrome. *Fertil Steril* **67**: 452–458.
24. Ehrmann DA, Rosenfield RL, Barnes RB, Brigell DF & Sheikh Z (1992) Detection of functional ovarian hyperandrogenism in women with androgen excess. *N Engl J Med* **327**: 157–162.
25. Dunaif A (1997) Insulin resistance and the polycystic ovary syndrome: mechanism and implications for pathogenesis. *Endocr Rev* **18**: 774–800.
26. Gilling-Smith C, Willis DS, Beard RW & Franks S (1994) Hypersecretion of androstenedione by isolated thecal cells from polycystic ovaries. *J Clin Endocrinol Metab* **79**: 1158–1165.
27. Gilling-Smith C, Story H, Rogers V & Franks S (1997) Evidence for a primary abnormality of thecal cell steroidogenesis in the polycystic ovary syndrome. *Clin Endocrinol* **47**: 93–99.
28. Conway GS, Honour JW & Jacobs HS (1989) Heterogeneity of the polycystic ovary syndrome: clinical, endocrine and ultrasound features in 556 patients. *Clin Endocrinol Oxf* **30**: 459–470.
29. Franks S (1989) Polycystic ovary syndrome: a changing perspective. *Clin Endocrinol Oxf* **31**: 87–120.
30. Goldzieher JW (1981) Polycystic ovarian disease. *Fertil Steril* **35**: 371–394.
31. Pache TD, de Jong FH, Hop WC & Fauser BCJM (1993) Association between ovarian changes assessed by transvaginal sonogrophy and clinical and endocrine signs of the polycystic ovary syndrome. *Fertil Steril* **59**: 544–549.
32. Dewailly D, Robert Y, Helin I, Ardaens Y *et al.* (1994) Ovarian stromal hypertrophy in hyperandrogenic women. *Clin Endocrinol* **41**: 557–562.
33. Gadir AA, Khatim MS, Mowafi RS, Alnaser HM, Muharib NS & Shaw RW (1992) Implications of ultrasonically diagnosed polycystic ovaries. I. Correlations with basal hormonal profiles. *Hum Reprod* **7**: 453–457.
34. O'Driscoll JB, Mamtora H, Higginson J, Pollock A, Kane J & Anderson DC (1994) A prospective study of the prevalence of clear-cut endocrine disorders and polycystic ovaries in 350 patients presenting with hirsutism or androgenic alopecia. *Clin Endocrinol Oxf* **41**: 231–236.
35. Peserico A, Angeloni G, Bertoli P *et al.* (1989) Prevalence of polycystic ovaries in women with acne. *Arch Dermatol Res* **281**: 502–503.
36. Knochenhauer ES, Key TJ, Kahsar-Miller M, Waggoner W, Boots LR & Azziz R (1998) Prevalence of the polycystic ovary syndrome in unselected black and white women of the southeastern United States: a prospective study. *J Clin Endocrinol Metab* **83**: 3078–3082.
37. Cresswell JL, Barker DJ, Osmond C, Egger P, Phillips DI & Fraser RB (1997) Fetal growth, length of gestation, and polycystic ovaries in adult life. *Lancet* **350**: 1131–1135.
38. Tayob Y, Robinson G, Adams J *et al.* (1990) Ultrasound appearance of the ovaries during the pill-free interval. *Br J Family Planning* **16**: 94–96.
39. Botsis D, Kassanos D, Pyrgiotis E & Zourlas PA (1995) Sonographic incidence of polycystic ovaries in a gynecological population. *Ultrasound Obstet Gynecol* **6**: 182–185.
40. Michelmore KF, Ong K, Mason S, Bennett S, Perry L, Vessey MP, Balen AH & Dunger DB (2001) Clinical features in women with polycystic ovaries: relationships to insulin sensitivity, insulin gene *VNTR* and birth weight. *Clin Endocrinol* **55**: 439–446.
41. Conway GS, Clark PM & Wong D (1993) Hyperinsulinaemia in the polycystic ovary syndrome confirmed with a specific immunoradiometric assay for insulin. *Clin Endocrinol Oxf* **38**: 219–222.

42. Waterworth DM, Bennett ST, Gharani N *et al.* (1997) Linkage and association of insulin gene VNTR regulatory polymorphism with polycystic ovary syndrome. *Lancet* **349**: 986–990.
43. Rodin DA, Bano G, Bland JM, Taylor K & Nussey SS (1998) Polycystic ovaries and associated metabolic abnormalities in Indian subcontinent Asian women. *Clin Endocrinol* **49**: 91–99.
44. Diamanti-Kandarakis E, Kouli CR, Bergiele AT *et al.* (1999) A survey of the polycystic ovary syndrome in the Greek island of Lesbos: hormonal and metabolic profile. *J Clin Endocrinol Metab* **84**: 4006–4011.
44a. Wijeyaratne CN, Balen AH, Barth J, Belchetz PE. Polycystic ovary syndrome in south Asian women: a case control study. *Clin Endocrinol*, 2002; **57**: 343–350.
45. Asunción M, Calvo R M, San Millán J L, Sancho J, Avila S & Escoar-Morreale H F (2000) A prospective study of the prevalence of the polycystic ovary syndrome in unselected Caucasian women in Spain. *J Clin Endocrinol Metab* **85**: 2434–2438.
46. Dunaif A, Sorbara L, Delson R *et al.* (1993) Ethnicity and polycystic ovary syndrome are associated with independent and additive decreases in insulin action in Caribbean Hispanic women. *Diabetes* **42**: 1462–1468.
47. Solomons CG (1999) The epidemiology of polycystic ovary syndrome – prevalence and associated disease risks. *Endocrinol Metab Clin North Am* **28**: 247–263.
48. Carmina E, Koyama T, Chang L, Stanczyk FZ & Lobo RA (1992) Does ethnicity influence the prevalence of adrenal hyperandrogenism and insulin resistance in polycystic ovary syndrome? *Am J Obstet Gynecol* **167**: 1807–1812.
49. Lapidus L (1986) Ischaemic heart disease, stroke and total mortality in women: results from a prospective population study in Gothenberg, Sweden. *Acta Med Scand* **705**(Suppl.): 1–42.
50. Reaven GM (1988) Role of insulin resistance in human disease. *Diabetes* **37**: 1595–1607.
51. Burghen GA, Givens JR & Kitabchi AE (1980) Correlation of hyperandrogenism with hyperinsulinism in polycystic ovarian disease. *J Clin Endocrinol Metab* **50**: 113–116.
52. Dahlgren E, Johansson S, Lindstedt G *et al.* (1992) Women with polycystic ovary syndrome wedge resected in 1956 to 1965 : a long term follow up focussing on natural history and circulating hormones. *Fertil Steril* **57**: 505–513.
53. Gjonnaess H (1989) The course and outcome of pregnancy after ovarian electrocautery in women with polycystic ovarian syndrome: the influence of body weight. *Br J Obstet Gynaecol* **96**: 714–719.
54. Rajkhowa M, Neary RH, Knmptala P *et al.* (1997) Altered composition of high density lipoproteins in women with polycystic ovary syndrome. *J Clin Endocrinol Metab* **82**: 3389–3394.
55. Norman RJ, Masters L, Milner CR, Wang JX & Davies MJ (2001) Relative risk of conversion from normoglycaemia to impaired glucose tolerance or non-insulin dependent diabetes mellitus in polycystic ovary syndrome. *Hum Reprod* **16**: 1995–1998.
56. Pierpoint T, McKeigue PM, Isaacs AJ, Wild SH & Jacobs HS (1998) Mortality of women with polycystic ovary syndrome at long-term follow-up. *J Clin Epidemiol* **51**: 581–586.
57. Elwood JM, Cole P, Rothman KJ *et al.* (1977) Epidemiology of endometrial cancer. *J Natl Cancer Inst* **59**: 1055–1060.
58. Coulam CB, Annegers JF & Kranz JS (1983) Chronic anovulation syndrome and associated neoplasia. *Obstet Gynecol* **61**: 403–407.

Acknowledgment

I am grateful to Dr K. Michelmore and Dr M. Rajkhowa for their assistance in the preparation of this chapter.

Chapter 8

Ovarian failure and resistant ovary syndrome

Premature Ovarian Failure

Premature ovarian failure (POF) occurs in approximately 1% of women and is defined as the cessation of ovarian function under the age of 40 years. The function of the ovary depends upon the total number of oocytes contained within primordial follicles. Primordial follicles and oocytes are derived during fetal life and the oogonial stem cell line is lost before birth.

The control of ovarian aging is still one of the biggest enigmas in reproductive biology. The function of the ovary depends upon the total number of oocytes contained within primordial follicles. Primordial follicles and oocytes are derived during fetal life and the oogonial stem cell line is lost before birth. In humans at approximately 4 weeks' gestation, the germ cells arise from the yolk sac and migrate along the hind gut to the genital ridge. The oogonia are able to move by pseudopodial amoeboid movements. Once the oogonia reach the genital ridge they become associated with cortical cords and lose their motility. From week 5 through to week 28 the oogonia undergo mitotic divisions. At the same time many oogonia are lost by atresia, some in their passage from the yolk sac and others once they have reached the gonad itself. Meiosis starts in approximately week 9 and the life cycle of the oocyte is such that it undergoes only part of the first meiotic division, entering meiotic arrest at the dictyate stage of prophase 1. The final number of oocytes is therefore determined by three factors: first, the maximum number achieved by mitotic divisions; second, the time at which they enter meiosis, thus preventing further increase in number; and third, the rate of atresia. The factors that affect the number of mitotic divisions and the transition from mitosis to meiosis are unknown.

From about 16 weeks' gestation the somatic pre-granulosa cells form in the genital ridge and differentiate into the granulosa cells lying on a basement membrane opposite theca cells. From about 16 weeks' gestation to 6 months postpartum the oocytes secrete their zona pellucida. Thus the primordial follicles begin to appear. The numbers of oogonia are maintained by cytokines and growth factors, in particular stem cell growth factor (*steel* factor) which has its own receptor (C-*kit*).

More germs cells die during fetal life than survive in primordial follicles. The maximum number of germs cells is approximately 7 million and this is achieved at 20 weeks' gestation.[1] By birth this is reduced to between 1 and 2 million. It is thought that the eliminated germ cells might have a higher rate of chromosomal abnormalities than those that remain, although this has never been conclusively proven.

The number of primordial follicles at puberty has been mathematically related to the final adult weight of a particular species. This has been expressed by the equation $N = 27\,700\, M^{0.47}$ with M being the adult weight in kilograms.[2] This equation remains true for different species and the life span of a species is related also to the number of primordial follicles at puberty and has been expressed as $N = 820\, L^{1.58}$.[2] In all species the primordial follicle number declines with age. In mice, for example, this is faster before than after puberty, while in humans the rate of disappearance of primordial follicles appears to be accelerated in later life. The size of the follicle store is not directly related to the rate of ovulation but the daily fraction recruited, which changes with age. Recruitment of primordial follicles occurs throughout life and is initially independent of follicle stimulating hormone (FSH) and the FSH receptor is expressed only at the primary follicle stage. The growing fraction of primordial follicles appears to be up-regulated when the total numbers are reduced and this explains the increased rate of loss in humans with age.[3] The accelerated rate of depletion in older ovaries is due more to the initiation of growth than atresia, although the control mechanisms are still to be elucidated. From birth to puberty approximately 75% of the follicle store is lost. At puberty about 250 000 follicles remain and between puberty and menopause there is the potential for up to about 500 ovulations.

Menopause occurs when there are approximately 1000 follicles left in the ovary. Post-menopausally, therefore, some follicles do remain but they do not grow to maturity, perhaps because high circulating levels of FSH cause receptor down-regulation. A number of mathematical models have been developed to express the rate of decline of primordial follicle number.[4–6] When 10 000 follicles remain the menopause will occur in approximately 5–10 years and when there are 100 000 remaining it will occur between 21.5 and 26.5 years. At the age of 25 approximately 37 follicles leave the human ovary by either growth or atresia daily (in other words, approximately 1000 per month), while at the age of 45 this has been reduced to approximately 2 per day. The rate of ovarian aging appears to be intrinsically determined and the half-life of the follicle population is approximately 7 years, increasing exponentially with a doubling of the exponential rate after the age of about 37.5 years.

If the rate of follicle loss did not increase then the menopause would be expected to occur at approximately 71 years of age. The reason for humans having a menopause is unclear and may actually represent an extension of life due to increased nutrition and well-being of the human population rather than as a physiological feature itself. With respect to the recruitment of the primordial follicles, this is due to unknown processes in cellular metabolism/signaling and no physiological interventions are able to halt recruitment. Thus recruitment occurs while an individual is pregnant and also while taking the contraceptive pill.

Richardson *et al.*[7] studied the number of follicles around the time of the menopause by looking at 17 women between the ages of 45 and 55 who had undergone a hysterectomy with bilateral salpingo-oophorectomy. Patients were divided into three groups depending upon their menstrual pattern. The mean age was similar in all groups and it was found that those who had regular menstrual cycles had a mean number of 1694 (SEM 460) follicles, while those who were perimenopausal with an erratic cycle had 181 (SEM 88) follicles and those who were menopausal had no follicles remaining. The frequency distribution of the age at menopause has been described by Treloar[8] in 763 American women. The age of menopause appears to be similar in all Western communities, although women in developing countries appear to have a menopause 5 or 6 years earlier and this may be a reflection of under-nutrition during fetal life as nutritional status during infant or adult life does not appear to have a direct bearing on ovarian aging.

Using mathematical models for the aging of the ovary, devised from data of follicle counts at different ages together with projected mean ages at menopause, Faddy and colleagues[4] have developed certain algorithms. For example, it has been suggested that the surgical loss of one ovary is not likely to hasten the menopause by more than 7 years (in other words, to the age of 44, by which time 5% of the population are menopausal). If 50% of the follicle store is lost by the age of 30 years then the expected age of menopause is 44 years and for each further year that a 50% reduction has occurred the menopause will be delayed by 0.6 years. Thus if 50% have been lost by the age of 37.5 years the menopause can be expected to occur at the age of 48. On the other hand, if 90% of the follicle store is lost by the age of 14 years, another 13 years of ovarian activity can be expected with a menopause occurring at the age of 27 years and for each further year that a 90% reduction has occurred, the menopause will be delayed by 0.6 of a year so that if 90% have been lost at the age of 37.5 years the menopause will be at the age of 41 years.

Atresia and apoptosis (that is, the programmed/physiological cell death) which is initiated by genes which code for effector proteins which lead to cell death in response to external stimuli occur once the follicle has passed its primary stage. Follicles that are not selected for ovulation undergo atresia at the later pre-antral or early antral stage (1 to 5 mm in diameter) when continued growth would be FSH dependent. Follicles destined for atresia can be rescued by FSH administration and the oocyte remains healthy until late stages of atresia, at which point it will resume meiosis due to loss of the cumulus complex.

The exact incidence of POF is unknown as many cases go unrecognized, but estimates vary between 1% and 5% of women.[9] In a study of 1858 women the incidence of POF was 1:1000 by age 30 and 1:100 by age 40.[9] Studies of amenorrheic women report the incidence of POF to be between 10% and 36%.[10,11]

Resistant Ovary Syndrome

Prior to the absolute cessation of periods of true premature ovarian failure, some women experience an intermittent return of menses, interspersed between variable periods of amenorrhea.[12] Gonadotropin levels usually remain moderately elevated during these spontaneous cycles, with plasma FSH concentrations of 15–20 i.u./L. This occult/incipient ovarian failure, or "resistant ovary syndrome," is associated with the presence of primordial follicles on ovarian biopsy. Ovarian biopsy is no longer recommended in the assessment of these cases because a single sample is not reliably representative and will not help with management. Occasionally pregnancies occur spontaneously in patients with resistant ovary syndrome. Ovulation induction therapy is of no benefit as the ovaries are usually as resistant to exogenous gonadotropins as they are to endogenous hormones.

In one series,[13] suppression of gonadotropin secretion with estradiol prior to human menopausal gonadotropin (hMG) stimulation was associated with ovulation in 68 of 361 cycles (19%), although there were only eight ongoing pregnancies. In our experience this approach has not been successful. In a few patients, immunosuppressive therapy has achieved limited success, but this is not a form of treatment that we can recommend, in the absence of a randomized controlled trial. It is probable that reports of pregnancy in women with POF or resistant ovary syndrome represent cases of fluctuating ovarian function rather than successes of treatment. There have been occasional reports of spontaneous resumption of ovulation and conception and it has been suggested that these cases may represent the fluctuating ovarian function of a "premature perimenopause" or transient ovarian failure caused by viral oophoritis. It has been found that most spontaneous remissions occur in patients in whom the ovaries can be visualized by ultrasound.

If a patient with resistant ovary syndrome and symptoms of estrogen deficiency wishes to conceive she should be advised to take a hormone replacement therapy (HRT) preparation, which will not inhibit ovulation (or adversely affect a pregnancy). On the other hand, if a pregnancy would be unwanted, it is important to advise the use of either an oral contraceptive preparation or contraception together with HRT.

Diagnosis of Premature Ovarian Failure

As women age, variability of intermenstrual interval increases but the mean interval falls (from 28 to 23 days). The mean age of the menopause in the UK is 50.6 years; we define a premature menopause as cessation of periods by 45 years and premature ovarian failure as cessation of periods by 40 years. The first endocrine change is an isolated elevation of FSH, followed by elevation of FSH and luteinizing hormone (LH), with a fall in serum estradiol concentrations with the development of amenorrhea. Over the next year there is a further fall of estradiol. The ultrasound shows normal, then small ovaries with few follicles, and then ovaries of less than 2 ml with no follicles.

If a woman has amenorrhea and an elevated serum FSH concentration (> 20 i.u./L) on more than two occasions, it is likely that she has POF. The longer the period of amenorrhea and the higher the FSH level, the greater the likelihood that the ovarian failure is permanent. A single elevated FSH level, even if greater than 40 i.u./L, should be treated with caution as spontaneous ovulation and pregnancy have still been observed. Once the diagnosis of POF has been made further specific endocrinological tests are unnecessary. Additional investigations include karyotype, screening for autoantibodies and associated autoimmune disease if relevant and a baseline assessment of bone mineral densitometry. A cardiovascular assessment is also important, including blood pressure and lipid profile. As always, a detailed history is important with particular attention to a family history of POF or autoimmune disease.

Causes of Premature Ovarian Failure (Table 8.1)

In approximately two-thirds of cases, the cause of ovarian failure cannot be identified.[14] It is unknown whether these cases are truly idiopathic or due to as yet undiscovered genetic, immunological, or

Table 8.1 Causes of premature ovarian failure
Idiopathic
Genetic: commonly Turner's syndrome, familial
Autoimmune
Pelvic surgery
Pelvic irradiation
Chemotherapy
Viral/bacterial infection
Galactosemia

environmental factors. A series of 323 women with POF attending an endocrinology clinic in London identified 23% with Turner's syndrome, 6% after chemotherapy, 4% with familial POF, and 2% each who had pelvic surgery, pelvic irradiation, galactosemia, and 46,XY gonadal dysgenesis.[14] Viral and bacterial infection may also lead to ovarian failure – thus infections such as mumps, cytomegalovirus, or HIV in adult life can adversely affect long-term ovarian function, as can severe pelvic inflammatory disease. Ovarian failure occurring before puberty is usually due to a chromosomal abnormality, or a childhood malignancy that required chemotherapy or radiotherapy. The likelihood of developing ovarian failure after therapy for cancer is difficult to predict but the age of the patient is a significant factor – the younger the patient, the greater the follicle pool and the better her chances of retaining ovarian function. The dose and type of chemotherapy are also important (see also Ch. 18). Environmental toxins might be a factor in causing POF. The best known toxin is of course smoking, which has been shown to lower the age of menopause.[15]

Genetic Causes of POF

Adolescents who lose ovarian function soon after menarche are often found to have a Turner's mosaic (46,XX/45,X) or an X-chromosome trisomy (47,XXX). There are many genes on the X chromosome that are essential for normal ovarian function. Two active X chromosomes are required during fetal life in order to lay down a normal follicle store. In fetuses with Turner's syndrome normal numbers of oocytes appear on the genital ridge but accelerated atresia takes place during late fetal life.[16] Thus streak gonads occur and it is only the mosaic form of Turner's syndrome that permits any possibility of ovarian function. X mosaicisms are the commonest chromosomal abnormality in reported series of POF, ranging from 5% to 40%.[11]

Turner's syndrome

Turner's syndrome is the commonest cause of gonadal dysgenesis. In its most severe form the 45,X genotype is associated with the classical Turner's features including short stature, webbing of the neck, cubitus valgus, widely spaced nipples, cardiac and renal abnormalities, and often autoimmune hypothyroidism. It is very important to detect coarctation of the aorta, as it is not safe to get pregnant by egg donation unless treated. Spontaneous menstruation may occur, particularly when there is mosaicism, but POF usually ensues. Management includes low dose estrogen therapy to promote breast development without further disturbing linear growth; cyclical estrogen plus progestogen may be used as maintenance therapy.

Fragile X syndrome

The fragile X syndrome is the commonest inherited cause of learning disability with a prevalence of 1:4000 males and 1:8000 females. It is characterized by a heterogeneous mixture of physical, behavioral, and cognitive features. Most published information refers to fragile X syndrome in males, of whom about 80% are moderately to severely mentally retarded, while females usually display a milder phenotype with a borderline IQ of 70–85. Fragile X syndrome is an X-linked dominant disorder with reduced penetrance. Unaffected carriers in a family have an increased risk of transmitting the disorder with successive generations. The disorder is due to a mutation in a gene on the long arm of the X chromosome, known as "fragile X mental retardation-1" (FMR-1, Xq27.3) which transcribes a cytoplasmic protein that is found in all cells but in higher concentration in ovary, brain, and testis. It is the absence of this protein that results in the fragile X syndrome phenotype. Affected families have mutations in the FMR-1 gene leading to hereditary instability. These mutations can be of variable sizes, the largest resulting in a "full mutation," while smaller mutations are known as "pre-mutations." As somatic cells in females have a randomly inactivated X chromosome, only half of females with the full mutation have a fragile X phenotype. Women with a pre-mutation are phenotypically normal but appear to have a significantly increased risk of POF. The largest series of 395 pre-mutation carriers found 16% with POF compared with 0.4% of a control population.[17]

Familial POF

There is evidence for strong genetic factors determining the age of the menopause. Interest has recently turned to specific familial forms of POF in which abnormalities are present in the critical region of the long arm of the X chromosome from Xq13 to Xq26. At least two genetic variants have been identified, the *POF 1* gene (Xq21.3-q27)[18] and the *POF 2* gene (Xq13.3-q21.1).[19] There are also a number of rare syndromes that are associated with premature ovarian failure, such as galactosemia.

Autoimmune Causes of POF

Ovarian autoantibodies have been found in up to 69% of cases of POF. However, the assays are expensive and not readily available in most units. It is therefore important to consider other autoimmune disorders, and screen for autoantibodies to the thyroid gland, gastric mucosa parietal cells, and adrenal gland if there is any clinical indication. There are a number of potential ovarian antigens and the potential for autoantibody formation has long been recognized. The clinical significance of antiovarian antibodies is uncertain, particularly as their concentrations fluctuate and do not always relate to the severity of disease. It is therefore uncertain whether antiovarian antibodies are pathogenic or secondary to antigen release after ovarian damage.[11]

Iatrogenic Causes of Premature Ovarian Failure

There are many iatrogenic causes of amenorrhea, which may be either temporary or permanent. These include malignant conditions that require either radiation to the abdomen/pelvis or chemotherapy. Both these treatments may result in permanent gonadal damage, the amount of damage being directly related to the age of the patient, the cumulative dose, and the patient's prior menstrual status. The likelihood of developing ovarian failure after therapy for cancer is difficult to predict but the younger the patient, the greater the follicle pool and the better her chances of retaining ovarian function. It is estimated that 1 in every 1000 adults are now survivors of childhood malignancy and for these women – and men – the cryopreservation of gonadal tissue prior to treatment might soon offer a real chance of restoring fertility, and, possibly, natural hormone replacement.

Gynecological procedures such as oophorectomy, hysterectomy, and endometrial resection inevitably result in amenorrhea. Hormone replacement should be prescribed for these patients where appropriate. Hormone therapy itself can be used to disrupt the menstrual cycle deliberately. However, iatrogenic causes of ovarian quiescence have the same consequences of estrogen deficiency due to any other etiology.

Management of Premature Ovarian Failure

The diagnosis and consequences of POF require careful counseling of the patient. It may be particularly difficult for a young women to accept the need to take estrogen preparations that are clearly labeled as being intended for older post-menopausal women, while at the same time having to come to terms with the inability to conceive naturally. The short- and long-term consequences of ovarian failure and estrogen deficiency are similar to those occurring in the fifth and sixth decade. However, the duration of the problem is much longer and therefore HRT is advisable to reduce the consequences of estrogen deficiency in the long term.

Younger women with premature loss of ovarian function have an increased risk of osteoporosis. A study of 200 amenorrheic women between the ages of 16 and 40 demonstrated a mean reduction in bone mineral density of 15% as compared with a control group and after correction for body weight, smoking, and exercise.[20] The degree of bone loss was correlated with the duration of the amenorrhea and the severity of the estrogen deficiency rather than the underlying diagnosis, and was worse in patients with primary amenorrhea compared with those with secondary amenorrhea. A return to normal estrogen status may improve bone mass density, but bone mineral density is unlikely to improve more than 5–10% and it probably does not return to its normal value. However, it is not certain if the radiological improvement seen will actually reduce the risk of fracture, as re-mineralization is not equivalent to the re-strengthening of bone. Early diagnosis and early correction of estrogen status are therefore important.

Women with POF have an increased risk of cardiovascular disease. Estrogens have been shown to have beneficial effects on cardiovascular status in women. They increase the levels of cardioprotective high density lipoprotein but also total triglyceride levels, while decreasing total cholesterol and low density lipoprotein levels. The overall effect should be of cardiovascular protection, although this has never been convincingly demonstrated.

Women with hypoestrogenic amenorrhea require hormone replacement. A cyclical estrogen/progestogen preparation is required for patients with a uterus in order to prevent endometrial hyperplasia. The HRT preparations prescribed for menopausal women are also preferred for young women as even modern low dose combined oral contraceptive (COC) preparations contain at least twice the amount of estrogen that is recommended for HRT. HRT also contains "natural" estrogens rather than the synthetic ethinylestradiol that is found in most oral contraceptives. A direct, long-term comparison, however, has not been performed.

The beneficial effects of hormone replacement in reducing osteoporosis and cardiovascular mortality are thought to outweigh the risk of breast cancer, particularly in women with POF. It is now thought necessary to perform annual breast examination only in women thought to be at high risk, for example those with a family history of breast cancer. Mammography in normal women, with active glandular breasts, is difficult to interpret, and so the use of mammography as a screening procedure in young women taking HRT is not recommended. It is the lifetime exposure to estrogen that is important and so young women with POF should be reassured that the use of HRT should not put them at increased risk of breast cancer at least until they reach the average age of menopause (i.e., 51 years) – and then only if they continue to take HRT for a further 5 years or more. Follow-up of patients with POF should be at least on an annual basis to monitor HRT, detect the development of associated diseases, and provide appropriate support and counseling.

Oocyte donation can be used to treat women with POF, of whatever cause, and for those who do not wish to use their oocytes for genetic reasons.[21] Oocyte donation may also have a place for women who do not respond to ovarian stimulation during IVF or whose oocytes repeatedly fail to fertilize in the presence of apparently normal sperm. More controversial is the use of donated eggs for post-menopausal women in their 50s and 60s – a practice that is not approved in the UK or by the European Society of Human Reproduction and Embryology (ESHRE). However, the outcomes to date have not demonstrated a detrimental effect on the recipients and it is a matter of ethical debate as to who should determine an individual couple's right to parenthood.

Implantation rates for the recipient are those appropriate for the age of the oocyte donor and usually about 30–40% per treatment cycle. Favorable results are thus widely achievable, although a downward trend in the birth rates, particularly above 40 years, suggests a small uterine effect on the outcome. An endometrial affect on implantation rates in patients having oocyte donation is apparent when one examines the etiology of the ovarian failure because the highest pregnancy rates are achieved in women with POF who have an anatomically normal uterus. Women with Turner's syndrome who have not had a spontaneous puberty and women who have received radiotherapy to the pelvis have reduced uterine blood flow and suboptimal endometrial development in response to exogenous estrogen therapy (sometimes radiotherapy destroys any subsequent endometrial function). These patients therefore do less well when undergoing oocyte donation. Furthermore, it would seem inadvisable to use the oocytes donated by a sister of a woman with POF as they also appear to do less well than those of anonymous fertile donors.[22]

It is necessary to provide the recipient with an artificial hormone replacement regimen (HRT), usually with increasing doses of oral estrogens,[23] with the addition of progesterone 3 days before embryo transfer (see Fig. 8.1). Recipients who have a spontaneous menstrual cycle require pituitary desensitization before commencing the hormone regimen, while amenorrheic women with ovarian failure do not. Interestingly, it is the latter group who appear to have better results, possibly because the HRT regimen has not been imposed on a pre-existing cycle. Close synchrony is required between the recipient's cycle and the donor's IVF cycle if fresh embryos – which provide better pregnancy rates than cryopreserved embryos – are to be transferred.

As with sperm donation (see Ch. 11), careful counseling is required for both partners and for the donor, who might be undergoing assisted conception herself or have an altruistic desire to donate eggs and thereby undergo an IVF cycle. Donor anonymity is usually preferred although known donation is not uncommon. The donor should be under the age of 36 in order to reduce the chance of age-related chromosomal problems.

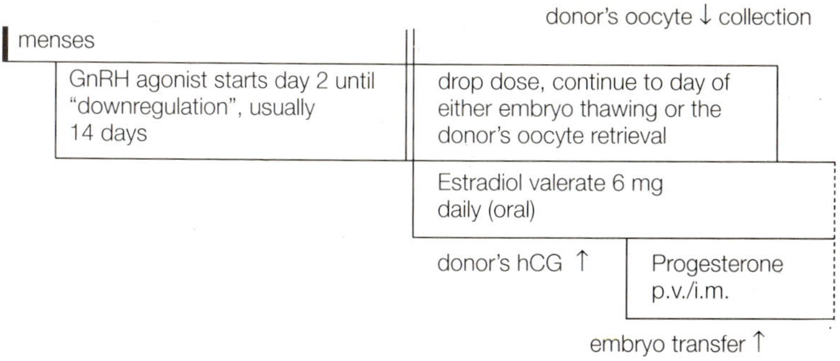

Figure 8.1 HRT regimen for frozen embryo replacement cycles or for oocyte donation. Women with a menstrual cycle should first undergo pituitary desensitization, while those with premature ovarian failure commence oral estradiol instead of their usual HRT regimen. It used to be thought that the estradiol valerate should be gradually increased in a stepwise fashion but it is now clear that a fixed dose of 6 mg from the start is satisfactory and can be continued for up to 100 days with no ill effect. The usual duration of estradiol therapy is 12–14 days before the commencement of progesterone. Progesterone should commence when endometrial thickness is at least 8 mm and the embryo transfer is performed on the fourth day of progesterone therapy (either vaginal Cyclogest (800 mg nocte), Uterogestan (300 mg micronized progesterone daily) or intramuscular injections of Gestone (100 mg daily)). Both progesterone and estradiol are continued beyond the positive pregnancy test and until the serum progesterone is > 127 nmol/L, usually at 7–8 weeks' gestation. The hormone support is then gradually withdrawn over the following 2 weeks. In reality the estradiol could be stopped on the day of embryo transfer and the progesterone could probably also be stopped once the pregnancy test is positive.

Egg sharing is an approach to egg donation that has gained popularity in recent years, whereby a woman requiring IVF who has insufficient funds for her own treatment donates some of her oocytes in return for free treatment. With appropriate counseling, egg sharing appears to work well, without adverse psychological consequences if the donor fails to conceive. A strict protocol is required to prevent unnecessary overstimulation of the donor's ovaries and also to ensure that surplus oocytes are donated only if a prerequisite number (usually 6–10) have been collected for the donor's own use.

Cryopreservation of Ovarian Tissue

Experimental work in animals has succeeded in transplanting primordial follicles into irradiated ovaries, with subsequent ovulation and normal pregnancy (see also Ch. 18).[24] An extension of this work has resulted in successful cryopreservation of human ovarian tissue[25] and reimplantation of the thawed tissue with resultant follicular growth, after stimulation with exogenous FSH. The methods employed were devised for the preservation of fertility and ovarian function in young women prior to sterilizing chemotherapy or radiotherapy. The potential exists for the cryopreservation of ovarian tissue for women destined to undergo ovarian failure – an event that might be predictable from genetic or family studies. Whether the cryopreserved ovarian tissue is genetically competent would, of course, be uncertain, but it is easy to foresee the day when women with fragile X pre-mutations or Turner's mosaicism might be asking for ovarian cryopreservation during their adolescent years. At the present time, however, appropriate advice would be for these women to aim for pregnancy using healthy donated oocytes.

References

1. Baker TG (1963) A quantitative and cytological study of germ cells in human ovaries. *Proc R Soc Lond B* **158**: 417–433.
2. Gosden RG & Telfer E (1987) Numbers of follicles in mammalian ovaries and their allometric relationships. *J Zool* **211**: 169–175.
3. Gougeon A, Ecochard R & Thalabard JC (1994) Age-related changes of the population of human ovarian follicles: increase in the disappearance rate of non-growing and early-growing follicles in aging women. *Biol Reprod* **50**: 653–663.
4. Faddy MJ, Gosden RG, Gougeon A, Richardson SJ & Nelson JF (1992) Accelerated disappearance of ovarian follicles in mid-life – implications for forecasting menopause. *Hum Reprod* **7**: 1342–1346.
5. Faddy MJ & Gosden RG (1995) A mathematical model for follicle dynamics in human ovaries. *Hum Reprod* **10**: 770–775.
6. Faddy MJ & Gosden RG (1996) A model confirming the decline in follicle numbers to the age of menopause in women. *Hum Reprod* **11**: 1484–1486.
7. Richardson SJ, Senikas V & Nelson JF (1987) Follicular depletion during the menopausal transition: evidence for accelerated loss and ultimate exhaustion. *J Clin Endocrinol Metab* **65**: 1231–1237.
8. Treloar AE (1981) Menstrual cyclicity and the pre-menopause. *Maturitas* **3**: 249–264.
9. Coulam CB, Adamson SC & Annegers JF (1986) Incidence of premature ovarian failure. *Obstet Gynecol* **67**: 604–606.
10. Balen AH, Shoham Z & Jacobs HS (1993) Amenorrhea – causes and consequences. In Asch RH & Studd JJW (eds) *Annual progress in reproductive medicine*. Parthenon Press, Carnforth, Lancashire, pp 205–234.
11. Anasti JN (1998) Premature ovarian failure: an update. *Fertil Steril* **70**: 1–15.
12. Cameron IT, O'Shea FC, Rolland JM, Hughes EG, de Kretser DM & Healy DL (1988) Occult ovarian failure: a syndrome of infertility, regular menses and elevated follicle-stimulating hormone concentrations. *J Clin Endocrinol Metab* **67**: 1190–1194.
13. Check JH, Nowroozi K, Chase JS, Nazari A, Shapse D & Vaze M (1990) Ovulation induction and pregnancies in 100 consecutive women with hypergonadotropic amenorrhoea. *Fertil Steril* **53**: 811–816.
14. Conway GS (1997) Premature ovarian failure. *Curr Opin Obstet Gynecol* **9**: 202–206.
15. Cooper GS, Baird DD, Hulka BS, Weinberg, CR, Savitz DA & Hughes CL (1995) Follicle-stimulating hormone concentrations in relation to active and passive smoking. *Obstet Gynecol* **85**: 407–411.
16. Singh RP & Carr DH (1966) The anatomy and histology of XO human embryos and fetuses. *Anat Rec* **155**: 369–383.
17. Allington-Hawkins DJ, Babul-Hirji R, Chitayat D *et al.* (1999) Fragile X premutation is a significant risk factor for premature ovarian failure: the International Collaborative Premature Ovarian Failure and Fragile X Study – preliminary data. *Am J Med Genet* **83**: 322–325.

18. Krauss CM, Turksoy RN, Atkins L, McLaughlin C, Brown LG & Page DC (1987) Familial premature ovarian failure due to an interstitial deletion of the long arm of the X chromosome. *N Engl J Med* **317**: 125–131.
19. Powell CM, Taggart RT, Drumheller TC *et al.* (1994) Molecular and cytogenetic studies of an X;autosome translocation in a patient with premature ovarian failure and review of the literature. *Am J Med Genet* **52**: 19–26.
20. Davies MC, Hall M & Davies HS (1990) Bone mineral density in young women with amenorrhoea. *Br Med J* **301**: 790–793.
21. Dean NL & Edwards RG (1994) Oocyte donation – implications for fertility treatment in the nineties. *Curr Opin Obstet Gynecol* **6**: 160–165.
22. Sung L, Sustillo M, Mukherjee T, Booth G, Karstaedt A & Coperman AB (1997) Sisters of women with premature ovarian failure may not be ideal ovum donors. *Fertil Steril* **67**: 912–916.
23. Lutjen P, Trounson A, Leeton J, Findlay J, Wood C & Renou P (1984) The establishment and maintenance of pregnancy using *in vitro* fertilisation and embryo donation in a patient with primary ovarian failure. *Nature* **307**: 174–175.
24. Gosden RG (1990) Restitution of fertility in sterilized mice by transferring primordial ovarian follicles. *Hum Reprod* **5**: 499–504.
25. Newton H, Aubard Y, Rutherford A, Sharma V & Gosden RG (1996) Low temperature storage and grafting of human ovarian tissue. *Hum Reprod* **11**: 1487–1491.

Chapter 9

Endometriosis

Introduction

Endometriosis can cause pelvic pain and infertility. In the context of the management of subfertility we have to ask what degree of endometriosis requires treatment? Treatment when it is advisable is best achieved with surgery without delaying the chance of conception by hormonal therapies that are contraceptive.

Diagnosis

Careful laparoscopic assessment of the pelvis reveals signs of endometriosis in up to 18% of women with proven fertility.[1] It is recognized that not all endometriotic lesions have the classic blue/black pigmented appearance. Atypical lesions consist of flame like blisters, clear nodules, white plaques, and peritoneal defects.[2] Endometrial glands have also been found after microscopic inspection of biopsies from macroscopically normal-looking peritoneum. Whether these changes represent pathology or simply one end of the normal spectrum is still a matter for debate (Fig. 9.1).

It has been suggested that the non-pigmented lesions are more common in younger women and that the darker lesions represent older or "burnt-out" disease.[3] Furthermore, endometriotic lesions change both in position and with time. It has been suggested that endometriosis is analogous to a field of mushrooms, with lesions appearing and disappearing at different times and in different places.

While a number of theories have been proposed for the pathogenesis of endometriosis, that of retrograde menstruation is the most popular and plausible. Retrograde menstruation is common, being seen in 75–90% of women who have had laparoscopies performed at the time of menstruation.[4] Menstrual blood does not always contain endometrial cells and the factors that influence implantation of ectopic endometrium are uncertain, for the prevalence of endometriosis has been estimated as 1–20%, not 75–90%. Women with endometriosis appear to have altered immune function, which may permit implantation of regurgitated endometrium. Abnormalities of cellular adhesion molecules, including the integrins and extracellular matrix proteins, are also thought to play a role in pathogenesis. The detection of endometriosis in women being investigated for subfertility is thought to

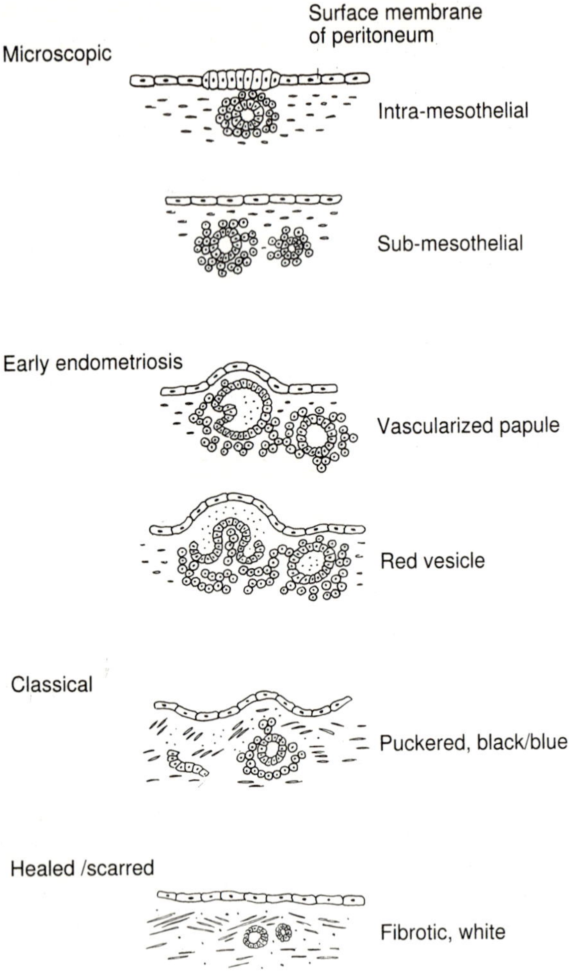

Figure 9.1 Development of peritoneal endometriosis (after Brosens *et al.* 1993 *Baillière's Clinical Obstetrics and Gynaecology* **7/4**: 741–757.)[2]

reflect their lack of conception and exposure to frequent menstruation rather than being a cause of the infertility. Indeed, the likelihood of finding evidence of endometriosis in women who attend for sterilization is increased in proportion to the interval since the birth of their last child.

Women with symptomatic endometriosis may have a genetic disposition to endometrial implantation on the peritoneum and a further disposition to an inflammatory response to the cyclical changes that occur in the ectopic endometrium. As is well known, the degree of endometriosis does not correlate with symptomatology: pelvic pain,

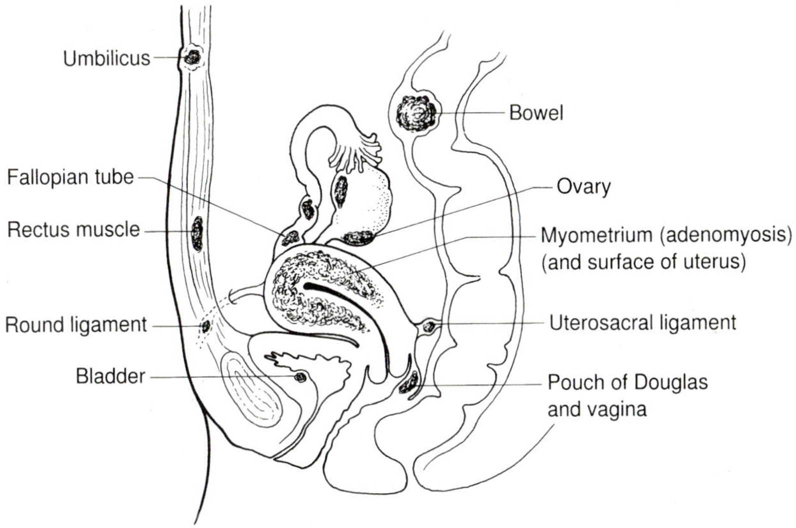

Figure 9.2 Sites of endometriosis.

dyspareunia, and dysmenorrhea. It is not possible, moreover, to predict which patients will develop progressive disease with resultant pelvic adhesions and ovarian cysts.

It is easy to envisage how severe endometriosis can affect fertility by distorting pelvic anatomy, with adhesions that smother the ovaries and tubes and with endometriotic ovarian cysts (Fig. 9.2). While endometriosis is found on the surface of the Fallopian tubes, it does not tend to affect the tubal lumen and typically the tubes are patent. Fertility can also be impaired by the dyspareunia that often accompanies the condition. There is still debate about the extent to which endometriosis affects fertility in the absence of pelvic deformity. It has been suggested that the peritoneal environment is altered, with an increased concentration of macrophages which impede sperm motility, phagocytose spermatozoa, and interfere both with oocyte pick-up by the Fallopian tube and with fertilization. However, while the relevance of these hypotheses was previously tempered by the failure of medical or surgical treatment to improve the pregnancy rates of women with minimal or mild endometriosis,[5,6] more recent evidence from two randomized trials has suggested a benefit from surgical ablation.[7,8]

Descriptive Classification of Endometriosis

Most investigative tests in reproductive medicine indicate reproductive function at the time of the test and give little information about the dynamics of the underlying problem. This is particularly the case with mild endometriosis, when diagnostic laparoscopy gives no indication about the possible progression of the disease.

Markers

A number of markers for endometriosis have been investigated, although more as non-invasive diagnostic tests rather than to monitor progression of the disease. Probably the most commonly used marker is the glycoprotein CA-125, an oncofetal celomic epithelium differentiation antigen. CA-125 levels in aspirates of peritoneal fluid and cysts of patients with endometriosis are much higher than in serum. Serum CA-125 concentrations are also elevated in patients with acute pelvic inflammatory disease and ovarian carcinoma and, while the levels tend to be higher than in patients with endometriosis, there is considerable overlap. It has been suggested that 35 U/ml be used as a cut-off serum concentration for CA-125, below which endometriosis is unlikely to be present. Unfortunately CA-125 measurements do not correlate well with either the progression of the disease or the response of endometriosis to treatment. However, the assessment of the CA-125 concentration may help distinguish cystic ovarian endometriosis from corpus luteum cysts, which may be difficult to discriminate by either ultrasonography or laparoscopy.

Antiendometrial Antibodies

Antiendometrial antibodies have been found to be significantly elevated in patients with endometriosis, although again this provides poor sensitivity or predictability of either severity or progression of the disease. This is particularly so as early lesions might elicit a stronger antibody response than older lesions and the techniques used to assay endometrial antibodies are not quantitative. The study of these and other markers for endometriosis continues but they are not in current use for the routine management of patients with the condition. We are not convinced that widespread screening for endometriosis will have a place in clinical practice, although there might be a place for screening in patients in whom there is a family history of endometriosis in order to help determine when more invasive investigations are indicated.

Laparoscopy

Laparoscopy is the mainstay of the classification of endometriosis and the best known system of classification is that of the American Fertility Society (AFS, now American Society of Reproductive Medicine, ASRM) (Table 9.1), in which the appearance of the disease, the degree of adhesions, and obliteration of the pouch of Douglas provide a score. It

Table 9.1 Modified American Fertility Society (AFS) scoring system for endometriosis

	Endometriosis	< 1 cm	1–3 cm	> 3 cm
Peritoneum	Superficial	1	2	4
	Deep	2	4	6
Ovary: R	Superficial	1	2	4
	Deep	4	16	20
Ovary: L	Superficial	1	2	4
	Deep	4	16	20
Posterior cul-de-sac Obliteration		Partial 4	Complete 40	
	Adhesions	<1/3 enclosure	1/3–2/3 enclosure	> 2/3 enclosure
Ovary: R	Filmy	1	2	4
	Dense	4	8	16
Ovary: L	Filmy	1	2	4
	Dense	4	8	16
Tube: R	Filmy	1	2	4
	Dense	4[a]	16	20
Tube: L	Filmy	1	2	4
	Dense	4[a]	8[a]	16

[a] *If the fimbrial end of the tube is completely enclosed, score 16.*

has been suggested that the AFS classification is limited by its inability to provide an indication of the activity of the disease and has no predictive value with respect to either pain or subfertility. We feel that there is no substitute for a careful descriptive record of the laparoscopic findings, together with photographs or a video if available (Fig. 9.3) (see also Table 9.2).

Biopsy

If there is doubt about the diagnosis at laparoscopy the lesions can be biopsied to provide a histological diagnosis, although in up to a third of clinically typical cases histological examination does not provide endometrial tissue. Furthermore, biopsy of the peritoneum can lead to bleeding and damage to other structures and so is not part of routine practice. Peritoneal lesions change with age, with clear papules usually being seen under the age of 25 years, followed by red (highly active), black (fibrotic, with old hemorrhage and intermediate activity), and white (scarred, inactive tissue) lesions – with a considerable degree of overlap between all types (Fig. 9.3).

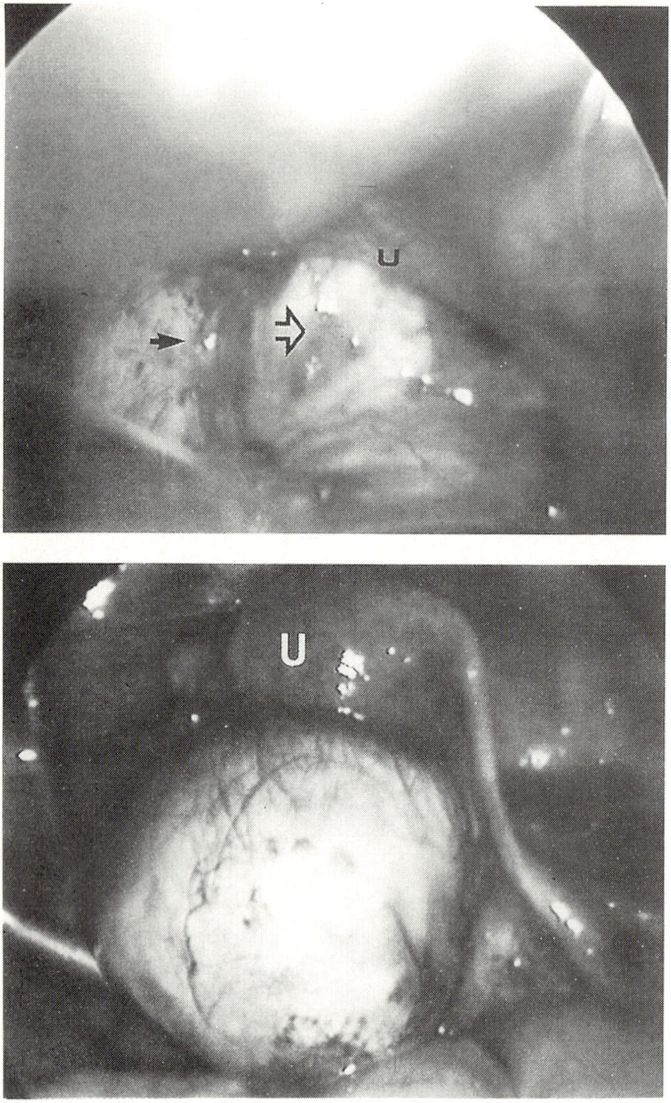

Figure 9.3a–b Endometriosis at laparoscopy. (**a**) Active spots of endometriosis are seen between the the uterosacral ligaments (u) and in the pouch of Douglas (open arrow) there is adjacent neovascularization and the new peritoneal formation (closed arrow). (**b**) The left ovary is supported behind the uterus (U) and is distended by a large endometriotic cyst (please refer to plate section for color figures).

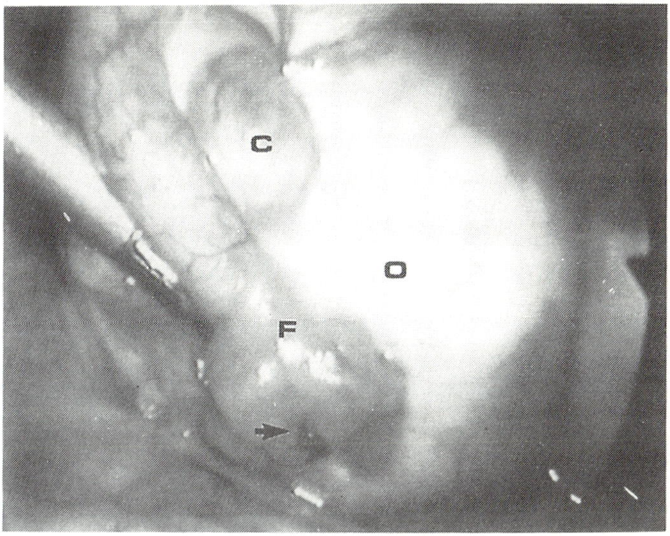

c

Figure 9.3c Endometriosis at laparoscopy. (**c**) Another view of the left ovary (O) indicates recent ovulation by virtue of a corpus luteum (C). The fimbrial end of the tube (F) appears reasonably healthy although there is an endometriotic deposit on its posterior margin (arrow) (please refer to plate section for color figure).

Table 9.2 Classification of endometriosis by severity (Acosta *et al.* 1993)[34]

Mild:	Scattered fresh lesions on peritoneal surfaces; minimal lesions on ovarian surfaces; no peritubal adhesions
Moderate:	Several surface lesions on one or both ovaries, with scarring, retraction or small endometriomata; minimal periovarian or peritubal adhesions; superficial implants in pouch of Douglas with scarring and retraction
Severe:	Involvement of one or both ovaries with endometriomata (>2 × 2 cm); one or both tubes bound down or obstructed by adhesions; obliteration of pouch of Douglas; thickening of uterosacral ligaments, bowel or ureteric involvement

Cysts

Some consider that ovarian endometriomata occur as a result of deposits on the surface of the ovary which cause invagination of the cortex, with adhesions over the surface which then result in an encapsulated cyst. Most endometriomata therefore represent relatively superficial disease and the appearance of these cysts can be misleading.

Management of Endometriosis

The management of endometriosis depends upon the wishes of the patient, specifically whether her predominant complaint is pain or infertility. If fertility is required but pain is also a problem then management is usually with analgesics, either alone or combined with surgical treatment. Appropriate analgesics include the non-steroidal anti-inflammatory drugs (NSAIDs); naproxen (250 mg t.i.d./q.d.s.) and mefenamic acid (500 mg t.i.d.) are particularly effective. There is some evidence that NSAIDs inhibit the process of ovulation through their antiprostaglandin action but endometriotic pain usually occurs at the time of menstruation rather than mid-cycle and so these drugs should be safe in women wishing to conceive.

When evaluating the outcome of therapy for endometriosis it is essential to distinguish between visible regression of the disease, as assessed by second-look laparoscopy, and the desired outcome, i.e., pregnancy and/or pain relief. Parenthetically, it is important to remember that post-treatment laparoscopic evaluation of the pelvis should be performed once the menstrual cycle has resumed rather than immediately the therapy has been discontinued, in order to obtain a representative assessment.[9] Second-look laparoscopies are usually reserved for patients within clinical trials rather than being part of routine clinical practice, which tends to be more orientated towards management of infertility.

Medical Therapy for Fertility

Controlled studies, with an untreated control group, have failed to demonstrate improvement in fertility with either medical or surgical therapy of mild endometriosis (in the absence of mechanical distortion). There is little to choose between the medical therapies with respect to subsequent fertility and a body of evidence that indicates no benefit when compared with expectant management.[6,10,11] These have been collected together in a systematic review[12] and combined in a meta-analysis in which the combined odds ratio for pregnancy was 0.83 (95% CI 0.59–1.39). This result indicates that treatment does not increase pregnancy rates and, if anything, may actually reduce them. This absence of demonstrable efficacy, together with the fact that the treatments are contraceptive, means that we do not therefore advocate the use of medical therapies for women who wish to conceive. Furthermore, medical therapy simply suppresses endometriosis for the duration of the therapy and does not prevent progression of the disease.

Endometriosis undergoes changes during the menstrual cycle, with age, and during hormonal therapy. Superficial endometriotic lesions, including those that underlie ovarian endometriomata, tend to undergo secretory changes during the luteal phase of the cycle, while enclosed nodular lesions are proliferative and do not undergo necrosis or shedding during menstruation. Endometriosis responds to the cyclical changes in ovarian hormones and regresses during pregnancy, when estrogen and progesterone serum concentrations are high. "Pseudo-pregnancy" treatment involves continuous administration of a combined oral contraceptive (COC) preparation and endometriotic implants eventually atrophy, although they tend to hypertrophy and undergo decidualization first.[13] There are fewer estrogen and progesterone receptors in endometriotic tissue than in the endometrium and so therapy should be continued for several months for the disease to become quiescent.

The initial studies involved higher doses of synthetic estrogens/progestogens than contained in low-dose COCs and were often discontinued because of side-effects. The use of continuous low-dose COCs has not been adequately studied for the treatment of endometriosis-related infertility. The COC does result in reduced menstrual bleeding and the rates of endometriosis in women who are either taking the COC or who have stopped recently are low compared with those who have stopped the COC for more than 12 months. Whether the COC should be prescribed prophylactically to women with a strong family history of endometriosis is uncertain.

Medroxyprogesterone Acetate

Progestrogens alone cause decidualization followed by atrophy. Oral medroxyprogesterone acetate (MPA) will induce amenorrhea and should be commenced at a dose of 30 mg/day.[14,15] If breakthrough bleeding occurs the dose can be increased to 50 mg/day. The main side-effects are weight gain, breast tenderness, mood changes, and fluid retention.

Gestrinone

Gestrinone provides a combination of the effects of an androgen, a progestogen and antiprogestogen, and an antiestrogen. It can be administered twice weekly (1.25–2.5 mg) and the dose titrated to induce amenorrhea. Side-effects include acne, oily skin, weight gain, nausea, and muscle cramps.

GnRH Agonists

Gonadotropin releasing hormone (GnRH) agonists cause pituitary desensitization and thereby induce amenorrhea. Depot preparations can be administered monthly and this aids adherence to treatment. Side-effects are those of estrogen deficiency: hot flushes, reduced libido, acne, and oily skin. Various regimens have been proposed in which "add-back" progestogens[16] or estrogen have been employed to prevent bone loss and other long-term effects of hypoestrogenism. Small doses are usually used, for example a daily tablet of tibolone, or ethinylestradiol 20 micrograms daily. We do not propose to discuss these further as they are more relevant to the chronic treatment of endometriosis in women who experience pain rather than for the treatment of infertility. Furthermore, we do not favor the *prolonged* use of GnRH agonists prior to IVF therapy, as there is no evidence of benefit (see below).

Danazol

Danazol is a synthetic anabolic steroid preparation which is also anti-progestogenic and antiestrogenic. It inhibits gonadotropin secretion and also has androgenic effects. Both danazol and GnRH agonists suppress disease activity and levels of anti-endometrial autoantibodies.[17] Efficacy correlates with achieving amenorrhea, which is usually induced within 8 weeks of administration, although the starting dose (400 mg/day) sometimes has to be increased to 600–800 mg/day. Side-effects can be troublesome and are secondary to the anabolic and androgenic properties of the drug. These include hot flushes, acne, oily skin, hirsutism, deepening of the voice, reduced libido, weight gain, nausea, headache, and muscle cramps. Because of the side-effects it is the authors' practice not to use danazol as a first-line therapy in the management of endometriosis.[18]

RU486

The antiprogestogen RU486 (mifepristone) inhibits ovulation, disrupts endometrial integrity, and antagonizes the mitogenic effect of estrogen on the endometrium; without producing a fall in mean serum estrogen concentrations. Long-term, low-dose daily administration induces amenorrhea and is being studied as a well-tolerated alternative therapy for the treatment of endometriosis.[19]

Efficacy

GnRH agonists and danazol have been compared in a number of prospective randomized studies and appear to be equally effective in reducing the endometriosis score by about 50% and achieving remission in about 25% of cases.[19,20–25] Both gestrinone[26,27] and MPA appear to be as effective as danazol[28] and GnRH agonists, with respect to post-treatment laparoscopy findings.

An issue of ongoing debate is the possible effects of severe endometriosis on the success of IVF therapy, as it has been suggested that rates of fertilization and implantation are impaired. It is reasonable to suppress active endometriosis with a GnRH agonist for 2–3 months prior to IVF, particularly if pituitary desensitization is part of the IVF treatment protocol.[29,30] Care should be taken, however, in those women who have had previous surgery to the ovaries or who have elevated basal serum follicle stimulating hormone (FSH) concentrations as prolonged suppression with a GnRH agonist might impede subsequent response to stimulation with gonadotropins.

Surgical Therapy

Surgical therapy for the treatment of endometriosis can be performed at the time of the diagnostic laparoscopy, although only if the diagnosis has been suspected and the patient has been given appropriate information and consent. It is our practice to consent women undergoing diagnostic laparoscopy for the possibility of ablation of minor endometriosis or adhesiolysis, which need not add more than 10–15 minutes to the procedure. Severe disease is sometimes apparent without pre-existing signs or symptoms and in these cases a detailed discussion with the patient is required before proceeding to more major surgery. Pre- or post-surgery medical suppression of endometriosis serves only to delay conception with only anecdotal evidence to suggest therapeutic benefit. Preoperative medical suppression of severe endometriosis reduces vascularity and might make surgery easier, but on the other hand estrogen-deficient tissues may become more friable and heal less well.[31] If the surgery has been aimed at removing active disease prior to IVF then it is advisable to continue GnRH agonist therapy after surgery, to reduce the risk of postoperative adhesion formation, and plan to commence superovulation therapy after 6–8 weeks (add-back therapy is not used at this time).

In considering surgery for endometriosis a distinction should be made between ovarian endometriomata and deeply infiltrating endometriosis, i.e., endometriosis that penetrates more than 5 mm below the peritoneal surface. Cystic ovarian endometriosis tends to be associated with adhesions, while deep infiltrating endometriosis is not and is often found in the pouch of Douglas, on the uterosacral ligaments, and in the uterovesical fold. Sometimes the lesions can be very deep yet have only a small visible surface area. Magnetic resonance imaging can be helpful in localizing the lesions and guiding the surgery. It is sometimes necessary to perform rectoscopy and an intravenous urogram prior to surgery. Where there is deeply infiltrating disease it is wise to prepare the bowel preoperatively. CO_2-laser excision appears to achieve better results than electrosurgery, as it has a minimal depth of penetration and provides greater control and precision. Laparoscopic surgery should only be performed by appropriately trained and skilled surgeons as endometriosis taxes the skill of the surgeon more than any other disease in the pelvis.

Aggressive treatment of deeply infiltrating endometriosis and cystic ovarian endometriosis is associated with cumulative pregnancy rates of up to 60% over 12 months, after which IVF will probably provide a greater chance of conception than a second-look procedure.[32] Large lesions often require laparotomy and sometimes bowel, or even ureteric, dissection. Such major surgery is usually reserved for patients with severe pain who have completed their family rather than for those with infertility, in whom GnRH agonist therapy combined with IVF is usually more appropriate.

Endometriomata can cause significant problems during IVF. Indeed, it is our experience that the only severe pelvic infections that have occurred after transvaginal ultrasound-guided oocyte collection have been when an endometriotic cyst has been entered accidentally. It has been suggested that pretreatment drainage of endometriomata increases the number of oocytes collected and enhances pregnancy rates. Medical therapy tends to have little effect on endometriotic cysts. We prefer to drain endometriotic cysts under direct visualization at the time of laparoscopic surgery rather than transvaginally, although others have reported good results with transvaginal aspiration of cysts. Laparoscopic drainage also enables definitive treatment to minimise recurrence. One should always remember that cysts can be malignant in women of any age and appropriate follow-up surveillance is required. Because of the risks of either laparoscopic surgery or transvaginal aspiration of endometriotic cysts our preferred strategy is not to interfere with a cyst in a woman with two functional ovaries and to avoid aspiration during the oocyte retrieval procedure. If there is an impaired ovarian response to stimulation we advise treatment of the cyst before further IVF therapy. If there are bilateral endometriomata we recommend surgery before IVF is commenced. If a cyst is entered accidentally during oocyte retrieval we attempt to drain it completely and provide prophylactic antibiotic therapy (Augmentin or a cephalosporin + metronidazole) for 7 days.

Surgery for mild endometriosis

In an attempt to answer whether mild/minimal endometriosis should be treated, the Endocan study, a multicenter randomized controlled trial, was conducted in Canada.[7] It aimed to establish whether the ablation or resection of endometriosis in minimal or mild (stage I or II) endometriosis improved the cumulative probability of pregnancy. The primary outcome was pregnancy with follow-up for 36 weeks. The study was well designed, with the exclusion of all other factors that might affect fertility and randomization at the time of laparoscopy.

Patients were not, however, blinded to randomization. Inclusion in the study depended on the visualization of typical blue–black endometriotic lesions and an AFS score of less than 16. This unfortunately meant that patients with adhesions were included in the study, so the intervention was not solely ablation of implants. At the end of the study, results in 341 patients were eligible for analysis: 172 patients underwent therapeutic laparoscopy and 169 had only a diagnostic laparoscopy. Those patients undergoing treatment had not only ablation of endometriotic deposits, usually with electrocautery, but also a division of adhesions. Thus, although the aim of the study was to investigate the effect of ablation or resection, in 9% of patients a significant co-intervention took place.

Patients treated at the time of laparoscopy had a significantly higher pregnancy rate than those who underwent only a diagnostic laparoscopy. Excluding those with adhesions, the odds ratio was still higher, but in both groups the confidence intervals were quite wide and the lower value approached 1. When patients who had adhesions were excluded, only 284 patients remained, and thus the study to consider the effect of ablation alone was underpowered (estimated requirement: 330 patients). It is interesting to note that despite a longer follow-up period than the 24 weeks seen in randomized controlled trials of medical therapy, the cumulative probability of pregnancy in the treated group was less than that observed in the expectant management group in the Cochrane review,[12] where pregnancy rates ranged from 23.5% to 47.2%. This may reflect the impact of the inclusion of patients with adhesions, but again questions the generalizability of the results of this trial and begs the question of whether the original aim has been adequately addressed.[33]

A smaller study by the Italian Group for the Study of Endometriosis[8] randomly assigned 54 patients to treatment of mild endometriosis and 47 to laparoscopy alone. After 1 year the pregnancy rates were no different at 24% and 29%, respectively. Thus, while treatment is unlikely to do harm and should not unduly lengthen the laparoscopic procedure, there is conflicting evidence of benefit.

Proposed Strategy for the Management of Endometriosis

Women with endometriosis-associated infertility have reduced fecundity of 1–3% per cycle yet, in the absence of mechanical distortion of pelvic organs, the mechanism is unclear. Medical therapy should be reserved for those women with moderate to severe endometriosis who are proceeding to assisted conception therapies within the following 2 months in order to render the endometriosis quiescent before commencing ovarian stimulation. Laparoscopic surgery should be performed at the time of the diagnostic procedure in mild cases and after careful preparation for moderate to severe cases with the aim of removing endometriomata and alleviating periovarian and peritubal adhesions. If conception does not occur within 6–12 months assisted conception in the form of IVF should be offered.

Endometriosis – key points

- Retrograde menstruation is the probable cause of most cases of endometriosis.
- The pathophysiology and time course of endometriosis are not fully understood.
- Minimal and mild endometriosis affect fertility and should be treated during the assessment laparoscopy.
- Moderate to severe endometriosis can result in infertility and may require more extensive surgery.
- The medical treatment of endometriosis is contraceptive and so appropriate for patients with pain but not infertility.
- Surgical treatment of endometriosis can improve the fertility of appropriately selected patients.
- Assisted reproduction technology is often required for those with severe endometriosis.
- Endometriomata may lead to severe pelvic infection if aspirated transvaginally, e.g., accidentally during oocyte collection for IVF.

References

1. Vessey MP, Villard-Macintosh L & Painter R (1993) Epidemiology of endometriosis in women attending family planning clinics. *Br Med J* **306**: 182–184.
2. Brosens I, Puttemans P & Deprest J (1993) Appearance of endometriosis. In Brosens I (ed) *Baillière's Clinical Obstetrics and Gynaecology* **7/4**: 741–757.
3. Redwine DB (1987). Age-related evolution in color appearance of endometriosis. *Fertil Steril* **48**: 1062–1063.
4. Kruitwagen R (1993) Menstruation as the pelvic aggressor. In: Brosens I (ed) *Baillière's Clinical Obstetrics and Gynaecology* **7/4**: 687–700.
5. Olive DL & Haney AF (1986) Endometriosis-associated infertility: a critical review of therapeutic approaches. *Obstet Gynaecol Surv* **41**: 538–555.
6. Thomas EJ & Cooke ID (1987) Successful treatment of asymptomatic endometriosis: does it benefit infertile women? *Br Med J* **294**: 1117–1119.
7. Marcoux S, Maheux R, Bérubé S & the Canadian Collaborative Group on Endometriosis (1997) Laparoscopic surgery in infertile women with minimal and mild endometriosis. *N Engl J Med* **97**: 212–222.
8. Parazzini F (1999) Ablation of lesions or no treatment in minimal–mild endometriosis in infertile women. A randomized trial. *Hum Reprod* **14**: 1332–1334.

9. Evers J (1987) The second look laparoscopy for the evaluation of the results of medical treatment of endometriosis should not be performed during ovarian suppression. *Fertil Steril* **47**: 502–504.
10. Badaway SZA, El Bakry MM, Samuel F & Dizier M (1988) Cumulative pregnancy rates in women with endometriosis. *J Reprod Med* **33**: 757–760.
11. Telimaa S (1988) Danazol and medroxyprogesterone acetate are inefficacious in the treatment of infertility in endometriosis. *Fertil Steril* **50**: 872–875.
12. Hughes E, Fedorkow D, Collins J & Vandekerckhove P (1999) Ovulation suppression for endometriosis (Cochrane Review). Cochrane Library, Issue 4. Update Software, Oxford.
13. Wingfield M & Healy DL (1993) Endometriosis: medical therapy. In Brosens I (ed) Endometriosis. *Baillière's Clinical Obstetrics and Gynaecology* 7:**4,** 813–838.
14. Luciano AA, Turskoy RN & Carleo J (1988) Evaluation of oral medroxyprogesterone acetate in the treatment of endometriosis. *Obstet Gynecol* **72**: 323–327.
15. Moghissi KS (1988) Treatment of endometriosis with estrogen–progestin combination and progestogens alone. *Clin Obstet Gynecol* **31**: 823–828.
16. Cedars MI, Lu JKH, Meldrum DR & Judd HL (1990) Treatment of endometriosis with a long-acting GnRH agonist plus medroxyprogesterone acetate. *Obstet Gynecol* **75**: 641–645.
17. Bayer SR, Seibel MM, Saffan DS, Berger MJ & Taymour ML (1988) Efficacy of danazol treatment for minimal endometriosis in infertile women. *J Reprod Fertil* **33**: 179–183.
18. Murphy AA & Castellano PZ (1994) RU486: pharmacology and potential use in the treatment of endometriosis and leiomyomata uteri. *Curr Opin Obstet Gynecol* **6**: 269–278.
19. Henzl MR, Corson SL, Moghissi K *et al.* (1988) Administration of nasal nafarelin as compared with oral danazol for endometriosis. *N Engl J Med* **318**: 485–489.
20. Dmowski WP, Radwanska E, Binmor Z, Tummon I & Pepping P (1989) Ovarian suppression induced with buserelin or danazol in the management of endometriosis: a randomised, comparative study. *Fertil Steril* **51**: 395–400.
21. Donnez J, Nisolle-Pochet M & Casanas-Roux F (1990) Endometriosis-associated infertility: evaluation of preoperative use of danazol, gestrinone and buserelin. *Int J Fertil* **35**: 297–301.
22. Fedele L, Bianchi S, Arcaini L, Vercellini P & Candiani GB (1989) Buserelin versus danazol in the treatment of endometriosis-associated infertility. *Am J Obstet Gynecol* **161**: 871–876.
23. Fraser IS, Shearman RP, Jansen RPS & Sutherland PD (1991) A comparative treatment trial of endometriosis using the GnRH agonist nafarelin and the synthetic steroid danazol. *Aust NZ J Obstet Gynaecol* **31**: 158–163.
24. Nafarelin European Endometriosis Trial (NEET) Group (1992) Nafarelin for endometriosis: a large scale, danazol-controlled trial of efficacy and safety, with 1 year follow up. *Fertil Steril* **57**: 514–522.
25. Shaw RW (1992) An open randomized comparative study of the effect of gosarelin depot and danazol in the treatment of endometriosis. *Fertil Steril* **58**: 265–272.
26. Fedele L, Bianchi S, Viezzoli T, Arcaini L & Candiani GB (1989) Gestrinone versus danazol in the treatment of endometriosis. *Fertil Steril* **51**: 781–785.
27. Hornstein MD, Gleason RE & Barbieri RL (1990) A randomised double-blind prospective trial of two doses of gestrinone in the treatment of endometriosis. *Fertil Steril* **53**: 237–241.
28. Telimaa S, Puolakka J, Ronnberg L & Kaupila A (1987) Placebo-controlled comparison of danazol and high-dose medroxyprogesterone acetate in the treatment of endometriosis. *Gynecol Endocrinol* **1**: 13–23.
29. Dicker D, Goldman JA, Levy T, Feldbert D & Ashkenazi J (1992) The impact of long term GnRH analogue treatment on preclinical abortions in patients with severe endometriosis undergoing *in vitro* fertilisation. *Fertil Steril* **57**: 597–600.

30. Nakamura K, Oosawa M, Kondou I *et al.* (1992) Menotropin stimulation after prolonged GnRH agonist pretreatment for *in vitro* fertilisation in patients with endometriosis. *J Assist Reprod Genetics* **9**: 113–117.
31. Thomas EJ (1992) Combining medical and surgical treatment for endometriosis: the best of both worlds? *Br J Obstet Gynaecol* **99**: 5–8.
32. Koninckx PR & Martin D (1994) Treatment of deeply infiltrating endometriosis (review). *Curr Opin Obstet Gynecol* **6**: 231–241.
33. Prentice A (2000) Endometriosis and infertility. In: Balen A (ed) *Infertility 2000*. Reed Healthcare Communications, Sutton, Surrey, pp 28–31.
34. Acosta AA, Puttram VC, Franklin RR & Besch PK (1993) A proposed classification of pelvic endometriosis. *Obstet Gynecol* **42**: 19–25.

Further Reading

Brosens I (ed) (1993) Endometriosis. *Baillière's Clinical Obstetrics and Gynaecology* 7: 4.

Hughes EG, Fedorkow DM & Collins JA (1993) A quantitative overview of controlled trials in endometriosis associated infertility. *Fertil Steril* **59**: 963–970.

Prentice A (2001) Endometriosis: clinical review. *BMJ* **323**: 93–95.

Thomas EJ & Rock JA (eds) (1991) *Modern approaches to endometriosis*. Kluwer, London.

Chapter 10

Tubal infertility and fibroids

Introduction

In vitro fertilization (IVF) has revolutionized many forms of fertility therapy, yet the question of IVF versus tubal surgery for mild to moderate tubal disease is still debated. IVF is a stressful and time-consuming treatment and each attempt offers only a single chance for pregnancy, unless embryos can be frozen for future use. Successful tubal surgery, on the other hand, can provide a permanent cure, with the possibility of more than one pregnancy. Furthermore, tubal surgery can be performed laparoscopically although there is still debate about the respective indications for open tubal microsurgery and laparoscopic tubal surgery. For example, the European Society of Human Reproduction and Embryology (ESHRE) Committee has suggested that the only indication for open tubal surgery is reversal of sterilization. In the UK tubal surgery is often funded by the National Health Service (although less so than 5 years ago), while IVF is not. In our initial discussion, however, we propose to set aside the matter of cost and select the appropriate treatment for the individual patient.

Techniques

The techniques employed in tubal surgery are of paramount importance and require adequate training, whether performed at laparotomy or laparoscopy. Open tubal surgery is optimally performed using an operating microscope. Magnification of the tube, usually 20–40×, allows inspection of the mucosa and the correct alignment of the canal during tubal reconstruction. Adequate access to the pelvic organs is required, although this does not always necessitate a large incision. The tissues should be handled carefully and continuous irrigation with a physiological solution (Ringer's lactate or Hartmann's solution, sometimes heparinized) should be employed.[1] Synthetic non-absorbable sutures (8–0 nylon) are usually used in order to minimize tissue reaction during healing, although some surgeons prefer synthetic absorbable sutures (e.g., Vicryl).

While some surgeons advocate the continued use of open microsurgery, the laparoscopic approach has gained favor in recent years.[2] Even after a four-portal procedure the patient recovers more rapidly than after a laparotomy and can usually return home the day following surgery or sometimes the same day. One study[3] compared the outcome of microsurgical and laparoscopic adhesiolysis and found no statistically significant difference in cumulative conception rates, which were a little over 40% after 12 months. The single most significant variable that affected the chance of a pregnancy was the duration of infertility and it was found that for each additional year of infertility the probability of a pregnancy was reduced by about 20%. The implications for delay through slowly moving waiting lists are profound.

The technique of laparoscopic surgery has to be meticulously executed and the limitations of the tools and risks of injury to adjacent structures appreciated, especially during use of laser or electrocoagulation. Follow-up studies have revealed no differences in the amount of tissue damage and adhesion reformation between CO_2 laser and electromicrosurgery (as assessed by measurement of residual particulate carbon, foreign body reaction, or tissue necrosis).

Endoscopic Tools

Electrosurgery is most commonly used and can be employed with a coagulating (intermittent) current, which results in cell dehydration, or a cutting (continuous) current that vaporizes the tissue; alternatively, the two modes can be blended. Unipolar diathermy produces a flow of electrons through tissue to the earth plate, while bipolar diathermy causes less adjacent tissue damage as the current flows between the two prongs of the forceps. Endocoagulation coagulates by heating tissue to 120°C without electrical energy escaping into the patient.

Laser therapy requires expensive equipment. Short wavelength lasers (KTP, Nd:YAG) coagulate well but cause poor vaporization. CO_2 lasers cut precisely as they vaporize well but coagulate less well, thereby causing wider areas of tissue damage when used to coagulate.

The ultrasonic vibrating scalpel vibrates at > 50 kHz, denatures proteins, and cuts tissue with minimal adjacent tissue injury compared with electrosurgery or lasers. As the protein cools it forms a hemostatic coagulum.

Presurgical Considerations

The couple will have been investigated thoroughly before the decision is made to perform tubal surgery. If there are coexisting fertility problems, for example sperm dysfunction, IVF should be recommended.[4] The patient's age is another important consideration, as the success rates of IVF decline with age and in women over the age of 38 it is prudent to move on to IVF quickly rather than wait for tubal surgery to have a chance to work.[5]

Presurgical investigations should include assessment of both the uterine cavity, by hysterosalpingography (HSG) or hysteroscopy, and the Fallopian tubes, usually by laparoscopy (see Ch. 4). Further assessment of the tube from within is offered by either salpingoscopy (via the laparoscope) or Falloposcopy (via the hysteroscope), both of which are still being evaluated (see Fig. 10.9). Selective salpingography and Fallopian tube cannulation can help distinguish the location of a proximal occlusion of the tube and are sometimes used to achieve recannulation without resort to surgery. Surgery is least likely to be of benefit when there is gross tubal damage with only a short length of normal tube or when there are extensive pelvic adhesions or an active disease such as endometriosis (see Ch. 9) (see Fig. 10.8).

Adhesiolysis (Figs 10.1 and 10.3)

Peritubal adhesions interfere with ovum pick-up and tubal transport, while periovarian adhesions may inhibit ovulation. When the tubes are patent and the ovaries freely mobile, adhesiolysis will result in good cumulative conception rates (60% in 24 months), although at second-look laparoscopy there is often a recurrence of the adhesions to some degree.[6,7] Dense adhesions carry a worse prognosis than fine, filmy adhesions. It is important to avoid producing raw areas of denuded peritoneum which will increase post-operative adhesion formation. Some advocate an early second-look laparoscopy, between 5 days and 2 months after the initial procedure, to allow further treatment of filmy adhesions before they become too dense (usually by 4–6 months after surgery).

The degree of magnification achieved during laparoscopy permits equivalent ease of surgery as with open microsurgery and the initial access to adherent pelvic organs is more easily achieved, without the need for macrodissection. The Canadian Infertility Evaluation Study Group performed a multicenter, randomized study[5] of laparoscopic salpingo-ovariolysis versus no treatment and found pregnancy rates at 12 months of 45% and 16%, respectively. The ectopic pregnancy rate after salpingoovariolysis is approximately 5% (compared with a population rate of 0.5–1%).[1,6 8] (See also Fig. 10.2.)

Salpingostomy

The mainstay of salpingostomy is the fashioning of a small ostium at the tip of the tube, with eversion of the tubal mucosa so that the reconstructed fimbriae are positioned to allow the ostium free movement

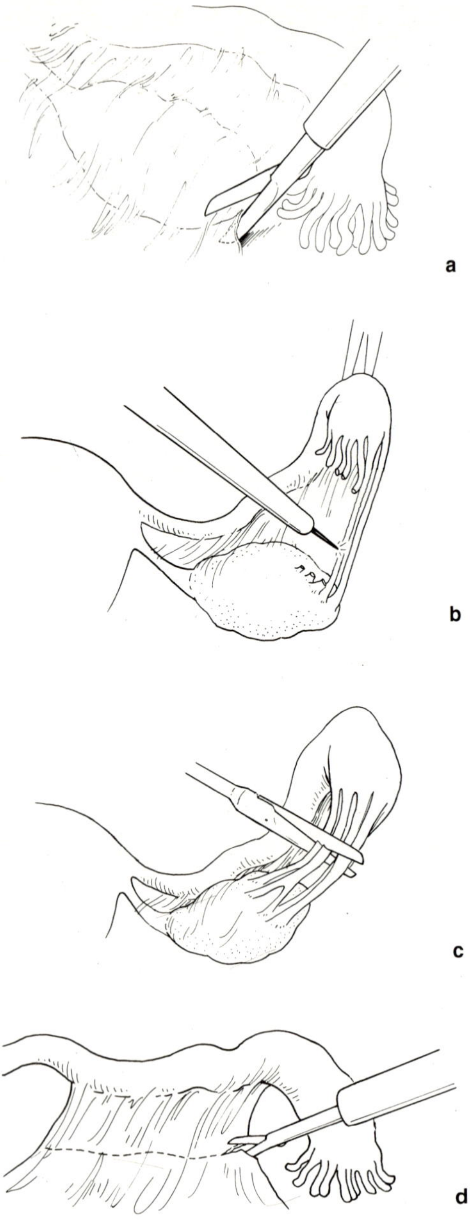

Figures 10.1a,b,c,d (**a**) Laparoscopic peritubal and periovarian adhesiolysis; (**b**) and (**c**) laparoscopic fimbriolysis (Winston & Margara[1], Wood[2]) and (**d**) salpingolysis.

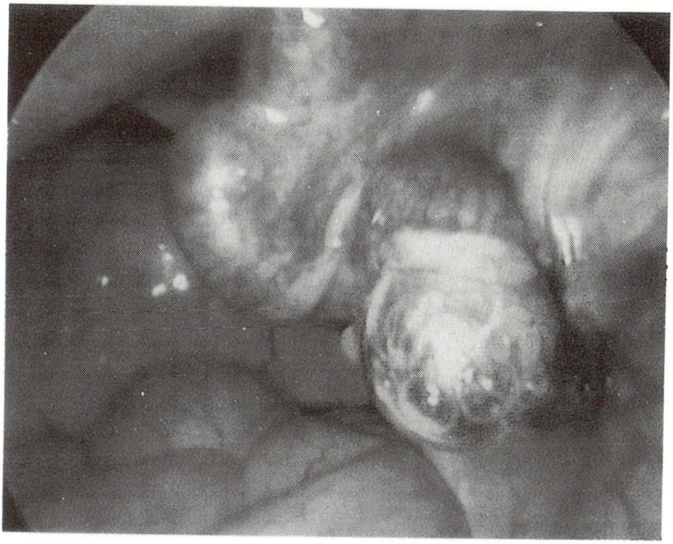

a

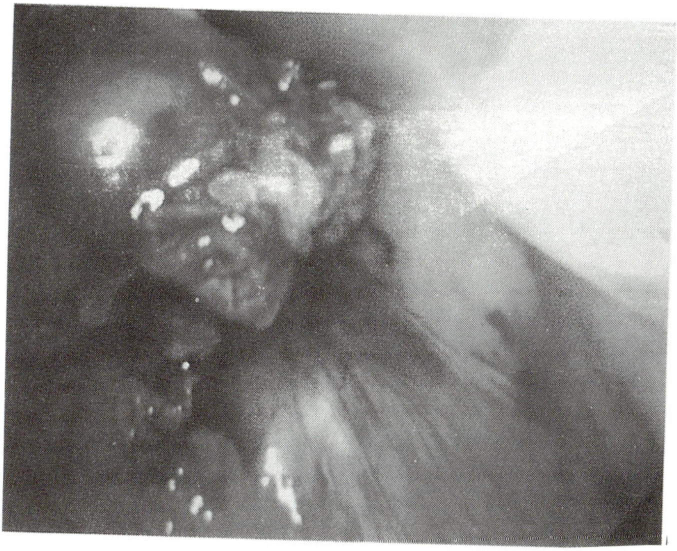

b

Figure 10.2a,b (**a**) Laparoscopy and dye: perifimbrial adhesions lead to loculation of the injected dye, yet there is some spill into the peritoneal cavity. In cases such as this an HSG examination can give the impression of normal tubal patency. (**b**) An adhesiolysis has been performed and the fimbrial end of the tube displayed to allow free flow of dye (please refer to plate section for color figures).

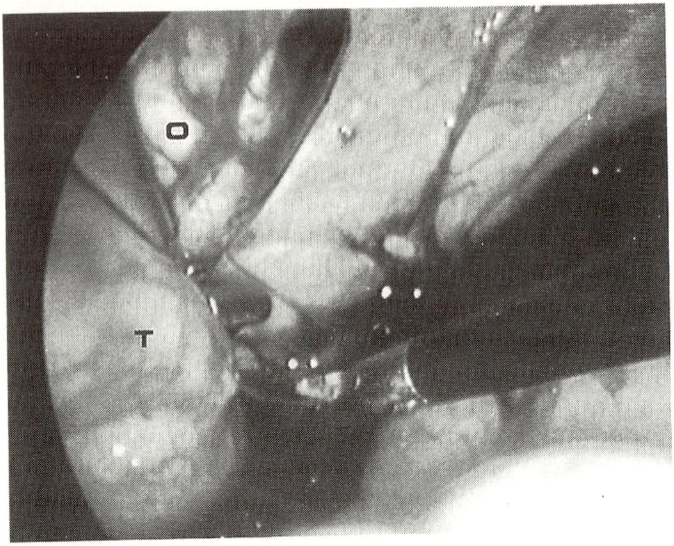

a

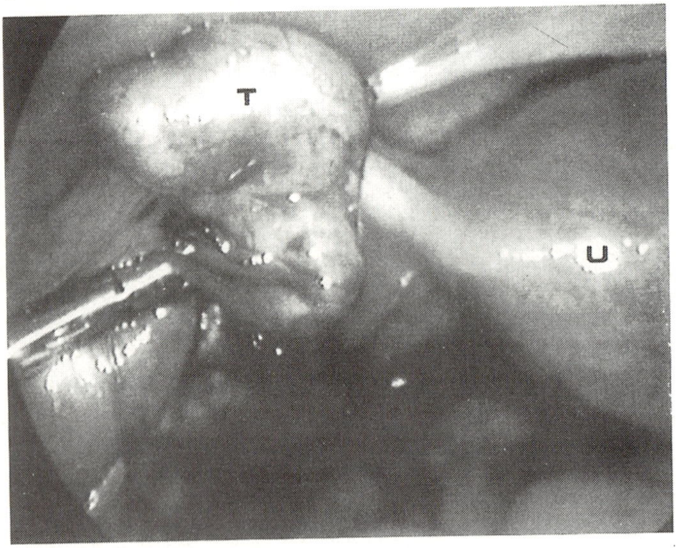

b

Figure 10.3a,b (**a**) Laparoscopy and dye: the left ovary (O) is tethered to the posterior leaf of the broad ligament and the tube (T) is adherent in the pouch of Douglas. Scissors are used to release the adhesions. (**b**) An adhesiolysis has been performed but the tube (T) is "retort" shaped, distended, and considerably damaged. The uterus (U) is seen to the right (please refer to plate section for color figures).

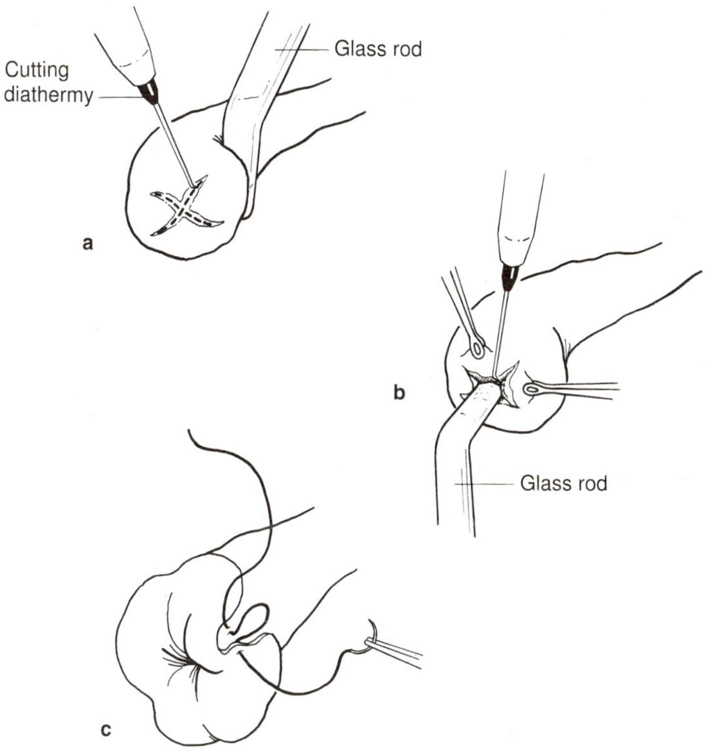

Figure 10.4 Open tubal microsurgery: salpingostomy; (**a**) a cruciate incision is made into the tube using cutting diathermy and (**b**) carefully extended; (**c**) the mucosal edges of the tube are then everted and sutured using a non-absorbable 6–0 suture.

over the ovary. Raw areas and linear incisions in the tube will heal over and should be avoided. The best cases to treat are those in which the tubes have thin walls, normal mucosa, and no periovarian adhesions, although when the distal end of the tube is blocked there are usually periovarian and peritubular adhesions. Large hydrosalpinges, greater than 1.5 cm in diameter, carry a worse prognosis.

Some advocate the insertion of a salpingoscope before deciding upon formal laparoscopic fimbrial reconstruction as the presence of intratubal adhesions or grossly damaged tubal mucosa will lead to abandonment of the procedure. While this has scientific logic, the tube has to be opened at its distal end in order to insert the salpingoscope and so there is little to be lost by proceeding with a fimbrioplasty. Pregnancy rates after salpingostomy range between 20% and 40%, with ectopic pregnancy rates of 5–20% (Figs 10.4–10.6).[1,6,7]

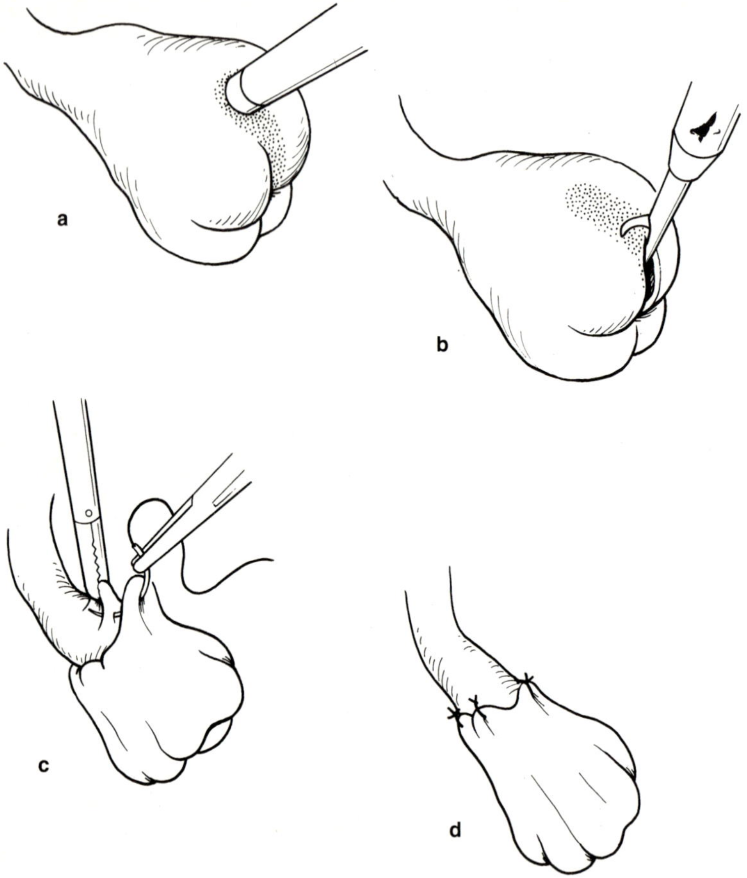

Figure 10.5 Laparoscopic salpingostomy with sutures using (**a**) laser or cutting diathermy; (**b**) sharp dissection; (**c**) and (**d**) laparoscopic sutures.

Cornual Occlusion

Tubocornual anastomosis is best achieved using open microsurgery. Advocates of laparoscopic surgery are, however, exploring the use of tubotubal anastomoses, but with variable results to date. Where there was damage to the intramural portion of the tube, reimplantation of the tube used to be practised. The results of tubal reimplantation are often poor and there is a risk of uterine rupture during pregnancy, so these cases are now best treated by IVF. Cornual occlusion due to infection (salpingitis isthmica nodosa, pelvic inflammatory disease, tuberculosis) is often associated with microscopic damage along the

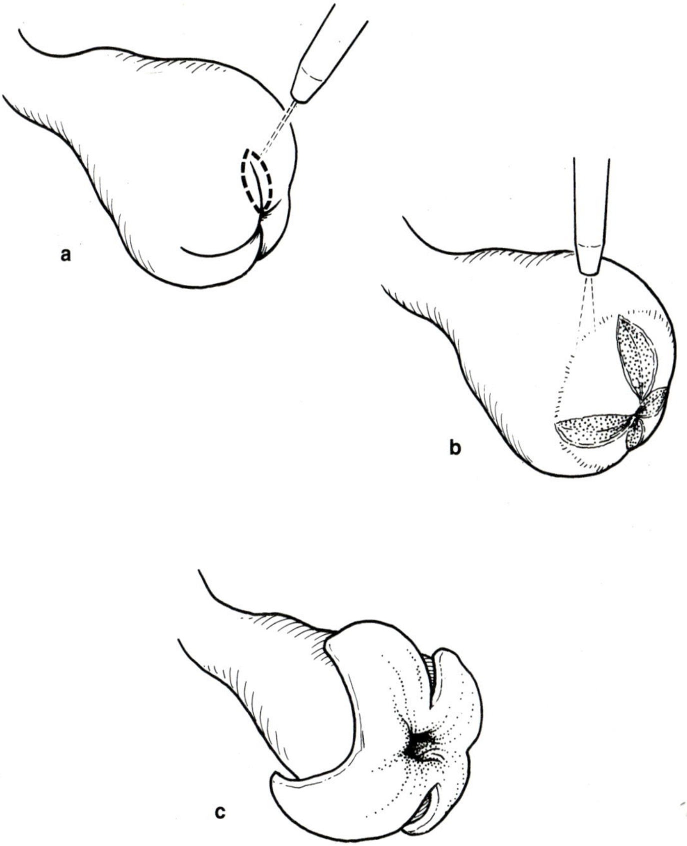

Figure 10.6 Laparoscopic salpingostomy with laser or diathermy to (**a**) incise the tube and (**b**) scar the serosa to cause (**c**) eversion of the mucosa.

length of the tube and so there is a worse prognosis and greater risk of ectopic pregnancy than after reversal of sterilization. The repair of the tube should be in two layers (muscularis with submucosa and serosa) using 8–0 non-absorbable synthetic sutures. Splinting of the tube may result in endothelial damage and is not recommended. It is important to remove an adequate section of the tube so that none of the diseased tube remains after surgery, as tubal patency, which results in 85% of cases, does not equate with tubal function or pregnancy, which occurs in approximately 50–60%. Post-surgery ectopic pregnancy rates are reported to be between 5% and 10%.[1,6,7]

Reversal of sterilization leads to the best results, not only because the patient is of proven fertility (although it is essential to check ovarian function and her new partner's semen analysis before embarking on

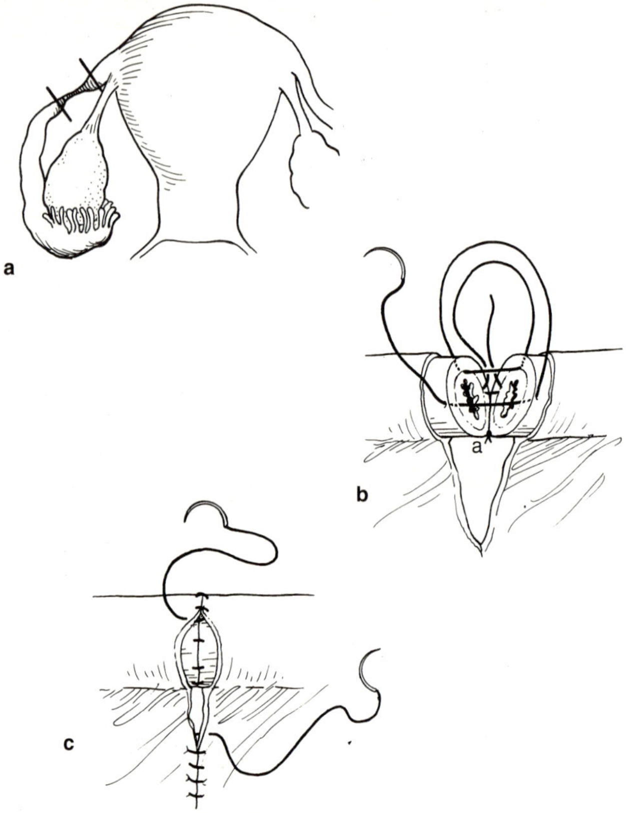

Figure 10.7 Open tubal microsurgery: tubocornual anastomosis: (**a**) after excising the stenosed segment of tube with a combination of cutting diathermy and sharp dissection, the clean edges are opposed using 8–0 nylon; (**b**) the first suture is placed at 6 o'clock (a) through the muscularis (not mucosa). Between 4 and 8 sutures are required. (**c**) The serosa and mesosalpinx are then repaired with 6–0 nylon.

surgery), but also because damage is to a very small portion of the tube. It is, however, essential to ascertain the method of sterilization as the older methods of Pomeroy ligation and tubal diathermy leave much less in the way of functional tube than the use of the Fallope ring, which in turn is more damaging than a clip. The best results are obtained if the reconstructed tube is longer than 4 cm, with at least 1 cm of distal ampulla. Pregnancy rates are between 60% and 80%, with ectopic pregnancy rates usually less than 5% (Fig. 10.7). While open laparotomy and microsurgical tubal reconstruction are still standard practice, some are achieving good results using laparoscopic techniques, sometimes robotically assisted.[9]

Reconstruction of Contralateral Tubes and Ovaries

In rare cases, when a tube has been lost from one side and the ovary lost from the other, it is necessary to mobilize the ovarian pedicle and bring it to the contralateral side to be close to the tube. In other cases a single tube has been fashioned from the remnants of two damaged tubes.

Transcervical Recannulation of the Tube

A false impression of tubal occlusion can be obtained during salpingography or laparoscopy because of either tubal spasm or the presence of viscous mucus plugs, which can be dislodged by either falloposcopy or selective salpingography. Transcervical cannulation of the tube using balloon tuboplasty, under fluoroscopic guidance, has been evaluated in recent years, with reports of tubal patency being achieved in approximately 80% of cases and pregnancy rates of 35%.[10,11] There are, to date, no controlled studies of these methods, but the best cases are likely to conceive and might even undergo spontaneous resolution of a functional blockage. (See also Fig. 10.8.)

Falloposcopy

The flexible falloposcope is inserted under hysteroscopic vision and provides both an image of the tubular lumen and the potential for recannulation by either flushing or tuboplasty.[12] Falloposcopic recannulation of the tube is likely to be successful only when there are minor intratubular adhesions or for the removal of mucus plugs and fibrinous deposits. The visualization of mucosal abnormalities might lead one to guide the patient to IVF sooner than if the architecture of the recannulated tube appeared normal (Fig. 10.9). Falloposcopy is limited by the optical systems available and, after early interest, has not become widely used. Furthermore, the product has been withdrawn from the market (see also p. 92)

Salpingoscopy

It has been suggested that the salpingoscope, inserted laparoscopically through the fimbrial end of the tube, provides clear visualization of the ampullary segment of the tube and is used more to guide decision making on the selection of patients for tubal surgery or IVF than for therapeutic procedures (Fig. 10.9).

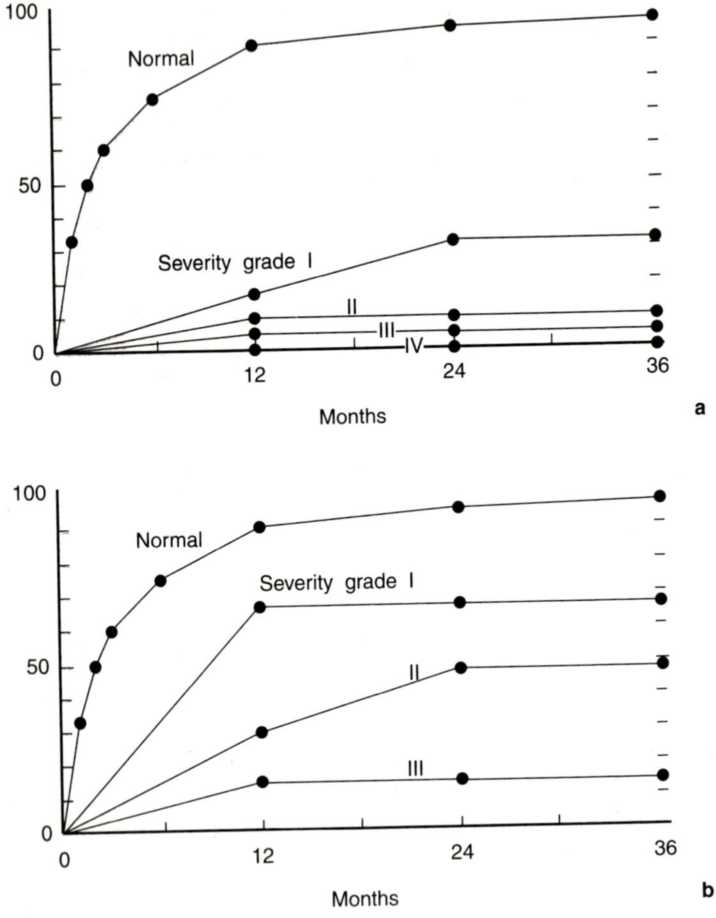

Figure 10.8 Cumulative conception rates (CCR) (**a**) before and (**b**) after tubal surgery related to severity of tubal disease (grade IV disease was not operated on).[13]

In Vitro Fertilization (see Ch. 13)

Most women with tubal infertility are optimally treated with IVF.[14,15] If they have a history of repeated ectopic pregnancy there is a case for performing a sterilization prior to IVF, as there is nothing more traumatic than developing a further ectopic pregnancy after the stresses of an IVF treatment cycle. The overall rate of ectopic pregnancy after IVF is 5% (i.e., higher than normal) because uterine transfer of the pre-embryo(s) does not ensure that it will remain in the uterine cavity. It is a big step to sterilize a woman who wishes to conceive

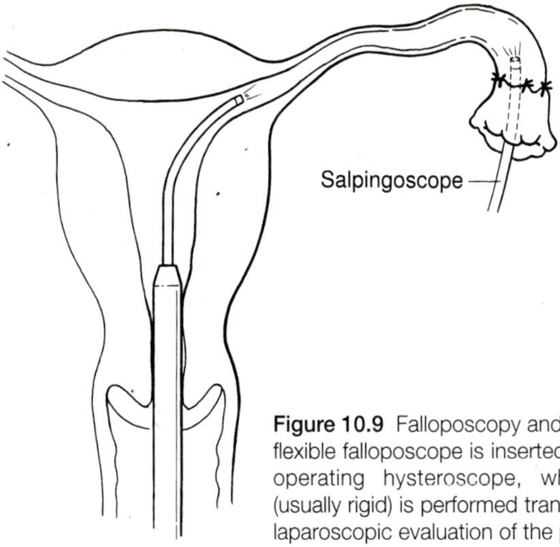

Figure 10.9 Falloposcopy and salpingoscopy. The flexible falloposcope is inserted via a channel in an operating hysteroscope, while salpingoscopy (usually rigid) is performed transabdominally during laparoscopic evaluation of the pelvis.

although those who have experienced ectopic pregnancies and have severe tubal damage will usually accept this. If an ectopic occurs after IVF in a patient with pre-existing tubal damage, the option of sterilization or salpingectomy should be discussed prior to surgery for the ectopic pregnancy.

There is good evidence to suggest that the presence of hydrosalpinges affects the outcome of IVF by having an effect on the endometrial environment, possibly through the passage of toxic fluid into the uterine cavity, which disrupts implantation.[16,17,18] If the tubes are completely blocked and there are large hydrosalpinges there is a case for their removal prior to IVF. In the largest prospective randomized controlled trial to date 204 patients were entered and 192 commenced IVF.[19] While there was no significant difference in the pregnancy rate between the salpingectomy group (36.6%) and the non-intervention group (23.9%), the live birth rates were increased (28.6% vs 16.3%, $p = 0.045$). The differences were more significant in the presence of bilateral hydrosalpinges and particularly so with ultrasound visible hydrosalpinges (Fig. 10.10) (clinical pregnancy rate 45.7% vs 22.5%, $p = 0.029$, live birth rate 40% vs 17.5%, $p = 0.038$). A systematic review of the three randomized controlled trials performed to date has produced an odds ratio of pregnancy (1.07, 95% CI 1.07–2.86) and live birth (2.13, 95% CI 1.24–3.65) in favor of salpingectomy, with no increase in complication rate during treatment.[20] Salpingectomy can usually be performed laparoscopically and while care should be taken not to compromise ovarian blood supply there is no evidence for an impairment of ovarian response in subsequent IVF.[21]

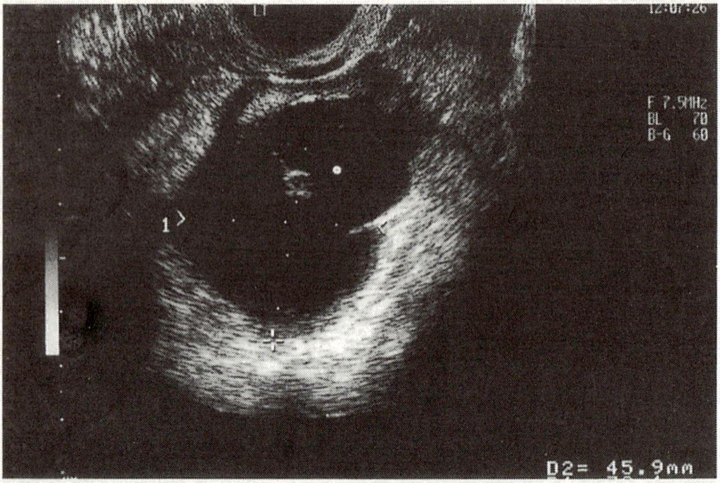

Figure 10.10 Transvaginal ultrasound scan of a hydrosalpinx. Courtesy of Mrs J. Smith, Assisted Conception Unit, Leeds General Infirmary.

Uterine Surgery

Myomectomy

Fibroids are often removed indiscriminately and myomectomy can result in extensive pelvic adhesion formation and damage to the integrity of the uterine cavity. Until recently it was thought that fibroids should only be removed if they are causing a significant distortion of the uterine cavity or if they are blocking the cornual region of the tube. Thus a study by Farhi *et al.*[23] demonstrated that implantation rates after IVF were not affected by the presence of fibroids unless the shape of the uterine cavity was altered. It is probably not the presence of fibroids that affects implantation rates but rather the distortion of the uterine cavity that they cause – perhaps by affecting endometrial proliferation and altering vascularization. Following more recent studies there is a vogue to remove fibroids of all sizes. There is increasing evidence that intramural fibroids affect implantation, even when there is no deformation of the uterine cavity.[24] A recent study found that fibroids of less than 5 cm diameter reduced ongoing pregnancy rates by a half following assisted conception.[25] Myomectomy is a major procedure with potential risks to the integrity and viability of the uterus. There has yet to be a randomized controlled study of myomectomy prior to assisted conception. Preoperative treatment with a gonadotropin releasing hormone agonist for 6–8 weeks will cause significant shrinkage of the fibroids and reduce vascularity and blood loss during surgery. Small submucosal

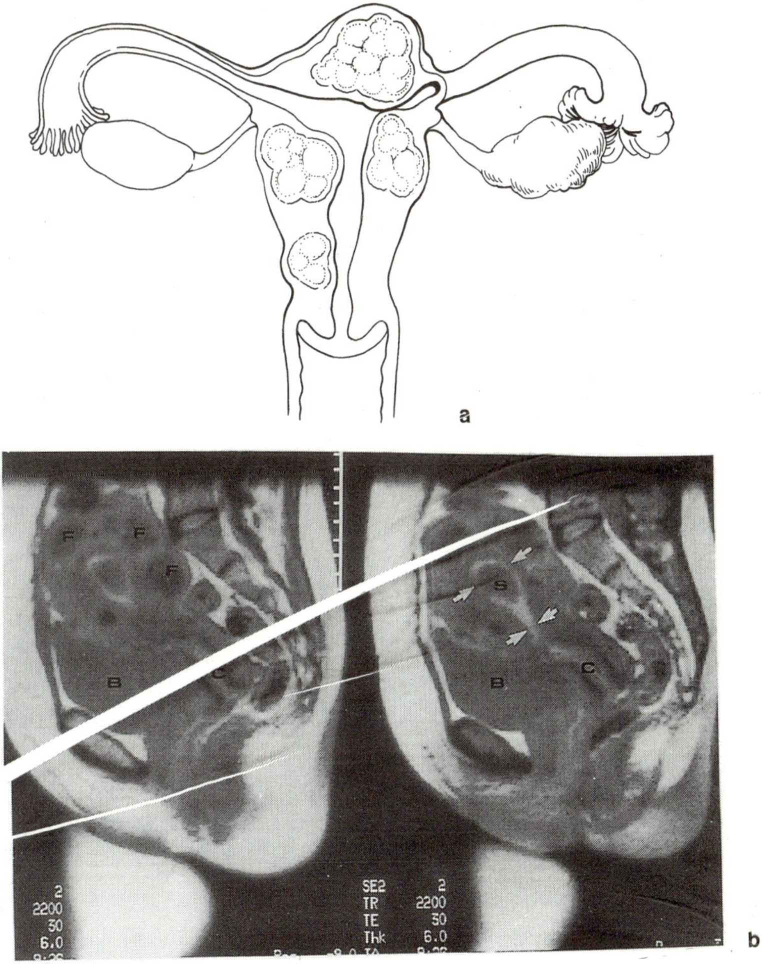

Figure 10.11a,b (**a**) Fibroids distorting the uterine cavity and causing tubocornual occlusion. (**b**) A proton density MRI scan showing two sagittal sections through the uterus, cervical canal (C) and bladder (B). Multiple intramural fibroids (F) can be seen. A large pedunculated submucosal fibroid (S) is outlined by the hyperintense (white) endometrium (arrow). This is the same patient as in Figure 4.30 (p. 89).

fibroids can be removed hysteroscopically, although whether they cause infertility is a matter of debate (Fig. 10.11).

Less invasive procedures than operative myomectomy are being evaluated for the management of fibroids, including uterine artery embolization and magnetic resonance imaging (MRI)-guided laser coagulative necrosis or high intensity focused ultrasound for the destruction of fibroids. The place of these techniques in the management of infertility is still being evaluated.[26]

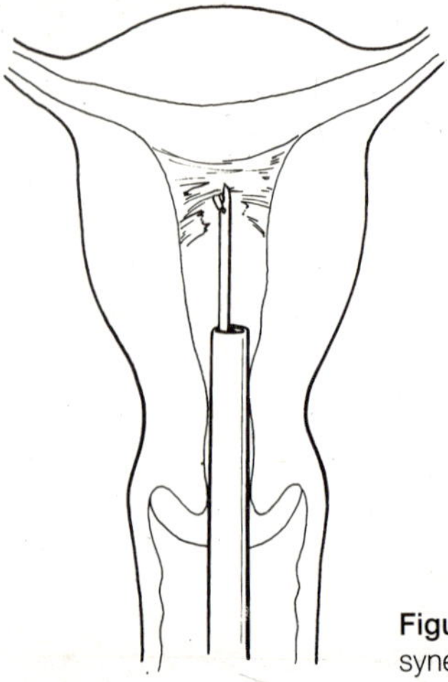

Figure 10.12 Hysteroscopic resection of intrauterine synechiae.

Intrauterine Polyps

Polyps are often found at the time of sonographic investigation of the uterine cavity, during an HSG or at the time of hysteroscopy. If the polyp appears to be blocking the cornual opening of the tube or if it is associated with an abnormal bleeding pattern it should be removed. If a hysteroscopy is being performed then polyps can be removed easily. If, however, the polyp is an incidental finding during imaging of the pelvis, in the absence of symptoms, surgery is not indicated as there is no clear evidence for an association between the presence of a polyp and infertility. If the patient is experiencing irregular bleeding or discharge, the polyp should be removed to exclude malignant change.

Intrauterine Synechiae

Hysteroscopic division of synechiae should be performed.. If the patient is amenorrheic with Asherman's syndrome the integrity of the cavity should be maintained using an indwelling intrauterine contraceptive device for 2 months, to allow the resumption of regular menstrual shedding, before it is removed and the patient allowed to conceive (Fig. 10.12).

Reconstruction of Uterine Anomalies

It is difficult to know which congenital uterine anomalies are associated with infertility as many women conceive and might only be found to have a uterine anomaly during incidental ultrasonography of the pregnancy or Cesarean delivery. Large intrauterine septa may result in an increased risk of miscarriage but probably do not affect implantation. If a septate uterus is found during routine investigations for infertility then one should question the need for surgery on the basis of whether the abnormality is having an effect on fertility. Is it reasonable, however, then to allow a patient who has been having difficulty in conceiving to continue with a high risk of miscarriage once she finally gets pregnant? As a miscarriage is by no means a certainty, we would counsel caution before performing major surgery on the uterus, which might in any case further disrupt the integrity of the uterus or lead to damaging adhesion formation.

The only chance of pregnancy for women with major uterine anomalies or congenital absence of the uterus (Mayer–Rokitansky–Küster–Hauser syndrome) is IVF surrogacy, in which the patient's oocytes are collected, usually by the transvaginal route (as these patients usually have a fully functional vagina), fertilized with her partner's sperm and then the embryos transferred to a surrogate host.

Management Strategy for Tubal Infertility

The practical management of tubal infertility is a choice between tubal surgery or IVF. If there are other factors in a couple's subfertility, such as sperm dysfunction or if the woman is over 38 years of age, it is logical to consider IVF rather than surgery. IVF is also indicated if there is moderate to severe tubal disease, i.e., distal tubal occlusion with hydrosalpinges, particularly if the latter are greater than 1.5 cm in diameter, thick walled and associated with extensive adnexal adhesions. Distortion of the intraluminal architecture or endotubal adhesions, detected by falloposcopy, salpingoscopy, or HSG, further worsens the prognosis for tubal surgery. Adhesiolysis is more likely to work in the presence of patent tubes and filmy adhesions, with dense adhesions being a poor prognosticator. Table 10.1 presents the British Fertility Society classification of pelvic disease related to the prognosis for natural conception following surgery.

Laparoscopic surgery is preferable to open microsurgery for all but tubal re-anastomoses and there is little to choose between the use of sharp dissection, laser, or electrosurgery. Constant irrigation of the tissues and good hemostasis are essential in order to minimize postoperative adhesion formation. Cumulative conception rates decline rapidly 12 months after tubal surgery and so IVF should then be advised.

Bilateral salpingectomy or tubal sterilization should be considered for women undergoing IVF who have tubal damage and a history of ectopic pregnancy (especially if the ectopic pregnancy has occurred as a result of IVF) because of the increased risk of a further ectopic pregnancy. The same applies for patients with hydrosalpinges, which adversely affect implantation rates during IVF, presumably because of antegrade flow of noxious fluid.

Table 10.1 British Fertility Society classification of tubal/pelvic infective damage

Minor (favorable surgical prognosis: > 50% over 2 years) Proximal occlusion without tubal fibrosis Distal occlusion without tubal distension Healthy mucosal appearance at HSG, salpingography Flimsy peritubal/ovarian adhesions
Intermediate (questionable surgical prognosis) Unilateral severe tubal damage Limited dense adhesions of tubes and ovaries, with otherwise normal tubes
Severe (poor prognosis: < 10% over 2 years) Bilateral severe tubal damage Extensive tubal fibrosis Tubal distension > 1.5 cm Abnormal mucosal appearance Bipolar occlusion Extensive dense adhesions

Tubal disease – key points

- Laparoscopic surgery has largely taken the place of open tubal microsurgery other than for reversal of sterilization.
- IVF is indicated if a pregnancy has not occurred within 6–9 months of tubal surgery.
- Bilateral salpingectomy or tubal sterilization should then be considered for women with tubal damage and a history of ectopic pregnancy and those with hydrosalpinges.

References

1. Winston RML & Margara RA (1992) The role of reproductive surgery. In: Templeton AA & Drife JO (eds) *Infertility*. RCOG/Springer-Verlag, London, pp 185–198.
2. Wood C (1994) Minimally invasive surgery in assisted conception. *Curr Opin Obstet Gynecol* **6**: 242–247.
3. Saravelos HG, Li T-C & Cooke ID (1995) An analysis of the outcome of microsurgical and laparoscopic adhesiolysis for infertility. *Hum Reprod* **10**: 2887–2894.
4. Van den Eede B (1995) Investigation and treatment of infertile couples: ESHRE guidelines for good clinical and laboratory practice. *Hum Reprod* **10**: 1246–1271.
5. Tulandi T, Collins JA, Burrows E *et al.* (1990) Treatment-dependent and treatment-independent pregnancy among women with periadnexal adhesions. *Am J Obstet Gynecol* **162**: 354–357.
6. Gomel V & Wang I (1994) Laparoscopic surgery for infertility therapy. *Curr Opin Obstet Gynecol* **6**: 141–148.
7. Graebe RA (1995) The role of endoscopy in the management of the infertile patient. *Curr Opin Obstet Gynecol* **7**: 265–272.

8. Maier DB, Nulsen JC, Klock A & Luciano AA (1992) Laser laparoscopy versus laparotomy in lysis of pelvic adhesions. *J Reprod Med* **37**: 965–968.
9. Falcone T, Goldberg J, Margossian H & Stevens L (2000) Robotic-assisted laparoscopic microsurgical tubal anastomosis: a human pilot study. *Fertil Steril* **73**: 1040–1042.
10. Gleicher N, Confino E, Corfman R *et al.* (1993) The multicentre transcervical balloon tuboplasty study: conclusions and comparisons to alternative technologies. *Hum Reprod* 8: 1264–1271.
11. Lederer KJ (1993) Transcervical tubal cannulation and salpingoscopy in the treatment of tubal infertility. *Curr Opin Obstet Gynecol* 5: 240–244.
12. Kerin JF, Williams DR, San Romano GA, Pearlstone AC, Grundfest WS & Surrey ES (1992) Falloposcopic classification and treatment of Fallopian tube lumenal disease. *Fertil Steril* **57**: 731–741.
13. Wu CH, Gocial B (1988) A pelvic scoring system for infertility surgery. *Int J Fertil* **33**: 341–346.
14. Gomel V & Taylor P (1992) IVF versus reconstructive tubal surgery. *J Assist Reprod Genet* 9: 306–309.
15. Hull MGR & Fleming CF (1995) Tubal surgery versus assisted reproduction: assessing their role in infertility therapy. *Curr Opin Obstet Gynecol* 7: 160–167.
16. Andersen AN, Yue Z, Meng FJ & Petersen K (1994) Low implantation rate after *in vitro* fertilisation in patients with hydrosalpinges diagnosed by ultrasonography. *Hum Reprod* 9: 1935–1938.
17. Fleming C & Hull MGR (1996) Impaired implantation after *in vitro* fertilisation treatment associated with hydrosalpinx. *Br J Obstet Gynaecol* **103**: 268–272.
18. Strandell A (2000) The influence of hydrosalpinx on IVF and embryo transfer: a review. *Hum Reprod Update* **6**: 387–395.
19. Strandell A, Lindhard A, Waldenstrom U, Thorburn J, Janson PO & Hamberger L (1999) Hydrosalpinx and IVF outcome: a prospective, randomized multicentre trial in Scandinavia on salpingectomy prior to IVF. *Hum Reprod* **14**: 2762–2769.
20. Johnson NP, Mak W & Sowter M (2002) Laparoscopic salpingectomy for women with hydrosalpinges enhances the success of IVF: a Cochrane review. *Hum Reprod* **17**: 543–548.
21. Strandell A, Lindhard A, Waldenstrom U & Thorburn J (2001) Prophylactic salpingectomy does not impair the ovarian response in IVF treatment. *Hum Reprod* **16**: 1135–1139.
22. Farhi J, Ashkenazi J, Feldberg D, Dicker D, Orvieto R & Ben Rafael Z (1995) Effect of uterine leiomyomata on the results of *in vitro* fertilisation treatment. *Hum Reprod* **10**: 2576–2578.
23. Eldar-Geva T, Meagher S, Healy DL, MacLachlan V, Breheny S & Wood C (1998) Effect of intramural, subserosal and submucosal uterine fibroids on the outcome of assisted reproductive technology treatment. *Fertil Steril* **70**: 687–691.
24. Hart R, Khalaf Y, Yeong C-T, Seed P, Taylor A & Braude P (2001) A prospective controlled study of the effect of intramural uterine fibroids on the outcome of assisted conception. *Hum Reprod* **16**: 2411–2417.
25. Management of Leiomyomata Mini-symposium (2000) *Hum Reprod Update* **6**: 587–620.

Chapter 11

Male factor infertility

Introduction

A clear diagnosis of the cause of male factor infertility can be made in only a small proportion of men who present with infertility.[1,2] Many will be labeled as having "idiopathic" male factor infertility for which there are no specific therapies. Indeed, a survey by the European Society of Human Reproduction and Embryology (ESHRE) of over 7000 men with male factor infertility revealed that there was no identifiable cause in 48.5%, "idiopathic" abnormal semen in 26% (12% oligozoospermia, 7% teratozoospermia, 4% asthenozoospermia), varicocele in 12% (and this is a disputed diagnosis), infection in 7%, immunological factors in 3%, congenital and sexual factors each 2%, and endocrine factors 0.6%.[3]

There is no single test that will predict the fertility potential of an individual. The semen analysis has little or no relation to the underlying etiology (see Ch. 4) and most treatments are based on enhancing sperm quality *in vitro* rather than treating the underlying dysfunction. Concern has been expressed that the evolution of microassisted techniques for IVF has led to a move away from trying to understand the causes of male infertility. We consider that our goal should be to give couples the possibility to conceive by natural intercourse rather than feed them into assisted conception programs, which are stressful, costly, and not without risks – risks largely borne by the female partner.

In addition to a thorough investigation of the man it is essential to ensure that his partner has normal reproductive function, as at least a third of couples with infertility have problems with both partners.

Cryptorchidism

The management of undescended testes has been discussed in Chapter 2.

Hypogonadism

Clinical Presentations

Endocrinological dysfunction as a cause of male infertility is uncommon but readily amenable to treatment. The causes of female hypogonadotropic hypogonadism have been described in Chapter 6 and apply equally to men. In addition to Kallmann's syndrome, other congenital disturbances of gonadotropin releasing hormone (GnRH) secretion include the Prader–Willi syndrome, the Laurence–Moon–Biedl syndrome, and familial cerebellar ataxia; all present with delayed puberty, as does "constitutional" delay of puberty.

Pituitary insufficiency is usually secondary to craniopharyngioma, pituitary adenomas, trauma, metastases, and hemochromatosis. Occasionally, congenital isolated deficiency of one of the gonadotropins occurs.

Treatment

The most physiological treatment for hypogonadotropic hypogonadism is replacement of pulsatile GnRH. The hormone is administered subcutaneously via a mini infusion pump at dose of 5–20 micrograms every 120 minutes. It can take several months for the testes to grow and produce sperm and so it may take a year or more before a pregnancy occurs. More practical than pulsatile GnRH is the use of parenteral (intramuscular or subcutaneous) gonadotropins, given two or three times a week.

Some men with hypogonadotropic hypogonadism can be resistant to treatment, particularly if they have a history of undescended testes. The association of hypogonadotropic hypogonadism with cryptorchidism is caused by the failure of neonatal hypersecretion of gonadotropins, which normally occurs as the pituitary of the newborn becomes free of negative feedback suppression by maternal/placental steroids – it is this mechanism that normally aids testicular descent.

Both follicle stimulating hormone (FSH) and testosterone are required for spermatogenesis. Testosterone administration at doses sufficient to achieve normal extratesticular functions does not, however, produce intratesticular levels that stimulate spermatogenesis. Thus if there is pituitary failure it is necessary to administer gonadotropin preparations that contain FSH and luteinizing hormone (LH) activity, for example human chorionic gonadotropin (hCG) 1500–2500 i.u./twice weekly or human menopausal gonadotropin (hMG) 150 i.u./2–3 times a week (some regimens add hMG after 8–12 weeks' treatment with hCG). Recombinantly derived FSH has also been used with some success. Some men with hypogonadotropic hypogonadism are also growth hormone deficient and they benefit from adjuvant growth hormone therapy.

If fertility is not required, or after a pregnancy has been achieved, it is important that hypogonadal men are given maintenance testosterone, usually as a monthly depot injection. Testosterone administration does not reduce the subsequent chance of stimulating spermatogenesis by either GnRH or gonadotropins, although spermatogenesis occurs more rapidly if it has already been achieved in the past. For this reason, it has been suggested that young men with newly diagnosed hypothalamic or pituitary hypogonadism should be given a course of GnRH/gonadotropin therapy to initiate spermatogenesis before commencing testosterone maintenance therapy. It would then be possible to cryopreserve sperm for use in future years.

General Health Factors

Alcohol can impair spermatogenesis and even a moderate intake (10 units a week) may further compromise the fertility of a man with pre-existing sperm dysfunction. Men with oligospermia should be counseled to reduce the amount they drink or stop altogether but should not expect to see an improvement for at least 3 months, and even then the change may be gradual. Cigarette smoking also impairs fertility and both partners should be encouraged to stop smoking, particularly while trying to conceive. Exposure of the testes to heat can have a detrimental effect, which is also likely to be more pronounced if there is already an underlying problem. Thus sitting in hot baths and wearing tight-fitting underpants and trousers should be avoided. We do not, however, recommend cold showers, as suggested by some.

We have seen a man with severely oligozoospermic semen demonstrate a complete recovery when the cycling season ended. His sperm count fell dramatically again a few weeks into the next season, when he resumed vigorous training wearing Lycra shorts. Athletes may also develop hypothalamic hypogonadism similar to the hypothalamic amenorrhea seen in sportswomen. There are well described seasonal variations in semen quality, with a decline during summer months which may be enough to render some men subfertile.

Chronic debilitating illness may lead to infertility. There are also a few notable conditions that particularly affect male fertility, namely diabetes, chronic renal failure, and thyrotoxicosis. As simple an acute illness as a streptococcal sore throat requiring penicillin can also result in a temporary azoospermia. It is therefore important to note any such illness in the past 3 months when reviewing the results of semen analyses.

A number of drugs and industrial toxins impair male fertility:

- Drugs: sulfasalazine (but not mesalazine), cimetidine, calcium antagonists, nitrofurantoin, spironolactone
- Radiotherapy and cytotoxic agents
- Occupational toxins: lead, arsenic, carbon disulfide, biphenyls, herbicides, insecticides, DDT, radiation
- Recreational drugs: alcohol, anabolic steroids, marijuana, opiates.

Oligoasthenozoospermia

The majority of men with subfertility have oligoasthenozoospermia of unknown cause. There is some evidence to suggest a familial tendency to subfertility in men, with an autosomal recessive mode of inheritance accounting for up to 60% of cases of male subfertility.[4] At present, little can be done in the way of direct treatment, although assisted conception procedures such as superovulation with intrauterine insemination (IUI) or IVF may be of benefit.

There are some chromosomal causes of azoospermia, such as Klinefelter's syndrome (47,XXY karyotype, 1:500 males) in which there is fibrosis of the seminiferous tubules and Leydig cell abnormalities. Men with Klinefelter's syndrome are infertile, although occasionally pregnancies have been reported using testicular sperm and intracytoplasmic injection of sperm (ICSI) and in Klinefelter variants, in which there is chromosomal mosaicism. The 47,XYY karyotype is associated with spermatogenic arrest and the Sertoli-cell-only syndrome, although some of these men do have normal spermatogenesis. Autosomal translocations may result in either azoospermia or severe impairment of fertility.

Genes responsible for spermatogenesis have recently been traced to an area on the long arm of the Y chromosome, azoospermia factor (AZF or DAZ – deleted in azoospermia – locus). The relative frequency and significance of Y-chromosome microdeletions in men with unexplained spermatogenic disorders is currently subject to intense scrutiny and likely to have a major impact on both diagnosis and therapy in the near future.

It is important to appreciate that many men apparently with azoospermia do have small foci of normal spermatogenesis within the testes. As many as 50% of men with supposed untreatable infertility (e.g., Sertoli-cell-only syndrome, maturation arrest) may produce sperm. Sperm may either be recovered from the ejaculate using special sperm preparation techniques (such as MERC – multiple ejaculation, resuspension, and centrifugation) or from the testes themselves, using multiple biopsy techniques that increase the likelihood of finding the normal foci. Although numbers of sperm found may be low, if mature sperm are present, there will usually be sufficient for ICSI. There is, however, a high rate of chromosomal abnormalities in the *sperm* when serum FSH concentrations are elevated or if testicular tissue is used for the extraction of sperm – and these may be transmitted to children conceived by ICSI (see Ch. 16).[5]

Frequency of Intercourse

The concentration of motile sperm in sequential ejaculates decreases in normospermic men but men with oligozoospermia or asthenozoospermia apparently benefit from sequential ejaculations, with intervals of either 1–4 hours or 24 hours producing either similar or more motile sperm in the second ejaculate when compared with the first (hence MERC preparation for assisted conception).[6,7] These observations suggest that impaired sperm transport through the male genital tract may have a role in causing reduced sperm motility.[8] Men with subfertility should therefore be advised to have intercourse at least daily, if not twice daily, around the time of ovulation rather than follow the usual advice given to normospermic men of alternate day intercourse. If assisted conception is required it may be beneficial to use pooled fresh ejaculates collected on the same day (see also Ch. 13).

Leukospermia

The finding of significant numbers of leukocytes ($> 10^6$/ml) in the semen analysis in a man without overt symptoms of genital tract infection may indicate subclinical infection, contamination by urethral commensal organisms, or misdiagnosis (immature germ cells can be mistaken for leukocytes by inexperienced laboratory scientists). Chlamydial epididymitis can result in either permanent damage or a prolonged inflammatory response in the absence of persistent organisms. There is evidence that the presence of leukocytes is associated with reduced fertilization capacity of sperm, mediated through the release of cytokines and reactive oxygen species (ROS). While the empirical use of antibiotics has been associated with a reduction in the concentration of leukocytes and improved sperm penetration assay scores (see Ch. 4), this does not always equate with improved fertilization *in vitro*. Methods of improving sperm dysfunction caused by ROS include the addition of superoxide dismutase during sperm processing for IVF and the use of pentoxifylline – again *in vitro*. The reason for the relative lack of success of antibiotics is that leukospermia is probably associated with viral rather than bacterial infection (for example, cytomegalovirus), so some have suggested that antiviral agents such as AZT be tried. Prospective randomized studies that have tested the use of antibiotics have also found a high spontaneous remission rate in the control groups.

Management

There is uncertainty about the optimum way to manage men with significant leukospermia: whether to give antibiotics and if so, which to prescribe and for how long. Early studies were promising but there is a high spontaneous remission rate in untreated patients.[2,9,10] Furthermore, seminal plasma contains natural antioxidants and so the effects of mild leukospermia on fertilization *in vivo* may not be as relevant as that seen *in vitro*.

In the presence of leukospermia it is our practice to prescribe either doxycycline (100 mg/day) or ciprofloxacin (500 mg/day) for 4–6 weeks and then to repeat the semen analysis. If there is an improvement we would repeat the semen analysis after 3 months without therapy and if the leukocytes have recurred we would advise long-term antibiotic therapy until a pregnancy has been achieved. If there has been no improvement with antibiotic therapy we discontinue the treatment in the absence of proven clinical infection. If the couple is undergoing assisted conception we advise antibiotic prophylaxis, commencing the day the female partner starts GnRH agonist therapy through to the day of oocyte retrieval. If significant leukospermia persists during an IVF cycle, leukocytes can be removed *in vitro* using dynabeads or their effects can be neutralized with antioxidants.

In our practice it is rare to see men with overt genital infections but historically, and in some parts of the world, sexually transmitted diseases such as gonorrhea are a major cause of occlusion of the spermatic tract.

Varicocele

Ligation of varicoceles is one of the most controversial areas in male infertility practice. Approximately 10–20% of the male population have a varicocele compared with 30–40% of men attending infertility clinics. Having detected a varicocele it can be graded (see Ch. 4) and further investigated by ultrasonography (± Doppler flow studies), nuclear scintigraphy, thermography, or venography. Varicoceles are associated with impaired seminal and hormonal parameters, which worsen with time, although the size of varicocele correlates poorly with the degree of spermatogenic dysfunction.[11,12] The presence of a varicocele is often associated with a reduction in the size of the ipsilateral testis and while the other testis can sometimes compensate, with time there can be a decline in spermatogenesis and testosterone production and an elevation in serum FSH concentration. In some cases both testes may be adversely affected by a unilateral varicocele. It appears that varicoceles may act as a "co-factor" in the pathophysiology of male infertility along with disruption of normal spermatogenesis and sperm head formation, increased levels of reactive oxygen species, and abnormal acrosome function.[13]

The development of varicoceles has been monitored in adolescent boys and a corresponding decline in the rate of testicular development observed. Varicocele ligation has been shown to reverse this trend, but the widespread use of surgery in teenage boys is not standard practice, particularly as there are no long-term follow-up data of either semen analyses or fertility.[14] There is also a school of thought that the varicocele is a progressive lesion in adult men, that left untreated might, in some cases, lead to increasing and irreversible infertility.[15] This is certainly a most contentious issue for which there is no clear consensus at present.

Varicocele Ligation

Varicocele ligation is usually performed via an inguinal incision, with ligation of the spermatic vein(s). As with virtually every surgical procedure nowadays, the laparoscopic approach has also been tried. Alternatively, embolization can be performed by an experienced radiologist and it is with this minimally invasive therapy that the future of varicocele treatment probably lies (Fig. 11.1).

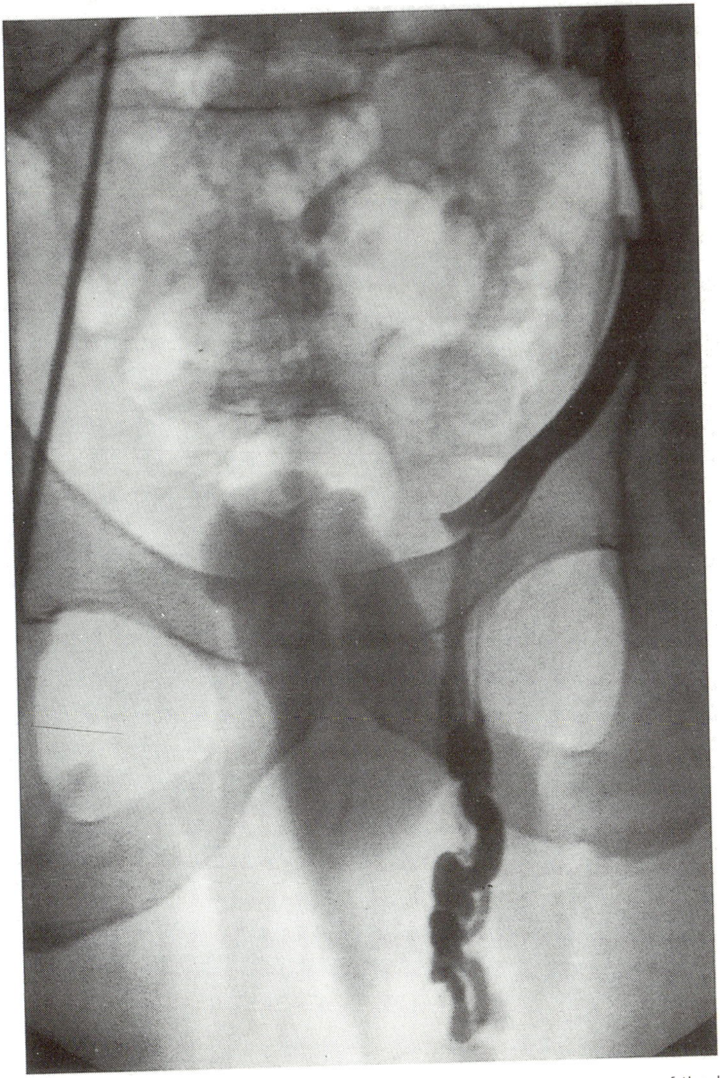

a

Figure 11.1 Embolization of varicocele. (**a**) Digital subtraction venogram of the left testicular vein showing a varicocele around the left testis.

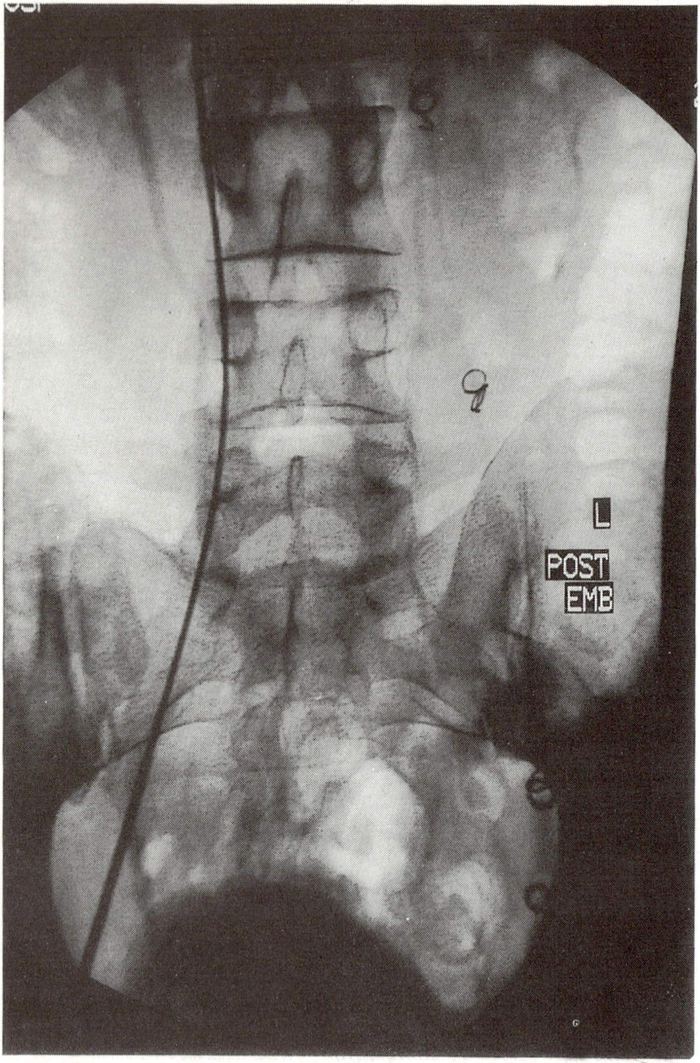

b

Figure 11.1 Embolization of varicocele. (**b**) After embolization there are multiple stainless-steel coils which have been placed via the angiographic catheter along the length of the left testicular vein up to the level of the left renal vein.

While a number of studies have observed an improvement in sperm parameters following varicocele ligation, most have used different definitions and there are no large studies that have been randomized to include an untreated group.[10,16] Furthermore, while semen parameters may improve there has been no evidence of an improvement in pregnancy rates. As varicocele size has a prognostic value, subclinical varicoceles should certainly not be treated. Two recent reviews have studied the current data and both conclude that even the best studies to date show conflicting results and there is no evidence from meta-analyses that occlusion of the spermatic vein improves fertility.[17,18] Treatment should therefore only be offered if symptomatic.

Antisperm Antibodies

Antisperm antibodies (ASABs) on the surface of sperm and in the cervical mucus are implicated as the cause of infertility in some couples, but there is lack of standardization of the assays and therapy is largely of unproven value. ASABs that interfere with fertility are heterogeneous and react with a number of epitopes on the sperm plasma membrane and acrosome. Assays for ASABs are discussed in Chapter 4.

Spermatozoa are protected from the circulation by tight inter-Sertoli junctions which develop behind the developing gametes and prevent the entry into the seminiferous tubules of blood components, such as immunoglobulins, macrophages, and leukocytes. The prevention of autoimmunity is further aided by the presence of T-suppressor lymphocytes in the epididymis and vas deferens. ASABs are thought to develop in men either when the blood–testis barrier breaks down or if there is a decrease in T-suppressor cell activity. Subfertility is thought to be caused more by IgA than IgG antibodies. Breaches in the blood–testis barrier occur with obstruction or injury to the reproductive ducts in the following situations:

- After vasectomy, at least 50% of men develop serum ASABs. The risk is increased in men with HLA-A28 and HLA-Bw22. Seminal plasma ASAB levels are low.
- Congenital obstruction of the vas deferens is associated with high serum, but low sperm-associated ASABs. Any cause of obstruction (e.g., after herniorrhaphy) can result in antibody formation and if there is unilateral obstruction, removal of the obstructed testis can lead to an improvement.
- Infection: chlamydial or gonoccocal.
- Testicular trauma such as biopsies and injury increases the likelihood of ASAB formation. Thus biopsies should only be performed after careful consideration in infertile men in units with the facility to perform ICSI (see Ch. 13). Prepubertal testicular torsion does not lead to antibody formation, because of the absence of sperm antigens.
- Idiopathic.

The development of ASABs in women could be due either to a deficient epithelial barrier in the genital tract, peritoneal cavity or gastrointestinal tract, or to inadequate immunosuppressive substances in the seminal plasma. Reassuringly, although perhaps surprisingly, there does not appear to be an increased rate of ASAB formation in women who have undergone IUI.

The rate of detection of ASABs in the serum, semen, and cervical mucus of infertile couples ranges from 5% to 25%, compared with less than 2% in fertile couples.[10] A wide range of tests is employed (see Ch. 4) and the cut-off levels of a significant concentration of antibodies are poorly defined. Furthermore, the detection of ASABs in the serum does not necessarily equate with a significant problem in the genital tract so the value of performing serum assays is uncertain.

ASABs impair sperm motility. Sperm-associated IgG activates complement and results in binding to polymorphonuclear leukocytes which then inactivate the sperm. IgA is secreted from the endocervix and Fallopian tubes and further affects sperm motility and, possibly, fertilization. There is a good correlation between the presence of cervical mucus ASABs and both sperm motility in cervical mucus and pregnancy rates. Fertilization rates are also reduced if more than 80% of sperm are bound with IgA ASABs, possibly by interfering with capacitation and the acrosome reaction. There are numerous publications that deal with the effects of ASABs but opinions still differ as to whether IgA or IgG antibodies are the more significant.[19–21] Furthermore, while some suggest that antibodies directed against the sperm head disrupt fertilization directly, others consider that antibodies directed to the tail are of greater significance because they interfere with sperm movement.

Management

The management of patients with ASABs is problematic. Corticosteroids are used widely in men and do suppress serum ASAB concentrations but appear to have less of an effect on sperm-bound ASABs. Corticosteroid therapy has a number of side-effects (mood changes, which can be severe, gastritis, weight gain) and complications (duodenal ulceration, hypertension, glucose intolerance, aseptic necrosis of the femoral neck). A suggested regimen is prednisolone 40 mg daily from days 1–10 of the partner's menstrual cycle, reducing to 20 mg on days 11–12 and then stopping (some use 5 mg or 10 mg per day for days 11–12).[22] It has been suggested that therapy should continue for at least 9 months to have a beneficial effect on pregnancy rates,[23,24] although some groups have found that steroids provide no benefit.[9,25] A prospective study by Sharma *et al.*[26] demonstrated that the men who gained most benefit from oral corticosteroids were those who started with significantly higher concentrations of IgG (tail) antibodies and grade I motility.

At present it is not possible to wash antibodies off sperm *in vitro* without damaging the sperm. Research is underway to investigate the effect of specific IgA proteases prior to IUI. Pregnancy rates tend to be low with IUI when there are associated ASABs.[27,28] IVF offers a better chance of a pregnancy, although it is important not to use the female partner's serum for incubation if she has a significant concentration of ASABs. There is conflicting evidence as to whether steroid therapy improves the outcome of IUI or IVF for men with ASABs. If these therapies are required, in our opinion it is probably the assisted conception rather than the steroids that enhances fecundity. Microinjection of spermatozoa into oocytes (ICSI) further enhances fertility and is usually used when IVF is required for men with significant ASABs.

Our approach to the finding of significant concentrations of ASABs, in the absence of any other cause of infertility, is to suggest a cycle of IVF (if this is a possible option). If fertilization is normal, superovulation with IUI is an alternative, less invasive treatment. If fertilization is abnormal, or ASAB levels high (particularly if to the sperm head), micromanipulation techniques are required (see Ch. 13). In our opinion, steroids do not have a major role in the current management of men with ASABs.

Obstructive Azoospermia

No underlying cause can be found in over half of patients with obstruction of the epididymis. The cause is often infective in origin, particularly in developing countries, though less so in the West; infective causes include gonorrhea, *Chlamydia*, filariasis, tuberculosis, bilharzia.

Congenital Bilateral Absence of the Vasa Deferentia (CBAVD)

In two-thirds of European men with CBAVD there are associated mutations of the genes that cause cystic fibrosis (CF). Pregnancies have been achieved using epididymal sperm but the fertilization rates are reduced. Furthermore, the CF gene complex mutations will be present in half of the children born by these techniques and we do not yet know how many of the male offspring will have the same problems as their fathers. Both partners should therefore undergo genetic screening before treatment, although at least two-thirds of men with isolated bilateral absence of the vas and point mutations of the CF gene complex do not have symptoms of CF. Sperm autoantibodies are often present when the vasa deferentia are absent.

Young's Syndrome

This involves a combination of chronic respiratory problems and obstructive azoospermia, secondary to inspissated epididymal secretions. The epididymes are often large and cystic, the vasa deferentia are normal, and there are no ASABs. There was an association between the development of this condition and the use of tooth powders containing mercury, which are no longer available. Young's syndrome overlaps both CF and Kartagener's syndrome.

Kartagener's Syndrome

Kartagener's syndrome, or the "immotile cilia syndrome," is an autosomal recessive condition in which male infertility caused by reduced sperm motility is associated with sinusitis, bronchiectasis, and transposition of viscera (e.g., dextrocardia). There is an ultrastructural defect in the dynein arms that create ciliary movements by causing movement between adjacent microtubules.

Surgical Trauma and Vasectomy

Surgical obstruction of the vas deferens may occur accidentally during childhood surgery for an inguinal hernia, during the repair of a hydrocele, or deliberately during vasectomy. The breach of the blood–testis barrier results in ASAB production only after puberty. Surgical reconstruction of the vasa in a man who requests reversal of vasectomy is associated with a significant rate of ASABs and the success of surgery declines with increasing time over 5 years post-vasectomy.[29]

Microsurgical Reconstruction of the Vasa

A vasovasostomy should only be undertaken by a skilled urologist using an operating microscope and 9–0/10–0 nylon sutures. The anastomosis is traditionally performed in two layers although this has been modified in some cases. In a review of nearly 1500 vasectomy reversals, the patency rate was 97% and the pregnancy rate 76% in those within 3 years of the vasectomy. The figures were 76% and 30% respectively if the vasectomy had been performed more than 15 years previously.[29] Even without the use of an operating microscope, patency has been achieved in up to 80% with pregnancy rates of 50% after 2–3 years.

Vasoepididymostomy is required if there is blockage in the epididymis and is most successful if the anastomosis (which can be end-to-end or end-to-side of a single epididymal tubule) is performed in the distal epididymis (Figs 11.2–11.4).[30]

Whenever any of these surgical procedures are performed it is essential to have the facilities available to collect a sample of sperm for cryopreservation, either from the epididymis or directly from the testis. Sperm stored in this way can be kept in reserve for future IVF/ICSI if the primary operation is unsuccessful.

If reconstructive surgery fails it may be possible to retrieve sperm surgically from either the epididymis or the testis. In simple cases, for example after vasectomy, a percutaneous epididymal sperm aspiration (PESA) can be performed under local anesthetic. If this fails a direct

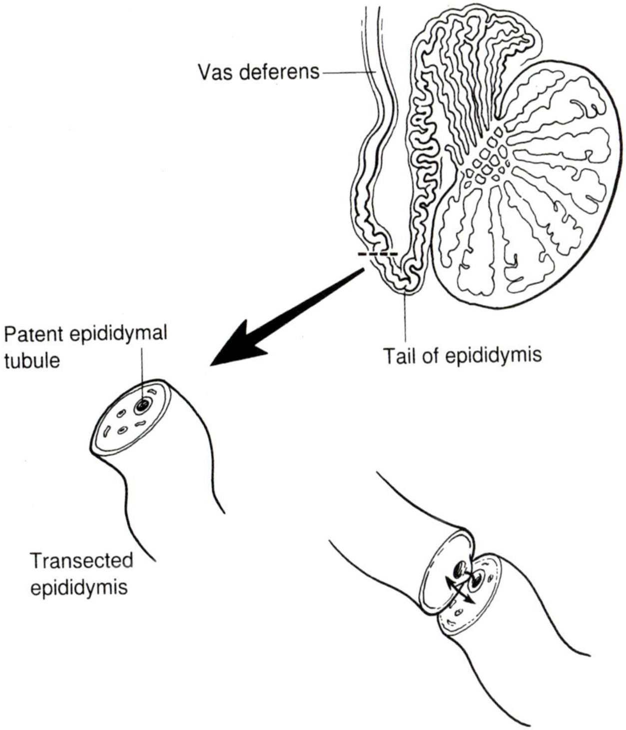

Figure 11.2 Microsurgical anastomosis: vasoepididymostomy. End-to-end anastomosis of a single epididymal tubule. The distal epididymis is transected and the obstructed area excised if necessary. After identifying a patent epididymal tubule, an anastomosis is performed to the vas.

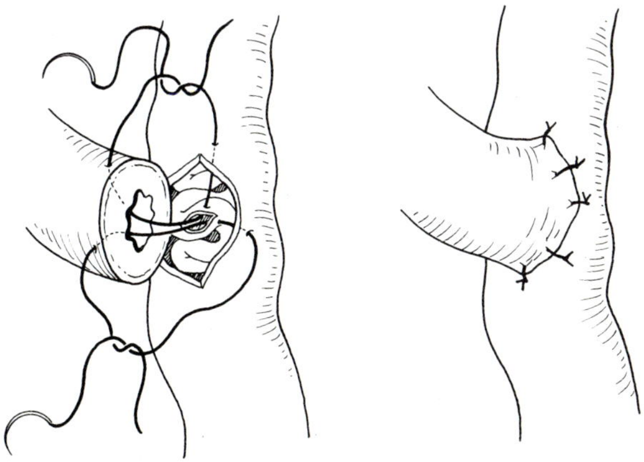

Figure 11.3 End-to-side anastomosis.

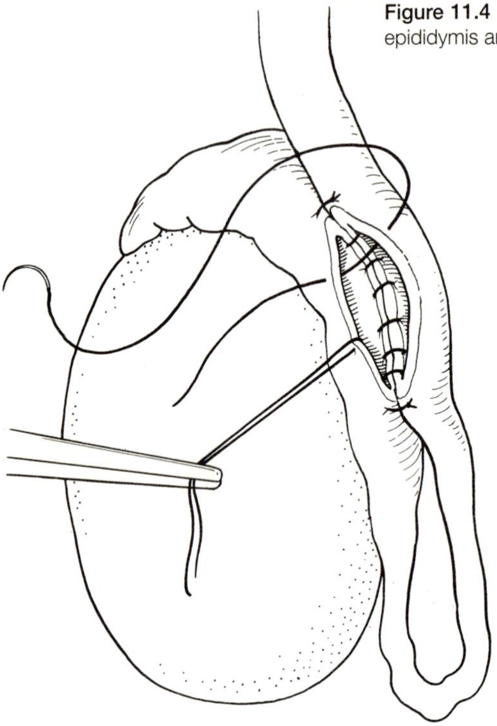
Figure 11.4 Side-to-side anastomosis of epididymis and vas deferens.

transcutaneous approach can be attempted (testicular sperm extraction – TESE). Alternatively, microsurgical epididymal sperm aspiration (MESA) may be performed (Fig. 11.5) under general anesthetic. Spermatozoa thus obtained are cryopreserved. They are usually of insufficient quantity or quality for either insemination or conventional IVF but may do well when ICSI is performed (see Ch. 13).

Idiopathic Male Factor Infertility

If there is no obvious reason for sperm dysfunction, as is the case in perhaps 50% of patients, the choice lies between assisted conception (superovulation/IUI or IVF ± micromanipulation techniques) or empirical treatments. A huge number of empirical treatments have been tried, none with any objectively demonstrated success. For completeness we list these therapies, before dismissing them:

- hCG, hMG, or antiestrogen (clomiphene citrate, tamoxifen) therapies are of no value in normogonadotropic idiopathic male infertility;[10,31,32] in some cases sperm numbers may be increased but most are abnormal.

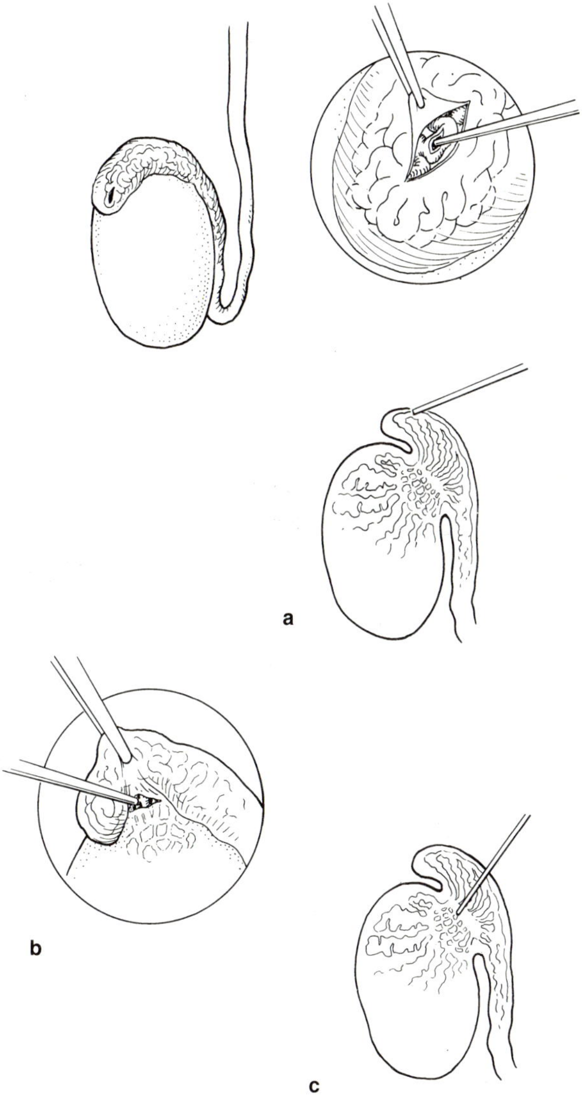

Figure 11.5 Microsurgical epididymal sperm aspiration (MESA) from (**a**) the proximal epididymis, (**b**) the vasa efferentia, (**c**) the rete testis.

- Testosterone administration is similarly ineffective and might be contraceptive.
- Testolactone increases serum FSH concentrations by inhibiting the conversion of testosterone to estradiol but is of unproven value in male infertility.

- Bromocriptine has been used unsuccessfully; if serum prolactin levels are elevated the consequence is usually impotence rather than infertility.
- Kallikrein: the results of individual trials show no real benefit, although when pooled there might be a slight beneficial effect. Kallikrein does not play a part in our clinical practice.
- Pentoxifylline: this caffeine derivative enhances sperm function *in vitro* but neither oral pentoxifylline nor caffeine aids natural conception.
- Vitamin E (100 mg three times daily): this might reduce reactive oxygen species and be of benefit to some men with asthenospermia and leukocytosis.
- Vitamin C (1 g four times daily) is said to reduce agglutination in uncontrolled trials.
- Zinc concentrations are reduced in the seminal fluid of men with chronic prostatitis but supplements do not improve fertility.
- Artificial vaginal insemination of an unprepared sample of the husband's sperm (AIH) is pointless.

Paternal Aging

There is an increased risk of congenital genetic defects with older fathers, just as there is with older mothers (see also Ch. 2). Such conditions include dominant disorders such as achondroplasia, myositis ossificans, Alpert's syndrome, Marfan's syndrome, Duchenne muscular dystrophy, hemophilia, and the sex-linked recessive bilateral retinoblastoma. It has been suggested that there is a link between male factor infertility and accelerated testicular aging, so that patients with infertility may have an increased risk of producing offspring with the above conditions.

Coital Dysfunction and Psychosexual Problems

Psychosexual Problems

It is self-evident that if there are problems with sexual function, fertility will be impaired. Furthermore, the desire for a child, which might be stronger in one partner, exacerbates psychosexual difficulties. These problems require a sympathetic approach, with counseling by trained personnel.

Erectile Dysfunction

Penile erection is under parasympathetic control (S2,3,4) and the rigidity of the corpora cavernosa requires testosterone, an intact arterial supply, and venous closure. The sympathetic nervous system initiates ejaculation (T10–L2) and closure of the internal sphincter of the bladder prevents retrograde ejaculation. The varied causes of impotence and failure to ejaculate are listed below. Approximately 80% of cases of erectile dysfunction have a cause, usually associated with reduced blood supply, and only 20% are "psychogenic."

- Impotence: psychogenic, anxiety, depression, peripheral arterial disease, diabetes mellitus, hyperprolactinemia, hypogonadism, antihypertensive and psychotropic drugs.
- Ejaculatory failure: psychogenic, hypogonadism, phenothiazines, alpha-blockers, aortic or abdominal surgery (e.g. AP resection), radial prostatectomy spinal cord injury, sympathetic nervous system injury, diabetes mellitus, multiple sclerosis.

Impotence/erectile dysfunction may be managed in primary care. Men and their partners will benefit from counseling and the role of negative and positive psychological, behavioral, and relationship influences on their sexual behavior. Treatment is initially with either sublingual apomorphine or oral sildenafil. Apomorphine acts within 20 minutes, while sildenafil takes an hour; both last for 3–5 hours. If oral medication has failed the next step is either an intracavernosal injection or an intraurethral pellet of prostaglandin E_1 (alprostadil) or papaverine. This must be performed with care and initially under medical supervision. Vascular microsurgery is indicated if there is vascular disease and localized arterial lesions. Inflatable penile prostheses have also been used with varying degrees of success.

It is important not to give testosterone to men with impotence caused by neuropathic lesions (for example, men with diabetes mellitus) as it increases libido, which cannot be satisfied, and worsens an already most distressing condition.

Many causes of ejaculatory failure can be treated using external vibratory massage, which can be performed by the patient or his partner placing a vibrator at the base of the penis and collecting semen for self-insemination. If this fails electroejaculation can be achieved using a rectal probe. This has to be performed by properly trained personnel because of the risk of autonomic dysreflexia and profound hypertension. Electroejaculation has been used for many spinal cord-injured men. Semen quality tends to decline with time after the injury and so the collected sperm often has to be used for IVF/ICSI rather than intravaginal or insemination or IUI. Sperm reservoirs have been used in some cases and these are surgically attached to the epididymis and sperm withdrawn transcutaneously when the reservoir is full but they frequently block and have not gained popularity. Recently aspiration of sperm from the vas has achieved success. Drug therapies include alpha-agonists, such as ephedrine hydrochloride (25 mg twice daily), although retrograde ejaculation is a common sequela.

Retrograde Ejaculation

This can occur after prostatectomy, bladder neck injury, sympathectomy, or with diabetes or multiple sclerosis. If the ejaculate is absent or of small volume (< 1 ml) with few or no sperm then the diagnosis should be suspected. The diagnosis is confirmed by finding sperm in a urine specimen collected after ejaculation. Alpha-agonistic drugs can be tried initially, such as ephedrine hydrochloride (25 mg twice daily). If this treatment fails the sperm can be collected by catheterization after ejaculation and washed immediately in IVF culture medium before insemination. It is important to alkalinize the urine; to achieve this oral sodium bicarbonate should be taken (1.3 g four times daily). An alternative approach is to fill the bladder in order to obstruct the retrograde passage of sperm and for the patient then to try to ejaculate.

Hypergonadotropic Testicular Failure

Hypergonadotropic testicular failure may be congenital (germ cell aplasia, the Sertoli-cell-only syndrome, germ cell arrest, or hypospermatogenesis) or acquired, for example as the result of viral orchitis (e.g., mumps), trauma, or toxins (Table 11.1). Some men with Klinefelter's mosaicism produce a few sperm intermittently, although most are sterile.

Evidence exists for the presence of an area on the long arm of the Y-chromosome that is involved in azoospermia and has been termed the AZF (or DAZ – deleted in azoospermia) locus. Point mutations or deletions in this area may lead to azoospermia (see also Ch. 4).

In some cases the serum FSH concentration alone is elevated, with normal concentrations of LH and testosterone; in other cases both elevated gonadotropins and low serum testosterone concentrations are present. Administration of testosterone will not achieve intratesticular levels sufficient to stimulate spermatogenesis and intratesticular injection

Table 11.1 Causes of hypergonadotropic testicular failure
Anorchism – fetal loss of testes, trauma, torsion, tumor
Infections – mumps, orchitis
Gonadal dysgenesis – defective Y chromosome
Persistent oviduct syndrome – lack of Mullerian inhibitory factor
Germ cell or Leydig cell aplasia
Klinefelter's syndrome
Cryptorchidism
Sickle cell disease
Noonan's syndrome
Myotonic muscular dystrophy

of testosterone, which has been successful in animal experiments, is of no benefit in humans.

In recent years there has been a change of policy toward men with azoospermia and elevated serum FSH concentrations, who previously would have been offered donor insemination. If the testes are not atrophic bilaterally and at least one is of a normal size it is worthwhile considering testicular exploration and biopsy as spermatozoa are often found and can be used for IVF + ICSI (see Ch. 13).[33] The elevated FSH level in these cases may be due to an overall reduction in functional testicular mass and the azoospermia due to obstruction somewhere along the spermatic duct. It is nowadays even worthwhile considering biopsy of bilaterally small testes as a few sperm can sometimes be obtained.

Micromanipulation Techniques (see Ch. 13)

The management of male factor infertility has been revolutionized over the last decade by the pioneering work of Van Steirteghem and colleagues in Brussels who developed the technique of ICSI, by which a single spermatozoon is injected into an oocyte to achieve a viable embryo and pregnancy. A number of techniques for the collection of sperm have evolved around ICSI so that fertility can be offered for men with obstructive azoospermia for whom surgery is either inappropriate or has already failed. Thus sperm can be aspirated from the epididymis, vas deferens, or the testis itself.

Androgen Insensitivity Syndromes (AIS)

Individuals with androgen insensitivity (testicular feminization syndrome – complete AIS; Reifenstein's syndrome – incomplete AIS) have a male genotype and abdominal testes but varying degrees of androgen target organ insensitivity. They have female external genitalia and are reared as girls, the diagnosis usually being made at puberty when there is primary amenorrhea, associated with lack of pubic hair. Sometimes inguinal herniae require surgery in infancy, when the diagnosis becomes apparent by the presence of testes in the hernia. The intra-abdominal testes should be removed because of the risk of malignancy, although there has been debate about the optimal timing of the operation. While fertility has not been possible, there has been discussion about retrieving genetic material from the gonads for possible use *in vitro*.

Donor Insemination

Despite the advent of microsurgical techniques for assisted conception, which has opened the possibilities for treatment for many men with either obstructive azoospermia or severe oligoasthenoteratozoospermia, there will always be a proportion of men who have complete azoospermia or genetic disease and therefore require donated gametes.

Selecting Donors

The selection and screening of sperm donors has to be scrupulous, not only to ensure that the frozen sperm has a good chance of achieving a pregnancy but also to prevent the transmission of disease to the recipient. While it is preferable to use donors with proven fertility, in reality the majority of donors have been students whose incentive is often the receipt of a small payment for "expenses" (a payment system which the Human Fertilisation and Embryology Authority (HFEA) wishes to abolish). In the UK the HFEA requires that donated sperm is cryopreserved for at least 6 months so that the donor can be tested for HIV after this period of time. Often part of the payment is held back as an incentive for the follow-up HIV test. Fresh sperm is no longer used for donor insemination treatment.

Spermatozoa are frozen in 7.5% glycerol at –196°C in liquid nitrogen. The pre-freezing sperm density should be at least 50×10^6/ml, with normal morphology and greater than 50% progressive motility. After thawing there should be at least 50% survival with 30% motility. If, however, sperm are being stored from a patient who requires cryopreservation prior to chemotherapy, these criteria can be relaxed, although when the sperm are required it might have to be used for assisted conception (possibly ICSI) rather than conventional insemination therapy.

Screening of donors should include a thorough medical history, including family history of genetic disease, clinical examination for herpes, human papillomavirus, urethral swab for *Chlamydia*, semen culture and blood screening for hepatitis B and C, HIV, syphilis, and cytomegalovirus. The donor's blood group (rhesus status) and chromosomal analysis are also assessed. Additional screening for CF is also performed.

Matching the Donor with the Recipient

Matching of the donor with the infertile male partner of the recipient is usually based on phenotypic characteristics (race, hair and eye color, height and build) and sometimes ABO and rhesus blood groups.

The fertility status of the female partner should be assessed. Investigations can be kept to a minimum if she is young and healthy, with a regular menstrual cycle and no history of gynecological disease: at the very least she should be immune to rubella and have an ovulatory luteal phase progesterone concentration. Unless there is a suggestion of tubal damage from the history, a test of tubal patency can be deferred until after six cycles of donor insemination. A pretreatment ultrasound scan of the pelvis is prudent to inspect ovarian morphology.

Timing

Monitoring for ovulation can be performed with kits that test for LH in the urine at the time of the mid-cycle surge. As soon as LH is detected the patient should contact the clinic and attend for donor insemination. We prefer to commence treatment by monitoring with serial ultrasonography. Once we have confirmed that ovulation is occurring we can then minimize the number of clinic attendances by using urinary LH kits. Ultrasonography not only provides an assessment of the developing follicle but also allows the administration of hCG to trigger ovulation and time insemination accurately. Ultrasound is particularly helpful if the woman has an erratic cycle; sometimes ovulation induction therapies (clomiphene citrate in the first instance) are also required.

Procedure

The nurse who performs the insemination procedure should assess the cervical mucus to ensure it has a well-estrogenized consistency. The sperm is loaded into a 1 ml syringe and insemination catheter and under direct vision deposited into the cervical canal or uterus. There is evidence from several prospective randomized studies, however, that IUI of donor sperm is more effective than intracervical insemination.[34] Clinics vary as to whether one or two inseminations are performed (on consecutive days).

Conception Rates (Figs 11.6 and 11.7)

Monthly conception rates using cryopreserved sperm are in the region of 10%, with an expected cumulative conception rate of 40–50% after 6 months and 70–80% after a year in women under the age of 35.[35] Conception rates tend to be higher in couples where the problem is azoospermia rather than oligozoospermia, as in the latter there are more likely to be adverse female factors as well. If a pregnancy has not occurred after 10–12 cycles of treatment it is appropriate to consider assisted conception techniques. Superovulation with IUI[36] requires a preparation of washed sperm and thus a higher initial number of motile sperm than simple donor insemination. IVF, on the other hand, requires fewer sperm but is of course more invasive than IUI.

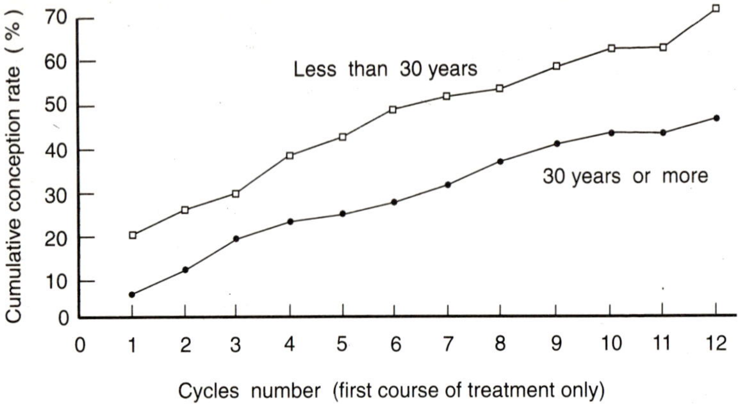

Figure 11.6 Cumulative conception rates for women aged under 30 years (diamond) and over 30 years (circle) undergoing donor insemination at the Middlesex Hospital, London. (From Shenfield *et al.* (1993) *Hum Reprod* **8**: 60, with permission.)[35]

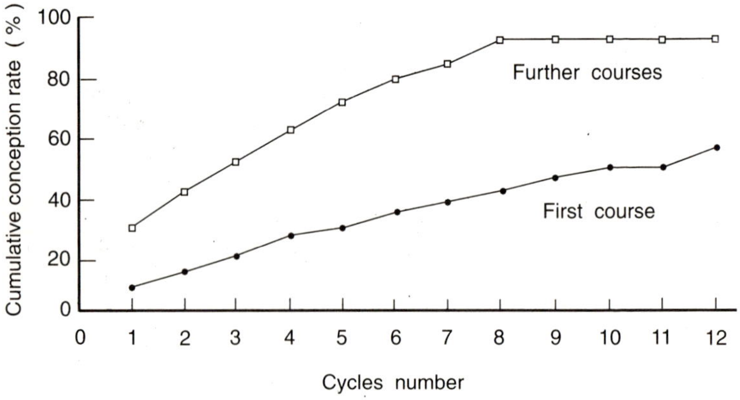

Figure 11.7 Cumulative conception rates for women undergoing donor insemination in their first course of treatment (circle) and in subsequent courses, after previous successful treatment (diamond). Thus, if treatment is successful patients are more likely to return for more treatment and have a good chance of further success. (From Shenfield *et al.* (1993) *Hum Reprod* **8**: 60, with permission.)[35]

Genetic Origins

The HFEA currently permits the storage of sperm for 10 years in the UK and prohibits the use of donated sperm once 10 pregnancies have been achieved, because of the putative risk of "paternal siblings" meeting in years to come and wishing to have children without knowing their own origins. The HFEA keeps a central record of all donors and resultant pregnancies but the genetic origins of the child are not recorded on the birth certificate. Non-identifying information about the donor is available to the offspring of donor insemination when they reach the age of 18 years. However, fewer than 20% of couples who use donated sperm actually tell their children how they were conceived. There is a groundswell of opinion in the UK that identifying information is important, particularly expressed by people who know the method by which they were conceived but wish to know their genetic origin. The matter is discussed further in Chapter 15.

Male infertility – key points

- Optimize health, limit alcohol and smoking.
- Hypogonadotropic hypogonadism responds to endocrine treatment.
- Idiopathic male factor infertility does not respond to hormones or other drugs.
- Infection should be treated with prolonged courses of antibiotics – doxycycline or ciprofloxacin – for at least 4–6 weeks.
- Varicocele ligation or embolization should not be recommended routinely.
- ASABs are a difficult problem. Some men respond to prolonged courses of high dose steroids but side-effects may be very severe and dangerous. We advise assisted reproduction technology (IVF ± ICSI).
- An elevated serum concentration of FSH no longer indicates the impossibility of conception as testicular exploration may yield small numbers of spermatozoa that can be used for ICSI.
- Donor insemination is still required for those with complete azoospermia or genetically transmissible conditions.

References

1. Cummins JM & Jequier AM (1994) Treating male infertility needs more clinical andrology, not less. *Hum Reprod* **9**: 1214–1219.
2. Skakkebaek NE, Giwercman A & de Kretser D (1994) Pathogenesis and management of male infertility. *Lancet* **343**: 1473–1478.
3. ESHRE (1994) Male sterility and subfertility: guidelines for management. *Hum Reprod* **9**: 1260–1264.
4. Lilford R, Jones AM, Bishop DT, Thornton J & Mueller R (1994) Case-control study of whether subfertility in men is familial. *Br Med J* **309**: 570–573.
5. Levron J, Aviram-Goldring A, Madgar I, Raviv G, Barkai G & Dor J (2001) Sperm chromosome abnormalities in men with severe male factor infertility who are undergoing *in vitro* fertilization with intracytoplasmic sperm injection. *Fertil Steril* **76**: 479–484.

6. Matilsky M, Battino S, Ben-Ami M, Gesleivich Y, Eyali V & Shalev E (1993) The effect of ejaculatory frequency on semen characteristics of normozoospermic and oligozoospermic men from an infertile population. *Hum Reprod* **8**: 71–73.
7. Tur-Kaspa I, Maor Y, Levran D, Yonish M, Mashiach S & Dor J (1994) How often should infertile men have intercourse to achieve conception? *Fertil Steril* **62**: 370–375.
8. Cooper TG, Keck C, Oberdieck U & Nieschlag E (1993) Effects of multiple ejaculations after extended periods of sexual abstinence on total, motile and normal sperm numbers, as well as accessory gland secretions, from healthy normal and oligozoospermic men. *Hum Reprod* **8**: 1251–1258.
9. Bhasin S, de Kretser DM & Baker HWG (1994) Pathophysiology and natural history of male infertility. *J Clin Endocrin Metab* **79**: 1525–1529.
10. Nieschlag E (1992) Care for the infertile male. *Clin Endocrinol* **38**: 123–133.
11. Chehval MJ & Purcell RN (1992) Deterioration of semen parameters over time in men with untreated varicocele: evidence of progressive testicular damage. *Fertil Steril* **57**: 174–177.
12. Nagao RR, Plymate SR, Berger RE, Perin EB & Paulsen CA (1986) Comparison of gonadal function between fertile and infertile men with varicoceles. *Fertil Steril* **46**: 930–933.
13. Marmar JL (2001) The pathophysiology of varicoceles in the light of current molecular and genetic information. *Hum Reprod Update* **7**: 461–472.
14. Laven JD, Haans LCF, Mali WPTh, Egbert RV, Wensing CJC & Eimers JM (1992) Effects of varicocele treatment in adolescents: a randomised study. *Fertil Steril* **58**: 756–762.
15. Cozzolino DJ & Lipshultz LI (2001) Varicocele as a progressive lesion: positive effect of varicocele repair. *Hum Reprod Update* **7**: 55–58.
16. O'Donovan PA, Vandekerckhove P, Lilford RJ & Hughes E (1993) Treatment of male infertility: is it effective? Review and meta-analysis of published randomized controlled trials. *Hum Reprod* **8**: 1209–1222.
17. Kamischke A & Nieschlag E (2001) Varicocele treatment in the light of evidence-based andrology. *Hum Reprod Update* **7**: 65–69.
18. Evers JLH (1998) Varicocele. In: Templeton A, Cooke I & O'Brien PMS (eds) *Evidence-based fertility treatment*. RCOG Press, London, pp 109–119.
19. Clarke GN, Lopata A, McBain JC, Baker HWG & Johnston WIH (1985) Effect of antisperm antibodies in males in human *in vitro* fertilisation. *Am J Reprod Immunol Microbiol* **8**: 62–66.
20. Hendry WF (1992) The significance of antisperm antibodies: measurements and management. *Clin Endocrinol* **36**: 219–221.
21. Marshburn PB & Kutteh WH (1994) The role of antisperm antibodies in infertility. *Fertil Steril* **61**: 799–811.
22. Hendry WF, Stedonska J, Parslow J & Hughes L (1981) The results of intermittent high dose steroid therapy for male infertility due to antisperm antibodies. *Fertil Steril* **36**: 351–355.
23. Haas GG & Manganiello P (1987) A double-blind, placebo-controlled study of the use of methylprednisolone in infertile men with sperm-associated immunoglobulins. *Fertil Steril* **47**: 295–301.
24. Hendry WF, Hughes L, Scammel G, Pryor JP & Hargreave TB (1990) Comparison of prednisolone and placebo in subfertile men with antibodies in spermatozoa. *Lancet* **335**: 85–88.
25. Lähteenmäki A, Räsänen M & Hovatta O (1995) Low dose prednisolone does not improve the outcome of *in vitro* fertilisation in male immunological infertility. *Hum Reprod* **10**: 3124–3129.
26. Sharma KK, Barratt CLR, Pearson MJ & Cooke ID (1995) Oral steroid therapy for subfertile men with antisperm antibodies in the semen: prediction of the responders. *Hum Reprod* **10**: 103–109.

27. Lähteenmäki A, Veilahti J & Hovatta O (1995) Intrauterine insemination versus cyclic low dose prednisolone in couples with male antisperm antibodies. *Hum Reprod* **10**: 142–147.
28. Robinson JN, Forman RG, Nicholson SC, Maciocia LR & Barlow DH (1995) A comparison of intrauterine insemination in superovulated cycles to intercourse in couples where the male is receiving steroids for the treatment of autoimmune infertility. *Fertil Steril* **63**: 1260–1266.
29. Belker AM, Thomas AJ, Fuchs EF, Konnak JW & Sharlip ID (1991) Results of 1,469 microsurgical vasectomy reversals by the Vasovasostomy Study Group. *J Urol* **145**: 505–511.
30. Schleigel PN & Goldstein M (1993) Microsurgical vasoepididymostomy: refinements and results. *J Urol* **150**: 1165–1168.
31. Sokol RZ, Steiner BS, Bustillo M, Petersen G & Swerdloff RS (1988) A controlled comparison of the efficacy of clomiphene citrate in male infertility. *Fertil Steril* **49**: 865–870.
32. World Health Organization (1992) A double-blind trial of clomiphene citrate for the treatment of idiopathic male infertility. *Int J Androl* **15**: 299–307.
33. Hauser R, Temple-Smith PD, Southwick GJ & de Kretser D (1995) Fertility in cases of hypergonadotropic azoospermia. *Fertil Steril* **63**: 631–636.
34. O'Brien P & Vandekerckhove P (2002) Intra-uterine versus cervical insemination of donor sperm for subfertility. Cochrane Database of Systematic Reviews.
35. Shenfield F, Doyle P, Valentine A, Steele SJ & Tan SL (1993) Effects of age, gravidity and male infertility status on cumulative conception rates following artificial insemination with cryopreserved donor semen: analysis of 2998 cycles of treatment in one centre over 10 years. *Hum Reprod* **8**: 60–64.
36. Patton PE, Burry KA, Thurmond A, Novy MJ & Wolf DP (1992) Intrauterine insemination outperforms intracervical insemination in a randomised controlled study with frozen donor semen. *Fertil Steril* **57**: 559–564.

Further Reading

Ombelet W, Vereecken A (eds) (1995) Modern andrology. *Hum Reprod* **10**(Suppl. 1). Oxford University Press, Oxford.

Varicocele and Male Infertility: Mini-Symposium (2001) *Hum Reprod Update* 7: 47–84, 461–486.

Chapter 12

Unexplained infertility

Introduction

One can consider two approaches to the diagnosis and management of unexplained infertility. The first is strictly scientific, with a quest for and exclusion of each known cause of infertility before the label "unexplained infertility" can be given. The second approach is a pragmatic one based upon a management-oriented policy, whereby treatment is commenced after the common obstacles to fertility have been excluded. The treatment of unexplained infertility essentially aims to boost fertility, usually by a combination of superovulation and close apposition of sperm and egg(s). Sometimes the use of assisted conception techniques provides clues to the underlying diagnosis, for example if there are problems with fertilization that can only be detected during *in vitro* fertilization (IVF) therapy.

Assessing the Cause of Infertility

Many centers have their own highly specialized areas of interest and research, which they then promote as the missing cause of unexplained infertility (Table 12.1). Thus it is possible to draw long lists of putative and subtle causes of infertility, many of which cannot be proven with certainty and few of which are actually amenable to a corrective remedy that has been shown to enhance fertility. One should also remember that couples with normal fertility can also have abnormal test results. Once the well-known and obvious causes of infertility have been excluded (see Ch. 4), the treatment of couples with unexplained infertility should follow clear protocols. The important tests are the assessment of ovulation (by serum progesterone), sperm function (basic semen analysis), and tubal patency (hysterosalpingogram). Supplementary investigations (e.g., follicular scanning, endometrial biopsy, laparoscopy/hysteroscopy, postcoital test, and complex sperm function tests) are useful in helping to predict the chance of conception but may not influence the outcome of treatment.

Studies of populations of patients with infertility indicate that approximately 10–25% have unexplained infertility, 20–30% ovulatory dysfunction, 20–35% tubal damage, 10–50% sperm dysfunction, 5–10% endometriosis, 5% cervical mucus problems, and 5% coital dysfunction.[1] A degree of subfertility is found in both partners in

Table 12.1 Subtle causes of subfertility that have been proposed as underlying "unexplained infertility," many of which have been found in couples of normal fertility (correction of the abnormality has not always been shown to improve fertility)

Ovarian and endocrine factors
Abnormal follicle growth
Luteinized unruptured follicles and functional ovarian cysts
Hypersecretion of LH
Hypersecretion of prolactin in the presence of ovulation
Reduced growth hormone secretion/sensitivity
Cytological abnormalities in oocytes
Genetic abnormalities in oocytes
Antibodies to zona pellucida
Peritoneal factors
Altered macrophage and immune activity
Mild endometriosis
Antichlamydial antibodies
Tubal factors
Abnormal peristaltic or cilial activity
Altered macrophage and immune activity
Endometrial factors
Abnormal secretion of endometrial proteins
Abnormal integrin/adhesion molecules
Abnormal T cell and natural killer cell activity
Secretion of embryotoxic factors
Abnormalities in uterine perfusion
Cervical factors
Altered cervical mucus
Increased immunogenicity
General immune factors
Altered cell-mediated immunity
Male factors
Reduction in motility, acrosome reaction, oocyte binding, and zona penetration
Ultrastructural abnormalities of head morphology
Embryological factors
Poor quality embryos
Reduced progression to blastocyst *in vitro*
Abnormal chromosomal complement – increased miscarriage rate

30–50% of couples, as usually a couple's subfertility is a relative rather than an absolute barrier to conception. It should be remembered that the greater the prevalence of a condition, the greater the predictive value of its screening test, so everyday tests are of most value in detecting the commonest causes of subfertility. The limitations of the various tests, however, should also be appreciated: tubal patency does not necessarily equate to normal function and an elevated luteal phase progesterone concentration does not confirm that an oocyte has been released from the follicle.

Unexplained infertility has been defined as the inability to conceive after 1 year in the absence of any abnormalities. Between 40% and 65% of couples given this label will conceive spontaneously over the following 3 years and it has been suggested that treatment should be deferred until the couple has been trying to conceive for at least 3 years, as before this time therapy does not confer any benefit over the natural chance of conception.[2,3]

It appears that the most important prognostic factors are the duration of infertility and the age of the female partner.[4] If the couple are experiencing secondary unexplained infertility, about half of those who have been trying for a year can expect to conceive within 3–6 months. In a study by Collins it was found that of those with primary infertility of 39 months' duration, the monthly chance of conception fell by about 2% as each month passed – a decrease of 10% per additional year of infertility.[5] Of course, the rate of progression to treatment and through the various therapies that are used to boost fertility will depend upon the age of the couple and their levels of anxiety together with the available (and affordable) resources. The management of unexplained infertility is usually empirical but couples undergoing treatment should always be treated as individuals (Fig. 12.1).

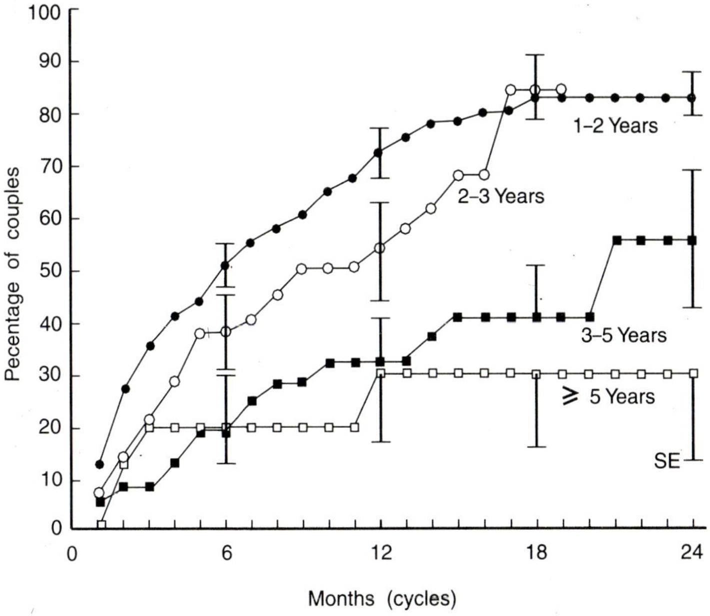

Figure 12.1 Cumulative conception rates in patients with unexplained infertility without any treatment related to the duration of infertility at the time of initial investigations. (From Hull *et al.* (1985) *Br Med J* **291**: 1693, with permission.) (Collins[1])

The Management of Unexplained Infertility

A number of approaches have been employed in the management of unexplained infertility.[6,7] We shall discuss some of the therapies that have been used and propose a stratified protocol, which we ourselves use in practice. Therapy should aim to boost the monthly pregnancy rate above the natural rate of 1.5–3% that is expected for couples who have been trying to conceive for over a year.

Clomiphene Citrate

It used to be thought that clomiphene enhanced fertility by correcting a subtle defect in ovarian function – either follicular development or luteal phase defect. It appears more likely, however, that stimulation of ovulation achieves its effect by increasing the number of follicles that develop and consequently oocytes that are released.

Glazener *et al.*[8] treated 118 women, 43% of whom were parous, with either 100 mg clomiphene citrate from days 2–6 or a placebo in a randomized crossover study. The overall pregnancy rates were significantly increased in the clomiphene-treated group after at least two cycles of treatment. Overall there was a 50% increase in pregnancy rates after three cycles of treatment. Benefit was only seen after 3 years' infertility and then more so in parous women. The cumulative conception rates after three cycles of treatment for those treated with clomiphene and placebo were 26% vs 20%, respectively, in the group with less than 3 years' infertility and 14% vs 3%, respectively, for those with more than 3 years' infertility, suggesting no benefit in treatment before this time. It was postulated that if these rates were maintained they would have reached 11% and 46% respectively after a year. There were no conceptions in the seven women older than 35, suggesting perhaps that older women should be treated more aggressively with assisted conception techniques. Serum progesterone concentrations in the luteal phase were significantly elevated in those women who benefited from treatment with clomiphene, although not at the expense of a high rate of multiple pregnancy.

Other studies have studied clomiphene combined with other treatments. Fisch *et al.*[9] performed a randomized, double-blind study comparing placebo with clomiphene (100 mg days 5–9) and placebo or human chorionic gonadotropin (hCG: 5000 i.u. days 19, 22, 25, and 28). The use of clomiphene alone significantly enhanced fertility (7/37 patients vs 0/36 controls) but hCG, either alone (4/36) or with clomiphene (3/39), conferred no extra benefit. Of the 148 couples with unexplained infertility, 39 conceived during the observation period before and after the trial – more than got pregnant during the study! Interestingly, 43% of those who failed to conceive and went on to have IVF were found to have a previously unrecognized male factor or fertilization defect.

In a study by Deaton *et al.*,[10] randomization was between timed intercourse or clomiphene (50 mg days 5–9) with intrauterine insemination (IUI) of a washed suspension of sperm. Ultrasound monitoring was used in the clomiphene-treated group, while the controls relied upon either basal body temperature or urinary assessment of luteinizing hormone (LH). The monthly fecundity was 9.5% in the treated group compared with 3.3% in the controls – a significant difference. There were no differences in the number of follicles between the conception and non-conception cycles, suggesting that it might have been the IUI that had a more important influence on outcome than the clomiphene. Another randomized study by Arici *et al.*[11] compared unstimulated IUI, timed by LH monitoring, with clomiphene stimulated IUI, timed by ultrasound monitoring and hCG to trigger ovulation. Pregnancy rates per cycle were 5% and 26% respectively.

Bringing all studies together in a recent systematic review, Hughes *et al.*[12] reported that treatment with clomiphene was superior to no treatment or placebo, with a common odds ratio per cycle of 2.5 (95% CI 1.35–4.62). While the studies performed to date appear to suggest a benefit from the empirical use of clomiphene in the treatment of unexplained infertility, a conclusive answer will only be provided if 2000 women are randomly allocated to either clomiphene or placebo. This is a study waiting to be done. When using clomiphene citrate one should always remember the side-effects of multiple pregnancy and the possible association between its prolonged use (greater than 12 cycles) and the possible risk of ovarian cancer (see Ch. 17).

Superovulation with Intrauterine Insemination

There are few prospective randomized studies[13] involving the use of gonadotropins alone in the treatment of unexplained infertility and most of those that have evaluated gonadotropins with IUI are retrospective analyses. Gonadotropin therapy requires careful monitoring with serial ultrasound scans in order to minimize the risks of ovarian hyperstimulation syndrome and multiple pregnancy (see Ch. 17). A non-randomized study by Mascarenhas *et al.*[14] demonstrated a significantly increased rate of pregnancy in women with unexplained infertility of more than 3 years' duration when superovulation with timed intercourse was compared with controls but at the expense of an 18% rate of multiple pregnancy.

It is reasonable to expect that the combination of gonadotropins to induce superovulation, with the release of two or three oocytes, with insemination of a prepared sample sperm into the uterine cavity should boost fertility.[15] There are, however, contrasting studies in the literature. Melis *et al.*[16] have reported a large prospective, randomized study comparing gonadotropin therapy and timed intercourse with gonadotropin therapy and IUI. Two hundred couples with at least 3 years' unexplained infertility received superovulation with follicle stimulating hormone (FSH) to produce at least two follicles. There was no significant difference in the outcome of the two groups, with a cumulative conception rate of approximately 43% after three cycles and a multiple pregnancy rate of 10%. A similar study from Glasgow[17] randomized 100 patients to receive ovulation induction, using pituitary desensitization with a gonadotropin releasing hormone (GnRH) agonist followed by FSH, with timed intercourse or IUI. There was a significant increase in the ongoing pregnancy rate after three cycles of 42% in the IUI group compared with 18% in the timed intercourse group. A meta-analysis by Hughes[18] has indicated that both superovulation with IUI and stimulation with FSH alone each increase fecundity two-fold, while combined there is a five-fold increase.

Superovulation with IUI protocols

The rationale behind superovulation with IUI encompasses the deposition of a prepared or enhanced preparation of sperm as close as possible to at least one oocyte (Fig. 12.2). Sperm can be prepared in a number of ways, the most common of which include simple sperm washing, swim-up techniques, and gradient separation techniques. Sperm washing is achieved by diluting a sample of liquefied sperm in culture medium, followed by centrifugation and resuspension in the medium, thereby removing seminal plasma but leaving bacteria and immotile spermatozoa in the preparation. The sample is enhanced further if the wash is repeated and the sperm then left to "swim up" to the surface of the media for 30–60 minutes, whence it is recovered, leaving debris, bacteria, and immotile spermatozoa at the bottom of the tube. The supernatant should now contain 80–100% motile sperm

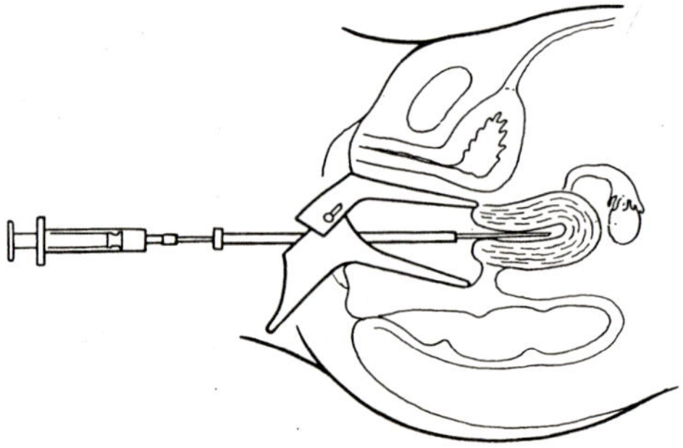

Figure 12.2 Intrauterine insemination.

and a significantly higher percentage with normal morphology. Alternatively sperm can be layered on an isotonic Percoll column, which provides a density gradient for the separation of morphologically normal, motile spermatozoa.

Ovarian stimulation is optimally achieved using gonadotropin injections without prior pituitary desensitization. We have found a step-down protocol to be of benefit, with the aim of recruiting two or three dominant follicles, using a starting dose of 150 units (75–100 units if under 30 years or polycystic ovary morphology on baseline ultrasound scan) and dropping to 75 (or 50–37.5) units after three doses. Treatment is started on day 2 of the cycle and ultrasound monitoring is commenced on day 8. Stimulation is continued and the dose adjusted as necessary, until there are two or three follicles of 16 mm diameter or more, with the largest follicle having a diameter of at least 18 mm and no more than three follicles in total greater than 14 mm. With this approach the monthly rate of conception is about 15–20% and the 4-month cumulative conception rate 40%. The risk of twins is in the region of 20% and the rate of triplet pregnancies < 1%.

Gamete Intrafallopian Transfer

Gamete intrafallopian transfer (GIFT) goes one step further than superovulation/IUI as it involves the collection of oocytes and the direct transfer of oocytes and sperm into a Fallopian tube (Fig. 12.3) (see Ch. 13). GIFT was evolved for the treatment of unexplained infertility because it was thought that the Fallopian tube provided a more physiological environment for fertilization than a dish in an incubator.[19] The main disadvantages compared with IUI are the need

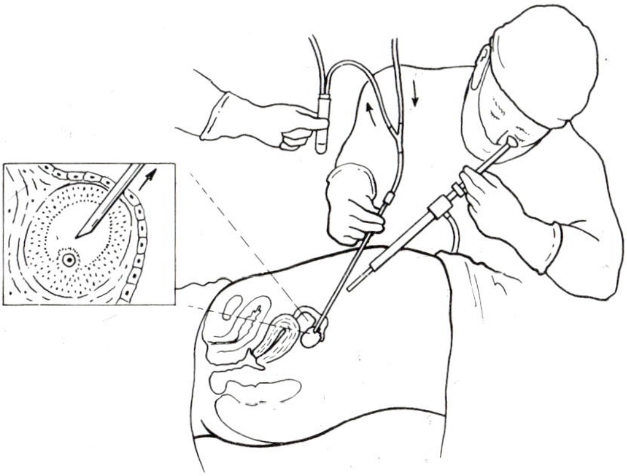

Figure 12.3 Gamete intrafallopian transfer (GIFT). Laparoscopic aspiration of oocytes prior to cannulation of the Fallopian tube and transfer of oocytes and sperm.

for a laparoscopy and a more complicated ovarian stimulation regimen (see Ch. 13).[1,20] Compared with IVF, GIFT fails to provide the couple with fertilized oocytes, although surplus oocytes can be fertilized *in vitro* and cryopreserved for future use.

A large multicenter randomized study was performed by the European Society of Human Reproduction and Embryology (ESHRE)[21] to study five treatments for unexplained infertility in 444 patients over 649 treatment cycles. There was no statistically significant difference in outcome between them (superovulation 15% per cycle, superovulation/IUI 27%, superovulation/intraperitoneal insemination 27%, GIFT 28%, and IVF 26%). This study can be criticized for a number of reasons, not least of which is the lack of a control group. Few centers in the UK still perform GIFT because of the greater advantages of IVF.

In Vitro Fertilization

IVF is a less invasive therapy than GIFT and confers the advantages of being able to study fertilization and the selection of good quality pre-embryos for transfer into the uterus. A prospective study by Ranieri *et al.*[22] showed that there was no difference in the rates of pregnancy when either GIFT or IVF was used after three failed cycles of superovulation/IUI for unexplained infertility. IVF has also been shown to be superior to no treatment in a randomized controlled trial[23] over one cycle of treatment. A systematic review is currently in progress by the Cochrane Collaboration, but has yet to report. It seems sensible to progress to IVF in couples with unexplained infertility after initial treatment with either clomiphene citrate or superovulation/IUI. In women over 35 years, IVF should be offered as first-line therapy.

Transcervical Cannulation of the Fallopian Tube

Transcervical cannulation of the Fallopian tube can be achieved using ultrasound guidance and cannulae that have a "memory" such that they can be straightened using an outer sheath to pass through the cervical canal and then, once inside the endometrial cavity, curve towards the tubal ostium. This technique can be used for insemination of prepared sperm, transfer of sperm and oocytes (i.e., transcervical GIFT), transfer of zygotes (i.e., transcervical ZIFT), or transcervical cannulation of the Fallopian tube for the transfer of pre-embryos on day 2 or 3 after IVF.

Strategy for the Management of Unexplained Infertility

In developing a strategy for the management of unexplained infertility one has to balance the efficacy of treatment, including cost-effectiveness,

Table 12.2 Management of unexplained infertility

< 35 years No treatment until 3 years' infertility		> 35 years Consider treatment after 1 year of infertility	
Primary infertility	*Secondary infertility*	*Primary infertility*	*Secondary infertility*
1. CC 6 cycles ±IUI	CC 6 cycles	IVF 1 cycle if fertilization, continue if problems discovered	CC 3 cycles ±IUI
2. Superovulation/IUI 3–4 cycles		If IVF OK superovulation/IUI 3–4 cycles	Superovulation/IUI 3 cycles
	IVF	Return to IVF	IVF

against the relative invasiveness of the various therapeutic options. The available evidence suggests that there is little to be gained by commencing therapy before a couple have been trying for at least 3 years. However, it is difficult to enforce this guideline in practice when confronted in the clinic by a distressed couple with "unexplained infertility." Furthermore, some of these couples will have as yet unidentified sperm, oocyte, or fertilization defects that will only be discovered during the process of IVF. There is a certain logic, therefore, in proceeding straight to IVF and if fertilization is normal, reverting to either no treatment until 3 years have elapsed or a less invasive treatment such as clomiphene citrate or superovulation/IUI. The age of the female partner should also be considered and there is a case for treating those over the age of 35 years more aggressively (Table 12.2).

The evidence to date indicates that empirical use of clomiphene citrate is superior to no treatment at all. Superovulation/IUI and GIFT appear to have a possible but unproven benefit. Furthermore, IVF may further enhance the chance of conception in selected patients and has been increasingly used for the management of unexplained infertility. The pace and intensity of treatment will often be governed by the couple's desires and anxiety, some wishing to proceed swiftly to assisted reproduction technology and others wanting to avoid high-tech treatments for as long as possible. It is essential to present the couple with a realistic appraisal of their chance of pregnancy with and without treatment and also to counsel them fully about the risks and side-effects of the various therapies.

If clomiphene citrate or gonadotropins are used we suggest careful monitoring with serial ultrasound scans of follicular development in order both to assess the response to treatment and to time intercourse/

insemination accurately. While ovulation will often occur spontaneously the timing of intercourse/insemination can be enhanced further by triggering ovulation with an injection of hCG (5000 i.u.).

References

1. Hull MGR, Glazener CMA, Kelly NJ *et al.*(1985) Population study of causes, treatment and outcome of infertility. *Br Med J* **291**: 1693–1697.
2. Rousseau S, Lord J, Lepage Y & van Campenhout J (1983) The expectancy of pregnancy for "normal" infertile couples. *Fertil Steril* **40**: 768.
3. Hull MGR (1992) Infertility treatment: relative effectiveness of conventional and assisted conception methods. *Hum Reprod* **7**: 785–796.
4. Collins JA, So Y, Wilson EH, Wrixon W & Casper RF (1984) Clinical factors affecting pregnancy rates among infertile couples. *Can Med Assoc J* **130**: 269–273.
5. Collins JA (1989) Natural course of unexplained infertility. *Proceedings of the Serono symposium on unexplained infertility: basic and clinical aspects*. Serono Aries Publishers, Rome, pp 71–85.
6. University of Leeds (1992) The management of subfertility. *Effective Health Care*, Bulletin Number 3.
7. Stovall DW & Guzick DS (1993) Current management of unexplained infertility. *Curr Opin Obstet Gynecol* **5**: 228–233.
8. Glazener CMA, Coulson C, Lambert PA *et al.*(1990) Clomiphene treatment for women with unexplained infertility: placebo-controlled study of hormonal responses and conception rates. *Gynecol Endocrinol* **4**: 75–83.
9. Fisch P, Casper RF, Brown SE *et al.*(1989) Unexplained infertility: evaluation of treatment with clomiphene citrate and human chorionic gonadotropin. *Fertil Steril* **51**: 828–833.
10. Deaton JL, Gibson M, Blackmer KM, Nakajima ST, Badger GJ & Brumsted JR (1990) A randomised, controlled trial of clomiphene citrate and intrauterine insemination in couples with unexplained infertility or surgically corrected endometriosis. *Fertil Steril* **54**: 1083–1088.
11. Arici A, Byrd W, Bradshaw K, Kutteh WH, Marshburn P & Carr BR (1994) Evaluation of clomiphene citrate and human chorionic gonadotropin treatment: a prospective, randomized, crossover study during intrauterine insemination cycles. *Fertil Steril* **61**: 314–318.
12. Hughes E, Collins J & Vandekerckhove P (2002) Clomiphene citrate for unexplained subfertility in women. Cochrane Database of Systematic Reviews, Issue 1, 2002.
13. Kirby CA, Flaherty SP, Godfrey BM, Warnes GM & Matthews CD (1991) A prospective trial of intrauterine insemination of motile spermatozoa versus timed intercourse. *Fertil Steril* **56**: 102–107.
14. Mascarenhas L, Khastgir G, Davies WAR & Lee S (1994) Superovulation and timed intercourse: can it provide a reasonable alternative for those unable to afford assisted conception? *Hum Reprod* **9**: 67–70.
15. Serhal PF, Katz M, Little V & Woronoski H (1988) Unexplained infertility – the value of Pergonal ovarian stimulation combined with intrauterine insemination. *Fertil Steril* **49**: 602–606.
16. Melis GB, Paoletti AM, Ajossa S, Guerriero S, Depau GF & Mais V (1995) Ovulation induction with gonadotropins as sole treatment in infertile couples with open tubes: a randomised prospective comparison between intrauterine insemination and timed vaginal intercourse. *Fertil Steril* **64**: 1088–1093.
17. Chung CC, Fleming R, Jamieson ME, Yates RSW & Coutts JRT (1995) Randomized comparison of ovulation induction with and without intrauterine insemination in the treatment of unexplained infertility. *Hum Reprod* **10**: 3139–3141.

18. Hughes EG (1997) The effectiveness of ovulation induction and intrauterine insemination in the treatment of persistent infertility: a meta-analysis. *Hum Reprod* **12**: 1865–1872.
19. Asch RH, Ellsworth LR, Balmaceda JP & Wong PC (1984) Pregnancy after translaparoscopic gamete intrafallopian transfer. *Lancet* **ii**: 1034–1035.
20. Leeton J, Healy D, Rogers P, Yates C & Caro C (1987) A controlled study between the use of gamete intrafallopian transfer and *in vitro* fertilisation and embryo transfer in the management of idiopathic and male infertility. *Fertil Steril* **48**: 605–607.
21. Crosignani PG, Walters DE & Soliani A (1991) ESHRE multicentre trial on the treatment of unexplained infertility: a preliminary report. *Hum Reprod* **6**: 953–958.
22. Ranieri M, Beckett VA, Marchant S, Kinis A & Serhal P (1995) Gamete intrafallopian transfer or *in vitro* fertilisation after failed ovarian stimulation and intrauterine insemination in unexplained infertility? *Hum Reprod* **10**: 2023–2026.
23. Soliman S, Daya S, Collins J & Jarrell J (1993) A randomized trial of *in vitro* fertilization versus conventional treatment for infertility. *Fertil Steril* **59**: 1239–1244.

Further Reading

Taylor PJ & Collins JA (1992) *Unexplained Infertility*. Oxford University Press, Oxford.

SECTION 3

Assisted conception, ethics, and the HFEA

Chapter 13

Assisted conception

Assisted conception techniques involve the laboratory preparation of gametes, artificially bringing them closer together and hence enhancing fertility by either bypassing an absolute obstruction to fertilization or boosting fecundity above that expected without treatment.

Assisted conception is used in the treatment of the following:

Tubal Damage

Assisted conception is indicated if the prognosis for tubal surgery is considered too poor or if conception has failed to occur within 12 months of tubal surgery (see Ch. 10). Consideration should be given to pre-treatment tubal sterilization, in order to minimize the risk of ectopic pregnancy after treatment. The presence of hydrosalpinges, if visible on a pelvic ultrasound scan, is associated with a reduced implantation rate, which has been shown to improve after salpingectomy (see Ch. 10).

Endometriosis

In vitro fertlization (IVF) is indicated for moderate to severe disease if conception has failed to occur within 12 months of ablative laparoscopic surgery (see Ch. 9). Consideration should be given to pre-treatment management of endometriotic cysts (see Ch. 9).

Male Factor Infertility

When there is severe sperm dysfunction and sperm preparation provides an inadequate specimen for superovulation intrauterine insemination (IUI: see Chs 11 and 12) or if conception has failed to occur after 3–4 cycles of superovulation/IUI, IVF should be offered. Micromanipulation techniques (i.e., intracytoplasmic sperm injection ICSI) are required to achieve fertilization if there is severe male factor infertility.

IVF is also indicated in couples in whom there is azoospermia and conception has not occurred with donor insemination (DI). The number of cycles of DI treatment should be governed by the female partner's age and other fertility problems: in women under 35 years it is reasonable to attempt 12 cycles, although conception should occur in 50–60% of couples by six cycles of treatment; women over the age of 35 may take longer to conceive but results of assisted conception treatments are also reduced and so the more successful therapies should not be delayed.

Unexplained Infertility

An argument can be made for a cycle of IVF in order to test the ability of the sperm to achieve fertilization, albeit in an artificial environment. If fertilization occurs and yet there is no pregnancy then a less high-tech treatment, such as superovulation/IUI (see Ch. 12), could be used for a few cycles before reverting to IVF. Some couples and clinicians, however, prefer a stepwise progression through therapies, culminating in IVF as the last resort. It is obviously appropriate to discuss the options with the couple and map out a management plan. Most couples feel more secure in the knowledge that they are to have a certain number of cycles of a particular treatment before moving on to another therapy, as sometimes the hardest part of fertility therapy, for both patients and clinician, is knowing when to move on, as there is a tantalizing uncertainty about the outcome if another cycle of a particular treatment is undertaken.

Cervical Infertility

This accounts for fewer than 5% of cases of infertility and is often overdiagnosed. Whether the real cause is "unexplained" or "cervical" infertility, the treatment of choice is superovulation/IUI (see Ch. 12), followed by IVF if it fails. So the diagnosis of cervical infertility and cervical mucus studies have become redundant.

Coital Dysfunction

Psychosexual counseling should be offered in the first instance (see Ch. 5) unless there is an organic cause for the sexual dysfunction (see Ch. 11). If assisted conception is required, then the treatment of choice is superovulation/IUI (see Ch. 12), followed by IVF if it fails.

Preimplantation Genetic Diagnosis (PGD)

IVF can be used to generate embryos from which single cells can be obtained for genetic studies or simple sexing in cases where there are life-threatening congenital diseases. Each cell in the pre-embryo is pluripotent and so a single cell can be removed up to the blastocyst stage without damaging the development of the fetus (see Ch. 18). Using this technique it is possible to transfer only healthy pre-embryos and avoid the risks of antenatal testing (chorion villus biopsy, amniocentesis) and the possibility of a termination should such tests prove positive. The number of conditions that can be detected is increasing the whole time, although only a handful of centers in the UK are currently performing PGD. In the future it may be possible to perform aneuploidy screening on all preimplantation embryos.

Assisted Conception Therapies

This book is not intended to provide a detailed account of all the various assisted conception techniques and we refer the reader who requires more information to the reference section. We outline current management strategies so that the interested gynecologist or general practitioner is well informed about assisted conception therapies. IVF is the most commonly performed assisted conception therapy and will be dealt with in greater detail at the end of this section.

Prior to assisted conception treatment, in addition to baseline infertility investigations, it is usual for most clinics to test couples for HIV, hepatitis B, and hepatitis C, in order to avoid iatrogenic transmission from one partner to the other and also to protect laboratory staff who are handling bodily fluids. Furthermore, cryopreserved gametes and embryos have the potential – albeit unproven – of cross-contamination through liquid nitrogen.

Superovulation/Intrauterine Insemination

Superovulation/IUI is indicated for couples with unexplained, mild to moderate male factor and cervical infertility. For a detailed account of superovulation/IUI, see Chapter 12.

Gamete Intrafallopian Transfer (GIFT)

GIFT[1] requires the presence of at least one functional Fallopian tube as 50 000–200 000 prepared sperm plus up to three oocytes are transferred into the tube, usually under direct laparoscopic visualization (see Fig. 12.3). Superovulation is achieved in an identical fashion to IVF and the oocyte retrieval procedure immediately precedes the GIFT. Some collect the oocytes laparoscopically, although it is our preference to perform an ultrasound-guided oocyte retrieval, as for IVF, because this permits a more reliable aspiration of all of the stimulated follicles.

The indications for GIFT are essentially those for superovulation/IUI, although it should not be performed as a first-line treatment when there is male infertility. The aim of the therapy is different, however, in that the gametes are placed directly into the Fallopian tube, the normal site of fertilization. Furthermore, there is a failsafe if more than three mature follicles develop, as they are all aspirated, whereas if this were to occur during superovulation/IUI the treatment would have to be canceled (or converted to an oocyte retrieval associated treatment at the last minute). Surplus oocytes can be fertilized with a view to cryopreservation of suitable pre-embryos.

GIFT evolved as a therapy that required little laboratory input, although if IVF is performed on the surplus oocytes this so-called advantage is lost. The disadvantages of GIFT compared with IVF are that a general anesthetic and laparoscopic procedure are required and the fate of the transferred gametes is unknown, with respect to fertilization. While GIFT has been attempted without laparoscopy, by way of transcervical cannulation of the Fallopian tube under ultrasound guidance, the results are not as good as conventional GIFT. Success rates with GIFT are certainly no better than with IVF and, in some cases, inferior. Thus, because of the more invasive nature of the procedure, GIFT is seldom performed these days in the UK. Our current practice would be to perform a laparoscopic transfer only when there is significant cervical stenosis (for example after cone biopsy) and in these rare cases we would prefer to perform ZIFT, after fertilization has occurred (see below). GIFT may also be performed if a couple has ethical or religious reasons against *in vitro* creation of embryos.

Zygote Intrafallopian Transfer (ZIFT), Pronuclear Stage Transfer (PROST), and Tubal Embryo Transfer (TET)[2,3]

This procedure goes one step further than GIFT by transferring fertilized oocytes at the pronuclear stage, usually 18–24 hours after insemination. TET is performed after 48 hours when the pre-embryo has cleaved. These techniques can be perfomed by either laparoscopy or retrograde transcervical cannulation of the tube (Fig. 13.1).[4]

The rates of ongoing intrauterine pregnancy and ectopic pregnancy are similar whether the gametes/pre-embryos are transferred into the uterine cavity or directly into the Fallopian tubes. Our experience is in favor of IVF rather than ZIFT (or related techniques) because of the avoidance of laparoscopy, which carries significant morbidity and

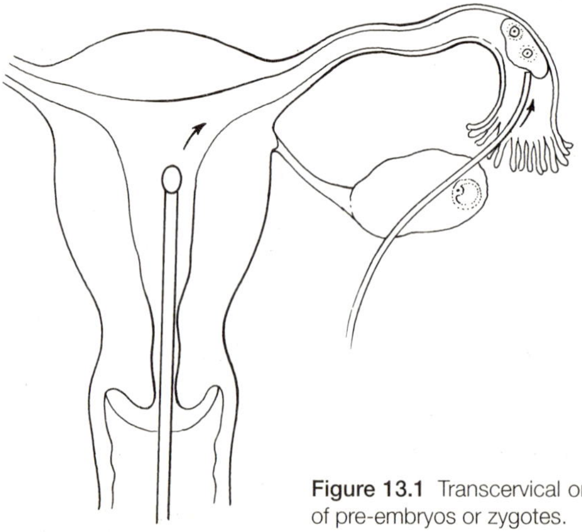

Figure 13.1 Transcervical or transfallopian transfer of pre-embryos or zygotes.

mortality. We would suggest that laparoscopic intrafallopian transfer be reserved for those very rare cases in which cannulation of the cervix is not possible, although even in these cases an alternative option is a transmyometrial embryo transfer.[5]

In Vitro Fertilization

The indications for assisted conception have been listed above. For a couple to undergo IVF, the female partner should have functioning ovaries and a normal uterus and the male partner at least one sperm per ejaculate. However, the lack of ovarian function can be bypassed with oocyte donation, the absence of sperm can be bypassed with sperm donation, and the absence of a uterus by IVF surrogacy. Sometimes both sperm and oocytes, or surplus embryos from another couple, are donated so that the resultant child has inherited no genetic material from either parent. Such parents have in reality "adopted" the embryos but do, of course, gain from the experience of pregnancy and childbirth.

It is the authors' opinion that IVF is sometimes embarked upon before all other treatment modalities have been exhausted and while we do not advocate unnecessary delay, particularly in older patients, the notion that IVF is the high-tech modern answer to every couple's subfertility is erroneous.[6] The stresses placed upon a couple by IVF (and other assisted conception procedures) are immense and the treatment has risks and complications (e.g., ovarian hyperstimulation syndrome (OHSS) and multiple pregnancy; see Ch. 17).

Regimens for IVF (Fig. 13.2)

IVF therapy has become increasingly simplified in recent years.[7–11] The use of gonadotropin-releasing hormone (GnRH) agonists with gonadotropins has resulted in greater ease of planning the superovulation stimulation than was possible with the earlier use of clomiphene citrate (CC) with gonadotropins.[12] That regimen had to be monitored carefully in order to predict and prevent the occurrence of an endogenous preovulatory LH surge. In the absence of GnRH analog controlled cycles there is a cancellation rate of 15–20% because oocyte retrieval has to be performed 26–28 hours after the detection of the endogenous surge and this often meant that oocyte collections were performed at night and at weekends.

When GnRH agonists are used (Table 13.1) the oocyte retrieval can be precisely timed to occur 34–38 hours after the administration of hCG. The latter acts as a surrogate for the normal mid-cycle LH surge and causes resumption of meiosis within the oocytes and their preparation for fertilization. Furthermore, there is good evidence that the oocytes do not become overmature within follicles that are considered to be ready for collection and so the administration of hCG

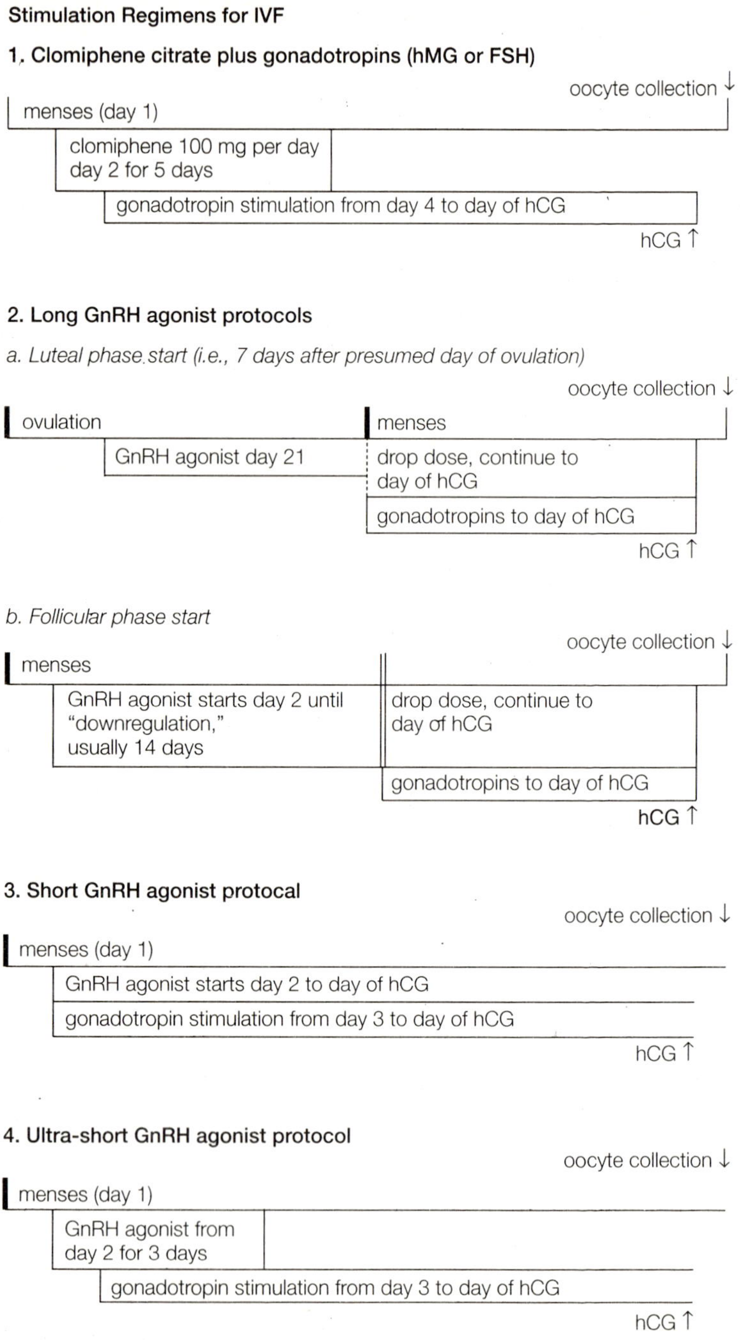

Figure 13.2 (cont'd opposite page)

5. GnRH antagonist protocol (a GnRH agonist can be given instead of hCG)

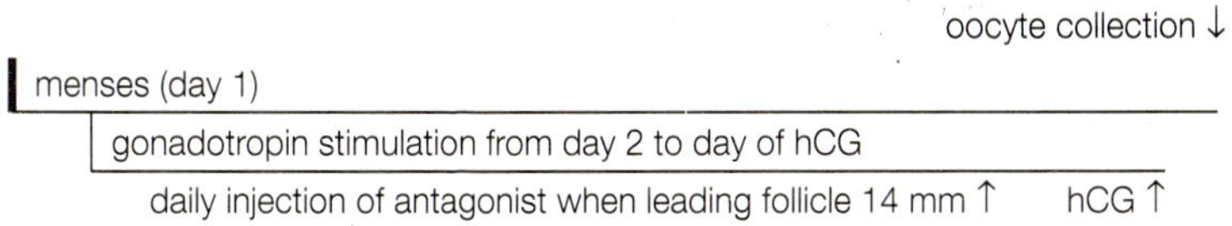

Figure 13.2 Most stimulation regimens commence the day after menses has started (i.e., day 2) for practical reasons. A day 1 start is acceptable but often not practical as most clinics like to communicate with their patients when they are about to start treatment. Alternatively, the combined oral contraceptive pill can be used to program the cycle (see text). Pituitary desensitization ("downregulation") has occurred when the serum concentration of LH is < 5 i.u./L and that of estradiol < 150 pmol/L (progesterone, if measured, should be < 3 nmol/L). Gonadotrophin preparations consist of hMG or FSH (see text). hCG or recombinant LH is given to trigger oocyte maturation when the largest follicle reaches at least 18 mm in diameter and there are at least two others > 17 mm. Oocyte collection is performed 35–36 hours later. Embryo transfer occurs approximately 48 hours after oocyte collection. Luteal support commences the day of embryo transfer and is usually given as progesterone suppositories (Cyclogest 200 mg nocte) or i.m. injections (Gestone 50–100 mg/day) and continued until the day of the pregnancy test. Some continue luteal support up to 12 weeks' gestation, although this is unnecessary.

can be delayed to avoid oocyte collection at weekends.[11] Indeed, by avoiding oocyte collections on Thursdays also, embryo transfer can be avoided at weekends and so the clinic can be run virtually on a weekday only basis. Most large clinics, however, provide flexibility and a 6 or 7 day service. Success rates appear to be better when GnRH agonists are used[13] and the rates of miscarriage, especially in patients with polycystic ovaries, appear to be reduced.[14]

A disadvantage of the use of GnRH agonists is the 2 weeks or more lead-in to the therapy during which pituitary desensitization ("downregulation") is achieved before stimulation with gonadotropins can be commenced. Pituitary desensitization is assessed by a combination of endometrial shedding and low serum concentrations of estradiol and LH (although ultrasound confirmation of a thin endometrium and quiescent ovaries is probably adequate). Some clinics prefer to commence agonist therapy on day 21 of the cycle and suggest that desensitization occurs more rapidly than if it is commenced during menstruation – usually day 2. A day 21 start, however, carries the risk of "rescuing" a corpus luteum with resultant functional cyst formation. A day 2 start virtually guarantees that the patient is not pregnant. We currently administer the combined oral contraceptive pill (COCP) for between 2 and 3 weeks commencing on day 1 of the menstrual cycle The pill is discontinued after 2–3 weeks and treatment with the agonist commenced. This regimen allows scheduling of cycles in a busy clinic and also the use of the COCP minimizes the occurrence of ovarian cysts resulting from

Table 13 .1 GnRH agonists

	Trade name	Structure	Relative potency	Dose
Native GnRH	–	Glu.His.Trp.Ser.Tyr. Gly.Leu.Arg.Pro.Gly. NH	1	
Buserelin	Suprecur	Glu.His.Trp.Ser.Tyr. **D-Ser9.(tBut).** Leu.Arg.Pro.**EA**	100	150 micrograms nasal spray (1 dose) 4 times/day
	Suprefact		100	500 micrograms s.c. drop to 200 micrograms
Nafarelin	Synarel	Glu.His.Trp.Ser. Tyr.**D.Nal(2)**. Leu.Arg.Pro. Gly.NH	100	200 micrograms nasal spray (2 doses) b.d.
Triptorelin	Decapeptyl	Glu.His.Trp.Ser. Tyr.**D.Trp**.Leu.Arg. Pro.Gly.NH	100	3 mg i.m. every 4 weeks
Goserelin	Zoladex	Glu.His.Trp.Ser. Tyr.**D.Ser.** **(+But)**.Leu.Arg.Pro. **Aza**.Gly.NH	50	3.6 mg s.c. every 4 weeks
Leuprorelin	Prostap	Glu.His.Trp.Ser.Tyr. **D.Leu**.Leu.Arg.Pro.**EA**	50	3.75 mg s.c. or i.m. every 4 weeks

The dose of the shorter acting preparations can be reduced once pituitary desensitization has been achieved.

the GnRH agonist "flare." The disadvantage, of course, is further prolongation of the treatment cycle.

The GnRH agonists can be administered intranasally, subcutaneously, or intramuscularly (by depot in some instances). The shorter acting preparations can be used to induce a flare response, being commenced on day 1 of the cycle, with gonadotropin stimulation starting the following day. The agonist is then either continued through to the day of hCG administration (the "short protocol") or given for 3 days only (the "ultrashort protocol"). The flare response can be utilized in those patients who have had a poor response in the past in order to try to maximize the response to stimulation – this it does to varying degrees. It is, in fact, difficult to predict an individual's response to stimulation: young women and those with polycystic ovaries tend to respond well, while older patients and those with elevated baseline serum concentrations of FSH (> 10 i.u./L on most assays) respond less well (see below). CC and GnRH stimulation tests (see p. 326) have been employed to improve the predictability of response but do not tend to be highly sensitive and are not popular in the UK. A more detailed account of GnRH agonist regimens may be found in reference 12, to which the interested reader is referred.

As with many aspects of current clinical practice, the evidence on which our therapy is based relies upon data from small trials. Furthermore, different preparations, criteria for treatment, and protocols have been used, making comparison of studies difficult. This has led to the use of meta-analyses of studies in order provide firmer conclusions. An early meta-analysis indicated that cycle cancellation rates had decreased and clinical pregnancy rates increased since the introduction of the "long" protocol of pituitary desensitization.[15] Ten studies were included in this analysis, with 914 agonist/gonadotropin cycles compared against 722 with CC and gonadotropins. The clinical pregnancy rates per cycle started were significantly greater with agonist treatment with an odds ratio for IVF of 1.8 (95% CI 1.33–2.44) and for GIFT 2.37 (95% CI 1.24–4.51). There were fewer canceled cycles (odds ratio 0.33, 95% CI 0.25–0.44) and more oocytes collected (odds ratio 1.5, 95% CI 1.18–1.87). With agonist use there was also a greater gonadotropin requirement by approximately 12 ampoules per cycle (in the days when an ampoule was universally 75 i.u.) and a trend towards a higher rate of ovarian hyperstimulation syndrome.[15] A more recent analysis of the different types of agonist regimen has been published in the Cochrane Database in which 26 trials met the inclusion criteria.[16] Those regimens that achieved pituitary desensitization produced the highest pregnancy rates and the luteal phase commencement of GnRH agonist was probably more advantageous than starting treatment in the follicular phase.

The advent of the third-generation GnRH *antagonists* enables us to dispense with pituitary desensitization and commence ovarian stimulation on day 2, with the daily administration of an antagonist once the leading follicle(s) has reached a diameter of 14 mm (usually day 6 or 7).[17] Alternatively, a single dose of a longer-acting antagonist may be given on about day 7–8. The GnRH antagonist acts immediately to inhibit pituitary secretion of follicle stimulating hormone (FSH) and luteinizing hormone (LH), without the flare effect of agonists or the need for 10–14 days' desensitization. An endogenous LH surge can be prevented, thereby allowing oocyte retrieval at the desired time. Oocyte maturation prior to collection may be initiated with a single shot of a GnRH *agonist* rather than human chorionic gonadotropin (hCG) – a strategy designed to reduce the risk of OHSS because of the shorter half-life of the agonist compared with hCG. The use of GnRH antagonists may also reduce the total requirements for gonadotropins and obviate any need for luteal support. GnRH antagonist cycles are certainly much shorter and more convenient for patients than the "long protocol" and many clinics are now increasingly using them. For an up-to-date review of GnRH antagonists, see Balen 2002.[18] It is our opinion that GnRH antagonist cycles are preferred by patients because of their short duration and minimal side-effects (for example, avoidance of symptoms of estrogen deficiency during pituitary desensitization). Initial studies found pregnancy rates were approximately 5% lower than with GnRH agonist cycles, although it has been suggested that there is a "learning curve" in appreciating the optimal time to plan oocyte retrieval. This is an area of ongoing research and we are certainly encouraged by recent data and are now using GnRH antagonists with increasing frequency.

Gonadotropin Therapy

Gonadotropin therapy for the stimulation of superovulation can be with either human menopausal gonadotropins (hMG), which contain urinary-derived FSH and LH in differing proportions depending on the preparation, or with urinary-derived FSH alone, which is available for administration subcutaneously because of its higher purity (see Table 6.9, p. 179). The advent of the recombinantly derived gonadotropins has broadened the scope of therapeutic agents and resulted in a potentially unlimited supply. There is evidence that recombinant FSH (rFSH) results in the production of more oocytes and embryos than the urinary-derived preparations and hence the potential for a greater overall pregnancy rate when pregnancies from subsequent frozen embryo replacement cycles (FERCs) are taken into consideration. The use of recombinant LH will provide a more physiological surrogate for the LH surge and, with a shorter half-life than hCG, should theoretically reduce the risk of OHSS.

To date there are two rFSH preparations: follitropin alfa (Gonal-F®, Serono Laboratories) and follitropin beta (Puregon®, Organon Laboratories). In discussing the benefits of a gonadotropin preparation one has to consider clinical efficacy, side-effects, and cost-effectiveness. Clinical efficacy includes the ability to stimulate folliculogenesis, the production of mature oocytes, appropriate steroidogenesis for endometrial development and, in the context of IVF, sufficient quality pre-embryos and, ultimately, good rates of pregnancy. The original sources of gonadotropins for therapeutic use were post-mortem pituitary extracts and the urine of postmenopausal women. The former source was withdrawn because of cases of Creutzfeldt–Jakob disease, which occurred predominantly in Australia but were also reported in Europe. The extraction and purification of postmenopausal urine were pioneered in Italy in the late 1940s to result in the production of hMG.[19] Twenty to thirty liters of postmenopausal urine were required to provide sufficient gonadotropin to treat one patient with one cycle of hMG. Through the 1960s the extraction process to remove non-specific co-purified proteins became more sophisticated, such that activity was increased 10-fold over the early preparations to 100–150 i.u. FSH/mg protein. Greater purity produced fewer hypersensitivity reactions and less discomfort from the smaller volume of the injection. Despite the increased purity of hMG (menotropin) and uFSH (urofollitropin) compared with the original preparations, their active ingredients only constituted 1–2% of the final product. The preparations still contain large amounts of urinary protein (including cytokines, growth factors, transferrins, and other proteins that might modulate ovarian activity) which makes uniform standardization very difficult, and leads to local reactions at the injection sites and occasionally systemic illness.

The use of monoclonal antibodies in the 1980s enabled further purification to be achieved by specifically selecting FSH out from the bulk hMG.[20] The extract was 95% pure with a several hundred-fold enhancement of specific gonadotropin bioactivity and was known as "highly purified urinary FSH" (u-hFSH HP; Metrodin HP®; Serono Laboratories, Switzerland). Extended clinical trials comparing uFSH (urofollitropin) and highly purified FSH demonstrated equivalent ovulation and pregnancy rates. Reduced hypersensitivity was reported, such that the subcutaneous route could be adopted for administration. However, the problems of supply, collection, transport, storage, and processing of an ever increasing requirement of urine remained and the pharmaceutical companies have now utilized the technology of genetic engineering to produce biosynthetic preparations. The genes for the alfa and beta subunits of FSH were incorporated into vectors which were then introduced into cells from a Chinese hamster ovary cell line. This process has resulted in an unlimited supply of highly stable therapeutic preparations with a high specific activity (reviewed by Hayden *et al.*).[21]

The biological activity of FSH is largely determined by the degree of glycosylation.[22] It can only be measured by bioassay and is not measurable by immunoassay. Pharmacopoeial monographs, taking account of the inherent precision of the methods in bioassays, allow 95% confidence limits of 80–125% of the stated dose on estimates of activity, in other words between 60 and 94 units of activity in a 75 unit ampoule (a potential variation of up to 57% between ampoules from different batches). The same pharmacopeial requirements have been applied to the recombinantly derived FSH preparations although in reality the variation is very much lower (± 2–3%). There is evidence that there is heterogeneity between the different recombinantly derived preparations, hence the nomenclature follitropin alfa and beta.

The relationship of isoform composition to function has been recently reviewed.[22] Data from *in vivo* bioassays suggest that one of the major factors which controls FSH action is the relative degree of clearance of different isoforms. It is interesting to note that those forms of FSH which are most potent *in vitro* tend to be least potent *in vivo*.[22]

A large number of intrinsic and extrinsic factors affect the performance of a drug *in vivo*. In the case of rFSH, the pattern of glycosylation, specifically terminal sialylation of the protein backbone, has excited much interest as it is crucial to the bioactivity of the hormone. Overall the isohormone composition of rFSH has proved to be very similar to pituitary extract but great effort has been spent establishing which forms have greatest bioactivity[23] in order to design the most specific and predictable drug. Sialylation determines acidity and isoelectric charge. Basic forms have higher receptor binding activity and therefore *in vitro* bioactivity but they are cleared more rapidly from the circulation than acidic forms. The more acidic isoforms have a 20-fold higher *in vivo* bioactivity, mainly due to their higher absorption, lower clearance rate, and longer elimination half-life. The pharmacokinetics of rFSH (Gonal-F®) are very similar to uFSH (Metrodin®).[24] In the future it is not unreasonable to foresee modifications to the molecular structure that lead to an extension of the half-life and *in vivo* bioactivity. This could enable the frequency of injections to be reduced, which would be greatly appreciated by the patient.

Advantages and disadvantages of recombinant FSH

There are a number of immediately apparent advantages of rFSH over its urinary predecessors. Aside from the improved logistics of the pharmaceutical process, controlled manufacture has led to a more homogeneous product with less inter-batch variability compared with the purification of enormous quantities of heterogeneous urine.[25] The supply is potentially unlimited and shortages should no longer be a threat to clinical practice. There is no risk of infection or contamination with drugs or their metabolites as there is with products from a human source. The manufacturers have also confirmed that there have been no reported cases of seroconversion to antigonadotropin antibodies.[26,27] The purity of the products has facilitated their administration which is effective, safe, and less traumatic when the subcutaneous route is used.[28] The most obvious advantages of rFSH are greater purity and specificity. It has been inferred that smaller doses and a more predictable response will result,[29] although this has not yet been confirmed.

Studies comparing the different gonadotropin preparations are varied and include a heterogeneous mix of protocols and various comparisons of hMG, purified urinary FSH, and recombinant FSH. An initial meta-analysis comparing urinary FSH with hMG claimed a higher clinical pregnancy rate with uFSH than with hMG.[30] This study implied that an adequate level of endogenous LH exists to achieve follicular and endometrial maturation, despite desensitization of the pituitary with a GnRH analog. It has also been suggested that exogenous LH supplementation in the form of hMG may be detrimental to the chances of achieving pregnancy.[31] Conversely a subsequent meta-analysis,[32] which included many additional studies, found no advantage with the use of urinary FSH over hMG. Furthermore, a recent series of publications have demonstrated improved fertilization and ongoing pregnancy rates in women who had serum LH concentrations greater than 0.5 i.u./L on the day of hCG compared with those whose LH concentrations were less than 0.5 i.u./L.[33] It appears that a low but critical level of LH is required throughout and towards the end of the follicular phase of the cycle and during superovulation regimens. The required LH need not necessarily be contained within the gonadotropin preparation that is administered provided that the level of pituitary desensitization is not too profound. The two recombinant FSH preparations (alfa and beta) are probably similar to each other, but studies comparing them are small. There is evidence that recombinant FSH preparations are more efficacious than urinary FSH and inherently we favor their use, if they are affordable. When not affordable we prescribe urinary hMG or urinary FSH.

CAUTIONARY NOTES: In assessing this debate it is essential to be aware of the interests of the pharmaceutical companies that manufacture gonadotropin preparations and to examine both authorship and sponsorship of the published studies. Note also that until about 5 years ago all gonadotropin preparations were produced with 75 international units of activity per ampoule. Now there is great variation in the way that the different products are packaged. It has become important, therefore, to refer to dosages in terms of units and not ampoules. For a list of currently available gonadotropin preparations see Table 6.9 (Ch. 6).

Ovarian reserve and prediction of response to stimulation

Ovarian reserve, or the number of releasable oocytes, declines with ovarian age, which does not always equate with the age of the woman. As ovarian reserve declines, so too does the chromosomal integrity of the ovulated oocytes, so that there is a rise in the rates of miscarriage and fetal chromosomal abnormalities. There are a number of tests of ovarian reserve but all have limitations. Measurement of ovarian hormones (e.g., estradiol, inhibin) to some degree reflects ovarian age (see Ch. 4). The response of the ovary to stimulation by gonadotropins is the essential test of ovarian function but provides only a retrospective analysis rather than a prospective indication of the likely response to treatment that can be used to determine the starting dose or stimulation regimen.

A baseline measurement of serum FSH concentration, usually on day 3 of the cycle, is a fairly good predictor of ovarian reserve. As the ovary fails, the FSH begins to rise in the follicular phase of the cycle. When the FSH is elevated there is a greater likelihood of monthly fluctuations in FSH concentration than when the FSH is normal. A fluctuating baseline FSH level is indicative of already compromised ovarian function. There is little to be gained by waiting to start treatment in a cycle in which the FSH level is closer to the normal range.

An ultrasound scan of the ovaries may also be helpful. Ovarian response has been positively correlated with ovarian volume and the number of antral follicles (see Ch. 4). The appearance of polycystic ovaries, whether or not there is overt polycystic ovary syndrome, indicates that the ovaries are likely to respond sensitively to stimulation, with the likely production of many follicles, although not necessarily with an equivalent number of oocytes of good quality. Patients with polycystic ovaries are at the greatest risk of OHSS (Ch. 17).

Stimulation tests have been evaluated with the aim of enhancing the predictability of ovarian response to superovulation. CC (100 mg) can be administered from days 5–9 and the serum FSH concentration measured on days 3 and 10. It is thought that in response to clomiphene the day 10 FSH rises before there is a rise in the basal day 3 FSH concentration. The clomiphene challenge test appears to be more useful in predicting reduced ovarian reserve when abnormal than in predicting normal ovarian function when the test is normal. Ovarian reserve can also be assessed by stimulation with a GnRH agonist. If these tests are used, normal ranges need to be developed for patients of different ages.

In practice a baseline serum FSH concentration on day 3 of the cycle usually suffices and if it is elevated it should be repeated on at least one occasion. We recommend that a baseline endocrine profile (FSH, LH, thyroid function) be repeated annually in women attending the fertility clinic, or more frequently if there is a change in the patient's menstrual cycle or an unexpectedly poor response to ovarian stimulation.

Our recommended starting dose for stimulation in superovulation regimens for IVF is 150 units of FSH or hMG in women with a normal serum FSH concentration under the age of 38 years. Women over the age of 38 years may be given 200–250 units, depending upon their baseline serum FSH concentration. In women with an elevated baseline FSH or those who have responded poorly in a previous cycle (i.e., fewer than 5 oocytes collected) we increase the dose to a maximum of 450 units. There appears to be no benefit in using higher doses, neither does there appear to be significant benefit in increasing the dose of stimulation mid-treatment after follicles have been recruited. If a baseline ultrasound scan indicates the presence of polycystic ovaries (whether or not there are signs of the polycystic ovary syndrome) we reduce the starting dose to 50–100 units, depending upon age and previous response to stimulation. If an exuberant response to stimulation is anticipated we commence ultrasound monitoring earlier (day 6 or 7 of stimulation) and may reduce the dose of FSH as soon as follicles greater than 10 mm in diameter have been recruited. The patient's response is reviewed after each cycle of treatment and the dose of stimulation adjusted according to the response obtained. We prefer to use the lowest dose that achieves the desired response and reduce the risk of ovarian hyperstimulation.

Ovarian cysts and IVF

The presence of simple cysts at the pretreatment scan should be noted and careful surveillance instituted to insure that they resolve spontaneously. Simple cysts do not require drainage before treatment provided they are not producing estrogen and preventing endometrial shedding. It is not unknown for ovarian malignancy to occur in young women and if there are any suspicious features (e.g., solid areas, multiple septa) the cysts should be treated before IVF is commenced. Transvaginal aspiration of complicated cysts should not be performed.

A study was performed in our clinic in which ovarian cysts that were encountered during IVF were divided into two categories: those present before and after GnRH agonist therapy was commenced.[34] The outcome of IVF was studied in both groups of patients who were randomly allocated either to having the cyst aspirated or having it left alone. In the patients who had a baseline cyst, unrelated to hormonal stimulation, the ovaries in which the cysts were aspirated developed a greater number of follicles and hence eggs than those which were not aspirated. There was, however, no difference in the total number of follicles or eggs between the two patient groups. On the other hand, the patients who developed cysts as a result of GnRH agonist therapy had a comparable response to treatment in both ovaries, irrespective of whether or not cyst aspiration was performed prior to ovarian stimulation. Aspiration of a unilateral cyst does not therefore appear to improve either folliculogenesis or oocyte recovery rates.

Monitoring therapy

Monitoring ovarian response to superovulation can be achieved by ultrasonography alone.[11] The dimensions of the growing follicles are plotted either daily or every other day, from around day 8 of stimulation, together with a measurement of endometrial thickness. The daily measurement of serum estradiol concentrations is of little help in the prediction of either success or the OHSS (see Ch. 17). Furthermore, serum estradiol concentrations appear to be proportional to the amount of LH in the gonadotropin preparation used in the stimulation regimen. When FSH alone is used to stimulate the ovaries, the serum estradiol concentration is approximately half the level found when hMG is used in the "long GnRH agonist protocol."

The preovulatory hCG "trigger" is usually administered when the leading follicle is at least 17–18 mm in diameter and there are at least three follicles greater than 17 mm (Fig. 13.3).

Oocyte retrieval

Ultrasound-guided oocyte retrieval is usually performed under light sedation plus analgesia; combinations of benzodiazepines, midazolam, and opiates are given intravenously or intramuscularly, with appropriate monitoring during and after the procedure. Administration of a local anesthetic (1% lidocaine (lignocaine)) into the vaginal fornices is of additional benefit.The procedure should be painfree. The patient is awake or lightly sedated and may be shown the oocytes on a closed-circuit video monitor attached to the embryologist's microscope. While it is possible for the patient's partner to be present, this is not the authors' current practice because of variable stress at seeing one's partner sedated. It is appropriate, however, that both partners are present at the embryo transfer. It is important that the patient is counseled carefully prior to oocyte retrieval as the procedure can

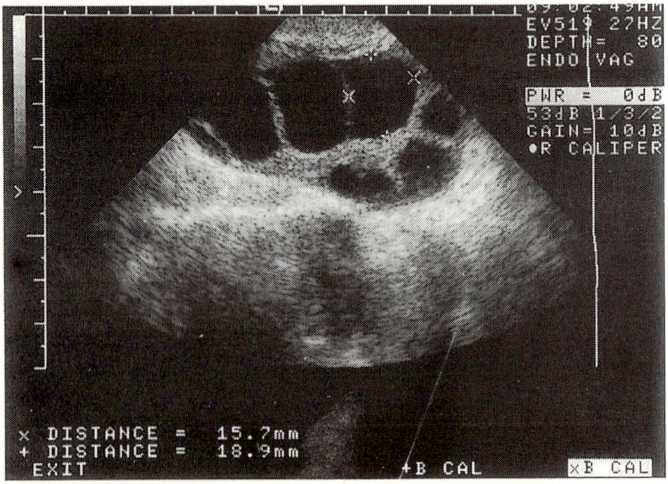

Figure 13.3 Transvaginal ultrasound scan of a stimulated ovary with three "mature" follicles seen in this plane.

occasionally be painful. Anxious patients may require heavy sedation or even general anesthesia with the attention of an anesthetist (Figs 13.4 and 13.5).

Oocyte retrieval should take about 20 minutes. We use a double lumen needle attached to an electronic pump, which enables rapid

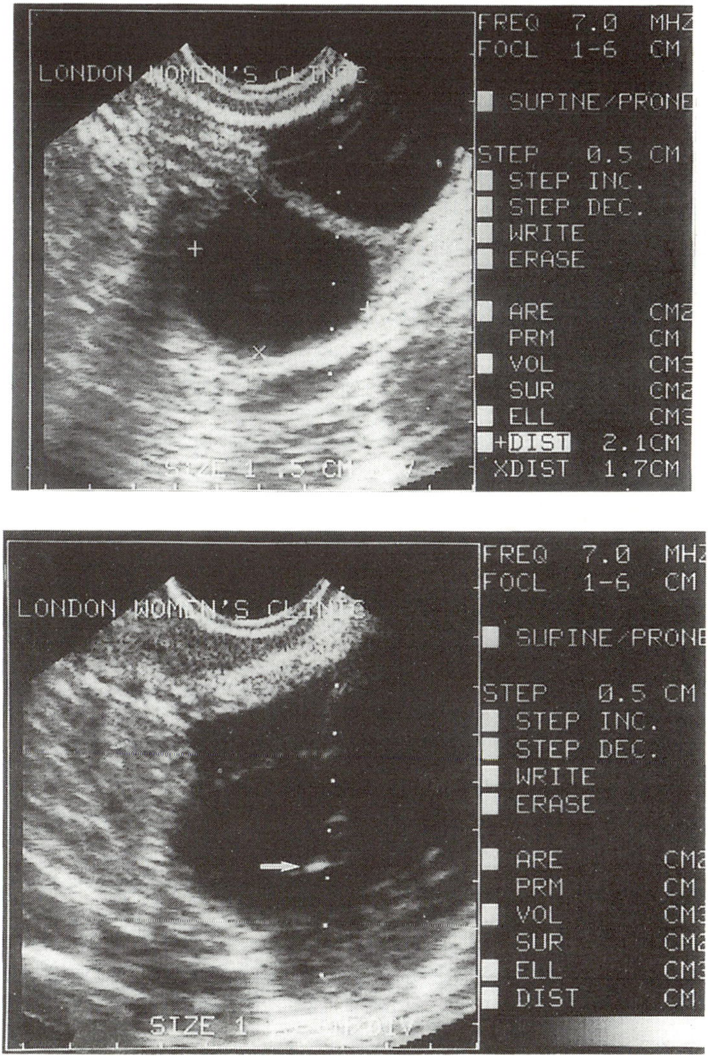

Figure 13.4a,b Oocyte retrieval. (**a**) During the oocyte collection procedure the ovary is magnified further and the needle guide (dotted line) indicates the track that the needle will take as it passes into the ovary. (**b**) The needle enters a follicle. Its tip is seen as a small echodense area (arrow).

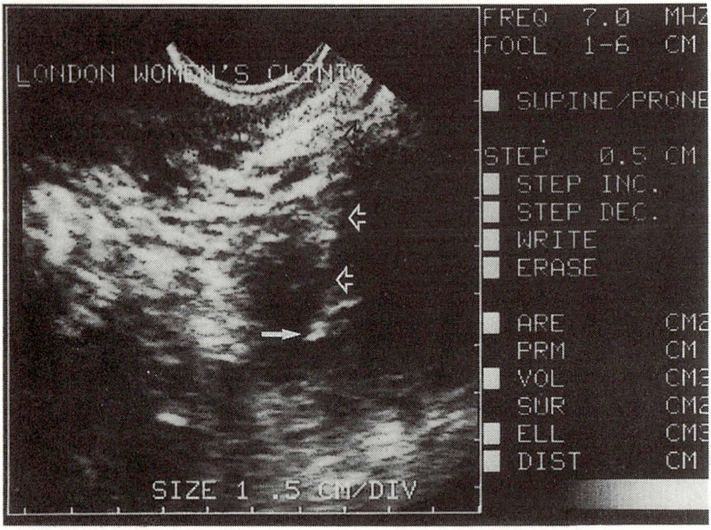

Figure 13.4c Oocyte retrieval. (**c**) As the follicular fluid is aspirated, the needle tip (arrow) can still be visualized within the collapsed follicle. It is also possible to see the dotted line of the needle if the needle guide is removed from the screen (open arrows).

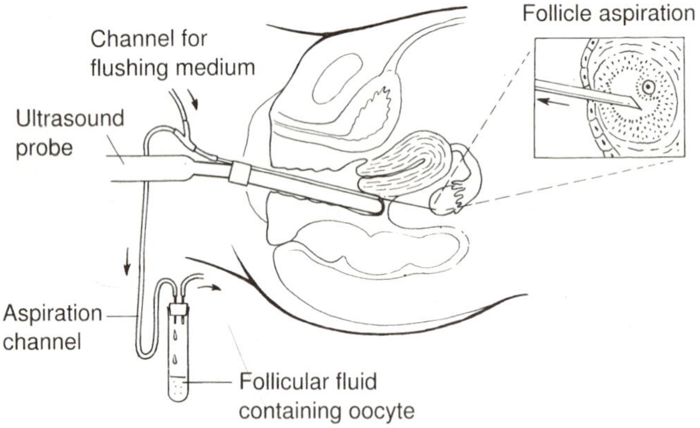

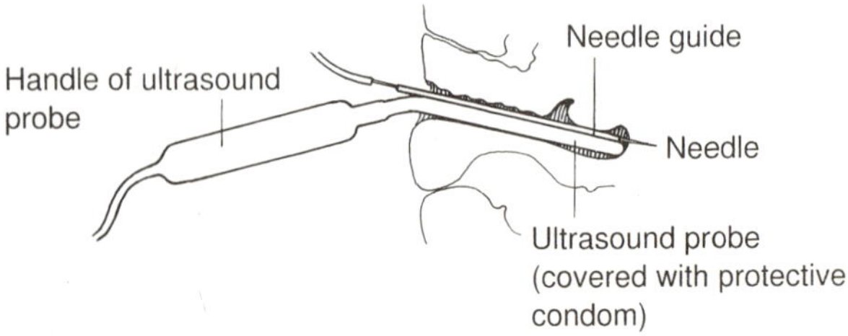

Figure 13.5 Oocyte collection.

aspiration of each follicle with minimal flushing. Indeed, we have found that repeated follicular flushing produces oocytes that fertilize less well and produce poorer quality embryos than those that appear in the initial follicular aspirate and first flush and so we have abandoned flushing, unless there are very few follicles and we are anticipating fewer than five oocytes.[35]

Patients considered to be at risk of developing the OHSS (see Ch. 17) must be given an information sheet warning them of the symptoms that can occur, because oral information will not suffice after sedative drugs have been given. It is also essential that arrangements be made for a follow-up assessment after 3 and 5 days, particularly if the plan is to freeze all pre-embryos and defer embryo transfer.

After oocyte retrieval, the semen is washed and prepared. Insemination is usually performed 1–6 hours after oocyte retrieval with 50–200 000 motile spermatozoa being placed with each oocyte; 16–18 hours later the oocytes are examined to ensure that correct fertilization has occurred, as defined by the presence of two pronuclei (see Figs 13.6–13.10). Multiple pronuclei indicate polyspermic fertilization or digyny (i.e., failure to extrude the second polar body) and are not suitable for transfer.

Embryo transfer (Figs 13.11–13.19)

Embryo transfer is usually performed 2–3 days after oocyte collection (at the 4–8 cell stage) (Figs 13.12 and 13.13). Research is under way to see if prolonged *in vitro* culture to the blastocyst stage (day 5) (Figs 13.14–13.17) improves the ability to select better quality pre-embryos for transfer (see Ch. 18). It may also enhance pregnancy rates and potentially reduce further the number of embryos transferred in order to minimize the rates of multiple pregnancy.[36,37] In the UK the Human Fertilisation and Embryology Authority (HFEA), which monitors the handling of all gametes for assisted conception, prohibits the transfer of more than three pre-embryos[39] and recommends the transfer of two in normal circumstances. There is a move in Europe, particularly Scandinavia, toward the transfer of a single embryo. Indeed many clinics are routinely transferring two, particularly in women under the age of 40, as there is no evidence that the transfer of three significantly increases the chance of pregnancy. It is important to aim for a healthy singleton pregnancy and be aware of the risks of multiple pregnancy (Ch. 17).

After embryo transfer the patient can go about her normal daily activities. Indeed, inactivity is best avoided as the 2 weeks up to the pregnancy test are hard for couples to cope with as they are no longer attending the clinic for regular scans and monitoring. It is usual to provide luteal support until the results of the pregnancy test are known and this itself can delay the onset of menstruation and give the couple

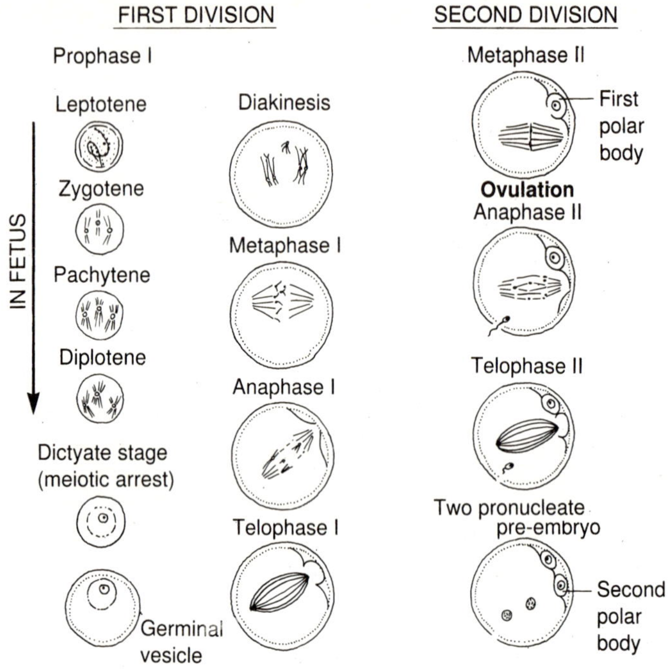

Figure 13.6 Meiotic division of the oocyte. Prophase commences in fetal life. During zygotene and pachytene the homologous chromosomes pair and then cleave longitudinally, with potential interchange of genetic material. During diplotene the chromosomes separate, except at the chiasmata, and enter first meiotic arrest. Meiosis is resumed at the time of the LH surge just before ovulation. The second meiotic division is then completed after fertilization.

false hope. Luteal support can be provided by either hCG or parenteral or vaginal progesterone (see Fig. 13.2 for regimens). The administration of hCG should be avoided if there is any risk of OHSS as it will continue to stimulate the ovaries, while exogenous progesterone will of course replace the secretion of the corpora lutea. Many clinics have now stopped giving hCG because OHSS is not always easy to predict.

There are a large number of protocols for luteal support, with hCG being given every 2–5 days at doses of 1000–5000 units s.c. and/or progesterone either 50–100 mg i.m. daily or 200–800 mg vaginally daily. No one regimen has been shown to be superior to another. Patients appear to prefer vaginal progesterone to injections. We administer vaginal progesterone 400 mg daily in all patients and stop on day 14 after embryo transfer whether the pregnancy test is positive or negative. There is now good evidence that luteal support improves outcome (for further discussion on luteal support in miscarriage, see Ch. 19).[40]

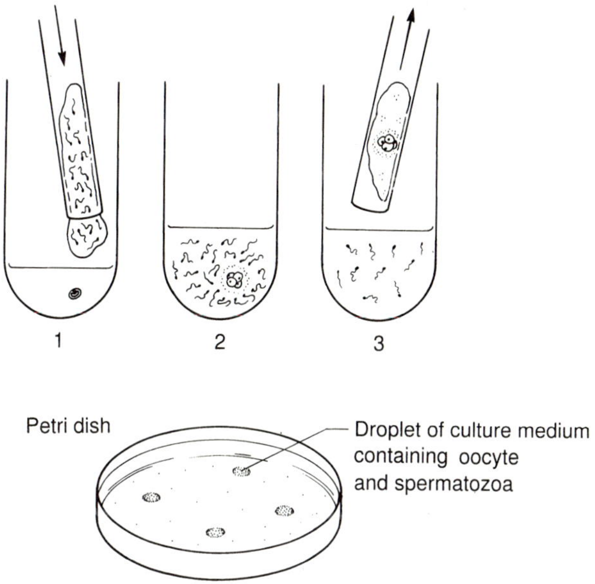

Figure 13.7 IVF. (1) The washed oocyte is exposed to sperm. (2) Fertilization is observed and (3) the pre-embryo is drawn into the embryo transfer catheter. IVF is performed either in a test tube or in a Petri dish in droplets of culture medium under a surface layer of oil.

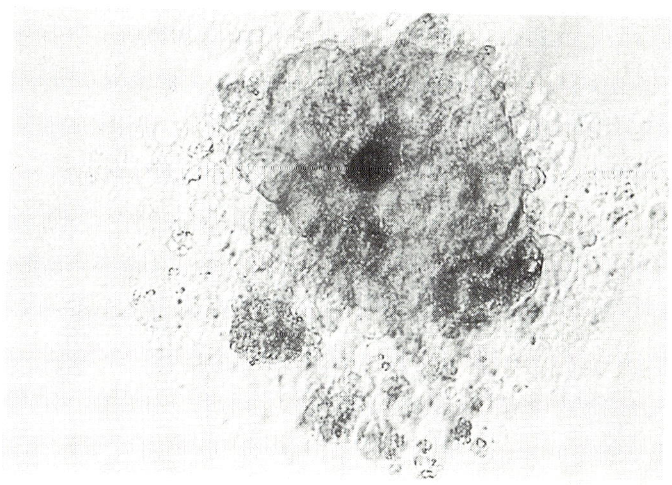

Figure 13.8 Oocyte immediately after follicular aspiration, covered in cumulus cells (please refer to plate section for color figure).

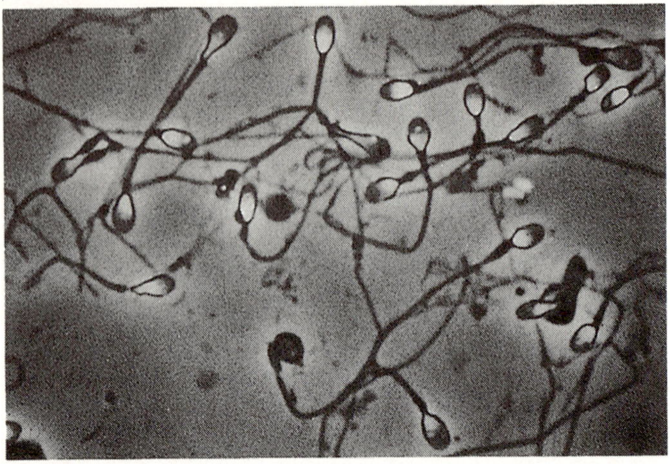

Figure 13.9 Phase contrast microscopy of normal spermatozoa (please refer to plate section for color figure).

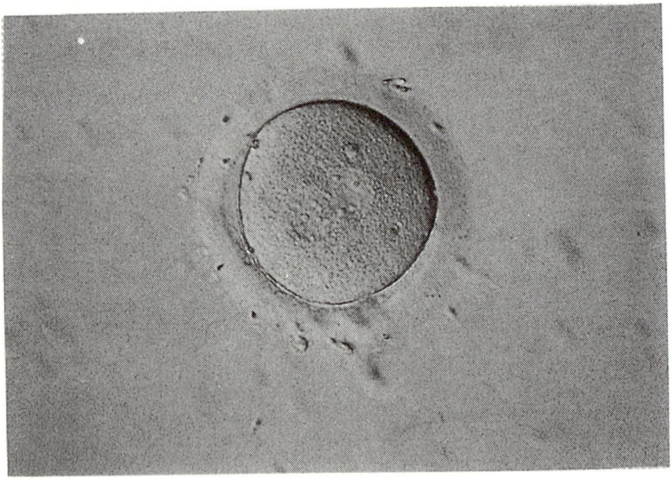

Figure 13.10 After fertlization two pronuclei can be seen clearly and spermatozoa can be seen attached to the outside of the zona pellucida (please refer to plate section for color figure).

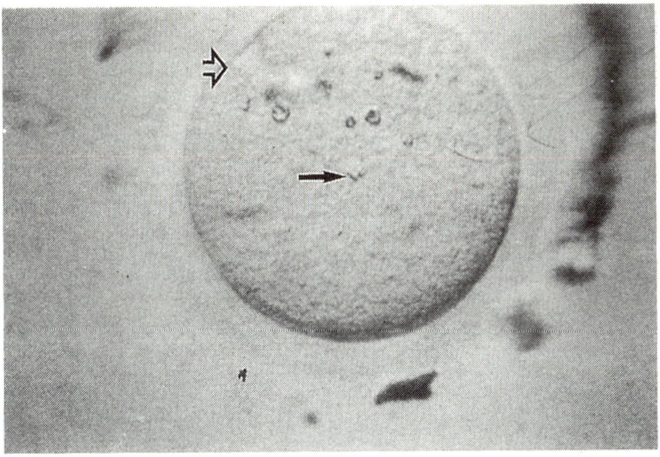

Figure 13.11 Oocyte immediately after ICSI has been performed. The site of the passage of the needle can be seen clearly (open arrow), as can the head of the spermatozoon (closed arrow) (please refer to plate section for color figure).

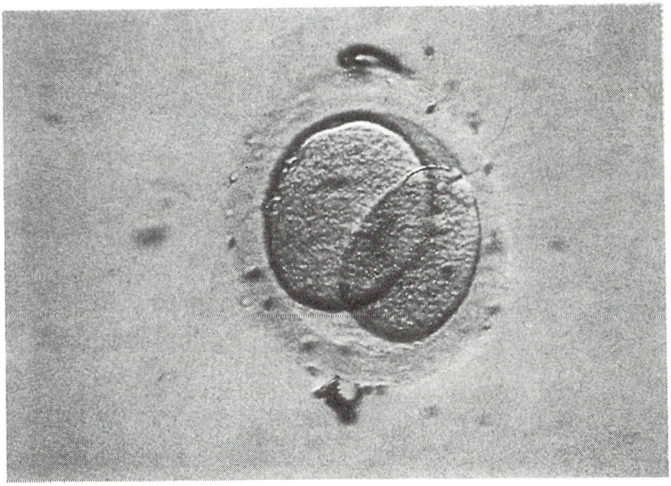

Figure 13.12 Two-cell pre-embryo (please refer to plate section for color figure).

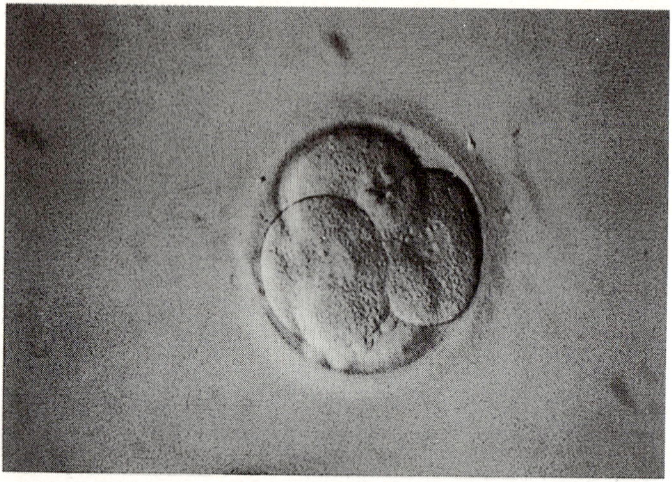

Figure 13.13 Four-cell pre-embryo (please refer to plate section for color figure).

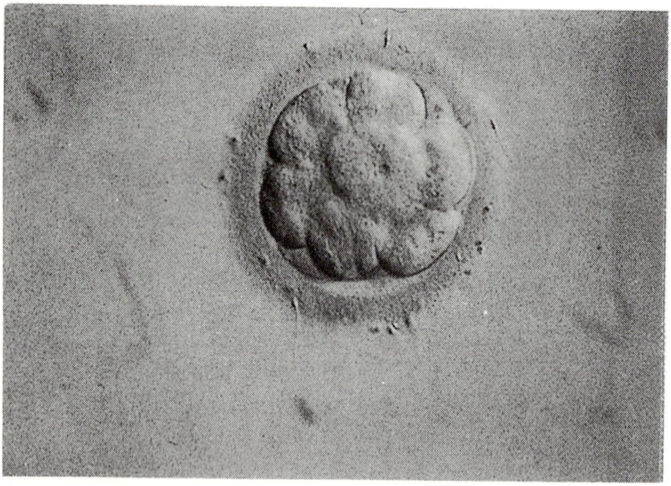

Figure 13.14 Morula stage (please refer to plate section for color figure).

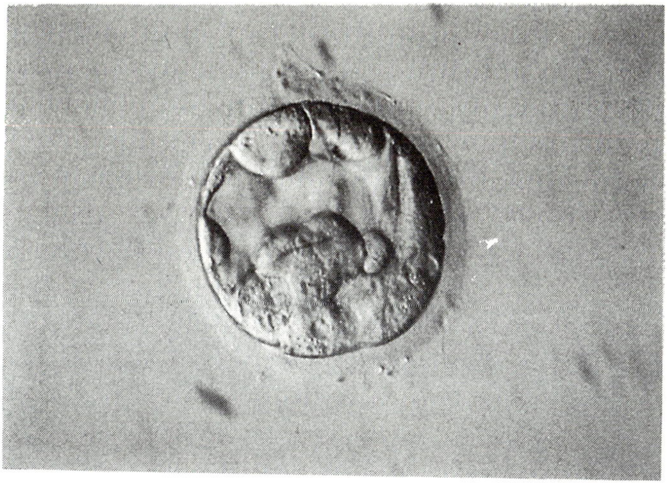

Figure 13.15 Blastocyst (please refer to plate section for color figure).

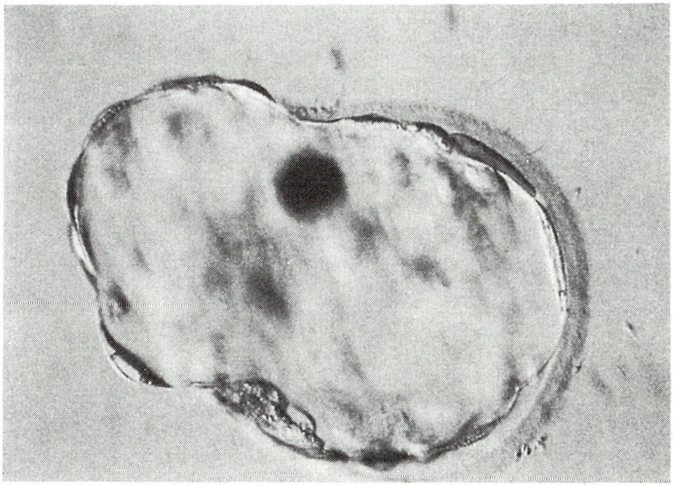

Figure 13.16 Blastocyst hatching (please refer to plate section for color figure).

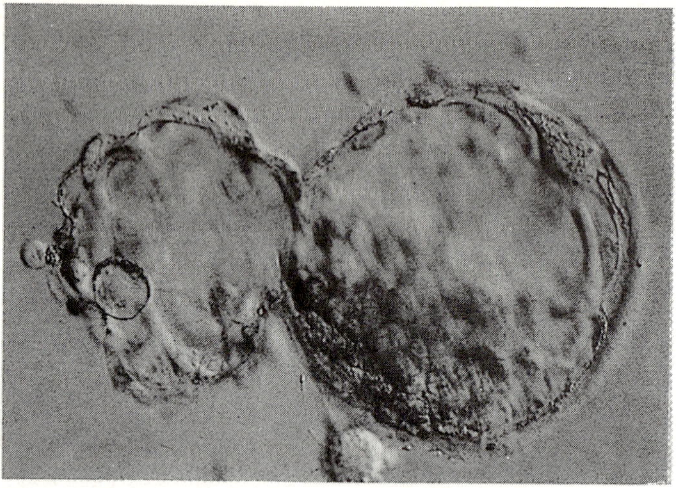

Figure 13.17 Hatched blastocyst (on right) (please refer to plate section for color figure).

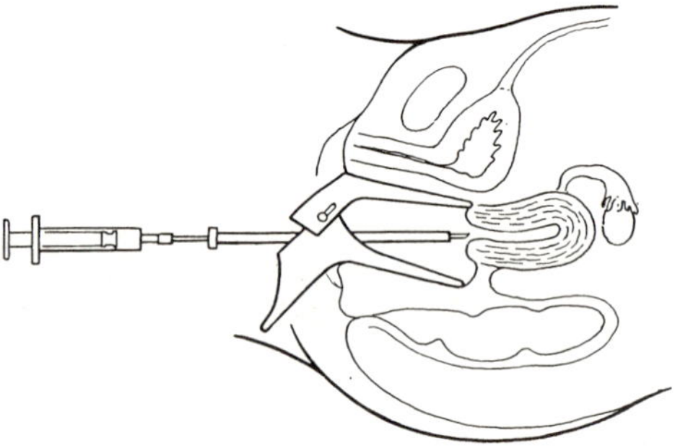

Figure 13.18 Embryo transfer.

Pregnancy rates after IVF (Figs 13.20–13.24)

A clinical pregnancy is defined as a rising level of hCG combined with ultrasound visualization of a gestational sac. Biochemical pregnancies are so named if hCG is present in the serum (in the absence of exogenously administered hCG for luteal support) yet bleeding occurs before a gestational sac is seen on ultrasound. It is a sensible convention not to include biochemical pregnancies in treatment results and care must be taken when comparing the results of different clinics or studies to ensure that the same definitions of pregnancy have been used.

The chance of a pregnancy following a single cycle of IVF is now approximately 35–40% in the larger units. There is no significant

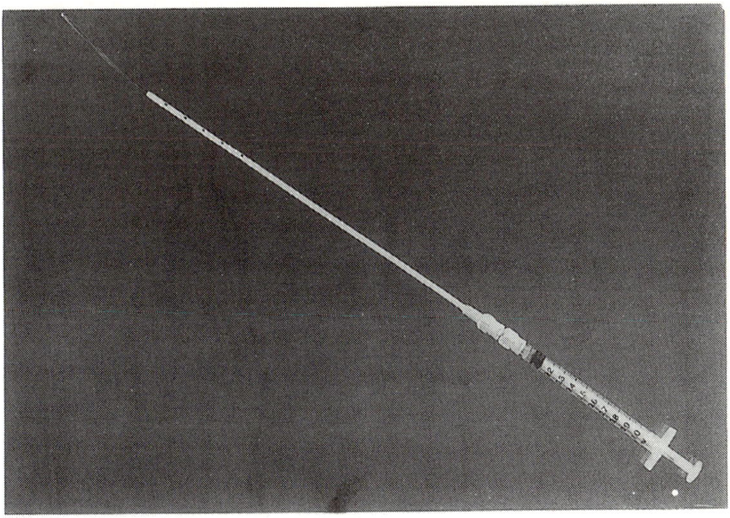

Figure 13.19 Embryo transfer catheter and syringe.

difference in pregnancy rates if two pre-embryos are transferred instead of three (which is the maximum permitted legally in the UK) but there is a reduced risk of multiple pregnancy. The overall chance of twins is about 20% and the chance of triplets is 5% when three pre-embryos are transferred. After the transfer of two pre-embryos the triplet rate is virtually abolished and the twin rate remains at 15–20%. The miscarriage rate is about 20% and the chance of an ectopic pregnancy is approximately 5%. In 2000 the most successful clinics in the UK achieved a live birth rate of about 30% per cycle started. The live birth rate for the UK was 19.5% for all age groups and 22.1% for women under the age of 38 (Table 13.2).[41]

The national results for 2000 are also depicted in Figure 13.20 which illustrates the multiple pregnancy rate of 7% of all cycles started, compared with a single pregnancy rate of 12%. Seventy-six per cent of cycles did not result in pregnancy.

The pregnancy rates achieved by IVF equate favorably with those expected for a couple without infertility when adjusted for the age of the female partner.[38,42] Cumulative conception and live birth rates, calculated by life table analysis, provide the best form of comparison between treatments, although they do not take into consideration couples who drop out of treatment because they are perceived as having a poor chance or because they cannot cope with the stresses of the therapy. The cumulative conception rates for a large clinic are shown in Figure 13.24.[38] There was a significant decline in success with increasing maternal age, such that the cumulative conception and live

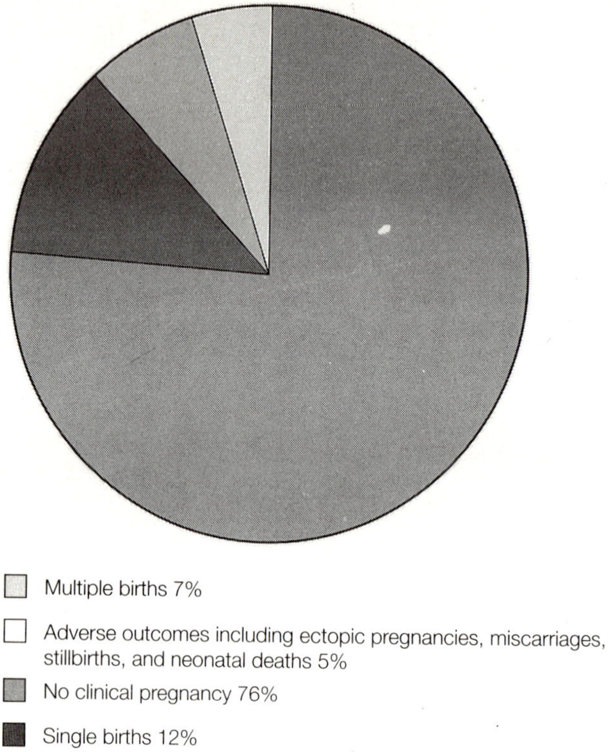

Figure 13.20 Results of assisted reproduction technology cycles.[41]

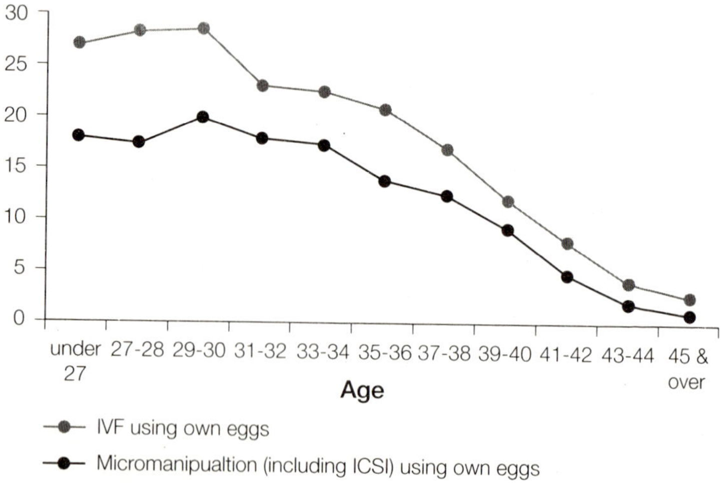

Figure 13.21 IVF live birth rate by woman's age (using own eggs).[41]

Live birth rates by duration of infertility				
		Live birth rate (%)		
Duration of infertility (years)	Number of cycles	Per treatment cycle	Per egg collection	Per embryo transfer
0	2258	13.3	15.6	17.9
1–3	8407	15.3	17.2	19.5
4–6	13483	14.0	15.7	18.3
7–9	7017	12.9	14.4	17.0
10–12	3701	12.4	13.9	16.4
over 12	2092	8.6	9.7	11.8
All results are adjusted for woman's age				

Figure 13.22 Live birth rates by duration of infertility.[41]

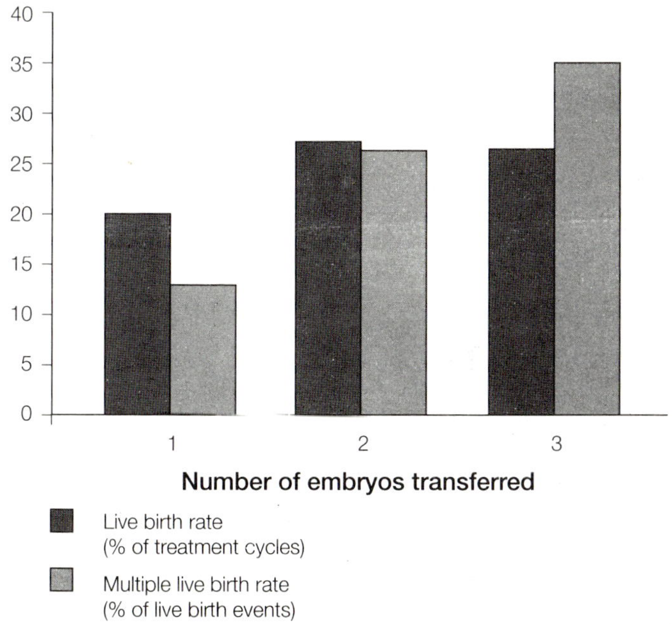

Figure 13.23 Live birth and multiple birth rates by number of embryos transferred.[41]

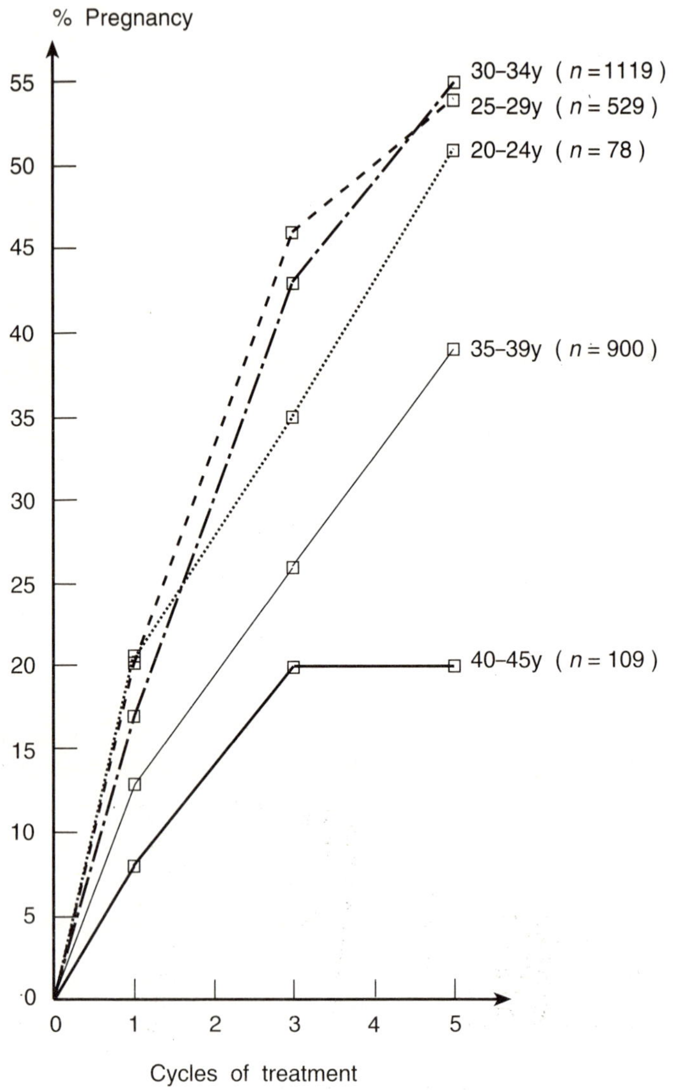

Figure 13.24a

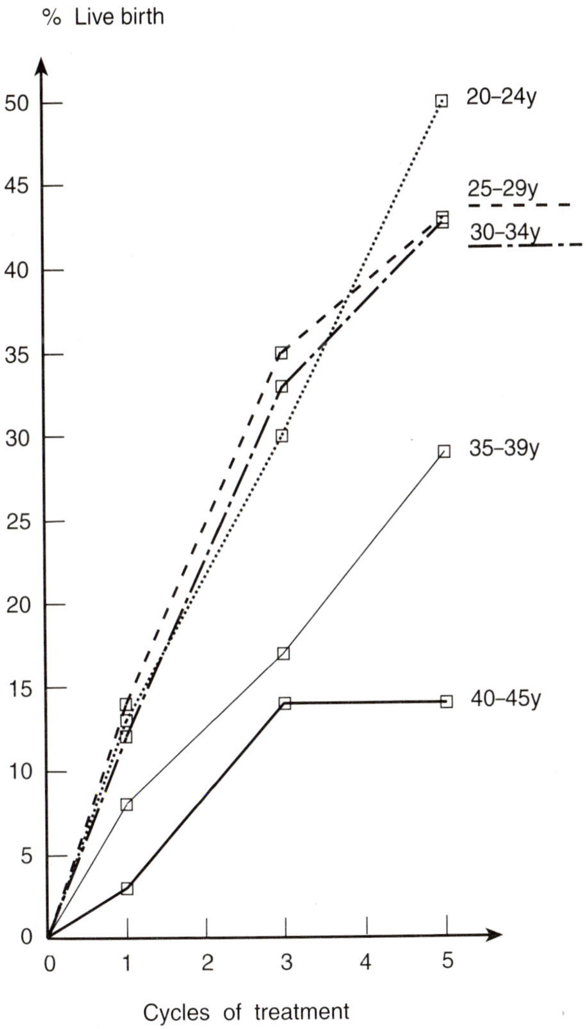

Figure 13.24b

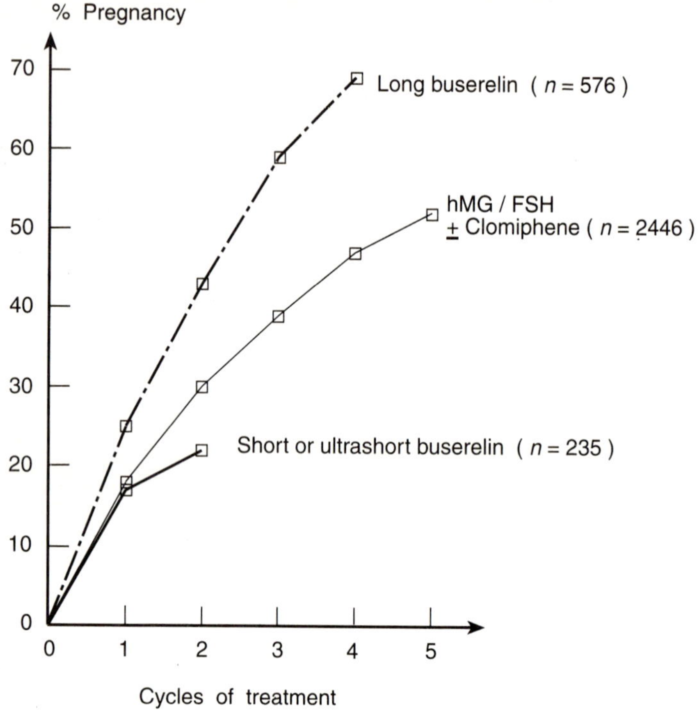

Figure 13.24c

birth rates after five cycles of treatment for women aged 34 or less were 54% and 45% respectively, compared with 39% and 29% for those aged 35–39 years and 20% and 14% for those over 40. An analysis of 36 961 cycles of IVF registered by the HFEA betweer August 1991 and April 1994 (excluding cycles involving gamete o embryo donation) showed the overall live birth rate per cycle to b 13.9%.[43] The highest live birth rates were in the age group 25–3(years. No pregnancies were recorded in women older than 45 years The most recent national statistics from the HFEA further illustrat the decline in live birth rates with both IVF and ICSI with increasin age of the female partner (Fig. 13.21 and Table 13.2[41]). There were nc significant differences in live birth rate per cycle by cause of infertility, although more women with unexplained infertility did not proceed to embryo transfer after egg recovery compared with women with tubal disease (23% compared to 14.1%), leading to a higher live birth rate per embryo transfer (19.7% compared to 16.5%, $p < 0.001$).[43]

The major factors that determine the chance of an ongoing pregnancy are the age of the woman, with rates declining over the age of

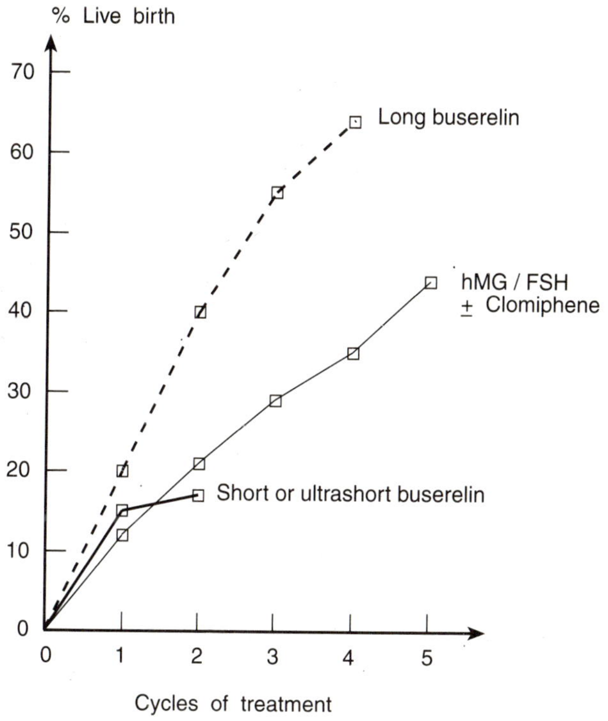

Figure 13.24a–d Cumulative conception rates (**a**) and live birth rates (**b**) after IVF in relation to the patient's age, irrespective of diagnosis of infertility. Both conception and live birth rates decline significantly with age, particularly in women over 34. (Data from Tan *et al.* (1992) *Lancet* **339**: 1390, with permission.)[38] Cumulative conception rates (**c**) and live birth rates (**d**) after IVF in relation to treatment regimen. Regimens with hMG and/or FSH, either alone or with clomiphene citrate, are compared with three different GnRH agonist regimens, using buserelin: ultrashort, short, and long (see text for details, p. 317). Both conception and live birth rates increase significantly with the use of the long buserelin protocol. (Data from Tan *et al.* (1994) *Am J Obstet Gynecol* **171**: 513, with permission.)[44]

35, increasing duration of infertility (Fig. 13.22), parity, and the number of oocytes collected. Not surprisingly, couples who have achieved a pregnancy are more likely to do so if they try again.[44] Indeed, many couples have now achieved their desired family size either through repeated attempts at IVF or by the transfer of cryopreserved pre-embryos obtained in a previously successful or unsuccessful cycle of treatment. In the UK now approximately 1% of babies are born as a result of assisted conception. In Europe, in 1998, there were over 230 000 assisted conception cycles – a rate of 3.2 cycles per 1000 women aged 15–49 years. The average clinical pregnancy rate per embryo transfer was 27% and the multiple pregnancy rate 26%.[45]

Table 13.2 Live birth rates		
	Below 38	All ages
Treatment cycles started (IVF and ICSI)	22.1% (4698/21 274)	19.5% (5304/27 230)
Egg collection	23.7% (4698/19 850)	21.1% (5304/25 171)
Embryo transfer	25.6% (4698/18 333)	22.9% (5304/23 171)
IVF only (per embryo transfer)	25.6% (2674/10 436)	22.7% (3072/13 523)
ICSI only (per embryo transfer)	25.6% (2024/7897)	23.1% (2232/9648)
Frozen embryo replacements (per embryo transfer)	14.3% (632/4406)	13.4% (733/5454)

Micromanipulation of Gametes for Severe Male Factor Infertility

Standard IVF requires the presence of more than 500 000 motile sperm in the total ejaculate. In cases where the sperm count is lower, fertilization can be assisted by a variety of micromanipulation techniques. Initial attempts involved either drilling through the zona with Tyrode solution (zona drilling) or by using a glass microneedle (partial zona dissection – PZD (see Fig. 13.26a). Alternatively, several spermatozoa were injected into the perivitelline space beneath the zona pellucida (subzonal insemination – SUZI (see Figs 13.25 and 13.26b). These techniques have been superseded by ICSI, the injection of a single spermatozoon directly into the cytoplasm (ooplasm) of the oocyte (Figs 13.11, 13.25 and 13.26c). ICSI, pioneered by

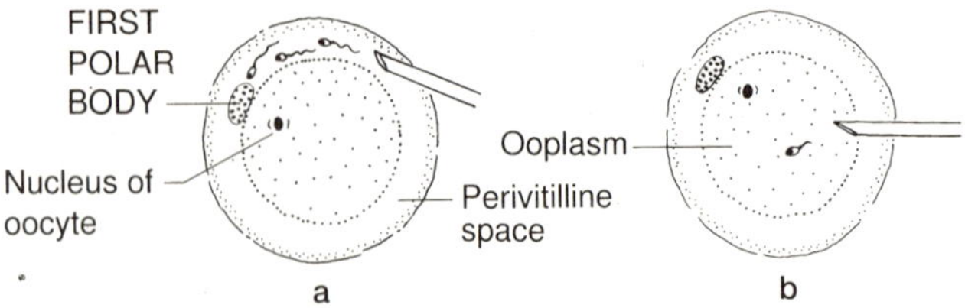

Figure 13.25 Microinjection of spermatozoa. (**a**) Subzonal insemination (SUZI). This was the original technique, now superseded by ICSI and no longer performed. (**b**) Intracytoplasmic sperm injection (ICSI).

Van Steirteghem and his team in Brussels, has revolutionized the management of male infertility and has provided the possibility of a pregnancy for men who previously would have required their partners to undergo donor insemination.[46–48]

ICSI can be used not only for men with profound oligozoospermia or asthenoteratozoospermia but also for those with obstructive azoospermia, after microsurgical or direct aspiration of sperm from either the epididymis or the testis. The spermatozoon is immobilized before ICSI, usually by breaking the tail, as flagellation within the

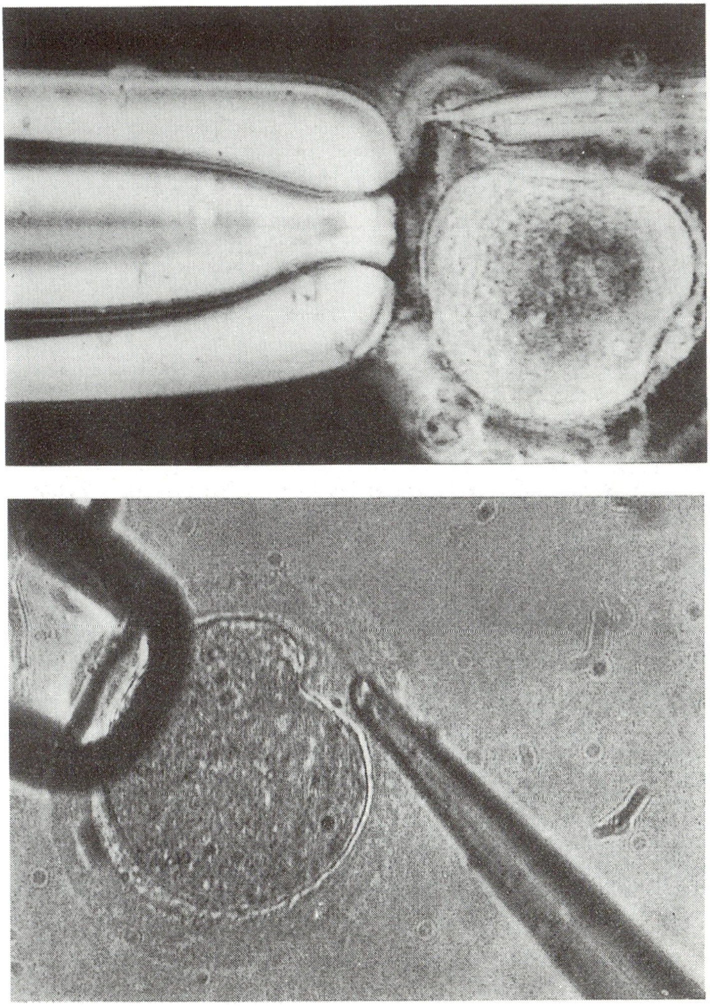

a

b

Figure 13.26

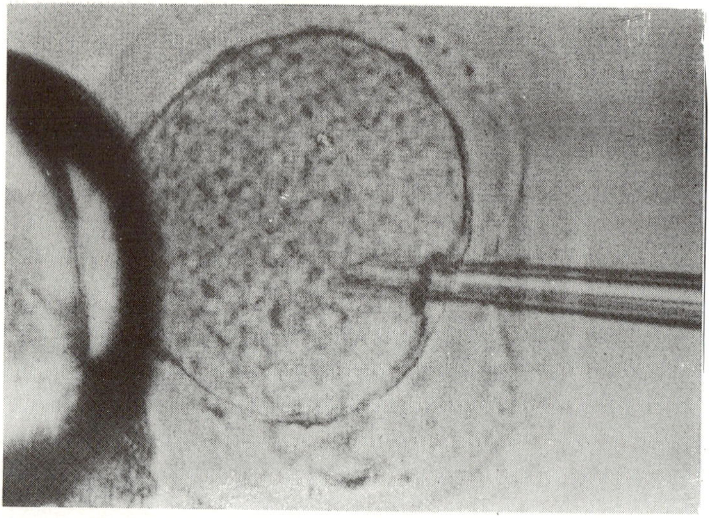

c

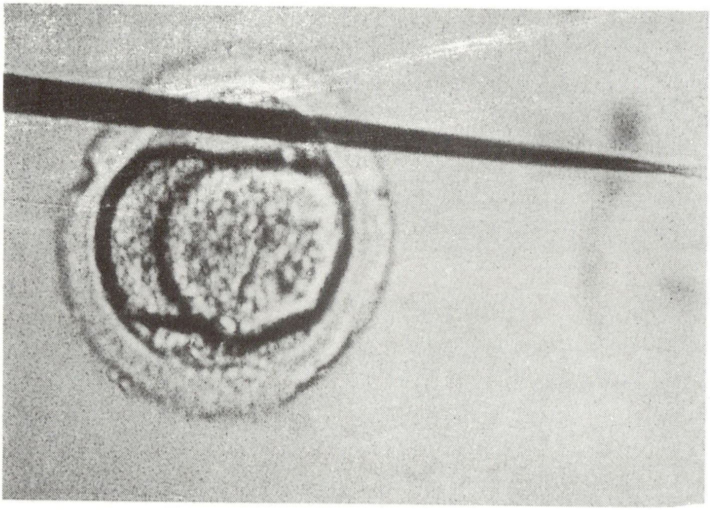

d

Figure 13.26a–d Micromanipulation techniques. (**a**) Partial zona dissection (PZD): the oocyte is held by a suction pipette while a glass needle is used to make a breach in the zona pellucida. Spermatozoa can then find their way in through the opening. (**b**) Subzonal insemination of sperm (SUZI). (**c**) Intracytoplasmic injection of sperm (ICSI) which is nowadays the preferred technique. (**d**) Assisted hatching of a pre-embryo, a technique in which PZD is employed to aid the later hatching of the blastocysts from embryos that have been generated *in vitro*.

ooplasm is undesirable and only the genetic contents of the sperm head are required.

Fertilization rates with ICSI are in the region of 60%, irrespective of the origin of the sperm, providing 90% of couples with an embryo transfer and chance of a pregnancy. Pregnancy rates after ICSI are the same as after IVF.[35] Furthermore, the elective transfer of two pre-embryos resulted in similar pregnancy rates as the transfer of three, after both IVF[37] and ICSI, confirming the effectiveness of a double embryo transfer, which should become more widely employed in order to reduce the risks of multiple pregnancy.[36] ICSI can be offered to couples in whom fertilization has failed during IVF in the absence of an apparent sperm problem, as assessed by standard sperm function tests. Transcription in the human embryo starts at the 4–8 cell stage[49] and so the signal for the first cleavage has to be provided by an extranuclear signal, which arises from the surface of the sperm (termed the cleavage signal (CS-1) protein). Thus, if fertilization occurs but cleavage fails, this might also be due to sperm dysfunction.

Micromanipulation of the embryo can also be performed in the form of "assisted hatching" (Fig. 13.26d) which is thought by some to improve implantation rates for patients with previous IVF failures.[50] There is no strong evidence, however, for its use.[51]

Important Considerations on the New Techniques

Recently, immature spermatids have been used for ICSI, thus opening up greater possibilities for men with testicular dysfunction. When round spermatid nuclei are injected into oocytes (ROSNI), spermatogenesis has not been completed and caution has been expressed about the genetic integrity of immature sperm. These techniques are not permitted in the UK. Various authorities have expressed concerns about the use of micromanipulation techniques because we have limited knowledge about the natural maturation process of spermatozoa and the ways in which sperm are naturally selected for fertilization. Most fertility therapies retain an element of natural selection, whether it be ovulation induction or IVF; that is, only "good eggs" are likely to become fertilized or result in good quality pre-embryos that are suitable for transfer. We are not able to distinguish between "good" and "poor" quality sperm other than by a crude assessment of morphology and nuclear condensation. There is some evidence for an increased rate of strand breakages in the DNA of sperm from men with subfertility, some of whom have cystic fibrosis or are carriers of cystic fibrosis mutations or other recessive gene anomalies. Furthermore, the stage at which genomic imprinting takes place is not known and there is a suggestion that genes may be modified in the epididymis – in other words, distal to the site of aspirated testicular sperm. The data on children born to date as a result of micromanipulation techniques are reassuring with respect to major congenital abnormalities[52] but there is an increased rate of sex chromosome anomalies and a suggestion that male children may have increased rates of infertility themselves (see more detailed overview in Ch. 16).

Cryopreservation of Gametes and Embryos

Cryopreservation of sperm is discussed in Chapter 11. Cryopreservation of oocytes has not been very successful to date, although pregnancies have been achieved, albeit with a low overall return rate for the number of oocytes frozen. It might be that cryopreservation of ovarian tissue followed by *in vitro* culture of follicles will provide a better chance of viable oocytes for women who are about to undergo chemo/radiotherapy or have an oophorectomy (see Ch. 18).

Embryos are stored in liquid nitrogen at −196°C, usually at the pronuclear or early cleavage stages. We prefer to store only good quality embryos (that is, grade 1 or 2 – out of a scale 1–5 – preferably four cell embryos). Embryo survival is in the region of 70% and if individual blastomeres are damaged, as each is pluripotent, there appears to be no harmful effect on the developing fetus. Thawed embryos are transferred 2–3 days after ovulation in carefully monitored natural cycles or 3 days after the commencement of progesterone therapy in artificial cycles in which pretreatment has been performed, first with a GnRH agonist and then with oral estradiol which is administered until the endometrium has developed adequately (Fig. 13.27). Doppler flow studies of the uterine vasculature have been used to optimize the timing of embryo transfer, although these techniques are still largely within the confines of research protocols.

Important Considerations

At the time of writing the HFEA permits embryo storage for 5 years in the first instance, with a possible extension for a further 5 years, although there is no evidence that deterioration occurs beyond this time. In fact, it has been estimated that it would take 2000 years for background cosmic radiation levels to have a detrimental effect on the genetic integrity of the cryopreserved cells. Children conceived from cryopreserved embryos have similar rates of minor and major congenital abnormalities as children conceived normally.[53,54] Furthermore, the rates of pregnancy, miscarriage, and congenital anomalies do not appear to be related to the duration of embryo storage. Despite this, couples with frozen embryos may have to face tough emotional decisions about how to dispose of them once they reach the time limit. The options include thawing for their own use, embryo donation to

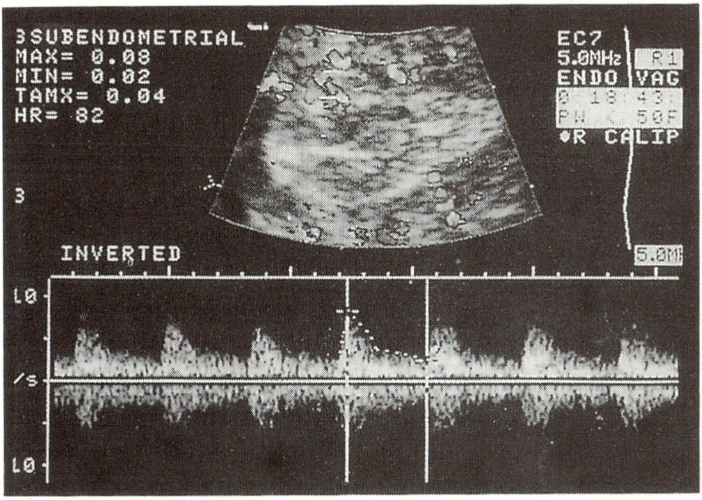

Figure 13.27 Color Doppler studies of the endometrium. Transvaginal ultrasound (5 MHz) with superimposed pulsed Doppler demonstrating flow through subendometrial vessels. Absent subendometrial or intraendometrial vascularization on the day of hCG administration during IVF appears to be a useful predictor of failure of implantation in IVF cycles, irrespective of the morphological appearance of the endometrium (with thanks to Dr J. Zaidi) (please refer to plate section for color figure).

couples with sperm and oocyte problems, embryo research, or discarding (i.e., destroying) the embryos.

Oocyte Donation

See Chapter 8 and Figure 13.28 for oocyte donation.

Surrogacy

IVF surrogacy is an option for women with ovaries but without a uterus, either because of a congenital absence (e.g., Rokitansky syndrome) or after hysterectomy (e.g., after severe obstetric hemorrhage or cervical carcinoma), or for women for whom a pregnancy would be a medical risk (e.g., severe heart or lung disease). Sperm must be frozen and quarantined for 6 months to reduce the risk of infection with HIV. A standard IVF regimen is used and the surrogate host prepared as for a frozen embryo replacement cycle. Egg collection can sometimes be difficult if the ovaries are situated high in the abdomen, in which case a transabdominal approach may be required.

Straight surrogacy is another option, less commonly performed, in which the surrogate host donates her own oocytes either to be inseminated *in vitro*, in a standard IVF protocol, or *in vivo*, in an IUI protocol.

There are strict regulations concerning surrogacy arrangements and few clinics offer this treatment because of ethical concerns and the complexities of the arrangements. It is our experience, and that of others,[50] that surrogacy can work extremely well and achieve higher success rates than standard IVF. Key components of a successful program are an experienced counselor and the selection of properly motivated surrogates who are fully informed of all of the IVF processes, their risks, and complications.

Assisted reproduction technology – key points

- IVF is the end-point treatment for many causes of infertility but should not be abused or embarked upon too early.
- Assisted reproduction technology is stressful, expensive, and carries certain risks, which should not be underestimated.
- IVF is a test of fertilization.
- Pituitary desensitization using a long regimen with a GnRH agonist provides the best results.
- GnRH antagonists may lead to shorter duration cycles.
- Age and baseline FSH are currently the best predictors of ovarian reserve.
- Micromanipulation techniques such as ICSI have revolutionized the treatment of severe male factor infertility and couples with a history of poor fertilization in previous cycles.

References

1. Asch R, Ellsworth L, Balmaceda J & Wong PC (1984) Pregnancy after translaparoscopic gamete intrafallopian transfer. *Lancet* **ii**: 1034–1035.
2. Devroey P, Staessen C, Camus M, de Grauwe E, Wisanto A & van Steirteghem AC (1989) Zygote intrafallopian transfer as a successful treatment for unexplained infertility. *Fertil Steril* **52**: 246–249.
3. Yovich JL, Blackledge DG, Richardson PA, Matson PL, Turner SR & Draper R (1987) Pregnancies following pronuclear stage tubal transfer. *Fertil Steril* **48**: 851–857.
4. Jansen RPS, Anderson JC & Sutherland PD (1988) Nonoperative embryo transfer to the Fallopian tube. *N Engl J Med* **319**: 288–291.
5. Kato I, Takatsuka R & Asch R (1993) Transvaginal–transmyometrial embryo transfer: the Towako method; experience of 104 cases. *Fertil Steril* **50**: 51–53.
6. Hull MGR (1992) Infertility treatment: relative effectiveness of conventional and assisted conception methods. *Hum Reprod* **7**: 785–796.
7. Edwards RG (1980) *Conception in the human female*. Academic Press, London.

8. Edwards RG, Steptoe PC & Purdy JM (1980) Establishing full-term human pregnancies using cleaving embryos grown in vivo. *Br J Obstet Gynaecol* **87**: 737–756.
9. Steptoe PC & Edwards RG (1976) Reimplanataion of a human embryo with subsequent tubal pregnancy. *Lancet* **i**: 880–882.
10. Steptoe PC, Edwards RG & Purdy JM (1980) Clinical aspects of pregnancies established with embryos grown *in vitro*. *Br J Obstet Gynaecol* **87**: 757–768.
11. Tan SL, Balen AH, Hussein EE *et al.* (1992) A prospective randomised study of the optimum timing of human chorionic gonadotropin administration after pituitary desensitisation in *in vitro* fertilisation. *Fertil Steril* **57**: 1259–1264.
12. Balen AH (2001) GnRH agonists and superovulation for assisted conception. In: Devroey P (ed) *Infertility and reproductive medicine clinics of North America*. WB Saunders, Philadelphia, vol 12, pp 89–104.
13. Tan SL, Doyle P, Maconochie N *et al.* (1994) Pregnancy and birth rates of live infants after *in vitro* fertilisation in women with and without previous IVF pregnancies. *Am J Obstet Gynecol* **170**: 34–40.
14. Balen AH, Tan SL, MacDougall J & Jacobs HS (1993) Miscarriage rates following *in vitro* fertilisation are increased in women with polycystic ovaries and reduced by pituitary desensitisation with buserelin. *Hum Reprod* **8**: 959–964.
15. Hughes EG, Fedorkow DM, Daya S, Sagle MA, Van de Koppel P & Collins JA (1992) The routine use of gonadotropin-releasing hormone agonists prior to *in vitro* fertilization and gamete intrafallopian transfer: a meta-analysis of randomized trials. *Fertil Steril* **58**: 888–896.
16. Daya S. Long versus short gonadotropin agonist protocols for pituitary desensitisation in assisted reproduction cycles. (Cochrane Review.) In The Cochrane Library, Issue 4, Oxford, 1999. Update Software 1999.
17. European Orgalutran® Study Group, Borm G & Mannaerts B (2000) Treatment with the gonadotropin-releasing hormone antagonist ganirelix in women undergoing controlled ovarian hyperstimulation with recombinant follicle stimulating hormone is effective, safe and convenient: results of a controlled, randomized, multicentre trial. *Hum Reprod* **15**: 1490–1498
18. Balen AH (ed) (2002) GnRH antagonist protocols in practice. *Hum Fertil* **5**: G1–48.
19. Donini P, Montezemolo R (1949) *Rassegna di clinica, terapia e scienze affini*. A publication of the Biologic Laboratories of the Instituto Serono **48**(143): 3–28.
20. Howles CM, Barri P, Cittadini E *et al.* Metrodin HP (1992) Clinical experiences with a new highly purified follicle stimulating hormone preparation suitable for subcutaneous administration. In: Lunenfeld B (ed) *FSH alone in ovulation induction*. Parthenon Publishing, New York, pp 45–61.
21. Hayden CJ, Balen AH & Rutherford AJ (1999) Recombinant gonadotropins. *Br J Obstet Gynaecol* **106**: 188–196.
22. Rose MP, Gaines Das RE & Balen AH (2000) Definition and measurement of FSH. *Endocrinol Rev* **21**: 5–22.
23. Lambert A, Rodgers M, Mitchell R *et al.* (1995) In-vitro biopotency and glycoform distribution of recombinant human follicle stimulating hormone (Org 32489), Metrodin and Metrodin-HP. *Mol Hum Reprod* **10**: 1928–1935.
24. Le Cotonnec, Porchet H, Beltrami V *et al.* (1994) Clinical pharmacology of recombinant human follicle-stimulating hormone (FSH) i. Comparative pharmacokinetics with urinary human FSH. *Fertil Steril* **61**: 669–678. ii. Single doses and steady state pharmacokinetics. *Fertil Steril* **61**: 679–686.
25. Loumaye E, Campbell R & Salat-Baroux J (1995) Human follicle stimulating hormone produced by recombinant DNA technology: a review for clinicians. *Hum Reprod Update* **1**: 188–199.
26. Recombinant Human FSH Study Group (1995) Clinical assessment of recombinant human follicle-stimulating hormone in stimulating ovarian follicular development before *in vitro* fertilsation. *Fertil Steril* **63**: 77–86.

27. Out HJ, Mannaerts BMJL, Driessen SGAJ & Coelingh Benninck HJT (1996) Recombinant follicle stimulating hormone (rFSH; Puregon) in assisted reproduction: more oocytes, more pregnancies. Results from five comparative studies. *Hum Reprod Update* **2**: 162–171.
28. Out HJ, Mannerts BMJL, Driessen SGAJ & Coelingh Benninck HJT (1995) A prospective randomised assessor-blind, multicentre study comparing recombinant and urinary follicle stimulating hormone (Puregon vs. Metrodin) in *in-vitro* fertilisation. *Hum Reprod* **10**: 2534–2540.
29. Bergh C, Howles C.M, Borg K *et al.* (1997) Recombinant human follicle stimulating hormone (r-hFSH; Gonal-F®): results of a randomized comparative study in women undergoing assisted reproductive techniques. *Hum Reprod* **12**: 2133–2139.
30. Daya S, Gunby J, Hughes EG, Collins JA & Sagle MA (1995) Follicle-stimulating hormone versus human menopausal gonadotropin for *in vitro* fertilisation cycles: a meta-analysis. *Fertil Steril* **64**: 347–354.
31. Loumaye E, Martineau I, Piazzi A *et al.* (1996) Clinical assessment of human gonadotropins produced by recombinant DNA technology. *Hum Reprod* **11**: 95–107.
32. Agrawal R, Holmes J & Jacobs HS (2000) Follicle stimulating hormone or human menopausal gonadotropin for ovarian stimulation in *in vitro* fertilization cycles: a meta-analysis. *Fertil Steril* 73: 338–343.
33. Westergaard LG, Laursen SB & Andersen CY (2000) Increased risk of early pregnancy loss by profound suppression of luteinising hormone during ovarian stimulation in normogonadotropic women undergoing assisted reproduction. *Hum Reprod* **15**: 1003–1008.
34. Rizk B, Tan SL, Kingsland C, Steer C, Mason BA & Campbell S (1990) Ovarian cyst aspiration and outcome of *in vitro* fertilisation. *Fertil Steril* **54**: 661–664.
35. Staessen C, Janssenswillen C, van den Abbeel E, Devroey P & van Steirteghem AC (1993) Avoidance of triplet pregnancies by elective transfer of two good quality embryos. *Hum Reprod* 8: 1650–1653.
36. Balen AH, MacDougall J & Tan SL (1993) The influence of the number of embryos transferred during *in-vitro* fertilization on pregnancy outcome. *Hum Reprod* 8: 1324–1328.
37. Staessen C, Nagy ZP, Liu J *et al.* (1995) One year's experience with elective transfer of two good quality embryos in the human *in vitro* fertilisation and intracytoplasmic sperm injection programmes. *Hum Reprod* **10**: 3305–3312.
38. Tan SL, Doyle P, Campbell S *et al.* (1992) Cumulative conception and livebirth rates after *in vitro* fertilisation. *Lancet* **339**: 1390–1394.
39. Human Fertilisation and Embryology Act (1990) HMSO, London.
40. Penzias AS (2002) Luteal phase support. *Fertil Steril* **77**: 318–323.
41. HFEA (2002) Annual Report. Reporting year 1999–2000. Website: www.hfea.gov.uk
42. Hull MGR, Eddowes HA, Fahy U *et al.* (1992) Expectations of assisted conception for infertility. *Br Med J* **304**: 1465–1469.
43. Templeton A, Morris JK & Parslow W (1996) Factors that affect outcome of *in-vitro* fertilization treatement. *Lancet* **348**: 1402
44. Tan SL, Maconochie N, Doyle P *et al.* (1994) Cumulative conception and livebirth rates after IVF, with and without pituitary desensitization with the gonadotropin-releasing hormone agonist, buserelin. *Am J Obstet Gynecol* **171**: 513–520.
45. Nygren KG & Andersen AN (2001) Assisted reproductive technology in Europe, 1998. Results generated from European registers by ESHRE. *Hum Reprod* **16**: 2459–2471.
46. Palermo G, Joris H, Devroey P & van Steirteghem AC (1992) Pregnancies after intracytoplasmic injection of a single spermatozoon into an oocyte. *Lancet* **340**: 17–18.
47. van Steirteghem A (1994) IVF and micromanipulation techniques for male factor infertility. *Curr Opin Obstet Gynecol* **6**: 173–177.

48. Alikani M, Cohen J & Palermo GD (1995) Enhancement of fertilisation by micromanipulation. *Curr Opin Obstet Gynecol* **7**: 182–187.
49. Braude P, Bolton V & Moore S (1988) Human gene expression first occurs between the four- and eight-cell stages of preimplantation development. *Nature* **332**: 459–461.
50. Brinsden PR, Appleton TC, Murray E, Hussein M, Akagboṣu F & Marcus SF (2000) Treatment by *in vitro* fertilisation with surrogacy: experience of one British centre. *BMJ* **320**: 924–929.
51. RCOG (2000) *The management of infertility in tertiary care.* RCOG Press, London.
52. Bonduelle M, Legein J, Derde M-P *et al.* (1995) Comparative follow-up study of 130 children born after intracytoplasmic sperm injection and 130 children born after *in vitro* fertilisation. *Hum Reprod* **10**: 3327–3331.
53. Sutcliffe AG, d'Souza SW, Cadman J, Richards B, McKinlay IA & Lieberman B (1995) Minor congenital anomalies, major congenital malformations and development in children conceived from cryopreserved embryos. *Hum Reprod* **10**: 3332–3337.
54. Tucker MJ, Morton PC, Sweitzer CL & Wright G (1995) Cryopreservation of human embryos and oocytes. *Curr Opin Obstet Gynecol* **7**: 188–192.

Further Reading

Devroey P (ed) (2001) *GnRH analogues.* Infertility and Reproductive Medicine Clinics of North America. WB Saunders, Philadelphia.

Chapter 14

The Human Fertilisation and Embryology Authority (HFEA)

Introduction

The Human Fertilisation and Embryology Authority (HFEA) of the UK was created in 1990 by the passage into law of the Human Fertilisation and Embryology (HFE) Act. Its principal tasks are to licence and monitor clinics that carry out IVF, donor insemination, and research on human embryos. The HFEA also regulates the storage of gametes (sperm and eggs) and embryos. By law, therefore, these procedures may only take place in clinics licenced by the HFEA.

The HFEA has other statutory functions. It must produce a Code of Practice which gives guidelines to clinics about the proper conduct of licenced activities, keep a formal register of information about donors, treatments, and children born from those treatments, publicize its own role, and provide relevant advice and information to patients, donors, and clinics. The HFEA must keep under review information about human embryos and their subsequent development and also the provision of treatment services and activities governed by the HFE Act.

The HFEA is a quasi-autonomous non-governmental organization (a quango) whose 24 members are appointed by the government of the day through the UK health ministers, according to Nolan guidelines. Its members are neither elected nor appointed as representatives of particular groups. By law, the chairman, deputy chairman, and at least half of the authority's members may not be involved in medical or scientific practice. The members determine the authority's policy and licence applications. The authority has an executive responsible for implementing its policy and licencing decisions and conducting its day-to-day activities. Seventy per cent of the HFEA's annual budget, presently capped at £1 559 000, is raised from license fees. Given the size of the industry the HFEA has been set up to regulate, this budget seems remarkably small. A recent business plan is set to increase both the fees and budget dramatically.

All licenced clinics require a "person responsible" who has specific responsibilities to ensure the conditions of its license are carried out. The centers must comply with a number of statutory requirements and with the HFEA's Code of Practice (see below). In evaluating a clinic, the HFEA is enjoined to consider all relevant interests – including those of patients, children, potential children, licenced clinics, and the wider public – and to take into account issues of safety, efficacy, and ethics. Licenses were originally renewed annually. However, the HFEA has now determined that established clinics can be issued with 3-year licenses, recognizing that a large proportion of clinics have been licenced for many years and that, in general, compliance with the law and the Code of Practice has been very good. A new clinic normally qualifies for a 3-year license only after it has achieved good compliance during its first 2 years.

Under the HFEA's 3-year inspection cycle, each center receives a broad-based general inspection by a full team once every 3 years, preceding renewal of its license. For interim or focused inspections, smaller teams are identified on a systematic basis, according to the nature and licencing history of the clinic. The team examines the clinic's compliance with the law, Code of Practice, and any directions previously made by the authority. It then submits a report to the license committee of the HFEA which determines whether or not a license is to be granted and whether any specific conditions are to be included. The authority may also undertake unannounced visits and visits arranged at short notice. There is not, however, a clearly defined structure for an inspection, neither do clinics have to adhere to nationally agreed clinical or laboratory operating protocols.

At the time of writing, 116 clinics are licenced by the HFEA for treatment and/or storage of gametes and embryos. Seventy-five are licenced for IVF and donor insemination (DI), 29 for DI alone. Nine clinics are licenced only for the storage of sperm. Satellite IVF (where clinical assessment, drug therapy, and monitoring take place at a secondary (satellite) center but egg retrieval, embryology, and embryo replacement are performed at a licenced primary center), and transport IVF (assessment, drug therapy, monitoring, and egg retrieval take place at the satellite center but embryology and embryo replacement at the primary center) do not in themselves require licencing. None the less centers offering these procedures need written agreements with each of the satellites defining which of them is responsible for assessment of welfare of the child, counseling, producing and providing patient information, as well as completion of the HFEA and other consent forms.

Practitioners should be aware of the implication of breaching the HFE Act, the directions of the HFEA, or the Code of Practice. Having made a preliminary inquiry about whether there is *prima facie* evidence of a breach, the HFEA may take specialist, including legal, advice. Its licence committee then decides on further action – and may refer matters to the Director of Public Prosecutions. At the time of writing, only two cases have been referred to the police and, one licence has been revoked, although several applications for new licences and variations to existing ones have been refused. There is an appeal procedure which takes the form of a re-hearing and both the clinic appealing and the licence committee can be represented. Ultimately there is right of appeal on points of law to the High Court.

The HFEA Register was started in 1991. It contains details of licenced treatments and patient characteristics for the whole of the UK and is now the largest database of its kind in the world. Since 1999 there has been a requirement to record additional information, especially regarding the storage of eggs and their subsequent use in treatment. Modification of its software is being introduced for secure electronic transfer of treatment data from clinics with a view to phasing out paper based input. The Register provides clinical data for the Annual Report, which, *inter alia*, provides an overview of national statistics of the outcome of licenced treatment. The Annual Report, Code of Practice and the HFEA's response to various issues are available free on its website (http://www.hfea.gov.uk). Publication of detailed, non-identifying data sets of treatments and their outcomes is planned for the near future. The HFEA has published a Patients' Guide to DI and IVF clinics since 1995. In response to requests from patients and others, the guide has been redesigned and separated into three booklets: *The Patients' Guide to Infertility and IVF*, *The Patients' Guide to IVF Clinics*, and *The Patients' Guide to DI*. The clinic data in these booklets are updated each year.

The HFEA maintains a manual for clinics, which provides guidance on completion of licence applications, details of the licencing process, representations and appeals procedures, the licence structures, Code of Practice, the information clinics are required to send to the HFEA, directions issued by the HFEA, and relevant regulations issued by Parliament. The Code of Practice is published, by law, by the HFEA, to guide clinics on how they should carry out their licenced activities. It includes guidance on: selection and screening of sperm donors; payment of expenses to donors; legal requirements for consent; handling and use of gametes and embryos; center staff and facilities; welfare of the child; and what information and counseling should be offered (Table 14.1).

The fifth revision of the Code of Practice was published in 2001. Each chapter of this comprehensive document is divided into a general section applicable to all individuals and specific sections for people seeking treatment, people providing gametes and embryos for donation, people seeking long-term storage of gametes, and people involved in egg sharing arrangements.

Embryo Research

All research on human embryos must be licenced by the HFEA. An application must be made for each project and applicants will need to

Table 14.1 HFEA Code of Practice

The headings in the fifth edition of the HFEA Code of Practice are as follows:
Staff Facilities Assessing people seeking treatment and welfare of the child Assessing and screening people considering donation Confidentiality Information Consent Counseling Use of gametes and embryos Storage of gametes and embryos Research Records Complaints

convince the HFEA that human embryos are necessary to fulfill the purposes of the investigation. Licences are only granted if the research is designed to promote advances in the treatment of infertility, increase knowledge about the causes of congenital disease, increase knowledge about the cause of miscarriage, develop more effective techniques for contraception or develop methods for detecting the presence of gene or chromosome abnormalities in embryos before implantation, increase knowledge about the development of embryos, increase knowledge about serious disease, or enable such knowledge to be applied in developing treatments for serious disease.

The following activities are prohibited by law: keeping or using an embryo after the appearance of the primitive streak or after 14 days, whichever is earlier; placing a human embryo in a non-human animal; replacing a nucleus of a cell of an embryo with a nucleus taken from the cell of another person or embryo; altering the genetic structure of any cell while it forms part of a human embryo.

As of August 2000, there had been 131 applications for research licenses since 1991; 31 of these were still ongoing. Most have been designed to improve treatment of infertility.

Social and Ethical Issues

Following public consultation, the HFEA concluded that, for infertility treatment, it is acceptable to use only tissue from live donors. It does not approve the use of oocytes obtained from adult cadavers nor the use of fetal ovarian tissue, although both sources are acceptable for embryo research. The ban on using fetal eggs and embryos in infertility treatment has been incorporated into the Criminal Justice and Public Order Bill so contravention of that ban would constitute a criminal offence.

The HFE Act states that no money or other benefit shall be given or received for the supply of gametes or embryos, unless authorized by directions. Donors may be paid up to £15 per donation (whether of sperm or oocytes) and reasonable expenses may be reimbursed. A maximum of 10 offspring may derived from a single sperm donor.

The statutory storage period for gametes and embryos is 10 and 5 years respectively. Regulations allow the storage period for sperm and embryos to be extended in certain circumstances.

Welfare of the Child

"The welfare of any child who may be born as a result of the treatment (including the need of that child for a father) and of any other child who may be affected by the birth" must be considered carefully before any treatment is offered. Although this injunction relates to the particular rules of licencing under the HFE Act, it is such an important position that in our opinion it should inform all types of infertility treatment. In the case of the HFE Act, the HFEA does not consider it precludes any particular category of patient from receiving treatment and so single or lesbian women, unmarried couples and postmenopausal women may all be treated. Factors that the HFEA, through its Code of Practice, recommends for consideration include:

1. The commitment of the woman and her partner to having and bringing up children
2. The ages and medical history of the partners
3. Risks, including inherited disorders, to the child to be born
4. The effect of a new baby on any existing child of the family.

Information

Licenced centers are obliged to provide details of treatment and its full cost, the likelihood of success, risks and side-effects, legal aspects (such as who will be the legal parents), availability of counseling and the need to consider the welfare of the child. One point that needs to be discussed about costs is who will pay for the drugs; many general practitioners now refuse to supply National Health Service prescriptions to patients undergoing IVF in private clinics.

Written information is essential and should be complemented by verbal explanation. The provision of understandable information is of course a prerequisite of obtaining informed consent.

Counseling

While there is an obligation on the clinics to provide counseling there is none on the patients to accept it. Counseling by trained professionals should be the aim. The Code recognizes three distinct types of counseling: implications counseling (to ensure the person understands the implications for themselves, their family, and for children born as a result of the proposed treatment), support counseling, and therapeutic counseling. The last includes helping people to adjust their expectations and to accept their situation. It may continue after the course of treatment has ended. Therapeutic counseling requires professional trained workers (see Ch. 5). The Code also recognizes the need for genetic counseling.

Consent

Written consent is required for centers to store gametes, to use them for IVF or the treatment of other women. Informed consent implies that the individual has been provided with relevant information and has had an opportunity to receive counseling. The HFEA has issued standard forms for consent both to treatment and for the use of gametes. In most cases it is appropriate to obtain consent from both partners. Anyone consenting to storage of gametes or embryos must specify the maximum period (normally 10 years) and what is to be done with the gametes or embryos if they themselves die or become incapable of varying or revoking their consent. Insemination with the late partner's or husband's sperm is permitted under the HFE Act but for it to take place the man must have given written consent for its posthumous use. It is important to realize that the Act states that such a man is not to be regarded in law as the father of offspring so produced.

Confidentiality

The HFE Act imposes a statutory limit on the disclosure of information so that, with a few exceptions, it is a criminal offence to disclose, without the consent of the individual, information about the treatment of any identifiable person by IVF or DI, storage of gametes or embryos from any identifiable person, or the identity of anyone born as a result of treatment. Information may, however, be disclosed in connection with legal proceedings, to the HFEA or to another licenced center in connection with treatment or to avert imminent danger to the health of the patient. The importance of the last reason is that it is permissible to supply information to the local hospital concerning the risks to a patient of developing, say, the ovarian hyperstimulation syndrome. Most clinics find it helpful to provide the couple with all the relevant information in the form of a letter which can then be used as they wish.

All personnel working in an assisted conception unit must be aware of the HFEA Code of Practice and, ideally, should have read it. Similarly all personnel who have access to identifying information have to appear on the clinic's licence, whether healthcare professional, scientist, administrator, secretary, receptionist, or cleaner.

Register of Information

The HFEA must by law keep a register of information about people undergoing licenced treatments and about donors. In order to compile this register, licenced clinics must provide the HFEA with specified information on all cycles of treatment by IVF or DI. The original purpose of this register was to inform adults (for these purposes defined as people over the age of 18, or 16 if they wish to marry) who ask whether they are related to someone they want to marry and to give people who are born as a result of the use of donated gametes some limited information about the donor.

Names of children born as a result of treatment are not collected. It is a criminal offense to reveal the identity of current or past donors, of patients, or their children.

Preimplantation Genetic Diagnosis (PGD)

PGD is used to detect whether an embryo created *in vitro* is carrying a genetic defect that will give rise to a serious inherited genetic disorder. It can also be used to determine the sex of an embryo where a family is at risk of passing on a serious sex-linked disorder, such as Duchenne's muscular dystrophy. Four centers are currently licenced to carry out PGD with one other center licenced only to carry out the embryo biopsy procedure.

The HFEA and the Advisory Committee on Genetic Testing (ACGT) (a body that has been absorbed by the newly created Human Genetics Commission (HGC)) issued a consultation paper on the issues surrounding the use of PGD at the end of 1999. In February 2002 the HFEA gave permission for an IVF clinic to use PGD and tissue typing to select an embryo free from a particular disease which would genetically match an existing relative. The particular circumstances of the case concerned the hopes of the parents of a 3-year-old boy with β thalassemia major, their wish being to create a child who could be a cell donor for his sick brother. The plan was to use PGD to select disease-free embryos followed by tissue typing to ensure a genetic match to the existing child. The parents' hope was that stem cells taken from the umbilical cord of the resulting baby could be transplanted into his brother to avoid his need for blood transfusion and marrow transplantation. While the outcome of the procedure is not known at the time of writing, several other couples have applied for permission to use these techniques for a variety of diseases. The HFEA plans to consider applications in which PGD is used for the sole benefit of a relative on a case by case basis.

Egg Freezing

The HFEA supports licencing of this procedure and allows frozen eggs to be used in IVF treatment. The HFEA has insisted that clinics offering this treatment must inform patients of any risks involved and also give clear information about the success rate (currently very low). Seven centers are currently licenced to carry out egg freezing.

Cloning (see also p. 373)

In 1998 the HFEA held a joint consultation with the Human Genetics Advisory Commission on human cloning. The ensuing report distinguished between reproductive cloning and *in vitro* work using cell nucleus replacement technology with a therapeutic aim. The report recommended that, while reproductive cloning should not take place, therapeutic cloning may hold promise for the treatment of serious illnesses. Specifically the report recommended to the Secretary of State that consideration should be given to specifying in regulations two further categories for which HFEA licenced embryo research may take place:

- Developing methods of therapy for mitochondrial diseases; and
- Developing methods of therapy for diseased or damaged tissues or organs.

In June 1999 the government announced the creation of an advisory group under the Chief Medical Officer to examine further the potential benefits, risks, and alternatives to therapeutic cloning. That group's recommendations were endorsed by the government in August 2000 and the following year Parliament agreed that its recommendations should be implemented.

Egg Sharing (see also p. 375)

Egg sharing is an arrangement whereby a woman receives free or subsidized IVF treatment in return for donating her surplus eggs. The HFEA permits egg sharing and has issued guidance on how it should be regulated. Its guidance is based on two general principles. The first requires that two separate agreements are prepared, one between the egg provider and the center and the other between the recipient and the center. The second principle concerns the treatment of the egg provider when only a few eggs are available. The guidance provides that, where there are fewer eggs collected than the minimum needed for sharing, the provider should be given the option of using all of her eggs at no additional cost to herself and with no further commitment. This principle must be reflected in the agreements between the center and the provider and recipient. The issues are discussed more fully in Chapter 15.

The address of the HFEA is: Paxton House, 30 Artillery Lane, London E1 7LS. Tel: 0207 377 5077 Fax: 0207 377 1871. Website: www.hfea.gov.uk

Chapter 15

Ethical issues

Introduction

In this book we do not offer a treatise on all aspects of the ethics of reproduction nor a prescription for each individual problem, but rather an attempt to indicate broad areas that are helpful to consider when responding to the ethical issues that often arise in infertility practice. Some of our discussion is general and reflects familiar issues of medical ethics. Some is particular to reproductive medicine and therefore requires knowledge of biology and reproductive technology.

The overall principles that inform any discussion of medical ethics include respect for the autonomy of the patient, together with the concepts of beneficence and justice. Respect for our patients' autonomy obliges us to ensure that those giving consent to treatment are fully informed and that confidentiality of their consultations is guaranteed. Beneficence involves considering the welfare of others and doing no harm. The problem, of course, is whose welfare we are talking about. For example, can zygotes and pre-embryos enjoy benefit or suffer harm? It is commonplace in infertility practice to place the physical harm risked by a potential mother against the psychological benefit that a successful outcome of treatment will bring to the couple, so we also have to think about the relative weight we apply to such benefit and harm.

When we turn to the issue of justice, we have to consider the fairness of the distribution of benefits and harm. We must also consider social and financial implications of fairness. Is a society behaving fairly when it makes the solution of a biological problem such as infertility only available to those who can afford it? There is no doubt that in the UK some health authorities regard IVF as a luxury form of treatment, on a parallel with the removal of tattoos and other cosmetic procedures.

Philosophically and politically speaking, beneficence is always uppermost for utilitarians. So far as the libertarian is concerned, the patient's autonomy dominates. For egalitarians justice is the driving force. Most people adopt a position that attempts to accommodate these principles in a kind of creative tension. Naturally, the extent to which any one of them is emphasized differs between individuals, groups and, indeed, countries. For example, in the USA, with its strong tradition of libertarianism, issues of autonomy often dominate over egalitarianism.

The overall feel of the American approach to infertility treatment is facilitative rather than regulatory and even now, so many years after the invention of IVF and with so many fertility-related ethical issues identified and medico-legal disputes exposed, the USA does not have a national agency for the regulation of assisted reproduction. On the other hand, policy in the UK has taken quite a proscriptive pathway and, as can be seen in Chapter 14, departures from the Code of Practice of the Human Fertilisation and Embryology Authority (HFEA) may breach the Criminal Justice Act and so be punishable under criminal law. It is worth reflecting on what has determined the difference between the increasingly regulated position developing in Europe compared with the situation in the USA and on whether the difference will have an impact on such vital subjects as the regulation of cloning and stem cell research.

Does Everyone Have a Right to Treatment?

Two issues that will always be central to any consideration of the ethics of reproduction are who has the right to reproduce and to what extent this right has to be balanced against the welfare of a child born as a result of the treatment. Generally speaking, in most societies a married heterosexual couple in a stable relationship is considered to provide the most appropriate environment for rearing children. On the other hand, most people recognize that legal marriage offers no guarantee of a suitable environment, and that couples and, some would argue, even individuals who are not married may not only assert a moral right to be parents but in fact provide a satisfactory environment in which to bring up children. While many people feel that some of the advanced technologies now employed in fertility therapy challenge the meaning of "family," the challenge does not really come from technology but rather from social changes which, in parts of the Western world, have resulted in divorce rates as high as 50%. There are increasing numbers of single parents who have conceived their children *per via naturalis*. The experience, therefore, of an increasing proportion of our population is of a family life that has not included all the traditional components. Increasingly fertility specialists are being asked to treat unmarried heterosexual couples, homosexual couples, and single women.

While few would wish to limit the rights of married couples to have children, concerns about duties to extracorporeal embryos and for the welfare of the offspring, the family, and the donors and surrogates have added strength when they also involve unmarried, single, or homosexual people requesting infertility treatment.[1–4] In the UK the view of the HFEA has been that, providing the medical team considers that the usual criteria in relation to the welfare of the child can be met (see

Ch. 14), there need be no proscription of such treatment for unmarried couples and single women. At the same time, it is also accepted that the moral discretion of those providing treatment has to be respected too and there is no legal obligation to treat.

Generally speaking, lesbian women have been refused fertility treatment (usually, of course, donor insemination) on the grounds that they would not provide an appropriate family environment because the child would have two mothers (but no father), would be genetically unrelated to one of the mothers, and the donor would be unknown to both of them. For single, heterosexual mothers, it has been argued that the lack of a father, together with the use of an anonymous donor, might lead to psychological difficulties for the child. People have questioned the suitability of a woman who is not involved in an intimate relationship with a man to be a mother. In fact, there are empirical data concerning these matters and the continuing studies of Golombok and Tasker have not indicated that such children are at any particular risk for psychological problems.[1] It is, after all, most likely that it is the quality of parenting that is important. In general, this seems very good in people undergoing fertility treatment. On the other hand, at present there are still few empirical data about the outcome of being conceived using semen from an anonymous donor or, indeed, from a known donor.

Biological Considerations

Much of the ethics of infertility therapy has been developed in response to advances in IVF technology. The principles are, none the less, firmly rooted and can often usefully be applied to other aspects of reproduction. It is necessary, however, to precede discussion with a brief reminder of the biology, so that the terminology clarifies rather than confuses. Such definition of terminology may also help in avoiding concepts that relate to a fetus (often derived from our thinking about termination of pregnancy) being applied to discussions about embryos and pre-embryos.

Fusion of *gametes* (sperm and egg) results in formation of the *zygote*, the fertilized egg which has the potential to develop into a human being to whom ultimately the full status and rights of a citizen are accorded. Only a quarter to a third of zygotes are thought to develop into a newborn infant. The full developmental potential of a zygote is therefore limited by the risks of prenatal development, childbirth, childhood, and early adult life. The statistics of these risks are, of course, influenced by many factors. Some of them are quite unknown but others are related to circumstances which are entirely within our own gift. Examples would be the extent to which a person's potential is eroded by poverty, an inclement environment, malnutrition, pollution, poor schooling, disease, etc.

The zygote undergoes cleavage to produce the eight cell *blastomere*, further development of which produces an outer layer, which is extraembryonic and becomes the placenta, and an inner layer, which becomes the embryo. It is the blastocyst whose outer layer loses its pluripotentiality first and interacts with the mother. In the second week after fertilization, the inner cell mass is organized first into two and then into three layers, with the development of the primitive streak. It is at this stage that the pre-embryo is committed, in the sense that it loses its capacity to undergo twinning. The zygote and early blastocyst are, therefore, pre-embryonic but it is the embryo which is the rudiment of the whole unique human being. Uniqueness is firmly established when the *embryonic axis* is formed about 2 weeks after fertilization and, after this, twinning and mosaicism are thought not to occur.

Moral Status of the Pre-embryo

When we consider the issue of the status to be accorded to the products of conception, it is clear that there are at least two opposed positions (by status, one means the accepted manner in which an individual is treated within society). In most pluralistic societies, status is progressive in the sense that a hierarchy is accepted in which progressive status is given to gametes, the zygote, the pre-embryo, the embryo, the fetus, and then finally to the newborn infant. In some traditions (notably the Roman Catholic Church) full status is accorded to the zygote. When the latter position is adopted, it becomes easy to understand why any kind of manipulation of pre-embryos is unacceptable.

The moral status of human pre-embryos may be viewed in three ways. The first, as mentioned immediately above, is that full human status is accorded from the moment of fertilization. The arguments in favor of this position are that a new genotype has been established at the point of fertilization and some of these zygotes will develop into full-term babies and adult humans whose autonomy requires protection throughout life. An alternative and equally polarized position is that the fertilized egg has no moral status whatsoever and that, of course, means we have no obligations to it at all. Arguments in favor of this point of view are that, at best, only 40% of pre-embryos that have been produced naturally develop into live infants; that, as described above, biological individuality is not established until the development of the primitive streak and, finally, that the pre-embryo is an undifferentiated entity, made up of cells which are each totipotent. This collection of cells is without limbs, organs, or sentience.

Not surprisingly, there is a third position which accords "some moral status" to the pre-embryo because of its unique genotype and its potential to develop into a sentient human being. This attitude differentiates the pre-embryo from a collection of cells that form a tissue, for example, a piece of skin (skin cells are not embryonic). It must be accepted, however, that this intermediate position is not without its own problems. While it obliges one to strive to improve the medicine of infertility therapy, the very notion of improvement implies a sense that we may value one pre-embryo over another. Life is, therefore, not seen as a gift with its own intrinsic value, but a gift of *potential* significance which can be modified or disposed of if it does not meet some notion of quality. From this perspective one can see how rapidly the very first elements of life may be developed into a commodity. That this is not merely a theoretical notion is illustrated by events that took place in the UK in the summer of 1996 when, as a result of fertility therapy (ovulation induction, not IVF), a woman became pregnant with eight fetuses. A contract between the pregnant woman and a national newspaper was made, such that in return for her story, she would receive £125 000 per delivered fetus. It is this fear that a fertilized human egg will become a means to another end, a commodity, rather than an end in itself (that is, a child wanted for its own sake) that underlies much public anxiety surrounding cloning and the use of embryonic stem cells.

Is IVF Ethical?

So far as the major religions are concerned, IVF and embryo transfer are acceptable within the framework of a marital relationship to Judaism, Islam, part of Christianity, Hinduism, and Buddhism. The Roman Catholic Church considers that, for the reasons indicated above, IVF involves a disregard for the sanctity of human life (life being defined here as starting at the moment of fertilization). Moreover, the IVF procedure separates procreation from sexual union, i.e., it takes it away from an act of love. Other objections that have been raised to the IVF procedure are that it involves the possibility of harm to the progeny, i.e., it involves exposing others (the pre-embryo) to a risk of harm for which consent has not (cannot) been obtained. Even if we apply the hierarchical view of the status of the products of conception elaborated above, we have to accept that the resulting child has accepted a risk, in part at least, for the benefit of its parents.

It has been argued that IVF is but one step down a slippery slope which will permit strange variants of the procedure which themselves will not prove acceptable. "Slippery slope" arguments are, of course, the very stuff of philosophy and, in our opinion, do not constitute a very powerful argument against IVF. They do, though, emphasize the importance of thinking through its implications. It has also been argued that since infertility is not life threatening, we should not permit medicalization of what is not seen as a medical problem. In our opinion, the view that medical therapy is only to be used for life-threatening conditions is nonsense. Few medical interventions are life saving, although it is to be hoped that all bring comfort. A general objection often raised is that IVF involves the use of medical resources to provide more offspring to an overpopulated world. In our view, this sets a perceived need of that vague entity, the world, to have fewer people against the immediate and actual right of an individual family to fulfill its reproductive potential.

In accord, then, with most of the major bodies that have offered opinions on the subject (the Ethical Committee of FIGO, the American Society of Reproductive Medicine,[5] the HFEA, and the majority of religions), we consider that IVF is ethically acceptable. It has to be recognized, though, that the major religions find third-party involvement in fertility therapy objectionable.

Experiments on Human Pre-embryos, Cloning and Stem Cell Research

No one approves of experiments on people who have not given their consent so one of the fundamental questions about research on pre-embryos is concerned with our notion of when the products of conception become human. For those who believe that the sanctity of human life begins with fertilization of an egg, experiments on pre-embryos cannot be considered. For those who consider that development of the primitive streak marks the stage at which the pre-embryo is committed (see p. 370) experimentation up to this stage – i.e. 14 days after fertilization – is acceptable. Differences between those who advocate and those who forbid experiments on the products of conception are therefore not so much ethical, more to do with when human life is perceived to have become established.

On the other hand, the possibility of creating children as a result of experimental manipulation of human gametes has alarmed most people and almost every country that has passed legislation on assisted human reproduction has banned human reproductive cloning on pain of severe penalties. There are several reasons underlying this fear, first and foremost of which is recognition that in the present state of knowledge it is not safe to use such techniques to create a human being. Even if our worries about safety could be resolved there remain significant concerns about the impact of cloning technology on individuals and society.

Clones are defined as a group of living organisms sharing the same nuclear gene set. They are essentially monozygotic twins formed by biological manipulation.[6] In animals two experimental methods have been used to produce cloned embryos: nuclear splitting and nuclear transfer. It is the latter which has been the subject of most of the published debate because it offers the possibility of creating a cloned embryo with a nucleus from a chosen source. The possibility therefore exists of manipulating the nuclear genome before transferring it to the enucleated oocyte, so creating an animal with a genome that can serve medical needs, for example one that produces large quantities of a protein needed for clinical purposes. The science of animal cloning is still in its infancy with many practical issues remaining unresolved at the time of writing.

Most countries have banned human reproductive cloning but the position with regard to the creation of cloned embryos for therapeutic purposes (essentially to obtain stem cells) is still evolving. Stem cells are tissue precursors which have two contrasting abilities: they can self renew and they can differentiate into more specialized cell types. In the embryo, stem cells are pluripotent, capable of giving rise to any of the 200 or so human cell types. In the adult, stem cells are more committed (termed multipotent) and their differentiation more restricted. In general their ability to self renew is inversely related to the degree of differentiation. Stem cell therapy is not new (it has been used in bone marrow transplantation and in the treatment of Parkinson's disease for some years), but it is the potential use of stem cells obtained from human blastocysts created *in vitro* that has occasioned concern. The debate is largely concerned with the extent to which we consider human embryos and fetuses have a right to protection, a debate that rehearses many of the issues raised earlier in this chapter concerning the moral status we accord the human embryo.[7,8] There is a further concern over the potential commercialization of unborn humans – creating human embryos to save lives is one thing, creating them to make money quite another.

While there are biological advantages of using fetal and embryonic stem cells (for example, they can be obtained relatively free of contamination from other cells, they have the potential to multiply indefinitely in the laboratory so one cell line might be able to treat many patients, theoretically they can be directed to differentiate into any of the cell types the patient might need), ethical and logistical concerns mean that studies of stem cells derived from adult tissues continue to be required. Stem cell research using human embryos was approved in the UK by Parliament in 2001 by an extension of the Human Fertility and Embryology Act; its regulation is currently being addressed by the HFEA.

Donors and Donation

Donor sperm, donor oocytes, and donor embryos have become an integral part of the modern management of infertility and nearly 18 000 babies have been born as a result of donations since the HFEA register was set up in 1991. Indications for the various donations go beyond the management of infertility and now include families with genetic disorders. Oocyte donation is usually performed for women without gonadal function (i.e., those with premature ovarian failure) or for those who do have intact gonadal function but who have inherited diseases that can be avoided by oocyte donation. Conditions requiring embryo donation include infertility, habitual abortion, and genetic diseases. The interests of the child, the recipients, and the donors must all be considered. In some countries donation of genetic material to single women is forbidden and, where the practice is allowed, regulations cover the relationships between biological and social parents, the banking and disposal of genetic material, the interests of the child, and the maintenance of medical records (see Ch. 14 for the position in the UK).

An important issue concerning third-party involvement in infertility treatment is that of payment to donors or, indeed, to surrogates.[4] A number of approaches can be considered. In France and New Zealand such donations are seen as genuine gifts, a public service performed with no thought of compensation either in the form of a reward or even for expenses. The position is similar to that for blood donation in the UK. An alternative is payment for expenses but not for the donation itself. Another possibility is that the donor receives a reasonable reward as recompense for the time, pain (egg donors only), and inconvenience of the donation, processes which clearly vary between men, women, and surrogates. Suggestions have been made that a reward be given for gametes, for pre-embryos or, indeed, for infants.

We think it unlikely that anyone would have difficulty in rejecting the idea of payment for an infant. Payment for a pre-embryo implies no respect for its humanity and payment for gametes dehumanizes them and turns them into a commodity. The Ethics Committee of the American Society of Reproductive Medicine accepts as ethical a reasonable reward for time and inconvenience, etc. In the UK payment may be made for reasonable expenses together with a small sum (£15) for the donation.

A recent development in the field of gamete provision is a procedure its originators have termed "egg sharing." This is an arrangement whereby a woman obtains free or subsidized IVF treatment in return for donating her surplus eggs. The procedure, which has been fueled by the universal scarcity of volunteer egg donors, has certainly resulted in an increase in the number of women who require egg donation being treated. Its proponents argue that since the donor is already undergoing treatment, egg sharing obviates the need for healthy volunteers to undergo ovarian stimulation and oocyte retrieval and so avoids placing them at risk from these procedures. Moreover, it is argued, the arrangement avoids "wasting" surplus but precious human eggs.

As mentioned in Chapter 14, the egg-sharing procedure is accepted by the HFEA, providing certain practical procedures are adhered to. We, however, do not find the arguments in favor of egg sharing particularly persuasive. First, the donor is required to provide her eggs in return for receiving a service she would otherwise have to pay for, raising straight away concern about the potential exploitation of those who yearn for a treatment they cannot afford. We cannot but note wryly its proponents' use of the term "sharing" to describe a situation in which a commodity is given as barter for a course of medical treatment. It does seem to us that at least some of the eggs retrieved (i.e., those provided in return for payment for the course of treatment the donor is undergoing) may be regarded as closer to means (in this case subsidized IVF) than to ends. The HFEA's guidelines do specifically address management of the case in which the donor's ovaries do not produce sufficient eggs for "sharing" to proceed (see Ch. 14). On the other hand, it is not difficult to imagine a scenario in which both doctor and potential egg provider might be tempted, albeit for different reasons, to elect for more powerful treatment than would have been required if simple IVF were being performed.

Gamete donation is anonymous in the UK, except when it has been intentionally undertaken between people who know each other. The Human Fertilisation and Embryology Act 1990 makes unauthorized disclosure of donors' names a criminal offense with a maximum penalty of 2 years' imprisonment and a fine. Moreover the law does not allow children who apply for information from the HFEA register to know the identity of current or past donors. The only people allowed to know a donor's name are members and employees of the HFEA and staff covered by an HFEA license at the clinic or storage center. In recent years, however, there has been considerable pressure from some of the people born as a result of donated gametes to learn more about their genetic origins. They point to the anomaly that adopted children gain the right of information about their birth parents but that children born from donor gametes are denied it. There can be little doubt that for some people their sense of personal identity is distressingly incomplete without this knowledge, a situation revealingly described by George Eliot in the Victorian novel *Daniel Deronda*. In present times one has only to consider the promises held out by the Human Genome Project to understand the health implications of withholding from people information about their genetic provenance. We find it difficult therefore to understand how the welfare of the child is best served by denying that person such fundamental information. Arguments about protecting the donor seem to have had little purchase when applied to birth parents of adoptees and there seems no reason why donors could not be afforded the same legal protection that they have. For many clinicians the most compelling reason for anonymity has been the fear that if donors were to have their identity revealed, they would cease to donate. This argument seems to us to prioritize the maintenance of a treatment program and the procreation of future children over the needs of existing people, to place the needs of the adults involved in assisted conception programs over the interests and rights of the children born through their efforts. There are, moreover, empirical data to show that, where access to donor information has been made available, the service has not collapsed, rather there has been a shift in the donor population away from students and toward older men who have completed their families. We would argue therefore for a change in the law to bring the right to information of children born as a result of donated gametes into line with that of adopted children. It goes without saying that this proposal refers only to future donors and that assurances of anonymity given to past and existing donors would continue to be honored.

Sex Selection

About 300 genetic diseases have thus far been linked to the X chromosome. Some are rare but others, like the fragile X syndrome, are among the most common genetic disorders causing mental retardation. Women carriers of an X-linked recessive disease have a one in four chance of having an affected child and a one in two chance if the child is a boy. If the child is a girl she would not be affected but would have a one in two chance of being a heterozygote and therefore a carrier of the disease.

Prenatal sex selection may be undertaken by sorting sperm, by preimplantation identification of the sex of the embryo, or by aborting a fetus of the sex which carries the disorder. While most people find sex selection for medical reasons acceptable, there are issues to be considered, such as the severity of the condition to be prevented.

Prenatal sex selection for non-medical reasons is a very different matter. The major religions oppose the procedure because, *inter alia*, it is seen to interfere with a divine plan. Two sets of non-religious arguments may also be considered. The first is, who has the right to decide what sort of people there should be? The second considers the consequences of sex selection: would it, for example, unbalance the sex ratio of the next generation? It would certainly have to be applied on a very wide scale to do so. We consider that in Western society more pressing arguments concern the commodification of life. Treating one sex as more desirable than another, to the point of prenatal sex selection, is to value one sex (the commodity) above life itself. It breaches the fundamental concept of equality of respect for men and women.

Fetal Reduction

The prognosis for a multiple pregnancy to be delivered successfully falls dramatically as the number of fetuses increases. Selective reduction of multifetal pregnancy is the procedure by which an attempt is made to save some of the fetuses by destruction of the others. It is usually performed in the first trimester. The associated rate of pregnancy loss is 8–15% in experienced centers. Controversy exists about the value of the procedure in triplet pregnancies but it clearly improves the perinatal outcome for women carrying four or more fetuses.

The use of the euphemistic term "selective reduction" rather than "selective abortion" indicates straight away how uncomfortable many people feel with this procedure.[9] None the less, it is important to bear in mind that, in the UK at least, some 400 abortions are performed every day. With fetal reduction the principle is to sacrifice one or more potentially normal lives so that the others will have a better chance to survive and lead healthy lives. The analogy of the overfilled lifeboat has been used – drowning people can legitimately be denied access to a dangerously filled lifeboat if bringing them aboard would result in the loss of additional lives. In the context of IVF, the number of multiple pregnancies and, therefore, the issue of selective abortion will be greatly reduced by adherence to the advice to transfer no more than 2–3 embryos. It is likely, however, that as a result of ovulation induction, cases where the procedure has to be considered will continue to occur.

Should Older Women be Offered IVF?

The most important determinant of the outcome of infertility treatment is the patient's age, so IVF becomes, like all other forms of treatment for infertility, less efficacious as the woman ages. The most important reason, therefore, for not offering older women IVF has little to do with ethics and everything to do with the very poor outcome of such treatment. The parallel is with not recommending coronary angioplasty to people who continue to smoke – there is no ethical objection to performing the procedure, merely the knowledge that continuing to smoke heavily so changes the ratio of risk to benefit that no advantage is gained from having the operation. In the case of IVF, a take-home baby rate of 1–3% is achieved in women over the age of 40.

The major debate about infertility treatment for older women concerns the issue of egg donation.[10] Here the impact of aging on fertility is avoided because that impact is predominantly exerted on the oocyte. The excellent results of oocyte donation in general have encouraged clinicians, and indeed patients, to believe that there need be no upper biological age limit to pregnancies achieved in this way.

There are empirical data describing the outcome of pregnancies achieved by oocyte donation in women past the usual age of the menopause. Broadly speaking, the risks to mother and baby are few and usually fully acceptable to the mother. So far as the child is concerned, the point is sometimes made that the life expectancy of its parents will be less than a child should normally expect. This argument should be seen in the context of children born into families of a more usual age, in which one or other of the parents dies.

Is it wrong for a woman to seek treatment if she knows that she will not be able to cope well with being a mother? We could consider it wrong if her becoming a mother is unjust, that is, if it infringes the child's rights. But the child is not really wronged because it cannot be born to other or better parents. The question that should be asked then is, "Are the interests of the potential child better served if he or she is born to a mother over the age of 50 or are they better served if the child never existed at all?" As there is no possibility of the potential child being born to any other parents, it becomes clear that there are very few situations indeed where it would be better not to be born. The very same argument applies to a reduced life expectancy resulting in the premature death of one's mother; to deny fertility treatment for that reason would be to suggest that it would be better never to have existed than for one's mother to have died when one was young. The conclusion then is that it is rarely right to withhold fertility treatment on the grounds of the interests of the potential child not being served.

Should People who are HIV Positive be Offered Infertility Therapy?

Most women who are HIV positive are of reproductive age and many of the risk factors that are linked to HIV infection (for example, unsafe sexual practices) may predispose them to infertility. In considering management of infertility in these patients, issues to be considered include the risk of mother-to-child transmission, the risk that the mother will die before the child reaches majority and, in couples who are discordant for the infection, the risk that the woman will become infected by intercourse with her partner without barrier protection (and then transmit the infection to her child).

In the early days of the AIDS epidemic around 25% of HIV positive women who gave birth transmitted the virus to their children. The prognosis for infected children was grim and those that were uninfected were likely to be orphaned very young. It seemed obvious then that treatment of infertility was inappropriate and guidelines issued by the American Society of Reproductive Medicine in the early 1990s reflected that point of view. Fortunately modern treatment for HIV infected women has changed the picture quite dramatically, although at the time of writing there has been no revision of the published advice not to treat the infertility of such patients. So what is the position now?

Recent studies indicate that when delivery by Cesarean section is combined with zidovudine therapy and the avoidance of breastfeeding, the rate of mother-to-child transmission falls to around 2%. The prognosis for infected children and infected mothers has improved substantially and will presumably continue to do so.[11] Seroconversion of women partners of HIV positive men who have had insemination with washed sperm has been reported only once and that many years ago. There are now reports of more than 2000 inseminations with washed sperm (pregnancy rate per insemination 14%) with no seroconversions in mother or child.[12] It is clear therefore that progress in the management of HIV infection in relation to infertility has been sufficiently reassuring to mean that for many patients in this situation indications for infertility treatment need not depart from those in uninfected couples. On the other hand, particularities of management will still have to take account of the severity of the HIV infection, co-morbidities such as infection, addiction, etc., and risks that the infection will be transmitted.

Conclusions

Many other ethical issues frequently arise in infertility practice but we do not consider their detailed discussion is feasible in a book primarily aimed at clinical management. Rather it is our hope that the discussions outlined here will provide a framework for considering the numerous ethical judgments that face us in everyday practice. A few examples: who owns gametes and embryos and who should decide their fate? What are the implications of the advances in preimplantation diagnosis; are there limits to the extent that we should change nature? Are there indeed limits to parental choice; what is our attitude, for example, to patients with say achondroplasia or congenital deafness who wish to have a child with the same condition? Should women be inseminated with their dead husband's sperm? To what extent should surrogacy be used to provide children for couples biologically unable to conceive, for example homosexual men? We may be sure that with the speed of developments in medical technology few of these problems will remain matters for armchair contemplation for very long. The reader is encouraged to prepare before such problems feature in the next consultation.

References

1. Golombok S & Tasker F (1994) Donor insemination for single heterosexual and lesbian women: issues concerning the welfare of the child. *Hum Reprod* **9**: 1972–1976.
2. Debate (1994) Artifical insemination of single women and lesbian women with donor sperm. *Hum Reprod* **9**: 1969–1971.
3. Englert Y (1994) Artificial insemination with donor semen: particular requests. *Hum Reprod* **9**: 1969–1971.
4. Shenfield F (1994) Particular requests in donor insemination: comments on the medical duty of care and the welfare of the child. *Hum Reprod* **9**: 1976–1977.
5. Ethics Committee of the American Fertility Society (1994) Ethical considerations of assisted reproductive technologies. *Fertil Steril* **62**(Suppl. 1).
6. Edwards RG & Beard HK (1998) How identical would cloned children be? An understanding essential to the ethical debate. *Hum Reprod Update* **4**: 791–811.
7. Weissman IH (2002) Stem cells – scientific, medical and political issues. *N Engl J Med* **346**: 1576–1579.
8. Evers K (2002) European perspectives on therapeutic cloning. *N Engl J Med* **346**: 1579–1582.
9. Birkowitz RL (1994) From twin to singleton. *Br Med J* **313**: 373–374.
10. Discussion (1994) An ethical debate: should older women be offered *in vitro* fertilisation? *Br Med J* **310**: 1455–1457.
11. Minkoff H & Santoro N (2000) Ethical considerations in the treatment of infertility in women with human immunodeficiency virus infection. *N Engl J Med* **342**: 1748–1750.
12. Gilling-Smith C (2000) Assisted reproduction in HIV discordant couples. *AIDS Reader* **10**: 581–587.

Further Reading

Boyle RJ & Savulescu J (2001) Ethics of using preimplantation genetic diagnosis to select a stem cell donor for an existing person. *Br Med J* **323**: 1240–1243.

Surean C & Shenfield F (1995) *Ethical aspects of human reproduction*. John Libbey & Co., London.

Chapter 16

Follow-up of children born from assisted reproduction techniques

Introduction

With approximately 1% of children in the developed world being born as a result of assisted reproduction techniques, it is essential that we evaluate their physical and emotional/psychological development. In so doing we must take into consideration their origins:

- Manipulated gametes, e.g., IVF itself, or intracytoplasmic sperm injection (ICSI)
- Cryopreserved gametes or embryos
- Donated gametes or embryos
- Surrogacy
- Non-heterosexual unions, e.g., donor insemination of single or lesbian women.

Manipulated Gametes

IVF and ICSI involve ovarian stimulation with collection of several oocytes, using drug regimens of variable complexity (see Ch. 13). The oocytes are then either placed together with sperm (IVF) or injected with sperm (ICSI). The gametes and consequent embryos are cultured, in specified culture media, usually for 2 days prior to embryo transfer, which may be changed and refreshed if culture is continued through to the blastocyst stage before embryo transfer.

The various drugs used in assisted conception have not been associated with congenital anomalies or adverse fetal outcome – and indeed result in healthy babies when used in the context of ovulation induction for anovulatory infertility. The main concern centers around the artificial selection of gametes and embryos, the effects of micromanipulation techniques, and the possible effects of embryo culture conditions.

In Vitro Fertilization

One of the difficulties when comparing the outcome of children born as a result of assisted conception with those conceived naturally is the high rate of multiple pregnancy with fertility treatments, which inevitably results in an increase in premature delivery and handicap (see Ch. 17). Some studies have, however, reported that even singleton IVF pregnancies have higher complication rates than natural singletons, although this may be secondary to maternal characteristics (e.g., increased age and underlying medical problems that resulted in subfertility) rather than the IVF technology itself. None the less, IVF singleton babies do appear to be at increased risk of being born prematurely and of being small for gestational age.[1,2]

A study from Sweden evaluated every child born as a result of IVF between 1982 and 1995.[3] There were approximately 6000 children, of whom 27% were from multiple pregnancies. Of the singleton pregnancies 2.6% were born before 32 weeks and 11.2% before 37 weeks, compared with 0.7% and 5.4% respectively in the general population. There was also a significantly smaller birthweight in the IVF babies when adjusted for duration of gestation. Interestingly, however, for a given birthweight, IVF babies were more likely to survive the perinatal period than naturally conceived babies. Twin IVF babies had similar outcomes to twin non-IVF babies.

Most studies from various countries (France, Israel, North America) have indicated that IVF does not increase the rate of congenital malformations or abnormal karyotype.[4–8] There was, however, a significantly increased risk of congenital malformations in the Swedish study,[3] with a risk ratio of 1.44 (95% CI 1.25–1.65) – with a risk ratio in singletons of 1.25 (1.07–1.46) and in multiples of 1.08 (0.93–1.25). There were more cases of neural-tube defects and esophageal atresia than expected, although the rate of neural tube defects was also higher in an Australian study[9] and esophageal atresia may be more prevalent in children of women with infertility for reasons that are unclear. These anomalies also appear more commonly in twins, irrespective of mode of conception.[10] A further study from Finland has reported a higher than expected rate of heart malformations – specifically septal defects – in IVF babies, when corrected for multiplicity, with a four-fold increase compared with a control group.[11] The authors suggest that reproductive ability with differing levels of maternal hormones may have an adverse effect on cardiac development. It is difficult to know how to interpret these studies, as surveillance of IVF pregnancies is often more intense than usual and couples who have conceived through assisted reproduction may be less inclined to terminate a pregnancy when an anomaly is detected antenatally. The overall conclusion is that it is probably maternal characteristics (age, subfertility factors, and concurrent disease) that influence the outcome of IVF rather than the IVF treatment itself.[12] It is essential that this topic continues to be kept under review.

When assessing the later development of children, it is first important to note that the rates of childhood cancer after IVF appear to be similar to the general population.[3,13] Most studies have reported psychomotor development in children to be normal (reviewed in Olivennes *et al.*).[12] Psychological development also appears to be normal and in some cases may be better than average, perhaps because of a higher level of parental input and/or expectation. Caution has been expressed, however, about over-protectiveness not always resulting in better well-being of the child.[14–16] A detailed study of children born from IVF at age 2–3 years, followed up to the age of 8–9 years, found no significant difference in psychosocial development when compared with a control group.[17] This and other studies dealt with singletons in order to make for easier comparison with controls. Twins and triplets of course bring with them additional problems for the family unit and can result in major stress, disharmony, and the potential for poor long-term outcome (see Ch. 17).

Intracytoplasmic Sperm Injection

As with standard IVF pregnancies, there is a high rate of multiple pregnancy with ICSI and this will have an adverse effect on perinatal outcome and congenital anomalies. The current evidence indicates that ICSI itself leads to a slight but statistically significant increase in de novo sex chromosome aneuploidy (0.6% rather than 0.2%), structural autosomal abnormalities (0.4% rather than 0.07%), and structural chromosomal aberrations inherited from the infertile father.[18] The rate of congenital malformations and developmental outcome of ICSI children appears to be the same as the normal and IVF populations.

The ICSI technique is of course usually used when there are significant male fertility problems, which may in themselves have genetic origins. Thus it is hardly surprising that structural chromosomal anomalies are transmitted from father to son. The ICSI process adds a further dimension, as a single spermatozoon are selected by the embryologist on morphological criteria, thereby bypassing the process of natural selection, which occurs both with spontaneous conception and with standard IVF. The ICSI technique may result in damage to the oocyte and also the injection of a small amount of culture medium along with the sperm. The unit in Brussels which developed ICSI has itself kept a comprehensive follow-up of children and co-ordinated a European database.[18] The incidence of major malformations in the general population is 2–3%. The Brussels survey has revealed an incidence of major malformations of 3.4% (96/2840 live born children) – 3.1% in singleton and 3.7% in multiple pregnancies.[19] When pregnancies that were terminated were included, the overall major malformation rate was 4.2%. There has been debate about this data, with a paper suggesting inappropriate classification of some cardiac anomalies as being minor rather than major,[20] yet these have been unsubstantiated.[19] Another large series, from Sweden, found a reassuring odds ratio of 1.19 (95% CI 0.79–1.81) for all minor and major malformations after stratification for maternal age and multiplicity of pregnancy.[21] There was, however, a slightly increased rate of hypospadias in male infants, which might relate to the underlying male factor problems.

With respect to longer-term development of children born from ICSI, the data are largely reassuring, with both the Belgian series[22] and a case control series of singleton children from the UK[23] indicating no difference from the normal or IVF conceived populations. A report from Australia, however, showed delayed development in memory, problem-solving, and language skills, particularly in boys[24] – although concerns were expressed about whether the control group was matched appropriately. In general the data are reassuring but long-term surveillance of outcome is obligatory.

Cryopreserved Gametes or Embryos

There is no evidence that the cryopreservation of gametes or embryos has a detrimental effect on subsequent fetal or childhood development.[12,25,26] Furthermore, it has been found that the risk for premature delivery is lower with cryopreserved than fresh embryos.[3]

Donated Gametes or Embryos

Physical development and the risk of congenital anomalies are the same as the general population. The main concerns center around lack of disclosure of parental origins, in which case there is only likely to be a problem if accidental disclosure occurs at some time in the future. Alternatively, when there has been disclosure there may be extreme unhappiness at not being able to trace one's genetic origins, as is currently the situation in the UK. This is a controversy which is yet to be resolved as it reaches to the core of current gamete donation practice, which is very much altruistic in the case of oocyte donation (other than when there is egg sharing – see Ch. 8) and often financially motivated in the case of sperm donation.

Surrogacy

As mentioned in Chapter 13, surrogacy works well provided thorough counseling is undertaken prior to the selection of the surrogate host. It is certainly our experience and that of others that outcomes are positive for both the surrogate's own family and that of the commissioning couple.

Non-heterosexual Unions, e.g., Donor Insemination of Single or Lesbian Women

In the UK, the Human Fertilisation and Embryology Authority (HFEA) states that when considering the welfare of children born as a result of assisted conception techniques, consideration should be given to the right for a child to have a father. This is not to say that single women or lesbian couples should not be treated with donor insemination but careful counseling should be provided first. The evidence to date indicates that children conceived in such circumstances are psychologically well adjusted, well cared for, and have the same rate of homosexuality as the general population (see recent review by Baetens & Brewaeys).[27]

Follow-up of children born from assisted reproduction techniques – key points

- The major causes of neonatal and developmental problems after assisted conception techniques are multiple pregnancy and prematurity.
- Minor and major congenital anomalies are similar to the normal population after IVF, ICSI, and the use of cryopreserved gametes and embryos.
- ICSI is associated with a slightly increased rate of chromosomal anomalies, which may be due both to the procedure and the underlying paternal abnormalities that necessitated ICSI.

References

1. Doyle P, Beral V & Maconochie N (1992) Preterm delivery, low birth weight and small for gestational weight in liveborn singleton babies resulting from *in vitro* fertilization. *Hum Reprod* **7**: 425–428.
2. Tanbo T, Dale P, Lunde O, Moe N & Abyholm T (1995) Obstetric outcome in singleton pregnancies after assisted reproduction. *Obstet Gynecol* **86**: 188–192.
3. Bergh T, Ericson A, Hillensjo T, Nygren K-G & Wennerholm U-B (1999) Deliveries and children born after *in vitro* fertilization in Sweden 1982–1995: a retrospective cohort study. *Lancet* **354**: 1579–1585.
4. FIVNAT (1995) Pregnancies and births resulting from *in vitro* fertilization: French national registry, analysis of data 1986–1990. *Fertil Steril* **64**: 746–756.
5. Friedler S, Mashiach S & Laufer N (1992) Births in Israel resulting from *in vitro* fertilization/embryo transfer, 1982–1989. National Registry of the Israeli Association for Fertility Research. *Hum Reprod* **7**: 1159–1163.
6. SART Registry (1999) Assisted reproductive technology in the United States: 1996 results generated from the American Society for Reproductive Medicine/Society for Assisted Reproductive Technology Registry. *Fertil Steril* **71**: 798–807.
7. Shoham Z, Zosmer A & Insler V (1991) Early miscarriage and fetal malformation after induction of ovulation by clomiphene citrate and/or human menotropins. *Fertil Steril* **55**: 1–11.
8. Westergard HB, Johansen AM, Erb K & Andersen AN (1999) Danish national *in vitro* fertilization registry 1994 and 1995: a controlled study of births, malformations and cytogenetic findings. *Hum Reprod* **14**: 1896–1902.
9. Lancaster P (1987) Congenital malformations after *in vitro* fertilization. *Lancet* **330**: 1392–1393.

10. Doyle P, Beral V, Botting B & Wale C (1991) Congenital malformations in twins in England and Wales. *J Epidemiol Commun Health* **45**: 43–48.
11. Koivurova S, Hartikainen A-L, Gissler M, Hemminki E, Sovio U & Jarvelin M-R (2002) Neonatal outcome and congenital malformations in children born after IVF. *Hum Reprod* **17**: 1391–1398.
12. Olivennes F, Fanchin R, Ledee N, Righini C, Kadoch IJ & Frydman R (2002) Perinatal outcome and developmental studies on children born after IVF. *Hum Reprod Update* **8**: 117–128.
13. Bruinsma F, Venn A, Lancaster P, Speirs A & Healy D (2000) Incidence of cancer in children born after *in vitro* fertilization. *Hum Reprod* **15**: 604–607.
14. Golombok S (1997) Parenting and secrecy issues related to children of assisted reproduction. *J Assist Reprod Genet* **14**: 375–378.
15. Golombok S, Cook R & Bish A (1995) Families created by the new reproduction technologies: quality of parenting and social and emotional development of the children. *Child Dev* **66**: 285–298.
16. Golombok S, Brewaeys A, Cook R *et al.* (1995) The European study of assisted reproduction families: family functioning and child development. *Hum Reprod* **11**: 2324–2331.
17. Colpin H & Soenen S (2002) Parenting and psychosocial development of IVF children: a follow-up study. *Hum Reprod* **17**: 1116–1123.
18. van Steirteghem A, Bonduelle M, Devroey P & Liebaers I (2002) Follow-up of children born after ICSI. *Hum Reprod Update* **8**: 111–116.
19. Bonduelle M, Liebaers I, Deketelaere V *et al.* (2002) Neonatal data on a cohort of 2889 infants born after ICSI (1991–1999) and of 2995 infants born after IVF (1983–1999). *Hum Reprod* (in press).
20. Kurinczuk J & Bower C (1997) Birth defects in infants conceived by intracytoplasmic sperm injection: an alternative explanation. *BMJ* **315**: 1260–1266.
21. Wennerholm UB, Bergh C, Hamberger L *et al.* (2000) Incidence of congenital malformations in children born after ICSI. *Hum Reprod* **15**: 944–948.
22. Bonduelle M, Joris H, Hofmans K *et al.* (1998) Mental development of 201 ICSI children at 2 years of age. *Lancet* **351**: 1553.
23. Sutcliffe AG, Taylor B, Li J, Thornton S, Grudzinskas JG & Lieberman BA (1999) Children born after intracytoplasmic sperm injection: population control study. *BMJ* **318**: 704–705.
24. Bowen JR, Gibson FL, Leslie GI *et al.* (1998) Medical and developmental outcome at 1 year for children conceived by intracytoplasmic sperm injection. *Lancet* **351**: 1529–1534.
25. Sutcliffe AF, D'Souza SW, Cadman J, Richards B, McKinlay IA & Lieberman B (1995) Minor congenital anomalies, major congenital malformations and development in children conceived from cryopreserved embryos. *Hum Reprod* **10**: 3332–3337.
26. Wennerholm U, Albertsson-Wikland K, Bergh C *et al.* (1998). Postnatal growth and health in children born after cryopreservation as embryos. *Lancet* **351**: 1085–1090.
27. Baetens P& Brewaeys A (2001) Lesbian couples requesting donor insemination: an update of the knowledge with regard to lesbian mother families. *Hum Reprod Update* **7**: 512–519.

Further Reading

Englert Y (ed) (1998) Gamete donation: current ethics in the European Union. *Hum Reprod* **13**(Suppl. 2). Oxford University Press, Oxford.

SECTION 4

Complications of treatment

Chapter 17

Complications of ovarian stimulation

The adverse effects of ovarian stimulation may be divided into immediate problems, such as drug-specific side-effects, the consequences of overstimulation of the ovaries, such as multiple pregnancy and the ovarian hyperstimulation syndrome (OHSS), and long-term problems such as the possible risk of ovarian cancer.

Drug-specific Side-effects

Clomiphene Citrate

Clomiphene induces ovulation by stimulating endogenous gonadotropin secretion but the drug is also concentrated in the ovaries and can, for instance, be detected in follicular fluid obtained at IVF. Clomiphene can cause overstimulation of the ovaries and during treatment many women notice breast tenderness and a feeling of bloatedness. OHSS has been recorded with clomiphene therapy but all but the very mildest cases are rare. Occasionally solitary ovarian cysts are formed. They usually resolve spontaneously, and aspiration is only rarely required. The overall risk of multiple pregnancy rises from the background rate of 1 in 80 to 1 in 10, an increase which is presumably more common in women receiving bigger doses and those with polycystic ovary syndrome.

Table 17.1 lists the adverse reactions reported to the Committee on Safety of Medicines (CSM) over the last 30 years. Given the extensive use of this drug, in terms of reports of immediate side-effects, it does seem remarkably safe. As with all spontaneous reporting, one cannot know how precisely the events are related to administration of the drug. It is worth noting, however, that neurological complaints feature strongly so complaints of dizziness, abnormalities of vision, and depression should be carefully evaluated. More worrying side-effects that have been reported are grand mal epilepsy and hallucinations. The risk of treatment with clomiphene in relation to the development of ovarian cancer is considered below.

Other side-effects are caused by expression of the antiestrogenic activity of clomiphene, namely flushing and sweating attacks. In doses above 100 mg per day for 5 days, the antiestrogen activity may adversely affect the endometrium and impair formation of cervical mucus and so reduce the chance of conception. Some women have reported transient loss of hair from the head.

Table 17.1 Adverse effects of clomiphene citrate (318 yellow cards, including six fatal reports between 1/7/63 and 10/7/95). Data from the Committee on Safety of Medicines

Abnormal vision	25
Nausea and vomiting	10
Dizziness	11
Diplopia	6
Grand mal epilepsy	5
Depression	8
Hallucinations	7
Ovarian cancer	2
Breast cancer	8

Tamoxifen

The main side-effects associated with tamoxifen have occurred with its long-term use in women with cancer of the breast (endometrial hyperplasia, polyps, and cancer). When used for induction of ovulation the immediate problems are similar to those of clomiphene, except that antiestrogenic effects in the genital tract do not seem to occur and the neurological problems of clomiphene have not been recorded.

Gonadotropin Preparations

Receptors for gonadotropins are found only in the gonads so that, other than overstimulation of the ovaries, side-effects caused by these preparations are essentially attributable to their non-hormonal content. The preparations derived from urine (Menogon, Metrodin) contain a substantial amount of urinary protein, itself containing various growth factors and other potential immunogens. Yet the remarkable fact is that, with the exception of causing reactions at injection sites, these compounds seem to have been free of immediate problems. The issue of long-term problems, e.g., ovarian cancer, is taken up below. The presence of the urinary proteins does mean, however, that these preparations have to be injected by the intramuscular route. Preparations purified by affinity chromatography (Metrodin HP and Menopur) or synthesized by recombinant technology (Gonal-F and Puregon) can be injected subcutaneously and local reactions are uncommon. It is, however, important that practitioners remain alive to the possibility of side-effects and that adverse reactions continue to be reported to the CSM, using the specific names of the compound involved – it should not be assumed that all recombinant preparations are identical.

Pituitary derived gonadotropins were used for induction of ovulation in a small number of women in the UK some 30 years ago. Following the discovery that a spongiform encephalopathy (Creutzfeldt–Jakob disease, CJD) could occur many years after treatment with pituitary derived growth hormone, concern developed that a similar complication might occur after treatment with pituitary derived gonadotropins. In Australia (where pituitary sourced gonadotropin was used in some 1500 women) four cases of CJD were identified. Despite a proactive campaign which succeeded in contacting 320 of the known 360 recipients of pituitary gonadotropin in the UK, no cases have so far been discovered. As the years pass the probability of cases occurring steadily declines.

Variant CJD (vCJD) can be transmitted to humans from cows affected by bovine spongiform encephalopathy (BSE). There has been some debate about whether human urine could be a potential source but the evidence to date is reassuring. There is no evidence to suggest that urinary-derived gonadotropin preparations are any less safe than recombinant follicle stimulating hormone (FSH).[1]

Gonadotropin Releasing Hormone

The chief side-effect of treatment with *pulsatile* gonadotropin releasing hormone (GnRH) is infection at the injection site. It has occurred in only two of more than 200 patients treated by us but is the main reason we have always favored the subcutaneous route of administration. An allergic reaction at the infusion site may occur; it is thought to be related to the intrinsic similarity of the tertiary structure of the GnRH molecule to the H_1 histamine receptor ligand.

OHSS is almost unknown as a result of treatment with GnRH. Multiple pregnancy (almost entirely twins) occurs in 5–6% of women treated with pulsatile GnRH, compared with 1.5% in the general population.

Gonadotropin Releasing Hormone Analogs

The GnRH superactive agonists initially stimulate gonadotropin release (agonistic phase). Pituitary desensitization then occurs, with the development of variable degrees of hypogonadotropic hypogonadism. Adverse effects are related to local problems at the sites of administration, to the consequences of the agonistic phase (e.g., expansion of solitary ovarian cysts), and to the consequences of overtreatment (e.g., estrogen deficiency) (see Ch. 13).

With the present generation of superactive agonists, the fundamental biochemical alterations to the GnRH molecule involve substitution of a D amino acid at the sixth position and variable changes to the tenth amino acid, changes which inhibit peptidase digestion of the molecule and therefore lead to its persistence at the pituitary GnRH receptor. A number of changes occur in the gonadotropin-secreting pituicyte, including loss (downregulation) of GnRH receptors. These cellular changes impair further secretion of luteinizing hormone (LH) and FSH.

Some of the analogs are administered by nasal insufflation (for example, buserelin, nafarelin) (see p. 320). Only about 4% of the nasal dose is absorbed and the compounds have to be sniffed between 2 and 6 times per day. They can produce local irritation and allergy, resulting in a stuffy and/or runny nose. Ordinary colds may impair absorption and lead to loss of efficacy. The analogs can be given by subcutaneous injection or as a long-acting depot preparation (goserelin) (p. 320). Few problems at the site of injection have been recorded.

During the initial (agonist) phase there is a striking increase of endogenous gonadotropins and not uncommonly ovarian cysts expand at this stage. We always precede treatment with a GnRH agonist with an immediate pretreatment ovarian ultrasound scan and if cysts of 10 mm diameter or more are seen, treatment is deferred. If cysts are present one can either await spontaneous resolution or give the patient a short course of treatment (3 weeks) with the birth control pill and then start the GnRH agonist when the repeat scan is clear. Indeed, we usually precede IVF treatment cycles with the oral contraceptive pill in order to minimize the risk of cyst development (see Ch. 13).

Many women using GnRH agonists for ovulation induction develop flushing and sweating attacks from the acute estrogen deficiency they provoke. Long-term complications of estrogen deficiency are only seen when these compounds are used for a long time as in the management of endometriosis. Using bone densitometry, numerous studies have shown varying degrees of skeletal decalcification. In our experience as much as a 10% fall in vertebral calcium may occur in 6 months. For this reason, and to prevent the acute symptomatology of estrogen deficiency, most clinicians offer "add back" treatment with low-dose estrogens (25–50 mg estrogen patch, 0.625 mg Premarin or tibolone) to patients using these analogs for prolonged ovarian suppression (for example in the medical treatment of endometriosis).

The GnRH *antagonists* are now being used increasingly. They achieve very rapid suppression of FSH and LH by competitive inhibition at the pituitary gonadotropin receptor. Because the antagonist is administered after ovarian stimulation with gonadotropins has commenced, there are no side-effects of estrogen deficiency and so the drugs are very well tolerated. Irritation at the injection site, which was a major problem with first and second generation antagonists due to histamine release, does not appear to be a problem with the third generation preparations that are in current use.

The Ovarian Hyperstimulation Syndrome

The pathophysiological hallmark of OHSS is a sudden increase of vascular permeability which results in the development of a massive

Table 17.2 Clinical grading of ovarian hyperstimulation syndrome

Mild
Weight gain, thirst, abdominal discomfort
Mild distension
Ovaries > 5 cm diameter
Moderate
Nausea and vomiting, distension and pain
Dyspnea
Abdomen distended but not tense
Ascites detected by ultrasound
Severe
Evidence of intravascular fluid loss
Third space fluid accumulation (tense ascites, hydrothorax)
Hemoconcentration, hypovolemia, oliguria, hepatorenal failure

extravascular exudate. This exudate accumulates primarily in the peritoneal cavity, causing a protein-rich ascites. Loss of *fluid* into the third space causes a profound fall in intravascular volume, hemoconcentration, and suppression of urine formation. Loss of *protein* into the third space causes a fall in plasma oncotic pressure which results in further loss of intravascular fluid. Secondary hyperaldosteronism occurs and causes salt retention. Eventually peripheral edema develops.

The syndrome is graded according to severity, as shown in Table 17.2. Mild ovarian hyperstimulation is characterized by fluid accumulation, as evidenced by weight gain, and abdominal distension and discomfort. Ultrasound examination shows enlarged ovaries with a diameter greater than 5 cm (Fig. 17.1). Grade 2 ovarian hyperstimulation is associated with the development of nausea and vomiting. The ovarian enlargement and abdominal distension are greater and cause more discomfort and dyspnea. Ascites can be detected by ultrasound. Grade 3 (severe) ovarian hyperstimulation syndrome is a life-threatening condition in which there is clinical evidence of contraction of the intravascular volume (subnormal central venous pressure with reduced cardiac output), severe expansion of the third space (tense ascites, pleural and pericardial effusions, all of which compromise the circulation and breathing), severe hemoconcentration, and the development of hepatorenal failure. In addition to the circulatory crisis, these patients are at risk from intravascular thrombosis. Deaths have been recorded in women with grade 3 OHSS, caused usually by cerebrovascular thrombosis, renal failure, or cardiac tamponade resulting from pericardial effusion.

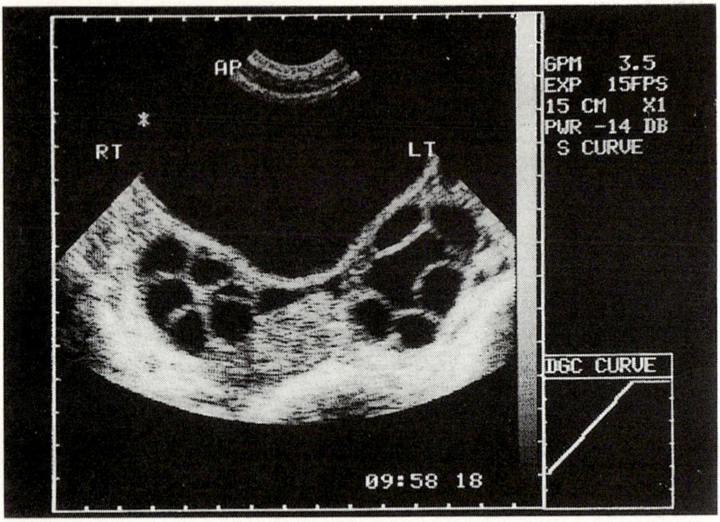

Figure 17.1 Transabdominal scan of overstimulated ovaries, with some free fluid seen around the uterus.

OHSS only occurs after overstimulated ovaries have been exposed to human chorionic gonadotropin (hCG). The condition therefore results most commonly when sensitive (i.e., polycystic) ovaries are exposed to excessive quantities of FSH and then to hCG; the finding that severe OHSS is often associated with pregnancy is probably related to the persistence of hCG in this situation. Even when the ovaries have been severely overstimulated, OHSS can generally be prevented by avoiding exposure of the ovaries to LH and/or hCG.

Prevalence

Most methods of ovarian stimulation can cause OHSS and the mild form may even result from the use of oral antiestrogens. In programs of ovulation induction the risk is related, *inter alia*, to the dose of gonadotropins (see below) and is rare with low-dose protocols (see Ch. 6). The overall risk is estimated to be about 4% and that of the severe form about 0.25%. In IVF the prevalence varies in published series from 1% to 10%, being highest in those combining gonadotropin stimulation with treatment with a GnRH analog. Severe cases occur in 0.25–2% of IVF cycles.

A distinction has been made between early and late OHSS,[2] with those presenting early (that is, 3–7 days after hCG administration) having significantly higher serum estradiol concentrations than those presenting late (12–17 days after hCG), while there is no difference in the number of oocytes collected. Those presenting late are more likely to be pregnant and have a severe form of the syndrome, due to persistent hCG stimulation of the ovaries.

Pathophysiology of the Ovarian Hyperstimulation Syndrome

While it has been known for many years that high circulating concentrations of estradiol are an immediate predictor of the syndrome, estrogen itself is not the cause of the sudden increase in vascular permeability. Such a change is not after all a feature of treatment with estrogen itself, even when the levels rise very abruptly, as after an implant. While numerous compounds, such as prostaglandins, kallikreins, etc., have been considered to mediate the process, the two prime movers in the development of OHSS are activation of the ovarian renin–angiotensin system and release of vascular endothelial growth factor (VEGF) from the ovary.

The follicle contains renin in an inactive form which is activated at mid-cycle (and by exposure of the ovary to hCG) and which then causes conversion of angiotensinogen to angiotensin I. This ovarian renin–angiotensin system is thought to be involved in the neovascularization which is so central a feature of the conversion of the avascular preovulatory follicle into the richly vascularized corpus luteum. Some years ago we reported excessive levels of renin activity in the plasma of a woman with severe, grade 3 OHSS at a stage of her illness when, as a consequence of treatment, the central venous pressure was several centimeters higher than normal (i.e., when secretion of *renal* renin would have been suppressed). Subsequent studies have shown that ascitic fluid in this syndrome contains very large amounts of angiotensin II compared with ascitic fluid obtained from women with liver failure. In rabbits angiotensin II increases peritoneal permeability and neovascularization. Moreover, in that species, treatment with an angiotensin-converting enzyme (ACE) inhibitor blocks the increase in peritoneal permeability that occurs in response to superovulation. Parallel studies have not, however, been performed in humans because of concerns over the use of ACE inhibitors in pregnancy. There is no doubt of the involvement of the renin–angiotensin system in the pathogenesis of OHSS, with hemotocrit concentrations being directly related to plasma renin activity and aldosterone concentrations.[3]

Vascular Endothelial Growth Factor

VEGF, also known as vascular permeability factor or vasculotropin, is a dimeric glycoprotein which promotes growth and cell division of vascular endothelial cells. It increases capillary permeability. VEGF is expressed in steroidogenic and steroid-responsive cells, such as those involved in repair of endometrial vessels and in implantation.[4] In primates, production of VEGF increases after the LH surge and is reduced by suppression of LH secretion during the luteal phase; VEGF production by human luteinized granulosa cells is increased by incubation *in vitro* with hCG, as detected by measuring messenger RNA (indicating synthesis by the luteal cells) and VEGF itself, as detected by an immunofluorescent assay. Using a bioassay which measured extravasation into the skin of an injected dye, McClure and colleagues[5] found increased amounts of VEGF in ascitic fluid obtained from patients with OHSS but not in ascitic fluid obtained from patients with liver failure. Most of the activity could be neutralized by incubation with an antiserum to recombinant human VEGF, indicating that VEGF is the major capillary permeability agent in OHSS. One might speculate that the activity that was not neutralized by the antiserum to VEGF was attributable to angiotensin II. Further studies have correlated follicular fluid concentrations of VEGF with OHSS and also with ovarian blood flow, as assessed by Doppler ultrasound flow studies.[6] Indeed serum VEGF concentrations have been proposed as a predictor for the development of the syndrome.[7]

The angiogenic response to LH or hCG is normally confined to a single dominant follicle. OHSS may be seen as an exaggeration of this response. Because of gonadotropin-stimulated overgrowth of follicles, VEGF, the major angiogenic mediator of vascularization of the corpus luteum, can no longer be confined to the ovary but spills over, first into the peritoneal cavity and then into the general circulation.

The Ovarian Hyperstimulation Syndrome and Thromboembolism

When considering the pathophysiology of the OHSS it is easy to appreciate the potential risk of deep venous thrombosis (DVT) and thromboembolic events. Indeed there has been an expanding literature on this association in recent years.[8] Not only is there a hypercoagulable state but also the combination of enlarged ovaries and ascites leads to reduced venous return from the lower limbs, which combined with immobility places the patient at risk of DVT. Furthermore, the thrombotic event need not only be in the lower limbs: a review of the world literature found that 75% of cases reported were in venous sites, with 60% in the upper limb, head and neck veins, with an associated risk of pulmonary embolism of 4–12%, while the remaining 25% were arterial thromboses and were mostly intracerebral.[8] It is difficult to give an explanation for these more unusual sites of thrombosis in young women, unless there is relative over-reporting because of their rarity.

The hypercoagulable state of OHSS may, in addition to the general vascular changes described in the previous section, relate to a change in clotting factors, which may be due to the recognized hematological changes of pregnancy:

- Increased concentrations of factors VII, VIII, IX, X, XII and fibrinogen
- Reduced concentrations of protein S, antithrombin III, and fibrinolysis.

Whether this thrombophilic state is secondary to high circulating estrogen concentrations is less clear, as the thrombophilic state of pregnancy tends to occur closer to term and post-partum. It is possible that women who develop OHSS have a tendency to thrombophilias (e.g., deficiency of protein C, S or antithrombin III or factor V Leiden expression), although the majority of women appear to screen negative after the event. An alternative theory is a leakage of factors such as antithrombin III into the ascitic fluid, thus resulting in a relative plasma deficiency.[9]

Venous thrombosis in the lower limb most often resolves without long-term sequelae, unless pulmonary embolism occurs, which may be fatal. Upper limb venous thrombosis may lead to disabling long-term disability, with persistent discomfort, cramp, weakness, and cold hands. Cerebral thrombosis may resolve completely but it can lead to various forms of long-term disability.

Risk Factors for the Development of the Ovarian Hyperstimulation Syndrome

Two of the important risk factors can be identified before treatment starts, the others as ovarian stimulation proceeds.

The presence of polycystic ovaries

Several studies have confirmed that patients most at risk are women with the characteristic appearance on ultrasound of polycystic ovaries. The essential point is that we are referring here to the presence of polycystic ovaries, as detected by ultrasound, not to the polycystic ovary syndrome. The polycystic appearance occurs in 20% of normal women but in 40% of patients undergoing IVF, irrespective of the indication for treatment. The significance of this finding is shown in Figure 17.2 which depicts the ovarian response to stimulation by gonadotropins in three groups of women with anovulatory infertility. In those with normal ovaries a unifollicular response was easy to obtain; in those with polycystic ovary syndrome, there was the familiar polyfollicular response. Women with polycystic ovaries on ultrasound but without the clinical features of the syndrome had a polyfollicular response that was indistinguishable from that seen in the patients with the clinical features of the syndrome.

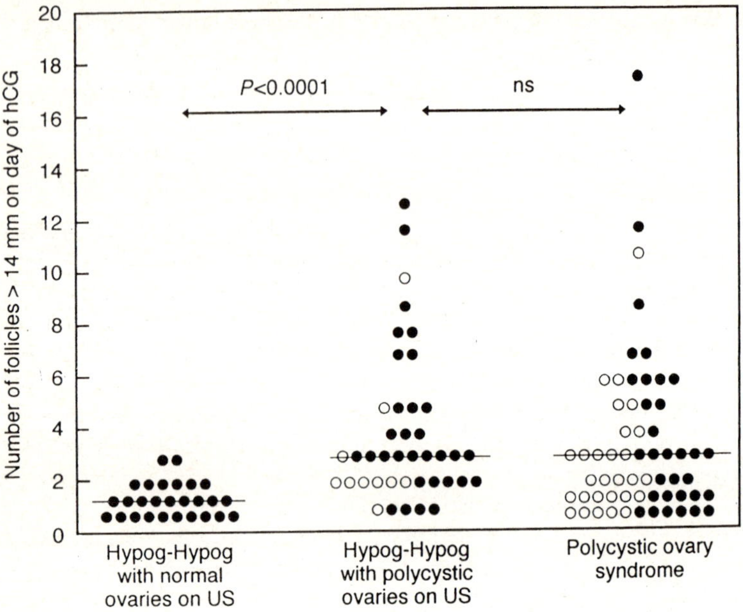

Figure 17.2 Each circle represents the number of follicles greater than 14 mm on the day of hCG in three groups of patients undergoing ovulation induction with hMG using either conventional (closed circles) or low dose (open circles) regimens. Patients with polycystic ovaries, whether they had hypogonadotropic hypogonadism (hypog-hypog) or polycystic ovary syndrome, exhibited the classic exuberant response to stimulation. (From Shoham *et al.* (1992) *Fertil Steril* **58**: 37, with permission.)[30]

These observations indicate the sensitivity of the polycystic ovary to gonadotropic stimulation. They emphasize the value of identifying polycystic ovaries before treatment starts so that the dose of gonadotropins can be adjusted appropriately.

The patient's age

Most cases of OHSS occur in younger women, consistent with the greater ovarian responsiveness in this group compared with older women.

Use of superactive GnRH agonists

Superactive GnRH agonists protect the ovary from an endogenous LH surge, so facilitating more convenient scheduling of ovum pick-up. The protection so afforded renders the ovary more amenable to stimulation of multifollicular development by high-dose gonadotropin treatment. Not surprisingly, this very advantage makes OHSS more common in treatment programs utilizing pituitary desensitization.

Development of multiple immature and intermediate-sized follicles during treatment

The development of large numbers of immature and intermediate follicles during treatment (see Fig. 17.2) indicates an exuberant response to gonadotropic stimulation, caused either by very sensitive, i.e., polycystic, ovaries (the usual situation) or too high a dose of gonadotropin in women with normal ovaries. This picture contrasts with that seen in women at risk from multiple pregnancy in whom the development of numerous *large* follicles (> 16 mm in diameter) is the marker of risk.

Exposure to LH/hCG

The clinical observation that exposure of the ovaries to LH, and usually to hCG, is a *sine qua non* of its development and that pregnancy is frequently associated with OHSS is consistent with the role of LH and hCG in stimulating the processes that mediate neovascularization and vascular permeability. These observations add plausibility to the clinical practice of attempting aspiration of all follicles in patients considered at risk because it is luteinized granulosa cells that are the source of the permeability factors.

Prevention of Ovarian Hyperstimulation Syndrome

Most of the maneuvers (Table 17.3) have been foreshadowed in the preceding discussion. All patients undergoing ovarian stimulation, whether to correct anovulation or for assisted fertility techniques, should have a pretreatment ultrasound scan and if polycystic ovaries are detected, the dose of gonadotropin should be lowered (see Ch. 6 for details of the low-dose protocol). If pituitary desensitization has been used one should be sensitive to the loss of the normal "protection" of the ovary caused by the block to estrogen-mediated positive feedback of LH release. If a long protocol of GnRH analog

Table 17.3 Prevention of ovarian hyperstimulation syndrome

- Pretreatment ultrasound assessment of ovaries: PCO?
- Care with gonadotropin administration: use low doses in women with PCO
- Care with GnRH analogs:
  (a) emphasize use of ultrasound rather than estradiol concentrations
  (b) note whether an LH-depleted gonadotropin preparation is being used
- Reduce use and dose of hCG:
  (a) consider withholding ovulatory dose of hCG
  (b) substitute progesterone for hCG in luteal phase
- Meticulous aspiration of all follicles
- Consider cryopreservation with deferred embryo transfer

treatment is followed by treatment with one of the pure FSH preparations, one must also be aware that the lack of LH changes the usual relationship of follicle maturation and number to circulating estradiol levels. In this situation measurement of serum estradiol concentrations underestimates follicle development. It is therefore essential that endocrine monitoring is supported by high-quality ultrasound, otherwise low circulating estradiol concentrations may encourage further and inappropriate gonadotropic stimulation despite adequate follicular development.

For the patient with overstimulated ovaries who is approaching the time of hCG administration, several strategies to make treatment safer may be considered. The first is to administer a low dose of hCG to initiate oocyte maturation and/or ovulation (i.e., not more than a single injection of 5000 i.u.) and, in patients receiving GnRH analog treatment and who therefore require luteal support, to give progesterone (400 mg per vagina for 14 days) rather than hCG. It is current practice now to use progesterone routinely for luteal support.

Recombinant LH has a shorter half-life than hCG and so may reduce the risk of short-term OHSS, although it will not influence OHSS resulting from hCG produced from the trophoblast of a developing pregnancy. In protocols where GnRH antagonists are used, the preovulatory trigger can be with a single dose of a GnRH agonist, instead of hCG – again a shorter acting preparation which should reduce the short term risk of OHSS.

In the treatment of anovulatory infertility there are two considerations. The first is the prevention of multiple pregnancy; if there are more than four follicles of 14 mm diameter or more in a young woman with polycystic ovaries, the safest course is either to withhold the hCG and advise the patient to avoid intercourse or, preferably, to convert the treatment to IVF-embryo transfer (ET) or gamete intrafallopian transfer (GIFT: see also Ch. 6). The second consideration is the prevention of OHSS. Here the issue is the development of multiple *small* follicles. Thus, if there are more than six follicles with a diameter of 12 mm or more we advise discontinuing treatment or converting it to IVF. In the latter situation, having meticulously aspirated as many follicles as possible, one may cryopreserve the embryos and defer their transfer to another cycle. Alternatively, one may withhold hCG, continue treatment with the GnRH analog, and restart gonadotropin stimulation at a lower dose.

In patients having IVF and using gonadotropin containing LH activity (i.e., hMG preparations), the following are conservative criteria for ovarian responses above which there is a significant risk of OHSS: a serum estradiol of greater than 10 000 pmol/L (3000 pg/ml) together with 20 or more follicles of 12 mm diameter or more. In the interpretation of estradiol concentrations one needs to recognize the aforementioned effects of using LH-depleted gonadotropin preparations in women receiving GnRH analogs in a "long" protocol (less estrogen than usual is made so estradiol concentrations underestimate the intensity of the ovarian response). For patients with a serum estradiol greater than 17 000 pmol/L (5500 pg/ml) with more than 40 follicles, hCG should be withheld and treatment abandoned. Treatment with the GnRH analog is, however, continued and when the ovaries regain their normal size, ovarian stimulation is resumed at a lower dose. When serum estradiol concentrations are 10 000–17 000 pmol/L with 20–40 follicles, hCG may be given but the embryos are cryopreserved and transferred at a later date.

Treatment with glucocorticoids does not prevent OHSS.[10] Prophylactic infusion of albumin has been investigated but personal experience has been disappointing[11] and unless its efficacy has been clearly demonstrated, we do not recommend its use.

Management of the Ovarian Hyperstimulation Syndrome[4,12,13]

Mild ovarian hyperstimulation is very common and is managed expectantly, its importance being that it should alert both patient and doctor to the risk of a more severe condition developing. The patient should be encouraged to weigh herself daily and take abundant fluids. A marked increase in weight (more than 5 kg) with the development of abdominal distension, nausea, and vomiting indicate the onset of grade 2 hyperstimulation and the need for hospitalization. Patients are often admitted to their nearest hospital and not the specialist unit providing ovarian stimulation, so good liaison is essential. We recommend patients are issued with an advice sheet concerning the symptoms of OHSS and what to do if they suspect it may be happening to them. The sheet should include the phone number and contact name of the liaison person in the treating clinic. In non-conception cycles, moderate ovarian hyperstimulation can be expected to resolve with the development of menstruation, although the ovarian cysts may persist for a month or so more.

Patients with grade 2 hyperstimulation need reassurance and explanation, together with hospitalization. Oral fluids are encouraged although vomiting may make an intravenous infusion necessary. If luteal support is required progesterone should be used. Full-length TED stockings and heparin 5000 i.u. b.d. s.c. are advised to reduce the risk of DVT. Adequate analgesia is required. Preferred drugs are paracetamol, with or without codeine, and pethidine for very severe pain. Non-steroidal anti-inflammatory drugs such as diclofenac should be avoided although indometacin has been used experimentally with good results. Antiemetics such as metoclopramide or Stemetil are given as needed. Table 17.4 indicates the surveillance that should be undertaken.

Table 17.4 Surveillance of moderate and severe ovarian hyperstimulation

Circulation • Intravascular contraction: (a) monitor CVP (consider administration of colloids) (b) look for pleural and pericardial effusion • Hemoconcentration: (a) measure hematocrit, white blood cell count, coagulation profile
Hepatic function Measure ascites (girth, ultrasound) and consider paracentesis Monitor liver function tests, in particular serum albumin
Renal function Monitor urine output (consider administration of crystalloids) Paracentesis, dialysis

The development of clinically detectable and usually painful ascites together with a deterioration in respiration, circulation, and renal function indicates the development of severe grade 3 hyperstimulation and, in most cases, the need for admission to an intensive care unit. The intravascular volume should be monitored by measurements of central venous pressure, renal function by meticulous attention to input and urine output, and hemoconcentration by measurement of hematocrit, whose level reflects intravascular volume depletion and blood viscosity. A hematocrit of over 45% is a serious warning sign and a measurement greater than 55% signals a life-threatening situation. There may be a striking leukocytosis, the white blood cell count rising to 40 000/cm^3. Measurement of body weight, serum urea, creatinine and electrolytes, together with serum albumin and liver function tests and periodic assessments of the coagulation profile, are mandatory.

Infusion of colloid is required to maintain intravascular volume, as indicated by restoration of normal central venous pressure. The choice lies between human albumin (50–100 g repeated as required) or intravenous dextran or hydroxyethyl starch, although the latter compounds carry the risk of anaphylactic reaction and dextran has been implicated in severe adult respiratory distress syndrome (ARDS). Crystalloid (normal saline usually) is administered for rehydration. If urine flow remains suppressed despite restoration of central venous pressure and rehydration, abdominal paracentesis, under ultrasound guidance, should be undertaken. The indications for this procedure are therefore the need for symptomatic relief of a tense ascites, oliguria, rising serum creatinine, falling creatinine clearance, and hemoconcentration unresponsive to medical therapy. Severe oliguria or renal failure persisting despite these measures usually necessitate dialysis.

Paracentesis of hydrothorax should be considered for relief of dyspnea. Cardiac tamponade from pericardial effusion may prove fatal if not rapidly relieved. Careful cardiological assessment together with cardiac ultrasound should therefore feature in the management of these patients. One must be aware of the possibility of reaccumulation of fluid in any of these cavities.

Surgery should be avoided in patients with OHSS unless there is evidence of ovarian torsion or marked hemorrhage or rupture of one of the ovarian cysts. Diuretics are contraindicated in these patients. Anticoagulation is indicated if there is evidence of thromboembolism or a deteriorating coagulation profile.

In summary, one should attempt to identify the patient at risk, consider the impact of the new gonadotropin preparations on the response to ovarian stimulation, and actively attempt to avoid trouble. Such an approach demands close contact with the patient and good liaison with colleagues in other centers who may be providing emergency care. Early referral to an intensive care unit will help to correct hemodynamic disturbances but the reproductive specialist must continue to play an active role in management, particularly concerning the issue of abdominal paracentesis and the evaluation of abdominal pain.

Multiple Pregnancy

The rate of multiple pregnancy has increased parallel to the introduction of assisted conception technologies, although now with greater awareness, the trend should be reversing. The avoidance of multiple pregnancy is now an issue of clinical governance, and the duty of responsible practitioners. Strict guidelines should be in place during ovulation induction protocols to ensure that the pre-ovulatory hCG trigger is only administered if there are no more than two mature follicles (see Ch. 6). Poorly monitored ovulation induction, whether by clomiphene citrate or gonadotropin therapy, is still the cause of the majority of multiple births. In IVF cycles the transfer of more than three pre-embryos is prohibited in the UK and there has been guidance advising the routine transfer of two (see Ch. 13). With further refinement of laboratory techniques (e.g., enhanced culture conditions, blastocysts transfer – see Ch. 18) it may soon be feasible to transfer a single pre-embryo without compromising success rates. In some countries, in particular North America, large numbers of embryos are transferred and fetal reduction offered at the end of the first trimester for high order multiples. Fetal reduction has a 15–25% chance of miscarriage and is a procedure that we prefer to avoid by reducing the multiple pregnancy rate in the first instance.

Multiple pregnancies carry increased risks (see also Ch. 16). Approximately 30% of twin pregnancies spontaneously reduce to singleton in the first trimester. Premature delivery is three times as common with twins as with singleton pregnancies and the risk of all other obstetric complications is increased (e.g., pre-eclampsia, abnormal bleeding, etc.). Triplet and quadruplet pregnancies further magnify the risks, with mean gestation at delivery of 33 and 31 weeks respectively and neonatal morbidity increased at least 20-fold. Cerebral palsy rates have been reported as 2.3 per 1000 singletons, 12.6 per 1000 surviving twins and 44.8 per 1000 triplets.[14] In addition to the increase in long-term morbidity in survivors of multiple gestation there are significant effects on family dynamics and the ability of parents to cope, as well as the potential detriment to any existing children.

Ovarian Cancer

Concern has developed over the last few years that women who have undergone ovarian stimulation may be at increased risk of developing ovarian cancer. Though the fourth commonest cause of death from cancer in the UK (after breast, lung, and colon cancers), ovarian cancer is still a relatively uncommon condition. When we also consider the very small proportion of the population that has received ovarian stimulation and the even smaller proportion that received it sufficiently long ago for it to be plausibly considered an etiological agent in any particular case, it becomes easy to see why it is proving difficult to evaluate the risk. Interpretation of the data has often been clouded by methodological flaws, as well as difficulties separating known risk factors, such as low parity and infertility, from any effect of ovulation induction and/or controlled ovarian stimulation.

Etiology of Ovarian Cancer

While an extensive discussion of the etiology of ovarian cancer is out of place in this book, certain factors are well recognized. The average age at diagnosis is 59–64 years; about 90% of cases arise from the ovarian epithelium and epidemiological studies indicate the importance of genetic, environmental, and endocrine factors. The incidence in women under the age of 30 years is approximately 5 per 100 000; age 30–50 years it is 21 per 100 000, rising to 46 per 100 000 at 60 years. Parity is protective, the effect increasing with each pregnancy. Protection from ovarian cancer is one of the non-contraceptive benefits of treatment with the oral contraceptive. Infertility and "incessant" ovulation are known to be associated with an increased risk. The question now is whether infertility treatment increases the risk compared with that associated with infertility itself, particularly when associated with low parity, e.g., failed treatment.

The most widely accepted model of ovarian cancer postulates that epithelial inclusion cysts, formed at each ovulation, are stimulated to undergo malignant transformation by gonadotropins that normally become elevated at the menopause. This model clearly predicts that agents which provoke multiple ovulation by gonadotropic stimulation will increase the risk of ovarian cancer. An alternative hypothesis, that gonadotropins may not only be mutagenic but mitogenic (i.e., provoke a pre-existing tumor), should also be considered. Finally, there have been reports of an association of infertility treatment with granulosa cell tumors. These will be reviewed below but they resonate with the finding that granulosa cell tumors develop in transgenic mice into which a gene encoding a long-acting form of LH has been introduced. These animals develop high serum LH concentrations and cystic ovaries, anovulation, and infertility together with granulosa and interstitial cell tumors.[15]

In considering the published studies it is important to recognize that only now are early users of infertility drugs reaching the age of the peak incidence of ovarian cancer. Because of the relative rarity of cases, the epidemiology is largely limited to case reports and case control studies. The sequence of infertility treatments must also be considered: until pretreatment with GnRH analogs was introduced into assisted fertility technology, most patients who received gonadotropin stimulation had already received (unsuccessful) treatment with clomiphene. Distinguishing between an effect of the various treatments and of persisting infertility is necessarily very difficult. For a more comprehensive review the reader is referred to Nugent *et al.*[16]

Clomiphene Citrate

An important case control study was published in 1994 by Rossing and colleagues.[17] These authors attempted to control for the confounding effect of infertility by analyzing cases and controls from a cohort of 3837 women evaluated in the Seattle area for infertility between 1974 and 1985. A total of 11 cases of ovarian cancer (four invasive epithelial carcinomas, five tumors of low malignant potential, and two granulosa cell tumors) were compared with 135 (infertile) controls. Clomiphene treatment had been taken by nine of the cases, five of whom had used it for 12 or more cycles. The authors found a significant association of clomiphene use for 12 or more cycles and the diagnosis of an ovarian tumor (relative risk 11.1, CI 1.5–82.3). The association was evident in women with and without ovulatory abnormalities and in parous and nulliparous women.

While this study has a number of limitations (set out clearly in the paper) it also has its strengths, such as obtaining the data from a review of case records rather than interview (thus avoiding recall bias), the use of a single cohort for cases and controls and the choice of a single agent to evaluate. The finding of an effect of the duration of treatment adds credence to the association. On the other hand it must be accepted that the women receiving prolonged treatment may represent a subgroup of patients with particularly refractory infertility and that it is the severe infertility that constitutes the predisposition to a high risk of ovarian tumor. Critics have noted the heterogeneity of the histological types and that only four of the tumors were invasive. The association with tumors of borderline malignancy is of interest because of a number of published case reports and the results in the case control study of Shushan *et al.* (see below).[18] That two of the lesions were granulosa cell tumors recalls to mind an earlier report by Willemsen *et al.*[19] of 12 such tumors associated with ovarian stimulation.

Is the association of treatment with clomiphene and this variety of ovarian tumors plausible? Given the lag time assumed to be necessary for a drug to act as a carcinogen, clomiphene has certainly been in use for long enough to exert a carcinogenic effect. It was after all the first real fertility drug and was introduced in the early 1960s. Clomiphene is concentrated in the ovary and has a very long biological half-life. It stimulates gonadotropin secretion and, in women with polycystic ovary syndrome, preferentially stimulates LH release. It is women with polycystic ovary syndrome with high LH concentrations who probably represent the majority of cases of recalcitrant infertility, which is intriguing given the findings in the transgenic mice with overexpression of the LH gene mentioned above: these animals have multicystic ovaries with persistent anovulation (which is, however, corrected by unilateral ovariectomy), together with granulosa (and interstitial) cell tumors. Perhaps the background to the granulosa cell tumors reported in women who had received infertility treatment is persistent hypersecretion of LH, made worse by clomiphene in women with polycystic ovary syndrome. The epithelial tumors are, one speculates, more likely to be related to stimulation of ovulation through the impact of clomiphene on pituitary secretion of both gonadotropins.

As a result of the Rossing paper, the Committee on Safety of Medicines recommended that clomiphene should not normally be used for more than six cycles. This in fact is no more than a reminder of its licenced use. In practical terms it also means that patients need to be counseled about the risk of ovarian cancer and treatment with clomiphene and reminded of the protective effect of a successful outcome (and previous or even future use of the contraceptive pill). Another implication is that there is now a great onus on the prescribing doctor to ensure maximum efficacy. This obligation raises the question as to whether it is wise to use clomiphene in general practice. We now consider that adequate surveillance can only be provided by reproductive medicine clinics with adequate monitoring facilities (see Ch. 6). The risks of second and third courses of treatment for subsequent pregnancies need to be evaluated in relation to the protective effect of pregnancy.

Gonadotropin Therapy

The first case report (in 1982) of an association of infertility treatment and ovarian cancer was with treatment with human menopausal gonadotropin (hMG) for 11 cycles. The issue has been studied in the context of a cohort study from Israel of 2632 women receiving treatment between 1964 and 1974.[20] No increased risk was detected but the power of this study was limited because of the variety of treatment regimens used. In 1992, Whittemore and colleagues[21] reported findings from a combined retrospective analysis of 12 US case control studies of ovarian cancer. While attracting considerable interest, this publication has been severely criticized; for example, it reported only 20 patients with invasive cancers who had received infertility treatment and these cases were derived from just three of the studies. On the other hand, a recent case control study from Israel[18] compared 200 women with ovarian cancer with 408 community controls. In this study there were 164 cases of invasive cancer and 36 of borderline malignancy. Compared with untreated women, women who reported using hMG, in any combination with other drugs and for any period, had a threefold higher risk of having epithelial ovarian cancer. Women with borderline tumors were significantly more likely to have been exposed to ovulation inducing agents (OR 3.52, 95% CI 1.23–10.09), particularly hMG (OR 9.38, CI 1.66–52.08). The association was not demonstrated when invasive tumors alone were considered. A number of subsequent studies have explored this issue further, with another Israeli study failing to demonstrate an increased risk for ovarian cancer in a series of 1197 infertile women with known drug history and a mean follow-up of 18 years.[22] A case control study of 1031 women with epithelial ovarian cancer from Italy was similarly reassuring.[23] A Danish case control study looking at 231 borderline ovarian tumors also failed to show an association with fertility drugs.[24] Furthermore, a Finnish study even suggested a falling rate of granulosa cell tumors concomitant with an increasing rate of ovarian stimulation.[25] There have also been studies looking at breast cancer risk, which have been equally reassuring.[22,26]

An important study from Australia investigated the incidence of invasive cancer of the breast, ovary, and uterus in 29 700 women, of whom 20 656 had been exposed to fertility drugs, while the remaining 9044 had been referred for fertility treatment but not received ovarian stimulation.[27] There were 143 breast cancers, 13 ovarian cancers, and 12 uterine cancers. In both those women exposed to ovarian stimulation and the unexposed group the incidence of breast and ovarian cancer was no higher than expected. Interestingly the incidence of uterine cancer, while not raised in the exposed group, was significantly higher than expected in the unexposed patients (OR 2.47, 95% CI 1.18–5.18). Taking the whole cohort together, women with unexplained infertility had more cases of ovarian and uterine cancer than expected (OR 2.64 [1.10–6.35] and 4.59 [1.91–11.0], respectively). Also, within 12 months of exposure to fertility drugs there was a higher than expected incidence of breast and uterine cancer, although this rise was transient and overall no greater than expected – perhaps there was greater surveillance in the immediate period after the treatment.

With respect to the question of ovarian cancer and gonadotropin therapy, we consider the current data to be largely reassuring (for contemporary reviews see references 16, 28 and 29). A cautionary note concerns the relatively short period of follow-up, considering that ovarian cancer is a disease with a peak incidence in a woman's seventh decade. If the aforementioned model of gonadotropin stimulation of epithelial cell proliferation has any value it seems plausible that substantial amounts of gonadotropins may have to be administered to have an adverse effect. None the less, it behoves us to counsel our patients about these putative risks, to use the smallest doses of ovarian stimulation for the shortest duration consistent with effective clinical practice, and to consider the follow-up assessment of women who have undergone unsuccessful infertility treatment.

References

1. Balen AH (2002) Is there a risk of prion disease after the administration of urinary-derived gonadotropins? Debate. *Hum Reprod* (in press).
2. Mathur R, Akande AV, Keay SD, Hunt LP & Jenkins JM (2000) Distinction between early and late ovarian hyperstimulation syndrome. *Fertil Steril* **73**: 901–907.
3. Fabregues F, Balasch J, Manau D *et al.* (1998) Haematocrit, leukocyte and platelet counts and the severity of ovarian hyperstimulation syndrome. *Hum Reprod* **13**: 2406–2410.
4. Shweiki D, Itin A, Neufeld G, Gitay-Goren H & Keshet E (1993) Patterns of expression of vascular endothelial growth factor (VEGF) and VEGF receptors in mice suggest a role in hormonally regulated angiogenesis. *J Clin Invest* **91**: 2235–2243.
5. McClure N, Healy DL, Rogers PAW *et al.* (1994) Vascular endothelial growth factor as capillary permeability agent in ovarian hyperstimulation syndrome. *Lancet* **34**: 235–236.

6. Agrawal R, Conway G, Sladkevicius P *et al.* (1998) Serum vascular endothelial growth factor and Doppler flow velocities in *in vitro* fertilization: relevance to ovarian hyperstimulation syndrome and polycystic ovaries. *Fertil Steril* **70**: 651–658.
7. Agrawal R, Tan SL, Wild S *et al.* (1999) Serum vascular endothelial growth factor concentrations in *in vitro* fertilization cycles predict the risk of ovarian hyperstimulation syndrome. *Fertil Steril* **71**: 287–293.
8. Stewart JA, Hamilton PJ & Murdoch AP (1997) Thromboembolic disease associated with ovarian stimulation and assisted conception techniques. *Hum Reprod* **12**: 2167–2173.
9. Ryo E, Hagino D, Yano N, Sento M, Nagasaka T & Taketani Y (1999) A case of ovarian hyperstimulation syndrome in which antithrombin III deficiency occurred because of its loss into ascites. *Fertil Steril* **71**: 860–862.
10. Tan SL, Balen A, Hussein EL, Campbell S & Jacobs HS (1992) The administration of glucocorticoids for the prevention of ovarian hyperstimulation in IVF: a prospective randomized study. *Fertil Steril* **57**: 378–383.
11. Shaker AG, Zosmer A, Dean N, Bekir, JS, Jacobs HS & Tan SL (1996) Comparison of intravenous albumin and transfer of fresh embryos with cryopreservation of all embryos for subsequent transfer in prevention of ovarian hyperstimulation syndrome. *Fertil Steril* **65**: 992–996.
12. Navot D, Bergh PA & Laufer N (1992) Ovarian hyperstimulation syndrome in novel reproductive technologies: prevention and treatment. *Fertil Steril* **58**: 249–261.
13. Brinsden PR, Wada I, Tan SL, Balen A & Jacobs HS (1995) Diagnosis, prevention and management of ovarian hyperstimulation syndrome. *Br J Obstet Gynaecol* **102**: 767–772.
14. Pharoah POD & Cooke T (1996) Cerebral palsy and multiple births. *Arch Dis Child* **75**: F174–177.
15. Risma KA, Clay CM, Nett TM, Wagner T, Yun J & Nilson JH (1995) Targeted overexpression of luteinizing hormone in transgenic mice leads to infertility, polycystic ovaries and ovarian tumors. *Proc Natl Acad Sci U S A* **92**: 1322–1326.
16. Nugent D, Salha O, Balen AH & Rutherford AJ (1998) Ovarian neoplasia and subfertility treatments. *Br J Obstet Gynaecol* **105**: 584–591.
17. Rossing MA, Daling JR, Weiss NS, Moore DE & Self SG (1994) Ovarian tumors in a cohort of infertile women. *N Engl J Med* **331**: 771–776.
18. Shushan A, Paltiel O, Iscovich J, Elchalal U, Pereetz T & Schenker JG (1996) Human menopausal gonadotropin and the risk of epithelial ovarian cancer. *Fertil Steril* **65**: 13–18.
19. Willemsen W, Kruittwagen R, Bastiaans B, Hanselaar T & Rolland R (1993) Ovarian stimulation and granulosa cell tumor. *Lancet* **341**: 986–988.
20. Ron E, Lunenfeld B, Menczer J *et al.* (1987) Cancer incidence in a cohort of infertile women. *Am J Epidemiol* **125**: 780–790.
21. Whittemore AS, Harris R, Intyre J & Collaborative Ovarian Cancer Group (1992) Characteristics relating to ovarian cancer risk: collaborative analysis of 12 US case-control studies. II Invasive epethelial ovarian cancers in white women. *Am J Epidemiol* **136**: 1184–1203.
22. Potashnik G, Lerner-Geva L, Genkin L, Chetrit A, Lunenfeld E & Porath A (1999) Fertility drugs and the risk of breast and ovarian cancers: results of a long-term follow-up study. *Fertil Steril* **71**: 853–859.
23. Parazzini F, Pelucchi C, Negri E *et al.* (2001) Use of fertility drugs and risk of ovarian cancer. *Hum Reprod* **16**: 1372–1375.
24. Mosgaard BJ, Lidegaard O, Kjaer SK, Schou G & Andersen AN (1998) Ovarian stimulation and borderline ovarian tumors: a case control study. *Fertil Steril* **70**: 1049–1055.

25. Unkila-Kallio L, Leminen A, Tiitinen A & Ylikarkala O (1998) Nationwide data on falling incidence of ovarian granulosa cell tumours concomitant with increasing use of ovulation inducers. *Hum Reprod* **13**: 2822–2830.
26. Ricci E, Parazzini F, Negri E, Marsico S & La Vecchia C (1999) Fertility drugs and the risk of breast cancer. *Hum Reprod* **14**: 1653–1655.
27. Venn A, Watson L, Bruinsma F, Giles G & Healy D (1999) Risk of cancer after use of fertility drugs with *in vitro* fertilization. *Lancet* **354**: 1586–1590.
28. Duckitt K, Templeton AA (1998) Cancer in women with infertility. *Curr Opin Obstet Gynecol* **10**: 199–203.
29. Dor J, Lerner-Geva L, Rabinovici J *et al.* (2002) Cancer incidence in a cohort of infertile women who underwent *in vitro* fertilization. *Fertil Steril* **77**: 324–327.
30. Shoham Z, Conway GS, Patel A & Jacobs HS (1992) Polycystic ovaries in patients with hypogonadotropic hypogonadism: similarity of ovarian response to gonadotropin stimulation in patients with polycystic ovarian syndrome. *Fertil Steril* **58**: 37–45.

Chapter 18

Emerging technologies

Introduction

It is important to appreciate the evolving field in which we work and the exciting advances that are occurring – many since the first edition of this book 5 years ago. We do not propose to present an exhaustive treatise of all areas of ongoing research in reproductive medicine. Instead we have highlighted a few important areas where recent research strategies are leading to changes in clinical practice. The interested reader is directed to the references which are largely reviews of the topics covered. The under-lying theme of the topics is in keeping with the theme of this book, namely the ability to help couples to achieve a healthy singleton baby.

Advances in the Laboratory

Blastocyst Transfer

The ultimate aim of IVF therapy is to achieve the birth of a health singleton baby. Yet it has been routine practice for multiple embryos to be transferred in attempts to increase the chance of getting pregnant at the risk of multiple pregnancy (Ch. 17). It is desirable to minimize the chance of a multiple pregnancy by transferring only a single embryo. By culturing embryos to the blastocyst stage (day 5) it may be possible to select a single embryo and even increase the prospect of getting pregnant. The difficulty is maintaining embryo viability in culture as studies have indicated that several embryos need to be formed so that there is a chance that one or two may be of good enough quality for transfer by day 5. It can be argued that if a patient produces a sufficient number of oocytes and embryos for blastocyst development to be feasible *in vitro* then this would probably have occurred *in vivo* after embryo transfer on day 2. In other words blastocyst culture may not help poor prognosis patients to conceive and may not necessarily aid those who would have conceived in any case – unless the transfer of a single blastocyst leads to a reduction of the multiple pregnancy rate. Despite these doubts there is continued interest in achieving blastocyst transfers and some groups have demonstrated significant success, good pregnancy rates and at the same time scoring systems to enable a single blastocyst to be selected for transfer.[1] Furthermore, prolonged embryo culture enables pre-implantation genetic diagnosis to be performed (see below).

Gardner and colleagues[1] have proposed "sequential culture media" to permit good rates of blastocyst development. Other groups, in particular that of Leese in York, in conjunction with ourselves, have also been looking at embryo culture conditions in order to improve embryo quality.[2] By analyzing the turnover of amino acids by single embryos in culture using high performance liquid chromatography it is possible to distinguish between those embryos which are destined to progress to blastocysts from those whose development will arrest, thereby enabling selection on day 2 or 3 for transfer.[2] This interesting finding is not only of clinical significance but also suggests that oocyte quality must play a major role in determining embryo viability as the activation of the zygotic genome does not occur until the 4–8 cell stage.[3]

In Vitro Maturation of Oocytes

In vitro maturation (IVM) of oocytes has been talked about for several years. The principle is to collect oocytes from unstimulated, or minimally stimulated, small follicles and then mature the oocytes *in vitro* prior to insemination, fertilization, and embryo transfer. Fully grown, germinal vesicle (GV)-stage oocytes once collected recommence meiosis and reach metaphase II over 24–48 hours of culture before fertilization by IVF or intracytoplasmic sperm injection (ICSI). The rationale is to minimize ovarian stimulation and hence reduce both the costs of IVF treatment and the potential risk of ovarian hyperstimulation syndrome (OHSS, Ch. 17). Furthermore, the costs of drugs required would be dramatically reduced. There is a particular attraction for using IVM in the management of anovulatory polycystic ovary syndrome (PCOS) as this is a group of patients who are at greatest risk of OHSS and who also produce oocytes of reduced quality and fertilizability.

There have been several studies looking at the feasibility of IVM and some pregnancies have been reported.[4–6] IVM, however, is still not a viable procedure for routine use, largely because relatively few immature oocytes will mature spontaneously *in vitro* and hence fertilization rates are disappointing. The process of oocyte maturation *in vivo* requires both the removal of an "oocyte maturation inhibitor" (OMI, which, although still to be identified, for many years has been thought to be cAMP) and a meiosis stimulating signal, which is thought to be follicular fluid meiosis-activating sterol (FF-MAS). Research is therefore pursuing the use of FF-MAS and other agents to enhance IVM protocols.

Other issues that need to be addressed if IVM is to become a clinical reality include adapting the oocyte collection procedure and priming the uterus. Mature IVF oocytes are surrounded by expanded and mucified cumulus granulosa cells, while GV oocytes collected for IVM are enclosed in tightly packed cumulus cells, which makes their collection far more difficult. A low aspiration pressure of 7.5–8.0 kPa (compared with 25 kPa for standard IVF) is required to enable transvaginal ultrasound-guided collection of immature oocytes from follicles of 3–10 mm diameter. The oocyte then matures *in vitro*, with first breakdown of the GV nucleus and then progression through metaphase I to metaphase II of the first meiotic division, ending with the extrusion of the first polar body. Concurrently, the oocytes must accumulate *in vitro* the quota of RNAs and proteins that are required to support early post-fertilization embryo development.[7] Hardening of the zona pellucida (outer membrane of the oocyte) may occur during culture of immature oocytes and so ICSI and assisted hatching may be required for fertilization and implantation, respectively. Parenthetically, assisted hatching has not been shown to be of significant benefit to the implantation of otherwise normal IVF embryos. We do not therefore recommend it, despite its widespread use in some parts of the world (e.g., North America).

Clinical protocols for IVM need also to take into consideration the requirement for exogenous steroid support to prime the uterus for implantation. Alternatively, embryos will need to be cryopreserved so that they can be replaced in a subsequent cycle.

In Vitro Maturation of Follicles

One stage earlier than the maturation of oocytes *in vitro* is the maturation of the follicles that contain them. The need for this technology arises from the options for obtaining oocytes after cryopreservation of ovarian tissue that has been performed prior to sterilizing chemo-/radiotherapy. Ovarian biopsies may also be used fresh, yielding a far greater number of follicles at the primordial or preantral stages than the number of oocytes that can be obtained for IVM. The *in vitro* culture of follicles is technically extremely challenging because of the complex changes that occur *in vivo* – many of which are not understood and probably take in the region of 6 months to develop from primordial follicle to the Graafian stage. In order to preserve the integrity of the oocyte/follicle unit it appears best to culture follicles within segments of ovarian cortex, rather than trying to dissect out individual follicles.[8,9] Once the follicle has matured, the oocyte within requires IVM prior to IVF/ICSI. To date, the mouse has been the only species in which live offspring have been produced by these methods and it will be a while before the technology can be successfully applied to humans.[10]

Cryopreservation of Oocytes and Ovarian Tissue (Fig. 18.1)

The ability to cryopreserve gametes has been available for many decades for a number of animals and for human spermatozoa – the latter both after donation for treatment of couples requiring donor insemination (see Ch. 11) or as an insurance before chemotherapy or vasectomy. In recent times there has been immense public interest in the potential for the freezing of oocytes and ovarian tissue – again predominantly for young women about to undergo sterilizing chemo-/radiotherapy. There has also been speculation that this technology could be used as an insurance against ovarian aging for career women who wish to delay child-bearing. While the authors are sympathetic with the pressures on women to succeed in a working environment that frequently shuns the needs of mothers, we feel that, in the first instance at least, the use of these emerging techniques should be focused on medical needs.

Oocyte cryopreservation

When a life-threatening disease such as cancer is diagnosed in a young person, fertility is seldom at the front of his/her mind. It is the responsibility of the physician to advise the patient of the possibility of fertility-preserving techniques prior to embarking upon potentially sterilizing therapy. For women the most realistic prospect of achieving future pregnancy is currently by cryopreservation of embryos generated during a quick IVF protocol (for example, using gonadotropins and a gonadotropin releasing hormone (GnRH) antagonist) which should be complete within 14 days. Relatively few embryos are likely to be generated in this way – on average 10. For religious or ethical reasons, some patients are unhappy to freeze embryos and in these cases oocytes could be frozen prior to insemination. This method may also be used for women without a partner. Presently the returns from oocyte cryopreservation are, however, very small. The patient would have to go through stimulation and oocyte retrieval as for IVF.

The oocyte is the largest single cell in the human and very sensitive to external insults. Few oocytes survive intact the process of freeze–thawing. The temperature sensitivities of the meiotic spindle and the mechanisms within the oocyte that regulate monospermic fertilization raise the risk of aneuploidy.[11] New and improved protocols for cryopreservation of mature oocytes, including storage of GV stage cells, and vitrification[12] are currently being developed. Some clinics have been offering oocyte preservation somewhat prematurely, in our view, without appropriate validation of the techniques and their subsequent safety.

Ovarian tissue cryopreservation (Fig. 18.1)

To date the only effective method of fertility preservation prior to therapy for cancer is sperm banking for postpubertal men, while cryopreservation of tissue containing immature gametes from both sexes is still only at the research stage. The ovarian cortex contains hundreds of thousands of primordial follicles at birth and several thousand for most of a woman's reproductive life. The number declines progressively and at a steady rate until the age of about 38 years, after which time the rate of loss doubles until the menopause occurs. The number of primordial follicles at a given age varies considerably between individuals. It is this number that constitutes a woman's "ovarian reserve" (see Chs 4, 8, and 13) and also reflects the ovaries' ability to withstand the insult of chemo-/radiotherapy in the treatment of cancer. Thus young women are more likely to retain fertility than older women.

There are a number of conditions in young women that may require potentially sterilizing treatment – not only malignant conditions such as Hodgkin's disease, sarcomas, germ cell tumors, lymphomas, and leukemias, but also some systemic conditions such as severe connective tissue diseases (e.g., systemic lupus erythematosus). There are an estimated 1 in 1000 young adults who are survivors of childhood malignancy and this figure is expected to rise. Treatments that are most likely to cause damage to the germ cells include:

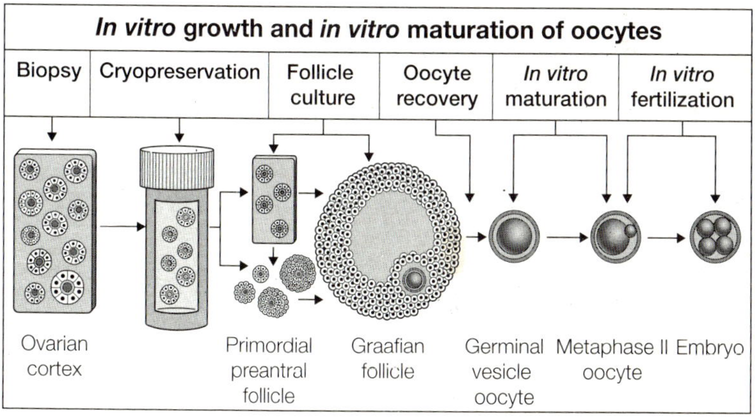

Figure 18.1 The principal steps involved in the *in vitro* growth (solid arrows) and *in vitro* maturation (open arrows) of oocytes. Courtesy of Dr Helen Picton, University of Leeds (in Balen A., *Fertility 2000*. Excerpta Medica, Amsterdam, pp 63–67).[16]

- Total body irradiation (prior to bone marrow or stem cell transplantation)
- Localized pelvic irradiation (without pre-therapy ovarian transposition)
- Chemotherapy: alkylating agents (cyclophosphamide, procarbazine, cisplatinum, lomustine, etc.), vinblastine, cytosine arabinoside.

Many regimens are evolving and so it is difficult to predict the long-term effects on fertility of some of the newer protocols.

Cryopreservation of ovarian cortical tissue offers the possibility of fertility preservation prior to sterilizing therapy for cancer. The technique is fraught with difficulty as the multicellular and heterogeneous nature of the follicle makes it hard to freeze.[10] The cells are protected from injury during the freezing process by replacing water with a cryoprotectant, such as ethylene glycol. All cryoprotectants are potentially toxic and work is still required to optimize the protocols. In order to obtain sufficient follicles for future use, we have found it necessary to take an entire ovary and dissect off the cortex, which is then frozen in strips. Thus we advise a laparoscopic oophorectomy for young women who stand a greater than 90% chance of being rendered sterile by chemo-/radiotherapy. Our current experience indicates that women over the age of 30 have too high a rate of attrition of follicles after the freezing and thawing of ovarian tissue for the procedure to be of benefit.

To date there has been limited success with reimplanting frozen–thawed ovarian tissue, with follicle growth demonstrated in autografts both under the skin of the forearm and in the pelvis. Viability has been short lived and ovulation has yet to be demonstrated. An alternative approach to autografting is *in vitro* growth of follicles followed by IVM of oocytes prior to IVF/ICSI. This would avoid the risk of reintroduction of malignant cells. Again the technology is a long way from being perfected. Furthermore, concerns have been expressed about the possible adverse effects of culture on genetic imprinting, which is a significant problem in animal models.[10]

It is anticipated that there are still many years of research before this technology becomes a reality. We therefore need to be cautious in our approach to the vulnerable patient confronted by the terrifying prospect of a life-threatening malignancy combined with the potential loss of fertility. On the one hand it is important that she is made aware of the options, but on the other counseled adequately about the realistic prospects of success. The British Fertility Society has produced a comprehensive document entitled *A strategy for future reproductive services for survivors of cancer*,[13] which discusses the psychological, ethical, and legal issues as well as the scientific possibilities.

Pre-implantation Genetic Diagnosis (Table 18.1)

Pre-implantation genetic diagnosis (PGD) involves the removal of one or more cells from the cleaving embryo in order to perform genetic testing to enable the subsequent transfer of only healthy embryos. PGD is indicated for couples who have had previous children/ pregnancies affected by life-threatening or major genetic disease, who otherwise would have to conceive naturally and undergo antenatal testing (e.g., chorionic villus sampling or amniocentesis) and a subsequent termination if tested positive. Controversial and ethical issues concern what constitutes a "major genetic disorder" and the possibility of "designer babies" now that the human genome has been mapped. Also there is a high frequency of chromosome or genetic abnormalities (40–50%) in human embryos, which increases with female age.[14] Aneuploidy screening can be performed to ensure that only genetically normal embryos are transferred during routine IVF in couples without a history of genetic disease – a potentially attractive option for older women who have a significantly increased risk of aneuploid embryos.[15] In the UK the Human Fertilisation and

Table 18.1 Common inherited conditions that can be screened by PGD

Single gene defects
Autosomal dominant:
Huntington's chorea
Autosomal recessive:
cystic fibrosis
Tay–Sachs disease
β-Thalassemia
sickle cell anemia
X-linked recessive:
Duchenne muscular dystrophy
hemophilia A
severe combined immune deficiency
Fragile X syndrome
Chromosomal disorders
Structural chromosome aberrations
Translocations
Inversions
Deletions
Aneuploidy risk:
trisomy syndromes: 21 (Down's); 18 (Edwards's); XXY (Klinefelter's)
monosomy syndromes: XO (Turner's)
tetraploidy

Courtesy of Dr Helen Picton, University of Leeds.[16]

Embryology Authority (HFEA) has restricted licenses for PGD to a handful of centers and then for specified and clearly defined conditions. Elsewhere, however, aneuploidy screening is becoming more widespread and unregulated.

Embryos are created in an IVF cycle (Ch. 13), although it is obligatory to perform ICSI to prevent contamination of the subsequent genetic analysis with surplus spermatozoa. The success of PGD relies upon the ability to culture embryos for up to 5 days *in vitro* and to use micromanipulation techniques to remove one or two blastomeres. Each blastomere is thought to be pluripotent and so those that remain have the potential to develop normally. Genetic analysis is performed by either the polymerase chain reaction (PCR) for DNA sequences or fluorescent *in situ* hybridization (FISH) for whole chromosomes or parts of chromosomes. Polar body biopsy can also be performed on oocytes prior to fertilization when the female is the carrier of the genetic defect.[16]

There are two main categories of genetic defects that cause inherited disease: those that affect chromosomes and those that affect single genes. To detect single gene defects in DNA extracted from single blastomeres, the DNA in the nucleus of the biopsied cell is rapidly amplified many times over by PCR.[17] The sensitivity of single-cell PCR may be further increased by the incorporation of fluorescently labeled primers into the PCR products.[16] This provides sufficient fluorescently labeled DNA for screening for defects such as cystic fibrosis. The multicolor FISH technique enables several chromosomes to be reliably detected simultaneously in a single cell to enable screening for the common aneuploidies of chromosomes 13, 18, 21, X, and Y. The major application of FISH in PGD has so far been for gender determination for the prevention of X-linked recessive disease. However, the development of probes for additional chromosomes will extend the application of FISH analysis for more general aneuploidy screening.[16] The technology for PGD is only available in a few centers worldwide and the number of children born as a result of these techniques is relatively few. For example, the large center in Brussels reported 183 cycles over 5 years with 29 ongoing pregnancies.[18]

Stem Cell Research, Cloning, Nuclear Transfer, and Cytoplasmic Transfer

The technology of stem cell culture has developed from the science of reproductive medicine, although does not apply specifically to the treatment of infertility. While stem cell culture may provide cell lines for the production of neurogenic tissue, hemopoietic tissues, and other cells for therapeutic purposes, further discussion of these emerging technologies is beyond the scope of this book. Similarly cloning is not a fertility treatment *per se*, although it could theoretically be used to create embryos from cells that are not gametes. Data from animal studies are presenting significant concerns about abnormal genomic imprinting and premature aging of offspring. It is therefore considered irresponsible by the majority of the scientific community to contemplate using this technology in humans, particularly as there is no clear indication. The transfer of cytoplasm from a "young" oocyte to an older one, or the transfer of a nucleus from an old oocyte into an enucleated younger one, have been proposed as a means of overcoming the affect of aging on mitochondrial function in the cytoplasm, which may in turn affect embryo function and fertility. These controversial techniques have not yet been accepted and could confer potential risks to offspring. The interested reader is referred to the list of further reading at the end of this chapter.

Advances in Therapeutics

FSH-CTP

In 1992, Fares *et al.* reported a new follitropin with a long half-life created by recombinant technology.[19] The longer half-life of human chorionic gonadotropin (hCG) compared with luteinizing hormone (LH) was recognized as being a function of the extra 30 amino acids and carbohydrate residues located at the carboxyl terminal which did not impede interaction with the LH receptor but did lead to persistence in the circulation and therefore a longer biological effect. The end of the beta-FSH gene was spliced off and discarded. The gene encoding the carboxy terminal portion (CTP) of the beta-hCG gene was spliced and introduced to the remaining portion of the beta-FSH gene. The new gene was transfected into a Chinese hamster ovary cell line and the resulting chimeric protein FSH-CTP extracted. Animal models have confirmed a longer lasting effect. This model is analogous to recombinant insulin analogs which can now be tailored to the individual patient with combinations of short-, medium-, and long-acting preparations. Eventually precise gonadotropin action might be dissected to the cellular level such that oligopeptides will be created to bind to specific receptors such as in the periovulatory follicle or corpus luteum.[20] Studies are currently taking place to explore the use of FSH-CTP both as a single injection in the management of anovulatory infertility and also to reduce the number of injections required for controlled ovarian stimulation.

Recombinant DNA technology has enabled the production of recombinant LH and hCG for clinical use, with the potential for tailoring the gonadotropin regimen much more precisely to the individual patient's needs. The degree to which this is both feasible and applicable is yet to be determined.

Needle-less Injector

As well as refinements in the drugs available for assisted reproduction treatments, there have been improvements in the ways in which they can be administered. Thus with increasing purity of gonadotropin preparations they can now be injected subcutaneously rather than intramuscularly, which is not only more comfortable for the patient but also makes self-administration easier. Automatic injecting devices, which administer a dose of FSH that can be adjusted according to patient need, further assist the injection process. A needle-free delivery system that delivers an aerosol of pre-dissolved rFSH through the skin surface in a single dose container powered by a compressed gas canister which is located behind the plunger. Still to come are oral preparations and analogs of drugs that at present can only be given parenterally.

Other Therapies

Since the first edition of this book was published 6 years ago a number of new therapies have begun to become established in clinical practice. The use of insulin sensitizing agents in the management of PCOS has become widespread (see Chs 6 and 7), and although the initial evidence is promising, we are still awaiting the results of adequately powered, placebo-controlled randomized controlled trials – such as the one we are coordinating from Leeds. The GnRH antagonists are another class of drugs that are now becoming established in our therapeutic armamentarium, and their use has been discussed in Chapter 13.

Gene therapies are being introduced gradually into clinical practice but have not yet been applied to reproductive medicine – possibilities include the manipulation of angiogenesis in the endometrium to aid implantation. These exciting prospects require much more research but may be in the realms of reality by the next edition of this book!

Acknowledgment

I am grateful to my colleague Dr Helen Picton PhD, Senior Lecturer, Department of Reproductive Medicine, Leeds University, for ideas and input to the text, tables and illustrations in this chapter.

References

1. Gardner DK, Lane M & Schoolcraft WB (2000) Culture and transfer of viable blastocysts: a feasible proposition for human IVF. In: Sjöberg N-O & Hamberger L (eds) Blastocyst development and early implantation. *Hum Reprod*, Suppl. 6. Oxford University Press, Oxford.
2. Houghton FD, Hawkhead JA, Humpherson PG *et al.* (2002) Non-invasive amino acid turnover predicts human embryo developmental capacity. *Hum Reprod* **17**: 999–1005.

3. Braude PR, Bolton VN & Moore S (1988) Human gene expression first occurs between the four- and eight-cell stages of preimplantation development. *Nature* **322**: 459–461.
4. Smith SD, Mikkelsen A & Lindenberg S (2000) Development of human oocytes matured *in vitro* for 28 or 36 h. *Fertil Steril* **73**: 541–544.
5. Trounson AO, Wood C & Kausche A (1994) *In vitro* maturation and the fertilisation and developmental competence of oocytes recovered from untreated polycystic ovarian patients. *Fertil Steril* **62**: 353–362.
6. Cha KY & Chian RC (1998) Maturation *in vitro* of immature human oocytes for clinical use. *Hum Reprod Update* **4**: 103–120.
7. Picton HM, Briggs D & Gosden RG (1998) The molecular basis of oocyte growth and development. *Mol Cell Endocrinol* **145**: 27–37.
8. Newton H, Picton H & Gosden RG (1999) *In vitro* growth of preantral follicles isolated from frozen/thawed ovine tissue. *J Reprod Fertil* **115**: 141–150.
9. Hartshorne GM (1997) *In vitro* culture of ovarian follicles. *Rev Reprod* **2**: 94–104.
10. Gosden RG, Mullan J, Picton HM, Yin H & Tan S-L (2002) Current perspective on primordial follicle cryopreservation and culture for reproductive medicine. *Hum Reprod Update* **8**: 105–110.
11. Gook DA & Edgar DH (1999) Cryopreservation of the human female gamete: current and future issues. *Hum Reprod* **14**: 2938–2940.
12. Kuleshova L, Gianaroli L, Magli C, Ferraretti A & Trounson A (1999) Birth following vitrification of a small number of human oocytes: case report. *Hum Reprod* **14**: 3077–3079.
13. Cooke I (ed) (2002) *A strategy for future reproductive services for survivors of cancer*. British Fertility Society, Bristol.
14. Wells D & Delhanty JDA (2000) Comprehensive chromosomal analysis of human preimplantation embryos using whole genome amplification and single cell comparative genomic hybridisation. *Mol Hum Reprod* **6**: 1055–1062.
15. Munne S, Grifo J, Alikani M, Cohen J & Tomkin G (1995) Embryo morphology, developmental rates, and maternal age are correlated with chromosomal abnormalities. *Fertil Steril* **64**: 382–391.
16. Picton HM (2000) Ongoing and future developments in infertility treatment. In Balen AH (ed) *Fertility 2000*. Excerpta Medica, Amsterdam, pp 63–67.
17. Handyside AH & Delhanty JDA (1997) Preimplantation genetic diagnosis: strategies and surprises. *Trends Genet* **13**: 270–275.
18. Vandervorst M, Staessen C, Sermon K *et al.* (2000) The Brussels experience of more than 5 years of clinical pre-implantation genetic diagnosis. *Hum Reprod Update* **6**: 364–373.
19. Fares FA, Suganuma N, Nishimori K, La Polt PS, Hsueh AJW & Boime I (1992) Design of a long-acting follitropin agonist by fusing the C-terminal sequence of the chorionic gonadotropin beta subunit to the follitropin beta subunit. *Proc Natl Acad Sci U S A* **89**: 4304–4308.
20. Gast MJ (1995) Evolution of clinical agents for ovulation induction. *Am J Obstet Gynecol* **172**: 753–759.

Further Reading

Edwards RG & Brody SA (1995) *Principles and practice of assisted human reproduction*. WB Saunders, London.

Fauser BCJM, Rutherford AJ, Strauss JF & van Steirteghem A (2002) *Molecular biology in reproductive medicine*. Parthenon Publishing, New York.

Gardner DK, Weissman A, Howles CM, Shoham Z (2001) *Textbook of assisted reproductive Techniques – laboratory and clinical perspectives*. Martin Dunitz, London.

Hillier SG, Kitchener HC & Nielson JP (1996) *Scientific essentials of reproductive medicine*. WB Saunders, London.

Sjöberg N-O & Hamberger L (eds) Blastocyst development and early implantation. *Hum Reprod*, Suppl. 6. Oxford University Press, Oxford.

Wolpert L (1998) *Principles of development*. Oxford University Press, Oxford.

Ziebe S & Hartshorne G (eds) (2000) Innovations and limitations in sssisted reproduction. *Hum Reprod*, Suppl. 5. Oxford University Press, Oxford.

SECTION 5

Pregnancy

Chapter 19

Miscarriage after fertility treatment

Introduction

Miscarriage is common, with a rate of between 10% and 30% of all spontaneous pregnancies.[1] Infertility is also common, affecting about 30% of couples.[2] The causes of infertility are multiple and diverse yet some, for example endometriosis and the polycystic ovary syndrome, (PCOS) may also affect successful implantation and pregnancy outcome. With the development of assisted conception it is now possible to overcome or circumvent many of the problems presented by the subfertile couple. The main questions arising from the various therapies available are: Do they increase the rate of miscarriage or fetal malformations? And if they are found to do so, is this caused by the treatment or is it a reflection of the underlying fertility disorder?

We address these questions by examining both the influence on miscarriage of the drugs used in ovulation induction and the effect of the different techniques employed in assisted conception. First it is important to consider special factors that pertain to miscarriage in the infertile couple.

Miscarriage in the Infertile Couple

Parental Age

Couples attending the infertility clinic tend to be older than the average couple attending an antenatal clinic. In a study of patients attending our unit, the mean age of female patients was 33 years, compared with a mean age of 28.8 years in women who give birth in England and Wales. Couples with subfertility may have tried for a pregnancy for several years before seeking medical advice and may then have attended both their general practitioner and gynecologist for investigation and possibly simple treatments before being referred for assisted conception. Women may also choose to delay starting a family, for example while establishing a career. Such a delay leads to a greater incidence of ovulatory dysfunction, endometriosis, and the possibility of developing gynecological pathology necessitating surgery, such as ovarian cysts, fibroids, and tubal damage.

In addition to the problem of becoming pregnant, the older woman has a high chance of miscarriage. In a series of 2730 sonographically confirmed pregnancies the overall first trimester spontaneous abortion rate was 14.6%.[3] The incidence of abortion in those women under 35 was 6.4%, rising to 14.7% in women between 35 and 40 years of age and to 23.1% in women over 40. The frequency of chromosomal abnormalities in abortuses was 82.7% and was greatest in the first 6–8 weeks (86.5%). There are extensive data that confirm a rising risk of chromosomal anomalies with maternal age[4–6] and this accounts, to a great extent, for the increasing miscarriage rate. If a pregnancy continues there appears to be no association between birth defects of unknown etiology and advancing maternal age.[7]

There has been disagreement in the literature concerning male factors in spontaneous abortion. Chromosomally abnormal spermatozoa that achieve fertilization may lead to the development of an abnormal fetus and the risk also increases with advancing paternal age. Polyploidy, however, is usually excluded during IVF procedures because embryos are screened at the pronuclear stage. If there are abnormal semen parameters severe enough to affect fertility there does not appear to be a correlation between abortion and sperm count or motility.[8] The use of donor sperm does not appear to have an adverse effect on miscarriage rate.[9]

Apart from the considerations of parental age, the couple with secondary infertility often presents with a poor obstetric history and with pregnancy losses prior to treatment, sometimes in as many as 70–80%.[9]

Hypersecretion of Luteinizing Hormone and Miscarriage

Hypersecretion of luteinizing hormone (LH) occurs only in the PCOS. There appears to be a strong association between elevated serum concentration of LH and miscarriage, possibly through an adverse effect on oocyte maturation.[10] A field study of 193 women planning to become pregnant showed that raised mid-follicular phase serum LH concentrations were associated with both a lower conception rate (67%) and a much higher miscarriage rate (65%), compared with those in women with normal serum LH concentrations (88% and 12% respectively).[11]

It was first demonstrated in 1985 that oocytes obtained from women undergoing IVF who had a serum LH value greater than one standard deviation above the mean on the day of administration of human chorionic gonadotropin (hCG) had a significantly reduced rate of fertilization and cleavage.[12] A study of women undergoing "natural cycle IVF" (that is, in unstimulated cycles) again found a reduction in fertilization rates in women who had elevated serum LH concentrations in either the early follicular (45.5%) or mid-follicular (50%) phase compared with an 87.5% fertilization rate in a control group who had normal serum LH concentrations.[13]

In a study of patients attending our clinic with amenorrhea who received treatment with pulsatile luteinizing hormone-releasing hormone (LHRH) for induction of ovulation, follicular phase plasma LH concentrations were significantly higher in those with PCOS than in those with other diagnoses.[14] In an extension of this study we found a miscarriage rate of 33% in women with PCOS compared with 10.6% in those with hypogonadotropic hypogonadism.[15] Furthermore, in women with PCOS there was a significantly reduced chance of conception and increased risk of miscarriage in those with an elevated follicular phase plasma LH concentration compared with those with PCOS and normal follicular phase LH levels.[15] The association of raised baseline and/or mid-follicular phase plasma LH concentrations with a poor response to treatment was also demonstrated in a series of 100 women with PCOS who were treated with low-dose gonadotropin therapy.[16] In this series, the patients with an elevated LH concentration also had a higher rate of miscarriage than the women with polycystic ovaries and normal LH levels.

LH has a role in the suppression of the oocyte maturation inhibitor (OMI). Oocytes are maintained in the first meiotic division from their appearance in the ovary during intrauterine life until just before ovulation, when oocyte maturation is completed, germinal vesicle breakdown occurs, and the first polar body is extruded (see Fig. 13.6). Since oocytes undergo maturation spontaneously when they are cultured outside the follicle, an intrafollicular OMI has been postulated, itself inhibited at mid-cycle by the ovulatory stimulus. The precise nature of OMI is uncertain. It is known, however, that cyclic adenosine monophosphate (cAMP) activates OMI or is itself OMI. One action of cAMP is to maintain meiotic arrest of the oocyte at the diplotene stage of prophase 1. The oocyte does not synthesize cAMP but obtains it from cumulus granulosa cells via processes that traverse the intercellular space. Stimulation by LH leads to disruption of these processes, loss of contact between granulosa cells and the oocyte, a fall in intraoocyte cAMP and then resumption of meiosis.

There appears to be a species-specific interval between ovulation and fertilization and if this interval is exceeded, physiologically aged oocytes are produced which may be subject to reproductive failure. Our hypothesis to explain the adverse effect of hypersecretion of LH on human fertility is therefore that hypersecretion of LH during the follicular phase results in an elevated concentration of intrafollicular LH which in turn results in premature oocyte maturation, with subsequent ovulation of a prematurely matured egg. Thus inappropriate release of LH may affect the timing of oocyte maturation such that the released egg is either unable to be fertilized or, if fertilized, miscarries.

A number of alternative "non-embryological" explanations of the association of hypersecretion of LH with reproductive disturbance have been offered. For example, it has been suggested that LH exerts its detrimental effect by causing oversecretion of ovarian androgens which suppress granulosa cell function and cause follicular atresia. In our experience elevated androgen levels in women with the PCOS are associated with symptoms of hyperandrogenism (hirsutism, acne) rather than infertility, which is instead positively correlated with LH excess. Furthermore, Shoham *et al.*[17] demonstrated that, in women treated with clomiphene citrate, high levels of LH during the follicular phase were associated with a reduced conception rate despite adequate follicular growth and corpus luteum function, as indicated by measurements of serum estradiol concentrations in the follicular phase and progesterone concentrations in the luteal phase.

Another explanation for the association of PCOS with miscarriage is an endometrial abnormality resulting from disordered prostaglandin synthesis.[18] Data in women having the transfer of frozen embryos in natural cycles, however, demonstrated no correlation between serum LH concentrations and the rates of conception and miscarriage.[19] The embryos in this study had been generated in IVF cycles in which pituitary desensitization had been used to achieve suppression of LH levels. Thus the elevated LH concentrations seen in the subsequent natural cycles of some of the women who received the frozen embryos could not have affected embryo quality and could only have exerted an effect by altering the endocrine or endometrial environments: in the event, no effect on outcome was detected.

Obesity is a common finding in women with the PCOS and a moderate elevation of body mass index to between 25 and 27.5 kg/m^2 is associated with an increased rate of miscarriage, independent of LH levels.[20] While these factors may be important for a healthy pregnancy outcome they do not explain the reduced fertilization rates observed with oocytes removed from women with high serum LH concentrations. Thus we have concluded that abnormal oocyte maturation is probably the main cause of reproductive failure in women who hypersecrete LH during the follicular phase of the ovulation cycle.

If hypersecretion of LH increases the risk of miscarriage, therapies that suppress serum LH concentrations might be expected to confer benefit. The use of GnRH agonists to achieve pituitary desensitization results in low serum LH levels, as does induction of ovulation using laparoscopic ovarian diathermy. Neither therapy has been shown conclusively to reduce miscarriage rates, although some studies have indicated that these are potentially promising treatments.

Diagnosis of Pregnancy

The intensity of early pregnancy monitoring is much greater in assisted than natural conceptions. Pregnancy can be diagnosed as early as 24 hours after conception, with the measurement of "early pregnancy factor." It is, however, hCG that is usually assayed. hCG can be measured in maternal serum and urine from between 8 and 11 days post-ovulation. It is therefore possible to determine the outcome of an assisted conception cycle in the late luteal phase and so women may know whether they are pregnant before the expected commencement of menses.

With the advent of sensitive assays for hCG it has been possible to obtain a better idea of the incidence of pregnancy failure in both natural and assisted conceptions. In 1967, Hertig[21] suggested that in natural cycles 85% of oocytes fertilize, 70% of these implant, yet only 58% of these survive until the end of the second week, and 16% of these are abnormal and abort shortly after this time. In a series of women trying to conceive, an elevated urinary hCG was found in 59.6% of 198 ovulatory cycles,[22] yet 62% of conceptuses were lost by 12 weeks and most of the losses (92%) were clinically undetected. The overall fecundity was therefore 22%, which is similar to that expected for a normal population.

It should be remembered that hCG is administered in most assisted conception regimens in order to mimic the mid-cycle LH surge. This is required in order to initiate oocyte maturation prior to a timed oocyte collection procedure. The injected hCG should have cleared from the circulation by 9–10 days after ovulation or oocyte retrieval, so hCG at a concentration of greater than 10 i.u./L on luteal days 11–13 indicates trophoblast development (one can be more certain if the hCG had been less than 5 i.u./L on days 9–10). Confusion because of exogenously administered hCG will disappear with the advent of recombinantly derived LH, which is now available but not widely used. Women who undergo assisted conception require luteal support, provided in the form of either progesterone or hCG. If the latter is used, a pregnancy can only be diagnosed by a rising concentration of serum hCG. We have found that when the serum hCG concentration is measured 12 days after embryo transfer, a value of greater than 50 i.u./L predicts a high likelihood of a normal ongoing pregnancy, while lower values suggest either miscarriage or ectopic pregnancy.

A pre-clinical or biochemical miscarriage occurs when there is a measurable serum hCG concentration, usually less than 50 i.u./L, which remains elevated for a few days only and results in a delay of menses of no more than 14 days. A clinical miscarriage occurs after the hCG has continued to rise to a time when an intrauterine gestation sac can be seen sonographically, either with or without a fetal pole or heart beat, but then a miscarriage occurs.

The phenomenon of the "vanishing embryo" has come to light since the advent of early pregnancy monitoring after assisted conception therapies. In one study early ultrasonography demonstrated spontaneous absorption of a gestation sac in 11 of 42 twin pregnancies and in five of 13 sets of triplets (in which two were reduced to singleton pregnancies).[23] In another study, 140 pregnancies were scanned weekly from the fifth to the thirteenth week of conception.[24] In the patients with one sac seen initially, 27% of the sacs disappeared; when there were two sacs, 25% disappeared, and with three sacs, 47% disappeared. The percentage of women who ended up with a viable pregnancy was 72%, 94%, and 100%, respectively, for those initially with one, two, and three sacs. The "vanishing embryo" can apply equally to spontaneous or artificially conceived pregnancies, although the risk of multiple pregnancy is of course greater after ovulation induction or assisted conception.

The Influence on Miscarriage of the Drugs Used in Fertility Therapy

Ovulatory failure accounts for about a fifth of cases of infertility. Over the last 30 years drug regimens of increasing complexity have evolved to induce ovulation. The drugs prescribed to anovulatory women are also used to induce multifollicular growth in women who ovulate normally. These women benefit from superovulation as the production of several oocytes increases the success of assisted conception therapies. The most commonly used preparations are the antiestrogens (e.g., clomiphene citrate), the gonadotropins and gonadotropin-releasing hormone analogs (see Chs 6 and 13). Information about the sequelae of the use of fertility drugs therefore chiefly refers to these three groups.

Antiestrogens

The most widely prescribed antiestrogen is clomiphene citrate. Its use in ovulation induction was first reported by Greenblatt *et al.*[25] at a time when human pituitary and menopausal urinary gonadotropins were also beginning to be extracted and standardized. In an early report of pregnancy outcome in a small number of women, Greenblatt *et al.* found the incidence of spontaneous abortion to be 22%.[26] Karow & Payne[27] reported on a heterogeneous group of 410 infertile women, in whom a pregnancy rate of 39.8% was achieved. The spontaneous abortion rate was 19%, similar to that seen in infertility patients prior to the advent of the drug. The incidence of twins was 8.6%, contributing to a premature delivery rate of 12%. There was no confirmation of an earlier theory that conception in the first treatment cycle resulted in an increased chance of miscarriage or multiple pregnancy. Also in 1968, a series of 2196 clomiphene-induced pregnancies was reported,[28] in which the miscarriage rate was 17.6%, the multiple pregnancy rate 10.2%, and the incidence of congenital anomalies 2.5%.

Although clomiphene was found to induce ovulation in about 90% of infertile women and pregnancy in 50%, the multiple pregnancy rate was sometimes as high as 50%. In general the miscarriage rate after clomiphene treatment has been reported to be between 20% and 27%, the rate of multiple pregnancy 10–15%, and the incidence of congenital abnormalities about 2–3%.[29–31]

One series reported an overall miscarriage rate of 9.3%, 28.1% if conception occurred during the first cycle of treatment, and as high as 70% if conception resulted after seven cycles. It was thought that prolonged usage of clomiphene might have a deleterious effect on the endometrium, causing atrophy and implantation failure. The relatively high miscarriage rate during the first cycle of treatment that was seen in this study was postulated as being secondary to the release of "overripe" oocytes after a prolonged period of anovulation. Interpreting data from the early use of clomiphene is complicated by the lack of uniformity in presenting details of maternal age and the cause of infertility. Monitoring was limited to measurement of urinary estrogens or vaginal cytology and often omitted. Pregnancy diagnosis was not as advanced as at present and so it is inappropriate to compare miscarriage data between the different series.

Most women who require clomiphene to induce ovulation have PCOS and are likely to have a tendency to hypersecrete LH. Clomiphene achieves its action through stimulation of both follicle stimulating hormone (FSH) and LH secretion by the pituitary and women with PCOS can respond with an exaggerated release of LH and a resultant reduction in the chance of conception and increase in the risk of miscarriage.[17,32]

Congenital Abnormalities with Clomiphene Citrate

The risk of congenital abnormalities and the physical development of infants born to mothers who have received clomiphene has not been found to be different to that of the general population, yet concern was expressed about the finding of an increased frequency of chromosomal abnormalities after induced ovulation,[33] an effect that appeared to persist during the subsequent, non-stimulated cycle. Following the report of two cases of neural tube defects after clomiphene therapy,[34] other isolated cases of congenital abnormalities appeared in the literature. Most have felt that factors related to infertility itself may be to blame, rather than ovulation induction, and that babies born after ovulation induction are no more at risk of being malformed than if they were conceived spontaneously.[35]

Whereas there continue to be reports that suggest a more than coincidental association between ovulation induction, specifically using clomiphene, and neural tube defects,[36] other reports are reassuring and suggest no evidence for this.[37] Shoham *et al.* reviewed 3751 births after clomiphene therapy and found an overall incidence of major and minor malformations of 32.5 per 1000 births),[1] this figure being within the range found among the normal population.[35]

Ovulation Induction with Gonadotropins

Women who do not respond to oral therapy may succeed in having ovulation induced with gonadotropin therapy. The preparations available either contain both LH and FSH or contain FSH alone (see Ch. 6). It was thought that the use of FSH alone would benefit women with the PCOS by minimizing circulating LH levels. However, these women are usually very sensitive to both forms of treatment and the use of FSH alone confers no advantage as serum concentrations of LH are still within the normal range when human menopausal gonadotropin (hMG) is used. The amount of LH in hMG preparations is small compared with the amount secreted by the pituitary and so is rapidly diluted after administration; furthermore, with unifollicular ovulation induction the developing follicle secretes hormones that feed back to the hypothalamus and pituitary and suppress endogenous LH secretion. Studies to date indicate that miscarriage rates are similar irrespective of the gonadotropin used.

As for the actual reported miscarriage rate after gonadotropin-induced ovulation, this varies between 11.3% and 27.5%. Lunenfeld *et al.* also reported an analysis of the abortion rates in both the first and subsequent treatment cycles and the first and subsequent pregnancies.[38] In this study it was found that whereas the abortion rate was 28.8% in a first pregnancy, it was only 12.8% in a second pregnancy. This figure is similar to the 13% of women who aborted after a spontaneous conception that followed a successful gonadotropin-induced pregnancy. There was no difference in the abortion rates of patients who became pregnant after the first or subsequent treatment cycles. This goes against a commonly proposed theory that anovulatory women release eggs of "poor quality" in their first ovulation induction cycle.[33]

Other groups have also found a higher miscarriage rate in the first gonadotropin-induced pregnancy. One series reported a reduction in miscarriage rate from 28.5% in first hMG pregnancies to 11.9% in those conceiving for a second time;[39] another series found these figures to be 33% and 9.8% respectively.[40] In contrast to these studies, a more recent paper reported an overall spontaneous abortion rate in 350 pregnancies after first treatment cycles of 24.2%, yet a 48% abortion rate in a subsequent pregnancy in women whose first hMG pregnancy ended in a spontaneous abortion; this compared to an incidence of abortion of 6.7% if the first hMG-induced pregnancy was normal.[41] These data are in keeping with the notion that the risk of miscarriage following a natural conception is directly related to a woman's past obstetric history.

We reported a retrospective analysis of all patients treated in the ovulation induction clinic at the Middlesex Hospital, London, from May 1982 to January 1993.[42] A total of 200 anovulatory patients were included in the analysis, 103 with clomiphene citrate-resistant PCOS, 77 with hypogonadotropic hypogonadism (HH), and 20 with weight-related amenorrhea (WRA). There was no difference in the mean age of the three groups. The cumulative conception rates (CCR) and cumulative live birth rates (CLBR) of the three groups in the first course of therapy and after 12 cycles of treatment are illustrated in Figures 6.8, 6.25 and 6.26. The miscarriage rates were 16.5% in PCOS patients, 22.9% in HH patients, and 32.3% in WRA patients and, while not statistically significantly different, this resulted in comparable CLBRs between the three groups.

Patients with amenorrhea secondary to weight loss respond well to ovulation induction therapy with normal or supranormal cumulative conception rates.[43–45] The miscarriage rate in these patients, however, was 32% and this resulted in a cumulative live birth rate that was similar to that of patients with PCOS and HH. Furthermore, women who conceived spontaneously and had a body mass index (BMI) of less than 19.1 kg/m^2 had twice the risk of delivering a low birthweight infant compared with women of normal weight ($p < 0.005$)[46] and they also had a higher incidence of preterm deliveries ($p < 0.01$). We have also reported previously that patients with WRA who conceive after treatment with pulsatile gonadotropin releasing hormone (GnRH) are more likely to deliver lighter babies than women of normal weight ($p < 0.001$).[47] Our current approach is therefore to encourage weight gain and not to induce ovulation in women with a BMI of less than 19.5 kg/m^2.

Congenital Abnormalities after Gonadotropin Treatment

An analysis of seven studies that addressed the outcome of gonadotropin-induced pregnancies concluded that this treatment results in the same incidence of congenital malformations expected for the general population.[1] These studies include a total of 1160 newborn infants, in whom the overall incidence of malformations was 54.3 per 1000 (21.6/1000 major and 32.7/1000 minor malformations).

Miscarriage after IVF and Related Procedures

The first published study of pregnancy outcome after IVF related to pregnancies that occurred after ovarian stimulation with clomiphene citrate or gonadotropins or a combination of both. In recent years there has been a move towards pituitary desensitization with a GnRH agonist (see Ch. 13).

The suppression of endogenous LH by GnRH agonists is of particular relevance and advantage to the woman with PCOS. Thus many oocyte-containing follicles may develop in the sensitive polycystic ovary free from the adverse environment of high tonic LH levels. These oocytes appear to fertilize better than those from cycles without pituitary desensitization, suggesting that it is indeed the abnormal hormonal milieu, rather than the polycystic ovary itself, that is the problem for women with PCOS.

Since the birth of Louise Brown in 1978, the first baby conceived by IVF (in an unstimulated, "natural" cycle), many groups worldwide have reported their experience with IVF and related procedures. It is only now, however, that we can get a realistic impression of miscarriage rates, because of the publication of series with large numbers of pregnancies, both from individual clinics and collated national statistics.

It is important to note the criteria used both to diagnose pregnancy and determine the gestational age at miscarriage, as these influence the interpretation of data from different series.[48] Some groups record biochemical pregnancies and miscarriage separately, while others classify both together under the heading "miscarriage." The mean age of patients and the methods used to stimulate follicular growth are not always recorded.

The first large series was the World Collaborative Report,[49] compiled from the results of 200 groups worldwide. There was a miscarriage rate of 29.9% in the 1084 pregnancies reported and the 1.5% incidence of congenital anomalies was considered to be similar to that occurring after natural conception. We reported a series of 1060 consecutive IVF pregnancies in which the rate of miscarriage was 26.6%, similar to the miscarriage rates of other large IVF series.[10] It is difficult to compare figures obtained after assisted conception procedures with miscarriage rates after spontaneous conceptions because of the more intensive early pregnancy monitoring and earlier diagnosis of pregnancy after IVF treatment. If one takes the timing of the miscarriage into account, the abortion rates that follow natural and assisted conception are similar.[48]

As expected, we found an increased risk of miscarriage with increasing maternal age. Women attending infertility clinics tend to be older than the average couple attending an antenatal clinic. The mean age of women giving birth in England and Wales is 28.8 years,[50] while the mean age of patients in our series was 32.2 years. As already discussed, there are extensive data that confirm a rising incidence of chromosomal anomalies with increasing maternal age and this accounts, in large part, for the increasing miscarriage rate. With respect to chromosomal abnormalities following assisted conception, Lower *et al.*[51] compared miscarriage following spontaneous and assisted conception and found no significant increase in the rate of chromosomal abnormalities after gamete manipulation. Thus the miscarriage rate is a reflection of maternal characteristics rather than of the gamete handling procedures.

We found that there was no relation between the miscarriage rate and the indication for IVF.[52] On the other hand, of the 538 patients in our series who had a pretreatment baseline ultrasound scan, those with normal ovaries had a 23.6% miscarriage rate compared with a rate of 35.8% in those with polycystic ovaries ($p = 0.0038$, 95% CI 4.68–23.10%). At the time of the study, a combination of clomiphene citrate and gonadotropins was still being used for some patients, whereas more recently GnRH agonists have been almost universally employed.

The rate of miscarriage in patients who received clomiphene citrate was 47.2% in those with polycystic ovaries and 20.3% in those with normal ovaries ($p < 0.00005$, 95% CI 15.59–38.33%). In patients who received buserelin in the long protocol, there was no significant difference in miscarriage rates between those with polycystic ovaries (20.3%) and those with normal ovaries (25.5%). There was also no difference in the miscarriage rates in women with normal ovaries who received clomiphene citrate (20.3%) or "long" buserelin (25.5%). There was, however, a highly significant difference ($p = 0.0003$, 95% CI 13.82–40.09%) in miscarriage rates in women with polycystic ovaries who received clomiphene (47.2%) and those who received "long" buserelin (20.3%).

These data supported the notion that it was the high level of LH in women with PCOS that was the adverse feature being ameliorated by treatment with the GnRH agonist. Miscarriage rates were not affected by treatment with hMG versus FSH in patients with normal (24.6% vs 28%) or polycystic ovaries (18% vs 25%) who were treated with "long" buserelin and similarly between hMG and FSH in patients with normal (19.3% vs 23.5%) or polycystic ovaries (47.6% vs 46.2%) who were treated with a clomiphene citrate regimen.

Several other studies have also examined the effect of pituitary desensitization on miscarriage rates after IVF and most report a beneficial effect of pituitary desensitization. This is perhaps most clearly demonstrated by an extension of the study by Tan *et al.*,[53] which examined the cumulative conception and live birth rates after IVF with successive cycles of treatment. In total, 4115 couples had undergone 7863 cycles of treatment which resulted in 1279 pregnancies. A multiple logistic regression analysis was performed to correct for the age of the patients, cause of infertility, year of treatment, and duration of infertility. The odds ratio of conception and live birth with pituitary desensitization compared with clomiphene citrate and gonadotropins were 1.63 (95% CI 1.31–2.03) and 1.88 (95% CI 1.39–2.55), respectively. The cumulative conception graphs are illustrated in Figure 13.24.

The high rate of miscarriage in those who had received clomiphene may be related to the deleterious effects of elevated serum LH levels. Clomiphene citrate causes an exaggerated early follicular phase release of both gonadotropins and the resultant elevated LH may reduce the chance of conception and increase the risk of miscarriage. The protective effect of GnRH agonists is presumably mediated by the functional HH and suppressed LH levels that they induce. Our study did not distinguish between the proposed beneficial effect of pituitary desensitization and the detrimental effect of clomiphene citrate. This issue has been clarified by Homburg *et al.*,[54] who studied the outcome of 97 pregnancies in women with PCOS, which was defined as ultrasound-detected polycystic ovaries plus anovulation and infertility and either oligo-/amenorrhea and/or hirsutism. The patients were treated by either ovulation induction or IVF with either hMG alone or hMG after pituitary desensitization with the GnRH agonist Decapeptyl. The miscarriage rate in the agonist-treated patients (17.6%) was significantly lower than the miscarriage rate in the women treated with hMG alone (39.1%, $p = 0.03$). The study demonstrates that pituitary desensitization is the important factor in reducing miscarriage rates in women with polycystic ovaries, rather than clomiphene citrate being the adverse factor, because clomiphene was not used in that study.

The use of a GnRH agonist to achieve pituitary desensitization has become popular in IVF clinics because of the flexibility it affords in programming oocyte recovery.[55] We have shown, however, that in women with an ultrasound diagnosis of polycystic ovaries, the use of buserelin is associated with a significant reduction in the rate of miscarriage in the group of women who are at greatest risk, though there appears to be no reduction in the rate of miscarriage for women with normal ovaries. Pretreatment pelvic ultrasonography is therefore important in order to select the treatment regimen that will lead to the best outcome.

A large study of women undergoing IVF found an increased rate of miscarriage in women with PCOS but suggested that this was caused by obesity rather than any other factors.[56] In this study the use of intracytoplasmic sperm injection (ICSI) was also associated with a lower risk of miscarriage – partly because of the younger age of the female partner and also possibly because oocyte factors play more of a role in the etiology of miscarriage and so couples undergoing ICSI may be less at risk.

When considering the different regimens for IVF it is important to appreciate the potential effects on endogenous hormone concentrations and endometrial receptivity. A recent series of publications has demonstrated improved fertilization and ongoing pregnancy rates in women who have serum LH concentrations > 0.5 i.u./L on the day of hCG compared with those whose LH concentrations are < 0.5 i.u./L.[57] It has been suggested also that high serum estradiol concentrations may be detrimental to uterine receptivity.[58] Thus a balance is required between the degree of suppression caused by the GnRH analogs and the steroidogenic potential of the gonadotropin preparations used to stimulate the ovaries (see also Ch. 13).

Luteal Support

A variety of regimens are used for supporting the luteal phase of assisted conception cycles (see Ch. 13). Published reports of randomized controlled trials assessing the use of progesterone or hCG have shown no significant differences in pregnancy rates.[59] There is strong evidence that luteal support is required, particularly when GnRH agonists have been used. Administration of progesterone is generally preferred to hCG because of the reduced risk of ovarian hyperstimulation syndrome. Luteal support does not affect rates of miscarriage.

There has been a vogue to advise low dose aspirin in order to increase pregnancy rates and reduce the risk of miscarriage. While aspirin therapy may have a role for some causes of recurrent miscarriage (see Ch. 20), there is no convincing evidence for its routine use and so at present we do not recommend it.

Management of Miscarriage

When a non-viable pregnancy has been diagnosed the management may be expectant or active, depending upon the clinical situation and the patient's wishes. Expectant management – in other words awaiting spontaneous and complete resolution of the miscarriage – does not affect future fertility any more than surgical evacuation of the uterus.[60] Active management is often offered to women who have a non-viable pregnancy after fertility treatment as the problem is usually detected before signs of impending miscarriage (e.g., bleeding or pain) and so expectant management could involve a wait of days or even weeks. The options for active management include surgical or medical evacuation of the uterus, the latter often favored these days because of the avoidance of a general anesthetic or instrumentation of the uterus. Couples who experience miscarriage should be offered support and counseling.

Summary

In conclusion, when one accounts for the intensity of early pregnancy monitoring after assisted conception procedures and hence the relatively frequent diagnosis of "biochemical" pregnancy, the overall spontaneous miscarriage rate is similar to that expected for the general population. Indeed, it has been pointed out that as a mean age of under 30 is usually quoted for patients in studies of miscarriage after spontaneous conception, the abortion rate in treated, subfertile women might be "even lower than that of the so-called normal population when adjusted for age."[1] It is also encouraging to note that the drugs used in assisted conception regimens do not appear to affect adversely the incidence of congenital abnormalities.

References

1. Shoham Z, Zosmer A & Insler V (1991) Early miscarriage and fetal malformations after induction of ovulation (by clomiphene citrate and/or human menotropins), *in vitro* fertilization, and gamete intrafallopian transfer. *Fertil Steril* **55**: 1–11.
2. Hull MGR, Glazener CMA, Kelly NJ *et al.* (1985) Population study of causes, treatment and outcome of infertility. *Br Med J* **291**: 1693–1697.
3. Brambati B (1990) Fate of human pregnancies. In: Edwards RG (ed) *Establishing a successful human pregnancy*. Serono Symposia, vol. 66. Raven Press, New York, pp 269–281.
4. Hassold T, Jacobs P, Kline J, Stein Z & Warburton D (1980) Effect of maternal age on autosomal trisomies. *Ann Hum Genet* **44**: 29–36.
5. Hook EB. Woodbury DF & Albright SG (1979) Rates of trisomy 18 in livebirths, stillbirths and at amniocentesis. *Birth Defects: Original Article Series*. AR Liss, New York, **15(5c)**: 81–89.
6. Trimble BK & Baird PA (1978) Maternal age and Down syndrome: age specific incidence rates by single year maternal age intervals. *Am J Med Genet* **1**: 1–5
7. Baird PA, Sadovnick AD & Yee IML (1991) Maternal age and birth defects: a population study. *Lancet* **337**: 527–530
8. Lev-Gur M, Rodriguez LJ, Smith KD & Steinberger E (1990) Risk factors for pregnancy loss apparent at conception in infertile couples. *Int J Fertil* **35**: 51–57.
9. Weir WC & Hendricks CH (1969) The reproductive capacity of an infertile population. *Fertil Steril* **20**: 289–298.
10. Balen AH, Tan SL & Jacobs HS (1993) Hypersecretion of luteinising hormone – a significant cause of subfertility and miscarriage. *Br J Obstet Gynaecol* **100**: 1082–1089.
11. Regan L, Owen EJ & Jacobs HS (1990) Hypersecretion of luteinising hormone, infertility and miscarriage. *Lancet* **336**: 1141–1144.
12. Stanger JD & Yovich JL (1985) Reduced in-vitro fertilisation of human oocyte from patients with raised basal luteinising hormone levels during the follicular phase. *Br J Obstet Gynaecol* **92**: 385–393.
13. Verma S *et al.* (1991) Influence of elevated LH during follicular phase on fertility as assessed in a natural IVF programme. Paper presented at the 7th Annual Meeting of the ESHRE.
14. Abdulwahid NA, Adams J, van der Spuy ZM & Jacobs HS (1985) Gonadotropin control of follicular development. *Clin Endocrinol* **23**: 613–626.
15. Homburg R, Armar NA, Eshel A, Adams J & Jacobs HS (1988) Influence of serum luteinising hormone concentrations on ovulation, conception and early pregnancy loss in polycystic ovary syndrome. *Br Med J* **297**: 1024–1026.
16. Hamilton-Fairley D , Kiddy D, Watson H, Sagle M & Franks S (1991) Low-dose gonadotropin therapy for induction of ovulation in 100 women with polycystic ovary syndrome. *Hum Reprod* **6**: 1095–1099.
17. Shoham Z, Borenstein R, Lunenfeld B & Pariente C (1990) Hormonal profiles following clomiphene citrate therapy in conception and nonconception cycles. *Clin Endocrinol* **33**: 271–278.
18. Bonney RC & Franks S (1990) The endocrinology of implantation and early pregnancy. *Baillière's Clin Endocrinol Metab* **4**: 207–231.
19. Polson DW *et al.* (1992) The effect of serum luteinising hormone concentrations on success rates of frozen embryo replacement into natural cycles. *Br Congress Obstet Gynaecol*, Abstract 152.
20. Hamilton-Fairley D, Kiddy D, Watson H, Paterson C & Franks S (1992) Association of moderate obesity with a poor pregnancy outcome in women with polycystic ovary syndrome treated with low dose gonadotropin. *Br J Obstet Gynaecol* **99**: 128–131.
21. Hertig AT (1967) The overall problem in man. In: Benirschke K (ed) *Comparative aspects of reproductive failure*. Springer-Verlag, New York, pp 11–41.

22. Edmonds DK, Lindsay KS, Miller JF, Williamson E & Wood PJ (1982) Early embryonic mortality in women. *Fertil Steril* **38**: 447–453.
23. Corson SL, Dickey RP, Gocial B *et al.* (1989) Outcome in 242 *in vitro* fertilization-embryo replacement or gamete intrafallopian transfer-induced pregnancies. *Fertil Steril* **51**: 644–650.
24. Tan SL, Riddle A, Sharma V, Mason B & Campbell S (1989) The relation between the number of gestation sacs seen after IVF-ET and outcome of pregnancy. *Proceedings of the XIIth Asian and Oceanic Congress of Obstetrics and Gynaecology*.
25. Greenblatt RB, Barfield WE, Jungck EC & Ray AW (1961) Induction of ovulation with MRL-41. *JAMA* **178**: 101.
26. Greenblatt RB, Roy S, Mahesh VB, Barfield W & Jungck EC (1962) Induction of ovulation. *Am J Obstet Gynecol* **84**: 900–907.
27. Karow WG & Payne SA (1968) Pregnancy after clomiphene citrate treatment. *Fertil Steril* **19**: 351–362.
28. MacGregor AH, Johnson JE & Bunde CA (1968) Further clinical experience with clomiphene citrate. *Fertil Steril* **19**: 616–622.
29. Adashi EY, Rock JA, Sapp KC, Martin EJ, Wentz AC & Jones GS (1979) Gestational outcome of clomiphene-related conceptions. *Fertil Steril* **31**: 620–626.
30. Garcia J, Jones GS & Wentz AC (1977) The use of clomiphene citrate. *Fertil Steril* **28**: 707–717.
31. Kurachi K, Aono T, Minagawa J & Miyake A (1983) Congenital malformations of newborn infants after clomiphene-induced ovulation. *Fertil Steril* **40**: 187–189.
32. Kousta E, White DM & Franks S (1997) Modern use of clomiphene citrate in induction of ovulation. *Hum Reprod Update* **3**: 359-365.
33. Boue JG & Boue A (1973) Increased frequency of chromosomal anomalies in abortions after induced ovulation. *Lancet* **i**: 679.
34. Dyson JL & Kohler HG (1973) Anencephaly and ovulation stimulation. *Lancet* **i**: 1256–1257.
35. Harlap S (1976) Ovulation induction and congenital malformations. *Lancet* **ii**: 961.
36. Cornel MC, Kate LPT, Dukes MN *et al.* (1989) Ovulation induction and neural tube defects. *Lancet* **i**: 1386.
37. Mills JL, Simpson JL, Rhoads GG *et al.* (1990) Risk of neural tube defects in relation to maternal fertility and fertility drug use. *Lancet* **336**: 103–104.
38. Lunenfeld B, Serr DM, Mashiach S *et al.* (1981) Therapy with gonadotropins: where are we today? Analysis of 2890 menotropin treatment cycles in 914 patients. In: Insler V, Bettendorf G (eds) *Advances in diagnosis and treatment of infertility*. Elsevier, Amsterdam, pp 27–31.
39. Ben-Rafael Z, Dor J, Mashiach S, Blankstein J, Lunenfeld B & Serr DM (1983) Abortion rate in pregnancies following ovulation induced by human menopausal gonadotropin/human chorionic gonadotropin. *Fertil Steril* **39**: 157.
40. Miyake A, Kurachi H, Wakimoto H, Hirota K, Terakawa N, Aono T & Tanizawa O (1988) Second pregnancy with spontaneous ovulation following clomiphene- or gonadotropin-induced pregnancy. *Eur J Obstet Gynecol Reprod Biol* **27**: 1–5.
41. Corsan GH & Kemmann E (1990) Risk of a second consecutive first-trimester spontaneous abortion in women who conceive with menotropins. *Fertil Steril* **53**: 817–821.
42. Balen AH, Braat DDM, West C, Patel A & Jacobs HS (1994) Cumulative conception and live birth rates after the treatment of anovulatory infertility. An analysis of the safety and efficacy of ovulation induction in 200 patients. *Hum Reprod* **9**: 1563–1570.
43. Homburg R, Eshel A, Armar NA *et al.* (1989) One hundred pregnancies after treatment with pulsatile luteinising hormone-releasing hormone to induce ovulation. *Br Med J* **298**: 809–812.
44. Nillius SJ & Wilde L (1978) Effects of prolonged luteinising hormone-releasing hormone therapy on follicular maturation, ovulation and corpus luteum function in amenorrheic women with anorexia nervosa. *Uppsala J Med Sci* **84**: 21–35.

45. Braat DDM, Schoemaker R & Schoemaker J (1991) Life table analysis of fecundity in intravenously treated gonadotropin-releasing hormone treated patients with normogonadotropic and hypogonadotropic amenorrhea. *Fertil Steril* **55**: 266–271.
46. Van der Spuy ZM, Steer PJ, McCusker M, Steele SJ & Jacobs HS (1988) Pregnancy outcome in underweight women following spontaneous and induced ovulation. *Br Med J* **296**: 962–965.
47. Armar NA, McGarrigle HHG, Honour JW, Holownia P, Jacobs HS & Lachelin GCL (1990) Laparoscopic ovarian diathermy in the management of anovulatory infertility in women with polycystic ovaries: endocrine changes and clinical outcome. *Fertil Steril* **53**: 45–49.
48. Steer C, Campbell S, Davies M, Mason B & Collins W (1989) Spontaneous abortion rates after natural and assisted conception. *Br Med J* **299**: 1317–1318.
49. Seppala M (1985) The World Collaborative Report on *in vitro* fertilization and embryo replacement: current state of the art in January 1984. *Ann N Y Acad Sci* **442**: 558–563.
50. Office of Population and Census Studies (OPCS) (1988) *Series FMI*. HMSO, London.
51. Lower AM, Mulcahy MT & Yovich JL (1991) Chromosome abnormalities detected in chorionic villus biopsies of failing pregnancies in a subfertile population. *Br J Obstet Gynaecol* **98**: 1228–1233.
52. Balen AH, Tan SL, MacDougall J & Jacobs HS (1993) Miscarriage rates following *in vitro* fertilisation are increased in women with polycystic ovaries and reduced by pituitary desensitisation with buserelin. *Hum Reprod* **8**: 959–964.
53. Tan SL, Maconochie N & Doyle P (1994) Cumulative conception and livebirth rates after IVF, with and without pituitary desensitization with the gonadotropin-releasing hormone agonist, buserelin. *Am J Obstet Gynecol* **171**: 513–520.
54. Homburg R, Levy T, Berkovitz *et al.* (1993) Gonadotropin releasing hormone agonist reduces the miscarriage rate for pregnancies achieved in women with polycystic ovaries. *Fertil Steril* **59**: 527–531.
55. Tan SL, Balen AH, Hussein EH, Mills C, Campbell S & Jacobs HS (1992) A prospective randomised study of the optimum timing of human chorionic gonadotropin administration after pituitary desensitisation in *in vitro* fertilisation. *Fertil Steril* **157**: 1259–1264.
56. Wang JX, Davies MJ & Norman RJ (2001) Polycystic ovarian syndrome and the risk of spontaneous abortion following assisted reproductive technology treatment. *Hum Reprod* **16**: 2606–2609.
57. Westergaard LG, Laursen SB & Andersen CY (2000) Increased risk of early pregnancy loss by profound suppression of luteinising hormone during ovarian stimulation in normogonadotropic women undergoing assisted reproduction. *Hum Reprod* **15**: 1003–1008.
58. Simon C, Garcia Velasco JJ, Valbuena D *et al.* (1998) Increasing uterine receptivity by decreasing estradiol levels during the preimplantation period in high responders with the use of FSH step-down regimen. *Fertil Steril* **70**: 234–239.
59. Penzias AS (2002) Luteal phase support. *Fertil Steril* **77**: 318–323.
60. Blohm F, Hahlin M, Nielsen S & Milsom I (1997) Fertility after a randomized trial of spontaneous abortion managed by surgical evacuation or expectant treatment. *Lancet* **349**: 995.

Chapter 20

Recurrent miscarriage

Introduction

Couples with recurrent miscarriage are fertile as, by definition, they will have experienced at least three consecutive miscarriages. Some, however, have coexistent subfertility and so the repeated loss of long-awaited pregnancies adds to the trauma that they have already experienced. The overall risk of miscarriage is between 15% and 25% and remains similar for women who have had any number of live born children.[1] After one miscarriage the risk of another miscarriage has been estimated as approximately 23%; after two consecutive miscarriages this increases to 29% and after three the risk is about 33% if a cause if found. In cases of idiopathic recurrent miscarriage the risk of a further miscarriage is 25%.[2] The risk of a second miscarriage after one or more live births is in the region of 20–25%. The majority of women who miscarry once, or even twice, after fertility treatment can be reassured that there is unlikely to be an underlying cause. Relatively few couples (approximately 1%) will experience recurrent miscarriages and they should be investigated further. It has been calculated that the chance of three consecutive miscarriages is 0.34%, which is lower than the observed rate of recurrent miscarriage, which suggests the possibility of an underlying cause.[3]

While up to a third of couples with recurrent miscarriage have experienced fertility problems at some time, we are often faced with couples attending the fertility clinic who have experienced one or two miscarriages. They might have undergone extensive fertility investigations and received various fertility therapies and so are naturally concerned that their next pregnancy is viable should they conceive after further treatment. Using the above criteria they do not have "recurrent" miscarriage and so would not usually warrant investigation. In the fertility clinic, however, it is unrealistic and unfeeling to expect subfertile couples to wait for their third lost pregnancy before they are investigated. It is therefore our practice to explain that while we are unlikely to find a cause, we advise a simple recurrent miscarriage screen (see below). Other groups are similarly sympathetic to such an approach.[2]

A tremendous amount of work has been performed in recent years in order to try to unravel the causes and treatment of recurrent miscarriage and to demystify some of the traditional remedies, which were of unproven benefit. The dedicated recurrent miscarriage clinic at

St Mary's Hospital, London, has gained considerable experience, being the largest such clinic in the UK, and produced many important publications, which will form the basis of this overview.[1,4]

Classification of Recurrent Miscarriage

An underlying cause is most likely to be found if the repeated miscarriages occur at a similar gestation. First trimester losses account for 75% of recurrent miscarriages and second trimester losses the remaining 25%. Even if a cause is found there is always the possibility that future miscarriages might be due to another cause, in other words they are of a sporadic nature and thus any treatment that is commenced has to allow for the fact that future miscarriages may not be due to the condition that has been treated.

The causes of recurrent miscarriage may have genetic, anatomical, infective, endocrine, or immune origins, but often no cause is found.

Genetic Causes

An abnormal fetal karyotype is found in about 60% of sporadic miscarriages and in about 30% of recurrent miscarriages.[5] Furthermore, only 3–5% of couples with recurrent miscarriage are found to have an obvious chromosomal abnormality, suggesting that the fetal abnormality is not secondary to a parental problem. It is always important to examine the fetal/placental chromosomes after a miscarriage, even if a non-genetic cause of recurrent miscarriage is suspected. The abnormalities that are sometimes found in parental chromosomes are usually balanced Robertsonian or reciprocal translocations (often between chromosomes 14 and 21). Additionally, chromosomal inversions or mosaics may be found but point mutations and lethal gene defects are not detected using routine testing.

Karyotyping the products of conception in cases of recurrent miscarriage may provide useful information for counseling and the future management of the couple.

Parental chromosomal abnormalities are not amenable to treatment. Genetic counseling should be provided and prenatal diagnosis offered for future pregnancies. Sometimes the use of donated gametes is appropriate.

Environmental Factors

While environmental factors such as radiation (but not working with VDUs), occupational exposure to chemicals (toluene, xylene, Formalin, some chemical disinfectants, glues, paints) and pollution may lead to an increased rate of sporadic miscarriage, there is no evidence that they are implicated in recurrent pregnancy loss. Alcohol and smoking also increase the risk of sporadic and possibly recurrent miscarriage.

Anatomical Abnormalities

An abnormal Mullerian tract, whether due to developmental anomalies (such as septate or bicornuate uteri) or acquired problems such as uterine synechiae or fibroids, is unlikely to lead to repeated pregnancy losses. The incidence of Mullerian duct abnormalities in women with normal pregnancies is approximately 3%, which is a similar rate to that found in women with recurrent miscarriage.[6] Furthermore, there is no evidence that the surgical treatment of uterine anomalies improves the chance of conception or the risk of miscarriage. There is evidence, however, that interventional surgery can cause peritubal and uterine scarring and so increase the chance of infertility. If a uterine septum is thought to be associated with recurrent miscarriage it is best excised hysteroscopically, although there are no prospective randomized controlled trials (RCTs) of such surgery.

Cervical incompetence may cause a second trimester miscarriage but is thought to be overdiagnosed and the use of cervical cerclage is widespread. The Medical Research Council/Royal College of Obstetricians and Gynaecologists (MRC/RCOG) study[7] of the use of cervical cerclage indicated that the rate of preterm deliveries could be reduced but without a significant improvement in neonatal outcome and there was no improvement in the rate of miscarriage. The large recurrent miscarriage study at St Mary's Hospital[8] found that almost half of the patients who had experienced second trimester losses had intrauterine deaths, 20% had contractions or bleeding, and a third had spontaneously ruptured membranes prior to the miscarriage. Cervical incompetence is associated with painless cervical dilatation prior to miscarriage and few women with recurrent miscarriage appear to fall into this category.

Infection

Intrauterine infection is a common cause of sporadic miscarriage, usually in the second trimester, but is not thought to result in recurrent miscarriage, other than in the rare situation of severe immunodeficient states. There has been much recent interest in the association of bacterial vaginosis (BV) with very early miscarriage after IVF, second trimester miscarriage and premature delivery, although no studies have found a role for BV in recurrent pregnancy loss.

Endocrine Abnormalities

Disturbances of the hypothalamic–pituitary–gonadal axis, in particular hypersecretion of luteinizing hormone (LH), can increase the risk of both sporadic and recurrent miscarriage (see below and Ch. 19). Other endocrine disorders can lead to infertility and pregnancy loss (see Ch. 3), although they do not cause recurrent miscarriage.[9] In particular, neither well-controlled diabetes mellitus nor thyroid disease is associated with recurrent pregnancy loss. It used to be common practice to assess glucose tolerance in women with recurrent miscarriage but this is no longer recommended. And while the assessment of thyroid status is simple and thyroid dysfunction is relatively common in women, it is not associated with recurrent miscarriage as such, unless there is a generalized underlying autoimmune disturbance.[10]

Luteal Phase Defects

Opinions on the role of a defective luteal phase in both infertility and miscarriage vary on either side of the Atlantic. The commonly held view in the UK is that a defective luteal phase is a reflection of inadequate follicular function and a "poor quality" ovulation. Luteal phase hormone concentrations do not correlate with the risk of miscarriage and luteal deficiency does not appear to be a recurrent phenomenon so is unlikely to cause recurrent miscarriage. A small study suggested that twice-weekly human chorionic gonadotropin (hCG) injections up to 14 weeks' gestation improved the chance of an ongoing pregnancy in women with oligomenorrhea and *two* previous miscarriages.[11] Our impression from available data, however, is that the use of luteal support, either with progesterone or hCG, does not reduce miscarriage rates for women with recurrent miscarriage (three or more consecutive miscarriages).[12,13] It is not recommended.

Hypersecretion of LH

Elevated follicular phase concentrations of LH are associated with an increased risk of infertility and miscarriage. In a series of 1537 women with recurrent miscarriage who attended the clinic at St Mary's Hospital, London, 52% were found to have polycystic ovary syndrome (PCOS) and of these 13% had an elevated serum LH concentration, 57% an elevated urinary excretion of LH, and 18% an elevated serum concentration of testosterone.[8] Despite having PCOS these women were fertile, with spontaneous ovulatory cycles and had experienced at least three first trimester miscarriages. Those with elevated LH levels (serum or urinary), who were under the age of 38 years, with normal karyotype and antiphospholipid antibody screening were randomly allocated into one of three treatment arms:

1. Spontaneous cycle with placebo luteal support
2. Spontaneous cycle with progesterone suppositories as luteal support
3. Treatment with a gonadotropin releasing hormone (GnRH) agonist followed by ovarian stimulation with human menopausal gonadotropins and progesterone suppositories as luteal support.

There was no benefit from the use of a GnRH agonist to suppress LH levels and this suggests that, at least in the case of recurrent miscarriage, hypersecretion of LH is not the cause of the problem but a marker for another reproductive abnormality. This may have an influence on the practice of fertility therapy when one considers the association between hypersecretion of LH, infertility, and miscarriage in women undergoing ovulation induction or IVF and the encouraging reports of an improvement in ongoing pregnancy rates when GnRH agonists are used (Chs 6 and 13). On the other hand, one should remember that in this study the selection of cases differed from all others and the measurement of LH in urine is very inaccurate. In reality GnRH agonists will continue to be used for assisted conception therapies as they provide tight control over the cycle, but their use in ovulation induction is less certain and probably unnecessary (see Ch. 6).

A more recent study from the same group studied 344 women who received no treatment and failed to identify a link between high serum LH or testosterone concentrations or body mass index in the 44% who miscarried.[14]

An elevated serum follicle stimulating hormone (FSH) concentration is found in 1–2% of women with recurrent miscarriage[4] and reflects reduced ovarian reserve and the possibility of premature ovarian failure (see Ch. 8). Counseling is required and oocyte donation may be indicated as the only potential treatment.

Immunological Causes of Recurrent Miscarriage

Immunological recognition and non-rejection of a pregnancy are fundamental to its survival. It has been suggested that recurrent miscarriage may result from a breakdown in the normal immune mechanisms, because of either autoimmune disease or the failure of the mother to produce a protective immune response for the genetically dissimilar pregnancy.

Autoimmunity

Approximately 2% of normal pregnant women and 15% of women with recurrent miscarriage have the lupus anticoagulant (LA) or anticardiolipin (aCL) antibody, both of which are antiphospholipid antibodies (aPL).[15,16] The primary antiphospholipid syndrome (PAPS) relates to recurrent miscarriage and/or a tendency to arterial and venous thrombosis or thrombocytopenia. Women with a normal obstetric history and aPL have a miscarriage rate of 50–75%, while those with recurrent miscarriage and aPL lose 90% of their pregnancies, and the miscarriage rate is even higher if the patient has systemic lupus erythematosus.[15] One should inquire about a history of migraine, epilepsy, arthralgia, and skin rashes and a family history of thrombosis, cerebrovascular accidents, and myocardial infarctions in relatives under the age of 50 years.

As with the assay of all biological markers for disease, it is essential to standardize the methodology of the laboratory protocols and this has been a particular issue with respect to aPL. The presence of the LA is assessed using tests of coagulation (the activated partial thromboplastin time (APTT), kaolin clotting time (KCT) and the dilute Russell's viper venom time (dRVVT)). The dRVVT is thought to be the best test for LA and is positive with a ratio of > 1.1. Blood for these tests should be collected with minimal stasis into a citrated bottle, using a 19 gauge butterfly needle, and measured within 2 hours. Both IgG and IgM anticardiolipin antibodies are assessed using an enzyme-linked immunosorbent assay (ELISA) and are abnormal if greater than 5 GPL or 3 MPL units, respectively. aPL have to be elevated on two occasions in order to make the diagnosis of the antiphospholipid syndrome.

A recent large study of 500 women with recurrent miscarriage[15] found that 26.4% were either LA or ACA positive. The dRVVT was positive in 14.6% of patients and after 8 weeks two-thirds of those who tested positive initially were still positive – 9.6% of the original study population. The levels of IgG and IgM aCL antibodies were elevated in 9.0% and 6.2%, respectively and remained positive 8 weeks later in just over a third of cases – 3.3% and 2.2%, respectively, of the whole study population. While many women appear to have transiently positive results, when the tests were performed on three occasions fewer than 0.5% of women had a positive result after it had been negative previously. Transiently positive results may be due to viral and other infections. Antinuclear factor titers were positive in approximately 8% of those who were either APA positive or negative and therefore not contributory. β_2-glycoprotein-I is an essential cofactor for ACA, which when bound together cause platelet aggregation. No differences in β_2-glycoprotein-I concentrations were found between normal women and women with recurrent miscarriages who were either APA negative or positive.

The majority of miscarriages in women with APAs occur in the first trimester and are thought to be caused by antibodies directed to the cytotrophoblast which disrupt implantation. Second trimester miscarriages in this group of patients are probably secondary to abnormal placentation with placental thrombosis and infarction. A prospective randomized study from the St Mary's group has indicated that aspirin (75 mg) combined with heparin (5000 units b.d.) significantly reduced the risk of miscarriage in women with aPL.[16] Indeed, with no treatment the live birth rate may be as low as 10%, with heparin alone 40%, and with heparin combined with aspirin 70%.[17] The treatment is discontinued at 34 weeks' gestation. The use of steroids is not recommended because, although levels of aCL fall, the rate of miscarriage is not helped and there is an increased risk of premature labor and pre-eclampsia.

Alloimmunity

For many years it was suggested that couples with recurrent miscarriage shared more human leukocyte antigen (HLA) alleles than expected. This was thought to lead to rejection of the conceptus (allograft) because the mother was unable to mount an adequate protective immune response. Immunotherapy has been performed using injections of paternal (or third party) lymphocytes into women with undetectable levels of antipaternal cytotoxic antibodies (APCA). However, levels of APCAs fluctuate, they are only measurable after 28 weeks' gestation and disappear between pregnancies and are therefore thought to be a poor indicator of alloimmune pregnancy failure. There is therefore no test that would identify couples at risk, even if alloimmune miscarriage exists as an entity. The Recurrent Miscarriage Immunotherapy Trialists Group published a worldwide collaborative observational study. They performed a meta-analysis on allogenic leukocyte immunotherapy for recurrent spontaneous abortion in 1994 and analyzed nine randomized and six non-randomized prospective studies.[18] A small improvement in live birth rate of 8–10% was found but the study group concluded that it was difficult to identify those patients most likely to benefit from immunotherapy and that a prospective placebo-controlled double-blind study is still required. Until then immunotherapy should be confined to research protocols. Furthermore, there are potential complications of immunotherapy, including transfusion reaction, anaphylactic shock, and hepatitis.

Thrombophilia

Women with thrombophilia may be at increased risk of recurrent miscarriage, although the efficacy of thromboprophylaxis is yet to be proven.[19,20] Thrombophilic conditions include deficiencies of antithrombin III, protein C and protein S, and activated protein C resistance which is secondary to a mutation in the factor V Leiden gene.

Table 20.1 Investigations for recurrent miscarriage	
First trimester miscarriages:	Chromosomal analysis of both partners Early and mid-follicular phase measurement of serum LH concentrations Measurement of lupus anticoagulant (dRVVT) and anticardiolipin antibodies (IgG and IgM)
Second trimester miscarriages:	Chromosomal analysis of both partners Measurement of lupus anticoagulant (dRVVT) and anticardiolipin antibodies (IgG and IgM) Ultrasound of the uterus followed by hysteroscopy and/or hysterosalpingogram if an abnormality is detected

Summary of the Investigation and Management of Couples with Recurrent Miscarriage (Table 20.1)

Recurrent miscarriage is defined as three or more consecutive miscarriages within a relationship.

Couples with repeated pregnancy losses need support within a specialized recurrent miscarriage clinic, which at the very least will be able to provide psychological support and serial ultrasound scans of the pregnancy. Of 114 women attending the St Mary's Hospital recurrent miscarriage clinic in whom no cause for the miscarriage was found, 71% who attended for supportive care during pregnancy had a successful outcome compared with 48% in those who did not attend ($p = 0.02$).

Genetic counseling should be offered to those with chromosomal abnormalities and preimplantation diagnosis or gamete donation considered. Women with the antiphospholipid syndrome should be treated with a combination of low-dose aspirin and heparin. Those who hypersecrete LH may benefit from treatment, although the correct management of these patients is still to be elucidated. If cervical incompetence is identified as the cause, cervical cerclage, by either a vaginal or sometimes an abdominal route, should be offered. The available data indicate that long-term antibiotic therapy is not justified.

References

1. Rai R, Clifford K & Regan L (1996) The modern preventative treatment of recurrent miscarriage. *Br J Obstet Gynaecol* **103**: 106–110.
2. Brigham SA, Conlon C & Farquharson RG (1999) A longitudinal study of pregnancy outcome following idiopathic recurrent miscarriage. *Hum Reprod* **14**: 2868–2871.

3. Rai R & Wakeford T (2001) Recurrent miscarriage. *Curr Obstet Gynaecol* **11**: 218–224.
4. Clifford K, Rai R, Watson H & Regan L (1994) An informative protocol for the investigation of recurrent miscarriage: preliminary experience of 500 consecutive cases. *Hum Reprod* **9**: 1328–1332.
5. Edmonds DK & Bennet MJ (1987) *Spontaneous and recurrent abortion.* Blackwell Scientific, Oxford.
6. Cook CL & Pridham DD (1995) Recurrent pregnancy loss. *Curr Opin Obstet Gynecol* **7**: 357–366.
7. MRC/RCOG Working Party on Cervical Cerclage (1993) Final report of the Medical Research Council/Royal College of Obstetricians and Gynaecologists multicentre randomised trial of cervical cerclage. *Br J Obstet Gynaecol* **100**: 516–523.
8. Clifford K, Rai R, Watson H, Franks S & Regan L (1996) Does suppressing LH secretion reduce the miscarriage rate? Results of a randomised controlled trial. *Br Med J* **312**: 1508–1511.
9. Baird DD, Weinberg CR, Wilcox AJ, McConnaughey DR, Musey PI & Collins DC (1991) Hormonal profiles of natural conception cycles ending in early, unrecognised pregnancy loss. *J Clin Endocrinol Metab* **72**: 793–800.
10. Coulam C & Stern J (1994) Endocrine factors associated with recurrent spontaneous abortion. *Clin Obstet Gynecol* **37**: 730–744.
11. Quenby S & Farquharson RG (1994) Human chorionic gonadotropin supplementation in recurring pregnancy loss: a controlled trial. *Fertil Steril* **62**: 708–710.
12. Goldstein P, Berrier J, Rosen S, Sacks HS & Chalmers TC (1989) A meta-analysis of randomized control trials of progestational agents in pregnancy. *Br J Obstet Gynaecol* **96**: 265–274.
13. Regan L (1997) Sporadic and recurrent miscarriage. In: Grudzinskas JG, O'Brien PMS (eds) *Problems in early pregnancy: advances in diagnosis and management*. RCOG Press, London, pp 31–52.
14. Nardo LG, Rai R, Backos M, El-Gaddal S, Regan L (2002) High serum luteinizing hormone and testosterone concentrations do not predict pregnancy outcome in women with recurrent miscarriage. *Fertil Steril* **77**: 348-352.
15. Rai R, Regan L, Clifford K *et al.* (1995) Antiphospholipid antibodies and β_2-glycoprotein-I in 500 women with recurrent miscarriage: results of a comprehensive screening approach. *Hum Reprod* **10**: 2001–2005.
16. Lockwood CJ, Romero R, Feinberg RF, Clyne LP, Coster B & Hobbins JC (1989) The prevalence and biologic significance of lupus anticoagulant and anticardiolipin antibodies in a general obstetric population. *Am J Obstet Gynecol* **161**: 369–373.
17. Rai R, Cohen H, Dave M & Regan L (1997) Randomised controlled trial of aspirin and aspirin plus heparin in pregnant women with recurrent miscarriage associated with phospholipid antibodies (or anti-phospholipid antibodies). *BMJ* **314**: 253–257.
18. Recurrent Miscarriage Immunotherapy Trialists Group (1994) Worldwide collaborative observational study and meta-analysis on allogenic leukocyte immunotherapy for recurrent spontaneous abortion. *Am J Reprod Immunol* **32**: 55–72.
19. Preston FE, Rosendaal FR, Walker ID *et al.* (1996) Increased fetal loss in women with heritable thrombophilia. *Lancet* **348**: 913–916.
20. Rai R, Regan L, Hadley E, Dave M & Cohen H (1996) Second-trimester pregnancy loss is associated with activated protein C resistance. *Br J Haematol* **92**: 489–490.

Chapter 21

Ectopic pregnancy

Introduction

Ectopic pregnancy occurs in approximately 0.5–1.0% of all pregnancies but this figure rises to about 5% after assisted conception therapies and to 20–30% in women with tubal damage after tubal surgery or a past history of ectopic pregnancy. A past history of pelvic infection accounts for about 40% of ectopic pregnancies. It has been argued that women with significant tubal damage should be sterilized before they commence IVF (see below). It is therefore important to understand the modern management of ectopic pregnancy in order to minimize any compromise of future fertility.

Diagnosis of Ectopic Pregnancy

A ruptured ectopic pregnancy is associated not only with impairment of future tubal function but also with significant mortality. It is essential to make the diagnosis of an ectopic pregnancy as early as possible so as to treat before rupture. An ultrasound scan should be performed at 5 weeks' gestation in a woman with a history of tubal damage or previous ectopic pregnancy or after fertility therapy. Transvaginal ultrasound should detect an intrauterine gestational sac and fetal cardiac activity at about 35 days from the previous menstrual period. If the picture is unclear and the patient is well clinically a repeat scan should be arranged for 1 week later. Serial ultrasound scans should then be performed until the location and viability of the pregnancy are confirmed. Sometimes an ectopic gestation can be seen clearly in the Fallopian tube, although this is the exception rather than the rule (Fig. 21.1a, b).

If the patient is experiencing pain or bleeding or if there are concerns about the possibility of an ectopic pregnancy, the serum concentration of human chorionic gonadotropin (hCG) should be measured. An ectopic pregnancy should be suspected if an intrauterine gestational sac cannot be detected by transvaginal or transabdominal ultrasound scan and the serum hCG level is greater than 1000 i.u./L or 1500 i.u./L, respectively. Serum hCG concentrations are higher in multiple pregnancy, and this is particularly relevant after fertility therapy when the risk of multiple gestation is increased. The gestational age is known fairly precisely after ovulation induction and even more accurately

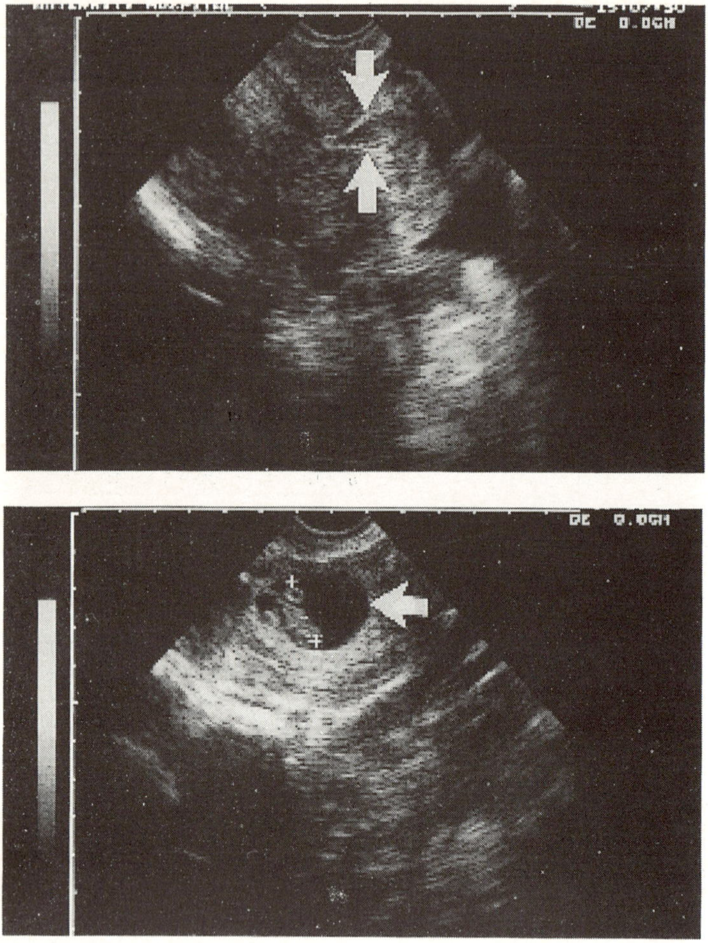

a

b

Figure 21.1a,b Transvaginal ultrasound scan demonstrating (**a**) an empty uterine cavity (between white arrows) and (**b**) an extrauterine (tubal) gestational sac with a live fetus within. See Figure 21.2 for laparoscopic findings.

after IVF. In these cases an intrauterine sac, or sacs, should be visualized by transvaginal ultrasound 24 days after conception. It is also important to remember the possibility of heterotopic pregnancy, particularly after IVF when two or three pre-embryos have been transferred. In a series of 1060 IVF pregnancies from our clinic there was an almost 5% rate of ectopic pregnancy and a 0.4% rate of heterotopic pregnancy.

A further guide to the nature of the pregnancy is provided by the rate of rise of hCG levels. In a normal pregnancy, the serum hCG concentration doubles every 2–3 days from 6 weeks' gestation. If the rise in hCG is less than 66% in a 48-hour period, a non-viable pregnancy (ectopic or miscarriage) is likely in 80% of cases.

Transvaginal ultrasound combined with studies of Doppler blood flow have enhanced the ability to distinguish intrauterine "pseudo sacs" from gestational sacs and have also been used to detect tubal pregnancies. The "pseudo sac" is usually a small area of fluid situated centrally within the uterine cavity as opposed to a pregnancy sac which implants in the endometrium lateral to the midline.

Treatment of Ectopic Pregnancy

Surgical Treatment of Ectopic Pregnancy

When there are signs suggestive of a ruptured ectopic pregnancy it is essential to perform a laparoscopy or laparotomy at once. The laparoscopic approach is preferred as minimal access surgery allows a swifter recovery time and the vast majority of ectopic pregnancies can be managed this way. It can sometimes be difficult to identify an early ectopic gestation during laparoscopic inspection of the pelvis and both Fallopian tubes should be inspected carefully before an incision is made into one. If there is any doubt about the site of the ectopic pregnancy or the completeness of its removal, careful follow-up is necessary with serial measurements of hCG (every 3–7 days) until the concentration has fallen to an undetectable level. One study[1] has indicated that the chance of a persistent ectopic pregnancy is low if there has been a fall of serum hCG concentration by 100 i.u./L or if there is a progesterone concentration of less than 33 nmol/L by 24 hours after surgery.

As little of the affected Fallopian tube as possible should be removed and care should be taken to conserve both ovaries. If the tubal pregnancy is unruptured, a linear salpingostomy may be performed (Figs 21.2 and 21.3).[2,3] The pregnancy is flushed from the tube and hemostasis secured using bipolar diathermy. It is not necessary to repair the tube because studies have demonstrated similar rates of tubal patency (75–85%), intrauterine pregnancy (50–60%), and recurrent ectopic pregnancy (10–20%) whether the tube is repaired or left to heal by itself after both laparoscopic and open surgery. In recent times there has been a vogue to perform a salpingectomy, taking care not to jeopardize ovarian blood supply.[4] However, a meta-analysis of retrospective studies of salpingectomy versus salpingostomy found similar rates of uterine pregnancy (46% vs 44%) and ectopic pregnancy (15% vs 10%).[5] The choice of procedure is often influenced by the state of the remaining Fallopian tube and past gynecological and obstetrical history.

A salpingectomy (Fig. 21.4) should be performed if there is extensive damage to the Fallopian tube from a ruptured ectopic pregnancy or if there are signs of pre-existing tubal damage that suggest a high risk

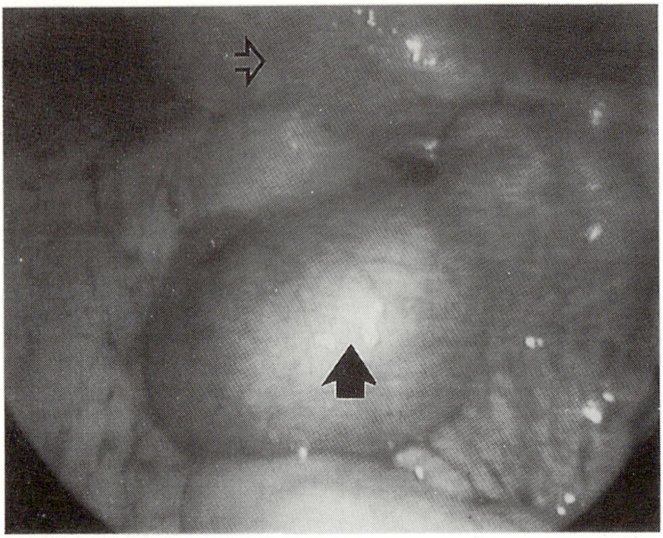

a

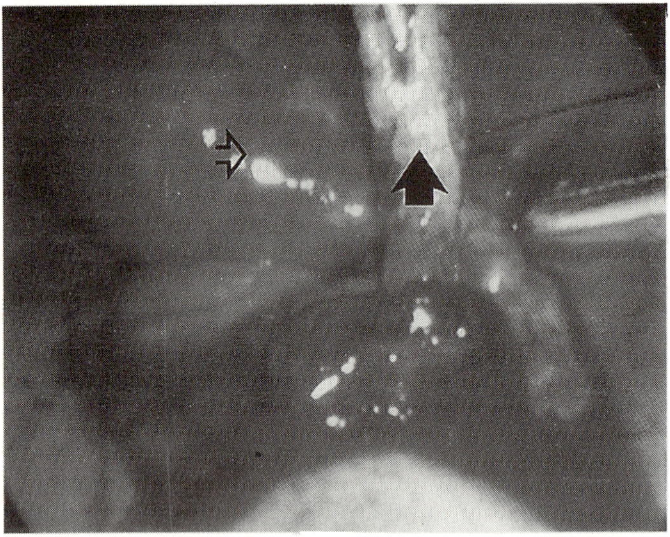

b

Figure 21.2a,b Laparoscopic findings of (**a**) an unruptured ectopic pregnancy (arrow) and (**b**) removal of the pregnancy through a linear salpingostomy. The uterus in (a) and (b) is denoted by an open arrow. (For the ultrasound findings of this case see Figure 21.1) (please refer to plate section for color figures).

a

b

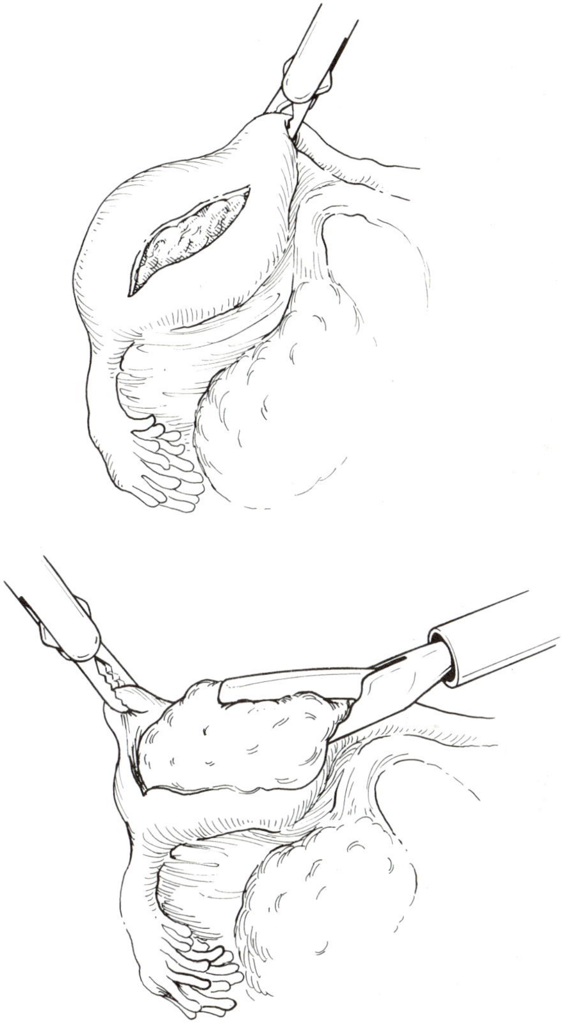

Figure 21.3a,b Laparoscopic treatment of ectopic pregnancy: linear salpingostomy. (**a**) The tube is incised along its antimesenteric border using cutting diathermy. (**b**) The ectopic pregnancy is removed and hemostasis achieved with bipolar diathermy. The tube is left open to heal, without the need for sutures (see also Fig. 21.2 a and b).

of loss of function. If the patient conceived after assisted conception for tubal disease she should be advised to consider either sterilization or bilateral salpingectomies in order to prevent further ectopic pregnancies. It can be extremely difficult to discuss sterilization with a couple who may have conceived after extensive fertility investigations and therapy and sometimes salpingectomy is best left as an interval

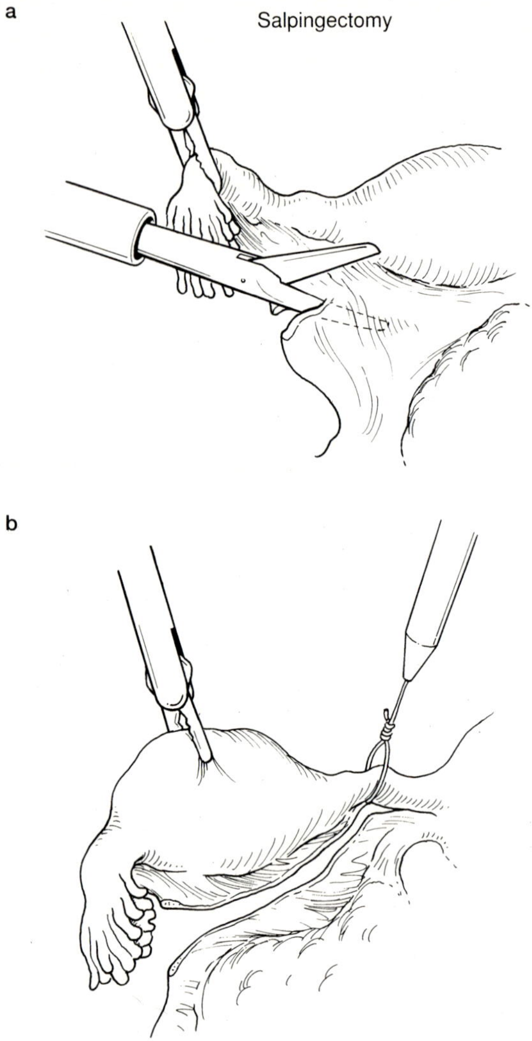

Figure 21.4a,b Laparoscopic treatment of ectopic pregnancy: salpingectomy. (**a**) The mesosalpinx is dissected with a combination of diathermy and sharp dissection. (**b**) An endoloop is placed around the tube and the tube is excised. Alternatively bipolar diathermy can be used to aid dissection from either end of the tube.

procedure. Even if a sterilization is performed, it does carry a failure rate (1:500–1000 sterilizations) and the couple must be counseled that there is still the possibility of a cornual ectopic pregnancy occurring in the future. Women who have hydrosalpinges may be advised to have bilateral salpingectomies because of the association between low implantation rates and a hydrosalpinx (see Ch. 10).

If the patient is asymptomatic and there is no obvious sign of an ectopic pregnancy, it is reasonable to perform serial measurements of hCG and a follow-up ultrasound scan after 1 week. If the hCG concentration is falling and the patient clinically stable it is sometimes possible to avoid surgery altogether, although the tube can still rupture after conservative treatment even when the hCG levels are falling.

Medical Treatment of Ectopic Pregnancy

Systemic methotrexate (usually 50 mg/m^2) has been used successfully to treat ectopic pregnancy.[6–8] Subsequent tubal patency rates appear to be similar after medical and surgical management. The patient requires careful observation and, in our experience, is often hospitalized for longer than after laparoscopic surgery, because the hCG level often rises before it begins to fall. It is essential once again to measure serum hCG concentrations until they are undetectable and this can take 30–90 days. The duration of stay in hospital depends upon the level of hCG, the patient's symptoms, the distance she lives from the hospital and her reliability to attend for regular follow up until the hCG levels have fallen. The advantage of medical treatment is the avoidance of surgery. On the other hand, laparoscopic appraisal of the pelvis at the time of surgery provides useful information for the patient about the extent of pre-existing and current damage. Methotrexate therapy is suitable when the serum hCG level is less than 2000 i.u./L and the diameter of the ectopic pregnancy less than 3 cm, in a patient who is otherwise stable.

In a series of 120 patients with ectopic pregnancy of less than 3.5 cm diameter, who were treated with a single dose of intramuscular methotrexate (50 mg/m^2), the side-effects were minimal.[7] Treatment was successful in 94% and 3% required a second dose, while 6% needed surgery. There were no cases of tubal rupture and 80% of those who tried subsequently conceived.

Sometimes it is necessary to give a second dose of methotrexate if hCG levels do not fall satisfactorily after 10–14 days. In our experience this is necessary in fewer than 5% of cases. If the ectopic pregnancy is more advanced and sited in a place that is less amenable to safe surgery (e.g., cornual ectopic or cervical ectopic) it is possible to give a higher dose of methotrexate (1 mg/kg per day) on alternate days with folinic acid "rescue" (calcium folinate 15 mg 6 hourly alternate days) over 8 days in total.

There has been one randomized study that compared a single dose of methotrexate (50 mg/m^2) with laparoscopic surgery, in patients with an unruptured tubal ectopic pregnancy of less than 3.5 cm diameter, with an hCG level of less than 5000 i.u./L.[9] Sixty-two patients were studied and, of those randomized to methotrexate, 35% required further treatment (further injections of methotrexate or surgery) compared with only 7% who received surgery ($p < 0.01$). These data are disappointing for those who advocate a medical approach. It is our experience that methotrexate is successful in 95% of patients who are diagnosed as having an early ectopic pregnancy after IVF, when the hCG levels are usually still less than 500. A more cautious approach is, however, required for the more advanced ectopic pregnancy. One must also always remember the possibility of heterotropic pregnancy, especially after IVF.

Methotrexate (1 mg/kg) can also be injected locally into the Fallopian tube, either by direct laparoscopic visualization of the tube or using ultrasound guidance – provided that the ectopic sac can be visualized. Alternatively, hypertonic glucose (50%) or prostaglandins can be used. We do not recommend these methods as they have only an 80% chance of success and are not as satisfactory as either systemic methotrexate or laparoscopic salpingostomy.[10]

References

1. Kadar N, Bohrer M, Kemmann E & Sheldon R (1994) The discriminatory human chorionic gonadotropin zone for endovaginal sonography: a prospective, randomized study. *Fertil Steril* **61**: 1016–1020.
2. Grainger DA & Seifer DB (1995) Laparoscopic management of ectopic pregnancy. *Curr Opin Obstet Gynecol* 7: 277–282.
3. Hagstrom HG, Hahlin M, Bennegard-Eben B, Sjoblom P, Thorburn J & Lindblom B (1994) Prediction of persistent ectopic pregnancy after laparoscopic salpingostomy. *Obstet Gynecol* **84**: 798–802.
4. Dubuisson JB, Morice P, Chapron C, De Gayffier A & Mouelhi T (1996) Salpingectomy – the laparoscopic surgical choice for ectopic pregnancy. *Hum Reprod* **11**: 1199–1203.
5. Claussen I (1996) Conservative versus radical surgery for tubal pregnancy: a review. *Acta Obstet Gynecol Scand* **75**: 8–12.
6. Goldenberg M, Bider D, Admon D, Mashiach S & Oelsner G (1993) Methotrexate therapy of tubal pregnancy. *Hum Reprod* 8: 660–666.
7. Stovall TG & Ling FW (1993) Single dose methotrexate: an expanded clinical trial. *Am J Obstet Gynecol* **168**: 1759–1765.
8. Stovall TG (1994) Medical management of ectopic pregnancy. *Curr Opin Obstet Gynecol* **6**: 510–515.
9. Sowter MC, Farquhar CM, Petrie KJ & Gudex G (2001) A randomized trial comparing single dose systemic methotrexate and laparoscopic surgery for the treatment of unruptured tubal pregnancy. *Br J Obstet Gynaecol* **108**: 192–203.
10. Tulandi T (1994) Medical and surgical treatment of ectopic pregnancy. *Curr Opin Obstet Gynecol* **6**: 149–152.

SECTION 6

Treatment failure

Chapter 22

When to stop treatment and other options

When to Stop Treatment

The most difficult part of fertility therapy is knowing when to stop. If there is an absolute cause of infertility, for example premature ovarian failure, when there is no possibility of becoming pregnant without treatment, stopping treatment is final. If, on the other hand, there are intermediate factors such as severe oligozoospermia, partial tubal damage, or unexplained infertility it is more difficult to stop treatment. There are two main reasons: firstly one can never be certain that the next cycle of treatment will not be the one in which a pregnancy occurs; secondly, there is always a chance of a spontaneous conception, albeit usually extremely slim by the time the couple has reached this stage. Of course, we are generally referring to IVF here as the couple is likely to have spent many years going through investigations, simple treatments, and then assisted conception. Some couples, however, do not wish to pursue high-tech assisted conception therapies and stop treatment at the point that IVF is advised.

There are several approaches to dealing with how many treatment cycles a couple should have. Integral to the process is a realistic appraisal of the couple's problems before they start and an honest view of their cumulative chance of a conception and live birth after a certain number of cycles. The appraisal will depend upon the individual couple's characteristics, age, duration of infertility, diagnosis, and the clinic's results. With all of this information the couple should at the outset have an understanding of what the treatment has to offer and hence realistic expectations. In reality, many couples have unrealistic expectations of treatment, an uncertain grasp of the statistics of cumulative conception rates, and an understandable feeling that they are special individuals rather than part of the population that make up the statistics. Indeed, cumulative conception statistics do apply to populations or groups of patients rather than individuals and can only be used to provide a rough guide of the efficacy of treatment.

Some couples drop out along the way because they find the treatment too difficult, unpleasant, painful, stressful, disruptive, or expensive. While couples who drop out would no doubt benefit from counseling and support, they are a different group from those who persevere and require guidance from the clinic about when to stop. We feel that if treatment is not working satisfactorily it is sensible to discuss its goal;

in other words to suggest how many more cycles the couple should undertake with the agreement to stop definitely after the agreed limit. It is our experience that this policy is generally better accepted than simply terminating treatment at the end of a cycle without prior discussion.

Most couples find stopping treatment extremely traumatic and the majority will always be deeply affected by their infertility. There are also those who have already got a child(ren) but are equally traumatized when they find they are unable to provide him/her with brothers or sisters and complete their family. Such couples deserve sympathy and support both when trying to conceive and when they eventually stop.

After stopping treatment some choose to forget all about having a family while others pursue other means of achieving one, such as adoption.

Adoption

It is very difficult to adopt a baby in the UK, largely because there are very few babies available. In the 1960s adopting a white baby in Britain was relatively easy, but the shortage began after the introduction of the contraceptive pill, legal abortion, and the greater acceptability of single motherhood. The adoption of mixed race babies has remained easier, although they are generally only offered – perhaps illogically – to black or mixed race parents because of the great controversy surrounding transracial adoption. It could be argued that any couple prepared to give a child a loving home environment should be able to adopt, irrespective of race or social background. The fact is, however, that there are now few babies for adoption and therefore certain – at times seemingly arbitrary – criteria are employed to select the "most suitable" prospective parents. There is tremendous geographical variation in the ease with which adoption can be achieved around Britain. The upper age limits vary from 34 to 38 years. Couples are also asked to stop any fertility treatment as soon as they embark upon the adoption process, because it is thought that if they were to conceive the adopted child might be made to feel unwelcome.

Adoption is controlled through adoption agencies which are either part of local authority social services departments or independent voluntary agencies, which are often connected with churches. The local social services adoption agencies often hold information evenings which prospective parents attend. Assuming that the local adoption agency's list is open, the couple are then allocated a social worker. It is the social worker's duty to ensure that the couple is suitable and can provide an appropriate family life for the adopted child(ren). There are no social workers who are dedicated to adoption full time and adoption is, unfortunately, usually bottom of their list of priorities. The couple need to obtain a medical record from their GP and a police check is performed to ensure that neither partner has a criminal record. References are also obtained from friends, employers, etc. The process can take between 9 months and 2 years, or more.

The social worker will by now have prepared a report for the adoption panel, which consists of members of the social services, police, and lay representatives. The panel tends to be quite authoritarian and has tight criteria, although there are no set standards around the country and there is some geographical variability. At the time of writing, there are plans to revise the rules governing adoption in the UK and to reduce the influence of social workers while increasing input from a panel of lay-people. If the couple is approved by the adoption panel they then go on a waiting list for a child. The birth parent(s) may express their wishes about the placement of their child(ren), for example with respect to religious upbringing, and this has to be considered by the adoption agency. Most agencies also place children into the same racial background as its birth parents, although controversial decisions have been made in the case of mixed race children.

It is very rare these days to be able to adopt a newborn baby and much easier to adopt an older child who might come from a disturbed background, from a children's home, or from a foster home. Agencies are more flexible with people who wish to adopt children with special needs, not only because they are harder to place but also because older parents, for example, might be better able to cope with more demanding youngsters than their younger counterparts. The adopting parents are given as much information as possible about the child's background, health, and former life, primarily so that this information can be passed on as the child grows and learns to understand his/her origins. It is considered essential to tell children that they are adopted so that they grow up with this knowledge rather than make the discovery when a lot older. Adopted children are permitted to see their birth certificate once they have reached the age of 18 and some then try to trace their original parents.

Once an adoption order has been granted it cannot be reversed and the adopted child becomes a full member of the new family, losing all legal ties with its birth parents. The child has to have lived with the adopters for at least 13 weeks before an adoption order can be made and this period cannot start until the child is at least 6 weeks old. The court appoints a reporting officer who checks that the birth parents understand what is taking place and both the mother and father (if the child is legitimate) have to sign their agreement to the adoption. If the birth parents do not agree to the adoption but have abandoned their child, the court can, in rare circumstances, make an adoption order without their agreement. It is also possible for the birth parents to transfer parenting rights to the adoption agency, by way of a "freeing order", which in turn is transferred to the adopting parents at the time of the adoption order. Once the adoption order has been made, the birth parents lose all rights over the child.

The cost of going through adoption is relatively low, as the agencies are not allowed to charge a fee and no money is allowed to pass from the adopters to the birth parents. The medical, police, and court certificates usually require a small fee. The adopting parents are allowed to claim child benefit from the social services department and other state benefits if the child has special needs.

It is interesting to note that while an immense effort is made in the screening of parents before they can adopt, there is no follow-up by the social workers who have made the decisions. We think this is a major failing, not only because there is no audit of the selection process but also because couples who have been trying hard to start a family for many years often require support and guidance once they have their first child; consider, for example, the support provided in the UK by the network of midwives and health visitors who regularly visit parents who go through a normal pregnancy. None the less, it appears that adoption tends to work well both for the adopting parents and the children, most of whom experience good family lives.

Adopting a Child from Overseas

Many countries have a central agency that coordinates inter-country adoption, although none exists in the UK. The Overseas Adoption Helpline has published a comprehensive procedural guide. An inspection has to be performed by the local social services department, in the same way as the standard adoption process, although the couple is required to pay for this and the costs can range from £2000 to £20 000. A detailed "home study" is performed by a social worker, who visits the home of the prospective adopters on more than one occasion and also speaks to the referees. Local authorities differ greatly with respect to the speed with which they organize the home study and the fee that they charge (up to £2000). Other expenses include travel, legal, and translation fees plus the possibility of donations to an orphanage.

The country from which the child is to be adopted often imposes strict criteria and sometimes communicates with the social services department. Countries that are sympathetic to overseas adoption of their children include Brazil, Bolivia, Chile, China, Colombia, Ecuador, El Salvador, Guatemala, Peru, the Philippines, Romania, Sri Lanka, and Thailand. Once the inspection process is complete and both health and police certificates have been obtained, an application is submitted to the Department of Health, which in turn puts the application to the Foreign and Commonwealth Office for legislation.

The Department of Health then coordinates the paperwork which has to be sent to the relevant embassy, which will translate the documents and forward them to the appropriate agency within their country. This local agency has then to approve the application and locate a suitable child, at which point the prospective parents can travel to meet the child. The adopters have then to apply for British entry clearance for the child (details of which are found in the Home Office document RON 117) and go through the relevant requirements for adoption in the child's country before being able to bring the child into Britain. Once home the adopters have to inform the social services department of their "intention to adopt" under British law and an adoption order is then made by a British court. When the adoption order is granted the child becomes a British citizen, provided that at least one of the adopting parents is British. Some countries stipulate, however, that the child should also retain his/her original nationality until aged 18 years, although such rules are not binding in Britain.

Fostering

It is in some ways easier to become a foster parent, although the social services still scrutinize foster parents very carefully. A fostering agency shares the responsibility for the child with the foster parents and an allowance is provided to help care for the child. Many foster parents have children of their own, while some have experienced infertility. Fostering is often open both to older parents and to less "socially acceptable" couples, such as lesbians and homosexual men. Fostering is generally for a limited period of time, until the child is able to return to its own family, be placed for adoption, or live independently. The temporary aspect of fostering can be especially emotionally traumatic for the couple who have no other children at home. Its effects on the child can be traumatic too.

Respite Care

An alternative to adoption and fostering is offering a place in the home for respite care of severely disabled children while their parents take a holiday. This can be extremely rewarding and many couples develop long-term relationships with the families that they help in this way.

Useful addresses

Androgen Insensitivity Support Group
2 Shirburn Avenue, Mansfield NG18 2BY
01623 661749

British Agencies for Adoption and Fostering
Skyline House, 200 Union Street, London SE1 01Y
0207 593 2000

British Fertility Society (National Society for Healthcare Professionals)
16 The Courtyard, Woodlands, Bradley Stoke, Bristol BS32 4NQ
01454 642211
www.bfs.co.uk

British Infertility Counselling Association (BICA)
69 Division Street, Sheffield S1 4GE
01342 843880
www.bica.net

CHILD (national support organisation with newsletter and helpline)
Charter House, 43 St Leonards Road,
Bexhill on Sea, E Sussex TN40 NJA
01424 732361
office@email2.child.org.uk
www.child.org.uk

Childlink Adoption Society
10 Lion Yard, Tremdoc Road, London SW4 7NQ
0207 498 1933

Cot Death Foundation
14 Halkin Street, London SWIX 7DP
0207 235 1721

COTS (Childlessness Overcome by Surrogacy)
Loandhu Cottage, Gruids,
Lairg, Sutherland, Scotland IV27 4EF
01549 402401

Daisy Network (premature menopause support group)
PO Box 392, High Wycombe, Bucks, HP15 7SH

Department of Health, Social Care Group
Wellington House, 133–155 Waterloo Road, London SE1 8UG
0207 972 4347/4084

Department of Health and Social Services, Child Care Branch
Dundonald House, Upper Newtownards Road, Belfast B24 3SF
01232 520000

Donor Conception Network
PO Box 265, Sheffield S3 7YX
0208 245 4369
www.dcnetwork.org

Home Office, Immigration and Nationality Department
Lunar House, Wellesley Road, Croydon, Surrey CR9 2BY
0208 686 0688

Human Fertilisation and Embryology Authority (HFEA)
Paxton House, 30 Artillery Lane, London E1 7LS
020 7377 5077
www.hfea.gov.uk

International Social Service of the UK
Cranmer House, 39 Brixton Road, London SW9 6DD
0207 735 8941

Issue (national fertility support organisation)
114 Lichfield Street, Walsall WS1 1SZ
01922 722888
webmaster@issue.co.uk
www.issue.co.uk

Miscarriage Association
c/o Clayton Hospital, Northgate, Wakefield WF1 3JS
01924 200700

Multiple Births Foundation
Hamm House, Hammersmith Hospital, Du Cane Road,
London W12 OHS
020 8383 3519

National Endometriosis Society
50 Westminster Palace Gardens, Artillery Row, London SW1P 1RL
020 7222 2776

Overseas Adoption Helpline
34 Upper Street, London N1 OPN
0207 226 7666

Overseas Adoption Support and Information Service (OASIS)
Dan y Craig Cottage, Balaclava Road, Glais, Swansea SA7 9HJ

Parent to Parent Information on Adoption Services
Lower Boddington, Daventry, Northants NN11 6YB
01327 260295

Scottish Office, Social Work Services Group
Room 43C, James Craig Walk, Edinburgh EH1 3BA
0131 244 5480

STORK (for families who have adopted from overseas)
71 Chelsham Road, South Croydon, Surrey CR2 6HZ
020 8680 5623

Turner Syndrome Support Society
1/8 Irving Court, Hardgate,
Clydebank G81 6BA
01389 380385
Turner.Syndrome@tss.org.uk
www.tsss.org.uk

Twins and Multiple Births Association (TAMBA)
PO Box 30, Little Sutton, South Wirral L66 1TH
01732 868000

Verity (National PCOS Support Group)
52–54 Featherstone Street, London EC1Y 8RT
enquiries@verity-pcos.org.uk
www.verity-pcos.org.uk

Welsh Office, Children and Families Unit,
Cathays Park, Cardiff CF1 3NQ
01222 823676

Further reading

Brinsden P (1999) *A Textbook of In Vitro Fertilization Assisted Reproduction.* Parthenon Publishing, New York.

A clinic-orientated text on ART.

Devroey P (ed) (2001) *Infertility and Reproductive Medicine Clinics of North America: GnRH Analogues.* WB Saunders, Philadelphia.

An update on the various uses of GnRH analogs.

Edwards RG & Brody SA (1995) *Principles and Practice of Assisted Human Reproduction.* WB Saunders, London.

A detailed scientific analysis of ART – science and practice.

Fauser BCJM, Rutherford AJ, Strauss JF & van Steirteghem A (1999) *Molecular Biology in Reproductive Medicine.* Parthenon Publishing, New York.

A detailed overview of molecular biology.

Gardner DK, Weissman A, Howles CM & Shoham Z (2001) *Textbook of Assisted Reproductive Techniques – Laboratory and Clinical Perspectives.* Martin Dunitz, London.

A comprehensive text on ART.

Hillier SG, Kitchener HC & Nielson JP (1996) *Scientific Essentials of Reproductive Medicine.* WB Saunders, London.

In depth scientific analysis of reproductive medicine.

Homburg R (2001) *Polycystic Ovary Syndrome.* Martin Dunitz, London.

A multi-author comprehensive overview of PCOS.

Kovacs GT (2000) *Polycystic Ovary Syndrome.* Cambridge University Press, Cambridge.

A multiauthor clinically orientated overview of PCOS.

RCOG (1998–2000) *The Management of Infertility in Primary, Secondary and Tertiary Care.* Three sets of guidelines. RCOG Press, London.

Shoham Z, Howles CM & Jacobs HS (1999) *Female Infertility Therapy: Current Practice.* Martin Dunitz, London.

An in depth overview of infertility therapy in practice.

Templeton A, Cooke I & O'Brien PMS (1998) *Evidence-based Fertility Treatment.* RCOG Press, London.

The proceedings of a RCOG scientific working party on infertility.

Wolpert L (1998) *Principles of Development.* Oxford University Press, Oxford.

Developmental biology and embryology.

Appendix 1

Daily Vitamin and Mineral Requirements

(see Ch. 3)

A healthy diet can be constructed by ensuring that the right amounts of the four main food groups are consumed. The following guidelines can be photocopied and given to your patients.

Group 1: Bread and Cereals

Bread contains B vitamins, calcium and iron; many cereals are fortified with vitamins and iron. Potatoes, rice, pasta, noodles, yam, and cassava are all good sources of fiber. At least four servings of these foods should be used every day as the main "bulk" of meals.

Group 2: Fruit and Vegetables

Fruit and vegetables provide a rich source of vitamins. Vitamins are lost by overboiling so vegetables should be cooked in a small amount of water or, alternatively, steamed. Dark green leafy vegetables (cabbage, spinach, sprouts, broccoli, watercress) are excellent sources of vitamins. At least four servings of fruit and vegetables should be consumed daily, one of which should be rich in vitamin C (large amounts of which are found in citrus fruit, fruit juice, blackcurrants, kiwi fruit, green peppers, and tomatoes). Women who change to a vegetarian diet sometimes become amenorrheic, secondary either to a reduction in the total calorie intake or to an increase in fecal excretion of estrogens.

Group 3: Dairy Products

Milk, milk products, cheeses, and yoghurt contain protein, minerals and vitamins (B group) and are the main source of dietary calcium. Three servings a day are recommended.

Group 4: Meat, Fish, Eggs, Beans, Nuts

These foods are rich sources of protein and contain a variety of minerals and vitamins. Two servings are recommended in a daily diet. Red meat is a good source of iron, which is also found in eggs, beans, lentils, nuts, green leafy vegetables, and fortified cereals. White fish is low in fat and high in protein.

Minerals and Salts

Iron (15 mg/day)

Red meat is the best source of iron; bread, pulses, and some vegetables (spinach) also contain iron, but most are low in iron. Vitamin C (see below) enhances iron absorption by the gut, while fibrous foods reduce iron absorption. Iron tablets usually contain 100–200 mg of iron; only a little of this is absorbed to give the correct daily requirement.

Calcium (700–1200 mg/day)

Half a liter of whole cow's milk contains 600 mg of calcium, as does a 48 g portion of cheddar cheese, 6 ounces (170 g) of fish or 400 g of yoghurt. Fortified breads and cereals, nuts, and fruit (apricots, oranges, figs) also contain moderate amounts of calcium.

Zinc (7 mg/day)

The best sources are red meat, liver, kidneys, wholegrain cereals, nuts, crustaceans, and cheese. Zinc deficiency is uncommon.

Sodium (1.6 g/day)

Sodium is found in plentiful amounts in the diet; indeed, it is best to avoid too much and to restrict your intake to less than 2.3 g daily (this is equivalent to 6.0 g of sodium chloride or salt). A high-sodium diet predisposes to hypertension (high blood pressure). One tenth of this daily requirement is found in a single portion of: ham, bacon, tongue, corned beef, sausage, smoked fish, breakfast cereals, pickles, tomato sauce, soy sauce, most biscuits, cheeses, yeast extract, canned vegetables, potato chips and many other foods. Low amounts of salt are found in rice, oatmeal, plain flour, fresh fruit and vegetables, fresh meat, fish, and poultry.

Iodine, magnesium, potassium, copper, and selenium

These are found in most foods and deficiency is very rare in the UK. A diet that contains potatoes, pulses, fresh/dried fruit, vegetables, fresh meat and fish, dairy products, and orange juice will provide sufficient minerals and salts.

Daily Requirements of Vitamins

The foods listed are the richest sources of vitamins and smaller amounts may be provided by other foods.

Vitamin A (700 mg/day)

Contained in carrots, spinach, broccoli, pumpkin, apricots, liver, kidney, eggs, dairy products, fish oils, margarine. Very high amounts are contained in liver, which should be avoided during pregnancy as it can be harmful to the developing baby.

Vitamin B_1, thiamin (1 mg)

Whole wheat, wheatgerm, yeast, pulses, nuts, pork, duck, yeast extract, oatmeal, fortified cereals, cod's roe, meats.

Riboflavin (1.1 mg)

Liver, kidney, milk, yoghurt, cheese, yeast extract, eggs, wheatgerm, mushrooms, fortified cereals.

Niacin (14 mg)

Meat, liver, kidney, fish, yeast products, yeast extract, peanuts, bran, pulses, wholemeal wheat.

Vitamin B_6 (1.2 mg)

Liver, wholegrain cereals, meat, fish, nuts, avocados, potatoes, eggs.

Vitamin B_{12} (1.5 mg)

Liver, kidney, sardines, meat, eggs, cheese, milk.

Vitamin C (40 mg)

Blackcurrants, guavas, oranges, citrus fruits, green peppers, rosehip syrup, cauliflower, broccoli, sprouts, cabbage, parsley, potatoes.

Vitamin D (3 mg)

Fish liver oils, fatty fish, fortified margarine, eggs, liver. Sunlight provides a sufficient source of vitamin D, even in the UK! Supplements are only required by those who are housebound.

Vitamin E (10 mg)

Wheatgerm and other vegetable oils, margarine, butter, eggs, wholemeal cereals, broccoli.

Vitamin K (100 mg)

Turnips, broccoli, cabbage, lettuce, liver.

Pantothenic acid, biotin, carnitine, inositol, aminobenzoic acid

These are often contained in multivitamin preparations but are widely distributed in foodstuffs and deficiency does not occur in the UK.

Index

Note: Page numbers is **bold** *refer to illustrations and tables.*

10